Rheumatological Medicine

Rheumatological Medicine

Paul A. Dieppe
BSC MB BS FRCP
Senior Lecturer, Bristol University and Honorary Consultant Rheumatologist, Bristol Royal Infirmary

Michael Doherty
MA MB BChir MRCP
Senior Lecturer, Nottingham University and Honorary Consultant Rheumatologist, City Hospital, Nottingham

Diana Macfarlane
MB BS MRCP
Consultant Rheumatologist, Lewisham Hospital, London

Peter Maddison
MA MB BChir MRCP
Consultant Rheumatologist, Royal National Hospital for Rheumatic Diseases, Bath

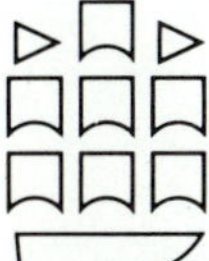

CHURCHILL LIVINGSTONE
EDINBURGH LONDON MELBOURNE AND NEW YORK 1985

CHURCHILL LIVINGSTONE
Medical Division of Longman Group Limited

Distributed in the United States of America by
Churchill Livingstone Inc., 1560 Broadway, New York,
N.Y. 10036, and by associated companies, branches
and representatives throughout the world.

First published 1985

ISBN 0 443 02524 X

British Library Cataloguing in Publication Data
Rheumatological medicine.
1. Rheumatism
I. Dieppe, P.A.
616.7'23 RC927

Library of Congress Cataloging in Publication Data
Rheumatological medicine.
Includes index.
1. Rheumatism. I. Dieppe, Paul. [DNLM: 1. Arthritis.
2. Rheumatism. WE 344 R472]
RC927.R478 1985 616.7'23 84-17070

Produced by Longman Group (F.E.) Ltd.
Printed in Hong Kong

Preface

In recent years rheumatology has emerged as a major branch of general medicine. The decline in infectious diseases, and increasing health demands of the community have contributed to the growth in numbers of patients presenting with rheumatic complaints. About 25% of general practice consultations now primarily concern the musculoskeletal system. Increasing awareness of the systemic nature of many rheumatic diseases and a rapid increase in the number and complexity of both diagnostic and therapeutic procedures have led to a huge expansion in "rheumatological medicine". Recent surveys of general medical beds in Great Britain show that the majority of patients admitted for acute disorders have a significant rheumatic problem.

Expansion of a discipline needs to be matched by an increase in published material. Several new journals of rheumatology have appeared over the last few years, and many excellent monographs have been published. Good student books and major works of reference are also available. However, there are few textbooks which are ideal for postgraduates as well as undergraduates, and hardly any that deal with rheumatology as a part of general medicine rather than as a separate discipline.

This book is an attempt to fill that gap. It has been written by four rheumatologists who are actively interested in the teaching and practice of general medicine as well as pursuing careers in academic rheumatology. The nature of the major rheumatic complaints and diseases have been described, and the available investigations and therapy are discussed. In addition, a major part of the book is concerned with the influence of rheumatic disorders on the whole body and on the relationship between systemic disorders and the musculoskeletal system. We hope that the book will therefore be useful to all postgraduates with an interest in medicine and a help to those preparing for the MRCP exam as well as to rheumatologists.

Bristol, Bath
and London,
1985

P. A. D.
M. D.
D. G. M.
P. J. M.

Contents

SECTION ONE

Introduction

1 The structure, function and breakdown of articular tissues

The musculoskeletal system contains the three main elements of connective tissue: cells, fibres and ground-substance. Bone and muscle are specialised connective tissues: in the former the matrix is mineralised to provide the rigid support the body needs; whereas the latter consists of specialised contractile cellular elements which produce movement. The joints and periarticular tissues provide the stable, weight-bearing links between bones, and the remainder of the body's connective tissue forms a supportive matrix for the limbs and internal organs of the body.

CONNECTIVE TISSUE

1. Cells

All the cellular elements of connective tissue are probably derived from the same primitive mesenchymal stem cell. Their main function is to synthesise and secrete the fibres and ground substance of supporting tissues; they are therefore similar and may be able to change function and morphology in response to alterations in the local environment (Fig. 1.1). There is increasing evidence for the existence of a number of local transmitter substances which act as chemical messengers between these cells, co-ordinating their activity in maintaining connective tissue integrity.

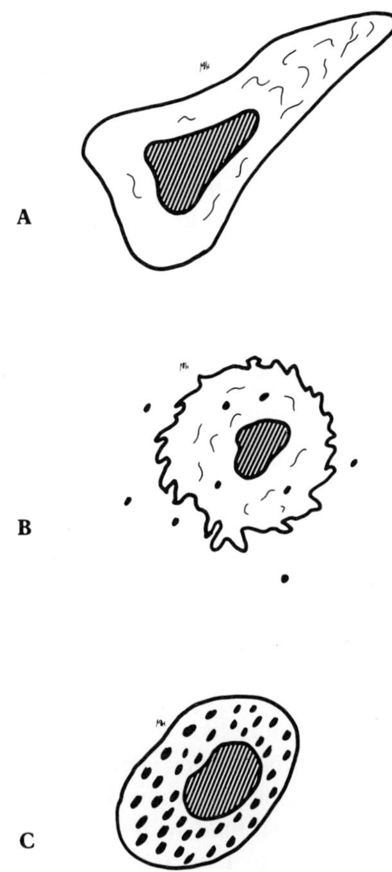

Fig. 1.1 Some connective tissue cells. **A.** Fibroblast: a triangular cell with an extensive Golgi apparatus. **B.** Chondrocyte: a cell with abundant Golgi apparatus, a few lysosomes and filaments which may bud off to form matrix vesicles. **C.** Mast cell: a cell full of large numbers of dark-staining granules containing heparin and other transmitters.

a) Fibroblasts

The fibroblast is a factory for production of collagen fibres and proteoglycans, and is present throughout all loose connective tissue. It is identified by its characteristic triangular, elongated shape, and has the ability to become motile and to contract, enhancing its ability to repair areas of tissue damage. Fibroblasts show some organ specificity in their secretory products, are metabolically very active and can replicate rapidly. They respond to many different local stimuli, including products of the macrophage and inflammatory mediators.

b) Chondrocytes

The chondrocyte can be defined as a cell producing type II collagen (see below) and proteoglycans; it is found within the firmer collagenous element of connective tissue, but is difficult to define morphologically. It has numerous processes on the cell surface which can bud off into the pericellular area to produce the matrix vesicles which are the initial sites of enchondral calcification and ossification. Like all connective tissue cells it has a Golgi apparatus to provide the secretory apparatus for its products, but chondrocytes also possess lysosomes containing destructive enzymes. They are metabolically active, but replicate relatively little. They secrete various cell–cell transmitters, probably including an endothelial inhibitory factor to prevent vascularisation of cartilage.

c) Synoviocytes

Synovial lining cells have been divided into three main types on morphological grounds. The numerous 'A' cells (about 60%) look like macrophages and are phagocytic; the 'type B' cells (about 30%) are more like fibroblasts and have an extensive Golgi apparatus. They are protein and carbohydrate factories, producing the secretory products of synovial fluid such as hyaluronate and other glycoproteins. The remaining 'C' cells are intermediate in type, and may be stem cells capable of dividing and transforming into synoviocytes. The ability of these cells to replicate is apparent in the synovial hypertrophy accompanying many rheumatic diseases. Specialised dendritic cells, which have an important role in immunological reactions, are also seen in the synovium.

d) Macrophages and mast cells

Connective tissues contain phagocytic scavenger cells (macrophages) as well as the synthetic elements. In addition to removing debris, these cells produce numerous intercellular transmitters and destructive products, and have a central role in both the initiation and repair phases of inflammation. They also have a central role in initiation and effector mechanisms of immunological reactions.

Mast cells are also numerous in connective tissue. These ovoid cells contain large numbers of darkly-staining granules, and a few surface microvilli; they look 'about to burst', and contain preformed packages of inflammatory mediators, including heparin and serotonin. As well as being receptors of inflammatory-stimuli-releasing mediators in response to trauma or IgE reactions, they also have a regulatory role in connective tissue metabolism.

2. Pleuripotential cells and intercellular communication

The interaction of the various cells in connective tissue has been mentioned. Some of the mediators which affect the destruction, repair and proliferation of connective tissue are illustrated. Of special interest are the relatively well-characterised connective-tissue-activating proteins (CTAPs), which increase the activity of synovial cells, and the monocyte-derived MCF Interleukin I and 'catabolin', which alter the activity of chondrocytes and other cells.

Some intercellular mediators (cytokines) involved in connective-tissue metabolism

1. Connective-tissue activating peptides
2. Interleukin 1
3. Osteoclast activating factor
4. Matrix factor
5. Catabolin
6. Monocyte co-culture factor (MCF)

3. Fibres

Three different types of fibre are described in connective tissue: a) the tough collagen bundles present in cartilage, ligaments, tendons and other connective tissues; b) the more extensible elastin fibres which predominate in blood vessels; and c) reticulin fibres: thin fibrils found in basement membrane and some loose connective tissue. Reticulin is similar to, and may be identical to, small collagen fibrils.

a) Collagen

Collagen accounts for about 30% of the total body protein. The basic unit is a long protein chain (approx length 300 nm) with a molecular weight of 285 000, and a natural tendency to exist in the solid phase. It is organised at several different levels: three fibres twist together to form a helix; and five of these helices are cross-linked to form a collagen fibril. Fibrils are further cross-linked to form the tough collagen fibres which give strength to cartilage, tendons and ligaments. This cross-linking is formed in a regular, reproducible way, so that the fibres look banded at a microscopic level (Fig. 1.2). Collagen is manufactured by cellular assembly of several separate protein chains; these are linked into triple helices and excreted from the cell as the soluble pro-collagen; the terminal portions of the proteins are then deleted by procollagen peptidase to produce insoluble collagen molecules.

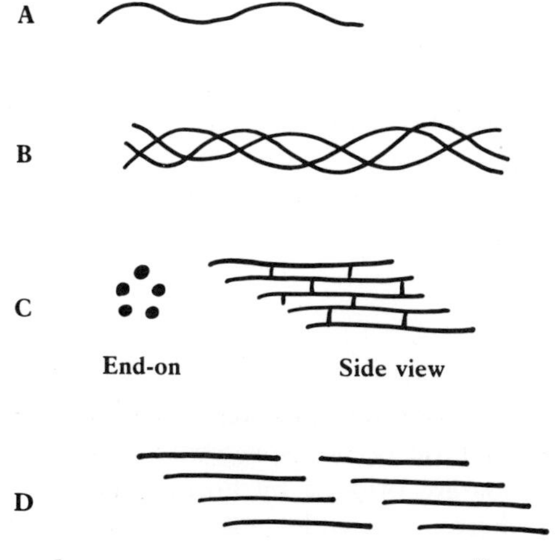

Fig. 1.2 The organisation of collagen fibres. A. Several different protein chains (α, β etc). **B**. Triple helix of protein chains forms collagen (e.g. α, $(II)_3$ in Type II collagen). **C**., Five helices form a fibril via cross-linking of collagen. **D**. Overlapping fibrils produce a 'banded' fibre of collagen.

The different types of collagen have slightly different amino-acid sequences in their constituent protein chains. As shown in Table 1.1, type II collagen (which has a relatively high content of hydroxylysine) is found in hyaline cartilage, type I collagen in most ligaments, tendons and periarticular tissue, and types III and IV in organs and basement membranes respectively. Other types of collagen have recently been described

Table 1.1 The main types of collagen

Type	Chain composition	Major sites
TYPE I	$[\alpha1\ (I)]_2\alpha2$	Bones, tendons, ligaments and elsewhere
TYPE II	$[\alpha1\ (II)]_3$	Cartilage
TYPE III	$[\alpha1\ (III)]_3$	Dermis, blood-vessels and elsewhere
TYPE IV	$[\alpha1\ (IV)]_3$	Basement membranes

b) Elastin

Fibres of elastin are found in vessel walls and in other tissue sites where elasticity is an important part of function. Elastin consists of long protein chains, but is less well-defined in its organisation than collagen. It is thought that numerous peptide chains link loosely together in spirals that can be stretched out to give the fibres their all-important elasticity.

4. Connective-tissue ground-substance

'Ground-substance' consists of complex sugars and proteins, usually linked together, filling the spaces between cells and fibres and playing a vital role in the regulation of tissue nutrition, support and water content. It is a remarkably complex, organised, dynamic and functionally important part of our connective tissues.

The basic subunits are proteoglycans and glycoproteins. The former consist of long-chain disaccharide sugar units linked to a central protein core, the latter of heterogenous polysaccharides linked to protein.

a) Proteoglycans

Glycosaminoglycans (GAG) are long-chain, unbranched polymers of repeating disaccharide units. They are linked by their terminal reducing sugars to protein-core molecules to form proteoglycans (PG). PG is the major constituent of the ground substance of cartilage and other articular and periarticular structures. The seven main sugar units (GAGs) are shown in Table 1.2. Hyaluronate is of major importance in synovial fluid and can form chains of very variable length, some of which are of massive proportions; chondroitin and keratin sulphate are found in cartilage proteoglycan, heparin in mast cells, and dermatan and heparan sulphate in other tissues.

Table 1.2 Major glycosaminoglycans of articular tissue

Compound	Molecular weight	Some sites of occurrence
Hyaluronic acid	4000–8000	Synovial fluid, cartilage
Chondroitin-4-sulphate	5–50	Cartilage
Chondroitin-6-sulphate	5–50	Vascular tissue
Dermatan sulphate	15–40	Skin, vascular tissue
Heparan sulphate	50	Lung, vascular tissue
Heparin	4–25	Mast cells
Keratan sulphate	4–20	Cartilage

The typical proteoglycan subunit of cartilage consists of a long-chain central protein core, with side-chains of keratin and chondroitin sulphate. These PGs may be further linked to a huge hyaluronate molecule to form an enormous proteoglycan aggregate, with a 'bottle-brush' structure (Fig. 1.3). These aggregates are strongly anionic and hydrophilic and have a strong influence on ionic concentrations, molecular transport, water content and swelling pressure of the tissues.

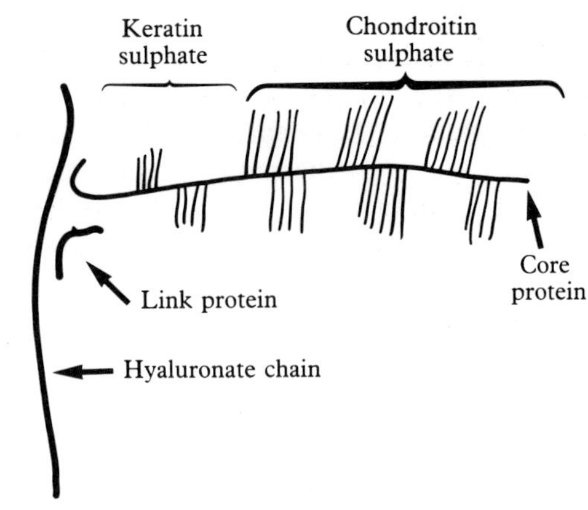

Fig. 1.3 Cartilage proteoglycans. Core protein has side chains of keratin sulphate and chondroitin-4-sulphate. In cartilage these proteoglycans are attached to long chains of hyaluronic acid via a link protein to form massive aggregates.

b) Glycoproteins

Glycoproteins are a diverse group of complex protein-sugar aggregates found in all connective tissues, basement membranes and cell surfaces. They form about 5% of cartilage dry weight and are widely distributed in other joint tissues. Other important examples of glycoproteins involved in joint disease include lysozyme, some of the acute-phase proteins, a lubricating glycoprotein recently identified in synovial fluid, cell-membrane antigens of the HLA system and blood-group specificity, and fibronectin. Fibronectin is a product of fibroblasts which occurs in the extracellular matrix, and has an apparent role to play in cell – cell attachment and in cell-collagen adhesion.

JOINTS

Joint structure depends on functional requirements; if little or no movement is necessary the bone-ends are bridged by fibrous tissue or cartilage, whereas if a wide range of movement is to occur a space must exist. Joints with cavities are bounded by a capsule which is lined by synovium which produces the lubricating fluid to fill the space. Joints are therefore classified as fibrous, cartilagenous or synovial.

Fibrous joints

These are articulations in which the bone-ends are fastened together by fibrous tissue (i.e. dense connective tissue containing a lot of collagen). They move very little. Examples include cranial sutures, tooth-to-jaw articulations (gomphoses) and the tibiofibular joint (a syndesmosis connected by an interosseous ligament).

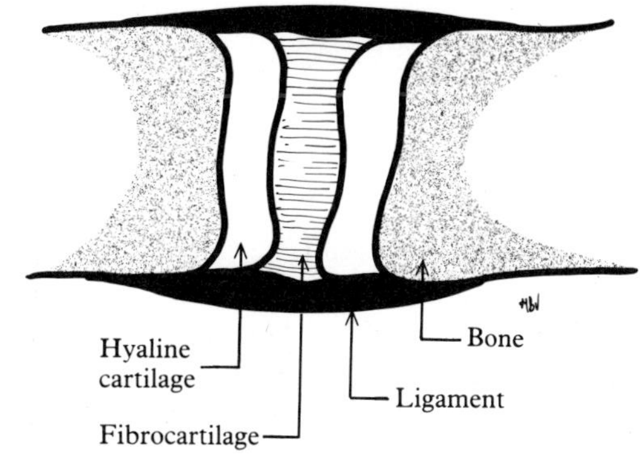

Fig. 1.4 Schematic cross-section of a fibrous joint

Cartilagenous joints

In these joints the bone-ends are connected to each other by cartilage and a limited amount of movement is possible. Primary cartilagenous joints are linked by hyaline cartilage, which eventually ossifies; such 'synchondroses' are found between the epiphyses and diaphyses of bones prior to epiphyseal fusion. Secondary cartilagenous joints (symphyses) usually have the structure shown in Figure 1.4. The bone-ends are covered with hyaline cartilage, and connected by flattened discs of fibrocartilage and fibrous bands (ligaments). The periphery of the cartilage and ligaments are richly innervated. Movement is allowed by compression of the relatively soft fibro-cartilage pad.

These joints occur in the axial skeleton rather than in the limbs; they include the manubrosternal joint, the pubic symphysis and the intervertebral joints.

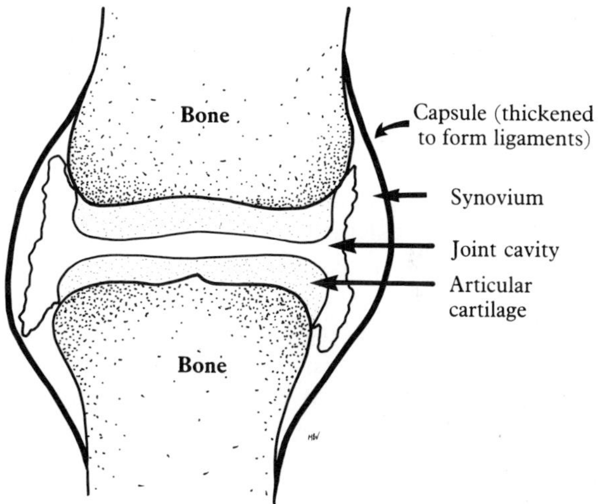

Fig. 1.5 Schematic cross-section of a synovial joint

Synovial joints

All the limb joints, as well as many axial ones, have a cavity, allowing free movement between the bone-ends; the stability of these articulations and limitation of movement therefore depends on muscles and ligaments surrounding them. The general structure is shown in Figure 1.5. The bone-ends are covered by a layer of hyaline cartilage; where this ends, synovial membrane is attached to the bone and reflected off it to surround the cavity; beneath the synovium is a thick tough fibrous capsule, which surrounds the joint and may be thickened to form ligaments. Some synovial joints have additional fibrocartilage pads dividing the cavity and attached to the capsule; the cavity itself is filled by a small volume of viscous synovial fluid.

a) Hyaline articular cartilage

The word *hyaline* is derived from the pearly-white, glistening appearance of the 2–4 mm thick structure which covers all articular surfaces. Hyaline cartilage is avascular, alymphatic and aneuronal; most of its dry weight comes from type II collagen and proteoglycans, and it contains relatively few cells (chondrocytes).

The zones, or strata, of articular cartilage are shown in Figure 1.6. The superficial zone contains collagen fibres lying tangentially to the surface,

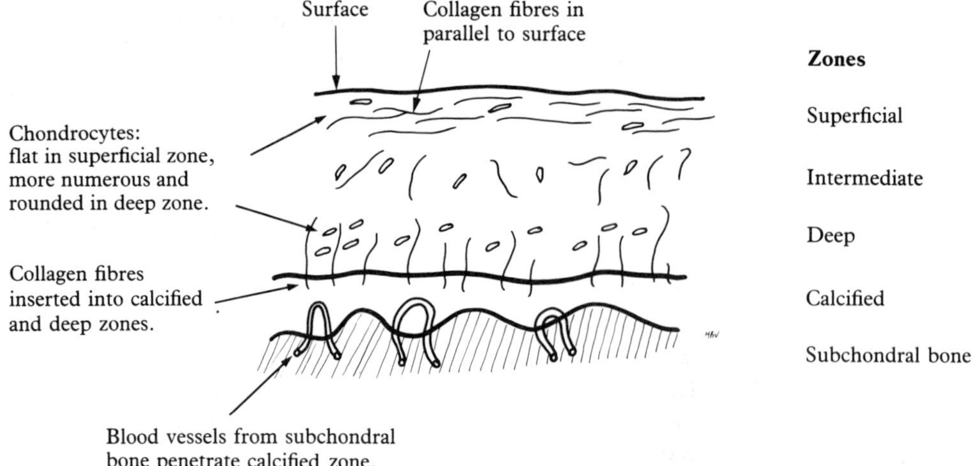

Fig. 1.6 Articular cartilage

criss-crossing fibres, and the deep zone has ovoid cells and fibres aligned perpendicular to the surface. The deep zone is demarcated by the 'tide-mark' from the calcified zone which interdigitates with bone.

The chondrocytes are surrounded by a clear zone of specialised ground-substance and often occur in groups of two or three. Nearly all the collagen is type II and the fibres form a tight meshwork which is interspersed with pressurised, hydrophilic proteoglycan molecules. The swelling pressure of the PGs gives the structure its rigidity. Conventional microscopy has suggested that the surface is not smooth, but many authors now believe that the ridges and pits seen are artifacts, and that *in vivo* articular cartilage does have a flat surface.

b) Fibrocartilage pads

These menisci occur in a few synovial joints and appear to divide the joint cavity and compensate for gross incongruity of joint surfaces. Fibrocartilage contains more collagen and less PG than hyaline cartilage, and type I as well as type II collagens are found. The whole tissue is softer and more pliable than hyaline cartilage because it lacks the same high content of pressurised PGs. Articular pads are usually attached to joint capsules, and may be covered with a synovial lining.

Joints containing fibrocartilage pads

1. Knee
2. Wrist
3. Tempero-mandibular joint
4. Sterno-clavicular joint
5. Acromio-clavicular joint

c) Synovial membrane

The synovial membrane is unusual as it has no true basement membrane. It consists of a loose connective-tissue stroma, interlaced with numerous capillaries, with a layer of one or two cells floating on its surface. There are very few nerve endings but numerous lymphatics. The capillary bed includes a deep layer of continuous vessels and a surface matrix of fenestrated capillaries with numerous gaps similar to those found in renal glomeruli (Fig. 1.7A).

Some authors distinguish three separate types of synovial tissue: areolar, fibrous and adipose. The fibrous type covers menisci and bone–cartilage junction areas; the areolar part is folded to allow movement and the adipose part covers subsynovial flat pads which extend into non-congruous areas of many joint cavities (Fig. 1.7B).

d) Capsule and ligaments

Subsynovial tissue merges with the joint capsule,

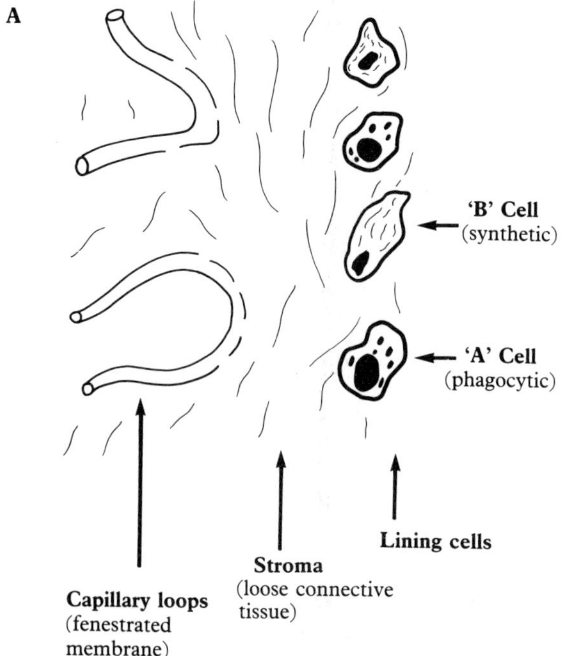

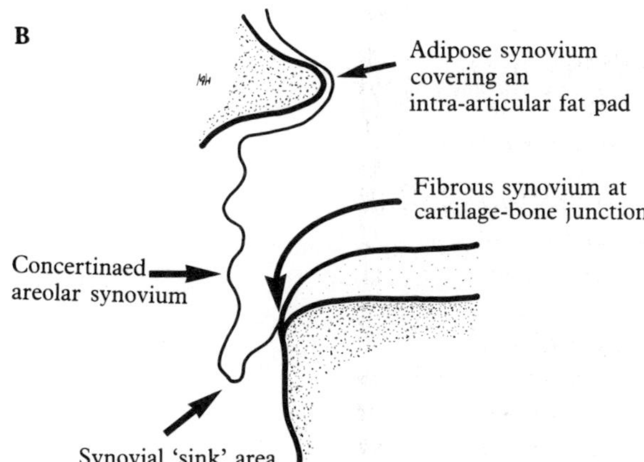

Fig. 1.7 A. The synovial lining of joints. **B.** Areas of joint synovium

which is a tough membrane encasing the joint cavity. Where joint movement needs to be limited, the capsule is thickened to form a ligament. Ligaments are fibrous bands of dense collagen bundles attached firmly to bone-ends; they tighten-up as the joint moves, thus preventing excess mobility. The capsule and ligaments, particularly where attached to bone, are the most innervated part of the joint, and contain numerous sensory and pain nerve endings.

e) The joint cavity and synovial fluid

The cavity of the joint contains synovial fluid. This is a viscous, clear, yellow substance containing very few cells and present in small volumes (large joints like the knee contain about 1 ml of fluid). Synovial fluid used to be thought of as a transudate of serum, to which synovial B cells added long chains of the GAG hyaluronate. It is now clear that the synovial membrane has a more active role and that various substances are transported more or less easily from serum to synovial fluid. The viscosity of the fluid is mainly due to the hyaluronate, but other substances, including some with probable lubricating function are added by the synoviocytes.

Nutrition of the avascular cartilage, as well as lubrication, is the main function of synovial fluid.

f) Bursae and tendons

Bursae are found throughout the body where movement causes friction between tissues. Deep bursae often overlie tendons or ligaments; superficial bursae usually overlie bony protruberances (examples include the olecranon, trochanteric and pre-patella bursae). The lining synovial tissue is like that of joint cavities and has a similar disease susceptibility.

Tendons are provided to transmit the movement of the contractile muscle tissue to the bone. Most of their dry weight is made up from type I collagen fibres arranged longitudinally. At one end these fibres are continuous with the fascial sheaths of muscle; at the other they merge into bone matrix through an area of partially mineralised fibrocartilage. The area of a tendon attachment to bone is richly innervated, well-vascularised and acts as a proprioceptive organ. Tendon and ligament insertions are also known as the 'entheses'.

g) Innervation and nutrition of joints

Nerve endings are found mainly in the capsule, ligaments and tendons of joints and in the enthesis. The cartilage is aneural and synovial tissue has very few nerve endings.

Four different morphological types of nerve ending are described and they have three main functions: nocioceptive (i.e. pain perception), proprioceptive (i.e. appreciation of joint position) and reflexogenic (i.e. reflex control of muscle tone around the joint).

The synovial membrane is richly vascularised from feeder vessels that enter at the joint margin. The bone end-plates also receive a good blood supply. However, the blood vessels end abruptly at the bone–cartilage junctions, and articular cartilage is avascular, perhaps due to the presence of an inhibitory factor that prevents vessels growing into the tissue. Cartilage nutrition is therefore dependent on the passage of molecules across the joint space or from the underlying bone. It seems likely that the synovial fluid composition and the proteoglycans of the cartilage facilitate transport of essential nutrients, but much remains to be learnt about nutrition and the passage of toxic and therapeutic substances into joints.

Joint function

The prime function of a joint is to allow controlled, stable movement. This requires well-lubricated surfaces that can withstand large stresses, and restraining factors to prevent instability.

a) Movement

Synovial joints can be classified according to their anatomy and the range of movement that this allows; ball-and-socket joints such as the hip allow much more movement than hinge joints such as the elbow, for example. The contour of the bones and the anatomy of the surrounding muscles, ligaments and other structures dictate movement, but the range or normal motion varies widely in different people and is affected by age, sex, race and occupation as well as by rheumatic disease.

b) Stability

Most movement is limited by ligaments becoming taut at the end of the normal range, or by the bony contour of the joint. Tendons and ligaments have a range of extensibility which rapidly decreases with increasing tension, providing flexible control of movement. Muscles, whose tension is partly controlled by proprioceptive information from tendon insertions, also provide stability. Thus if the quadriceps muscles around the knee are weak, the knee tends to 'give way' on use.

c) Lubrication

Synovial joint lubrication is excellent, the coefficient of friction being about 0.02 (less than that of a skate on ice). It increases with prolonged loading, but can withstand both sudden impulses and more sustained forces across the joint. Lubrication is probably facilitated by special glycoproteins such as 'lubricin', synthesised by the synovial membrane and attaching itself to the cartilage surface to aid boundary lubrication. Fluid is also forced out of the loaded cartilage to assist movement (boosted lubrication).

d) Biomechanics of joints

Articular cartilage has to withstand shear forces, impulse loading, and sustained pressure. Normal joints are not congruous (Fig. 1.8) so that weight-bearing is limited to a small area of the surface. Load-bearing may alter the contact areas by causing deformation of the cartilage and underlying bone. The rate of change of these forces is

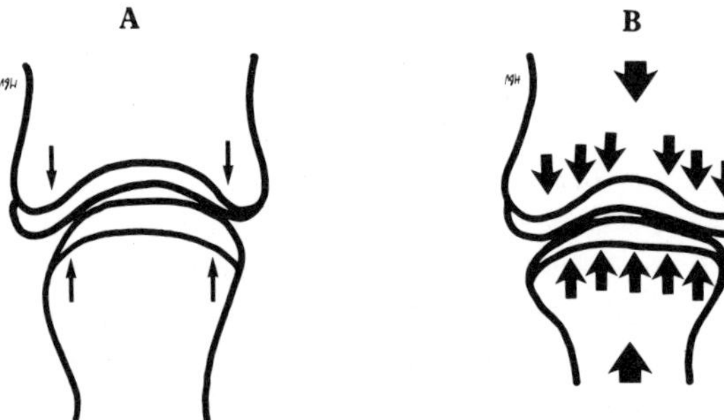

Fig. 1.8 Joint congruity and load-bearing areas. Joints are normally incongruous (**A**), small areas of weight-bearing occurring at the joint margin. Heavy loading (**B**) increases the areas of contact.

enormous; the load on the hip joint, for example, may increase to about five times body weight on heel strike, and then become negative as the foot is lifted off the ground. In rheumatic disease these forces and their distribution may be altered considerably and joint congruity is often changed.

e) Synthetic function of joint tissue

The synovial membrane and articular cartilage both have important synthetic functions as well as providing smooth, stable movement. The membrane produces the hyaluronate and other glycoproteins of synovial fluid, and the chondrocytes are constantly renewing the cartilage matrix. The rate of turnover of the proteoglycans and collagen is slow (particularly that of collagen), but may be of importance in chronic rheumatic disease.

f) Reticuloendothelial function of joints

The phagocytic cells of the synovial membrane are scavengers able to remove debris from the joint space quickly and efficiently. There are also specialised immunoreactive cells in the membrane, which respond briskly to the presence of foreign antigens. The membrane can rapidly transform into tissue like that seen in lymph nodes. This aspect of joint function has protective value, but is also important in the pathogenesis of joint disease (Chapter 2).

DISEASE OF THE MUSCULOSKELETAL SYSTEM

The WHO has defined rheumatology as that branch of medicine concerned with disorders of the musculoskeletal or locomotor system, including inflammatory and other joint diseases, generalised connective-tissue disorders, back problems and disorders of the periarticular tissues. Rheumatic diseases can be further subdivided or classified according to their aetiology, pathology, anatomical structures involved or clinical features.

Different structures may be damaged in rheumatic disease. Some conditions are limited to one site; for example many bone and periarticular lesions remain anatomically localised. Disorders of the subchondral bone, articular cartilage or synovial tissues tend to interact because of the close anatomical and functional relationship of these tissues. Thus Paget's disease of bone (affecting the subchondral bone) often causes a secondary arthritis, and synovitis of any cause may result in secondary damage to the articular cartilage. Many other disorders affect the connective tissues more generally, although they may be localised in their clinical expression due to the influence of other local factors.

Several different aetiological factors have been identified in rheumatic disease. Most current classifications are based on aetiology, and in this book separate chapters are devoted to infectious diseases, crystal deposition disease, neoplasia,

Anatomical structures affected in the rheumatic diseases

1. Localised disorders, e.g.
   a) Some bone disorders
   b) Many periarticular lesions
2. Joint disease involves
   a) Subchondral bone
   b) Articular cartilage
   c) Synovium
3. Generalised, e.g.
   Abnormalities of connective tissue

Aetiological factors in rheumatic disease

1. Congenital abnormalities in connective-tissue structure or function
2. Physical trauma
3. Infection
4. Immunopathogenic mechanisms
5. Nutritional deficiency
6. Chemical injury
7. Crystal deposition and the presence of particles
8. Neoplastic changes
9. Ageing of connective tissues

nutritional and toxic disorders and inherited abnormalities of connective tissue. However, many of the most important rheumatic diseases including rheumatoid arthritis, osteoarthritis and systemic lupus erythematosus remain idiopathic. In some synovial inflammation and immunopathogenic mechanisms dominate the pathology (Chapter 2), in others age-related changes in the connective tissues appear to be important. Several other idiopathic diseases can only be defined on a clinical basis: polymyalgia rheumatica for example, is recognised and diagnosed on the basis of a characteristic symptom complex but its aetiology and pathology remain obscure.

Ageing of connective tissue

All elements of connective tissue change continually throughout life; the rapid change in structure and function during growth being followed by a slower phase of gradual change in later years.

As age increases there may be a gradual loss in the cellular elements of connective tissues such as the articular cartilage, which also loses water in its deeper zones. Collagen changes little, although cross-linking may alter. Proteoglycan aggregation changes and the glycosaminoglycan content of different tissues alters with age; there is an increase in chondroitin-6-sulphate at the expense of chondroitin-4-sulphate for example. At the macroscopic level, cartilage thins a little and gains a yellow colour (an age-related pigment). Other tissues such as bone and skin may show more dramatic loss of thickness and substance. Age is also associated with changes in other systems, including renal and hepatic function and immune surveillance.

The influence of these age-related changes on the pathogenesis of joint disease in unclear. Some disorders, such as rheumatic fever, are most prevalent in childhood; others, like ankylosing spondylitis chiefly affect young adults; increasing age apparently protects against the onset of these conditions. Other diseases increase in prevalence with age or occur mainly in the elderly; examples include osteoarthritis, crystal deposition diseases and polymyalgia rheumatica, although age alone is an insufficient explanation for their pathogenesis.

Connective-tissue breakdown

Connective-tissue destruction can be produced mechanically by physical disruption of bones or joints or chemically by proteolytic enzymes released during inflammation (Table 1.3).

Table 1.3 Two 'final common pathways' in the breakdown of articular tissue

1. Physical disruption
   Balance: Mechanical forces — v — Tissue resistance
2. Inflammation
   Balance: Autodigestion — v — Tissue repair

The joints and periarticular tissues are subjected to repetitive mechanical stress and only survive if the connective-tissue matrix can cope with the forces applied. Abnormal stress or excessive use can destory tissue; obvious examples include bone fractures due to trauma of to overuse (stress fractures). If the connective tissue matrix is weakened, due to loss of proteoglycan or abnormal collagen for example, normal joint use may cause mechanical damage.

Chemical disruption of connective tissues can result from extraneous toxins but is much more commonly due to the proteases released from macrophages, polymorphonuclear leucocytes and other cells found in inflamed tissue. Inflammation can also lead to the generation of increased levels of destructive enzymes from connective-tissue cells such as the chondrocyte, which may then destroy rather than maintain the tissue matrix. Inflammation is the most important single pathogenic mechanism known in the rheumatic diseases and is the final common pathway causing both symptoms and tissue damage in many different disorders.

Inflammation

Inflammation can be defined as the response of living tissue to injury. It is a protective response which mobilises phagocytic cells to remove the injurious stimuli, brings antibody and other humoral antitoxins to the site of damage and activates the repair process. However, in many rheumatic diseases inflammation appears to be

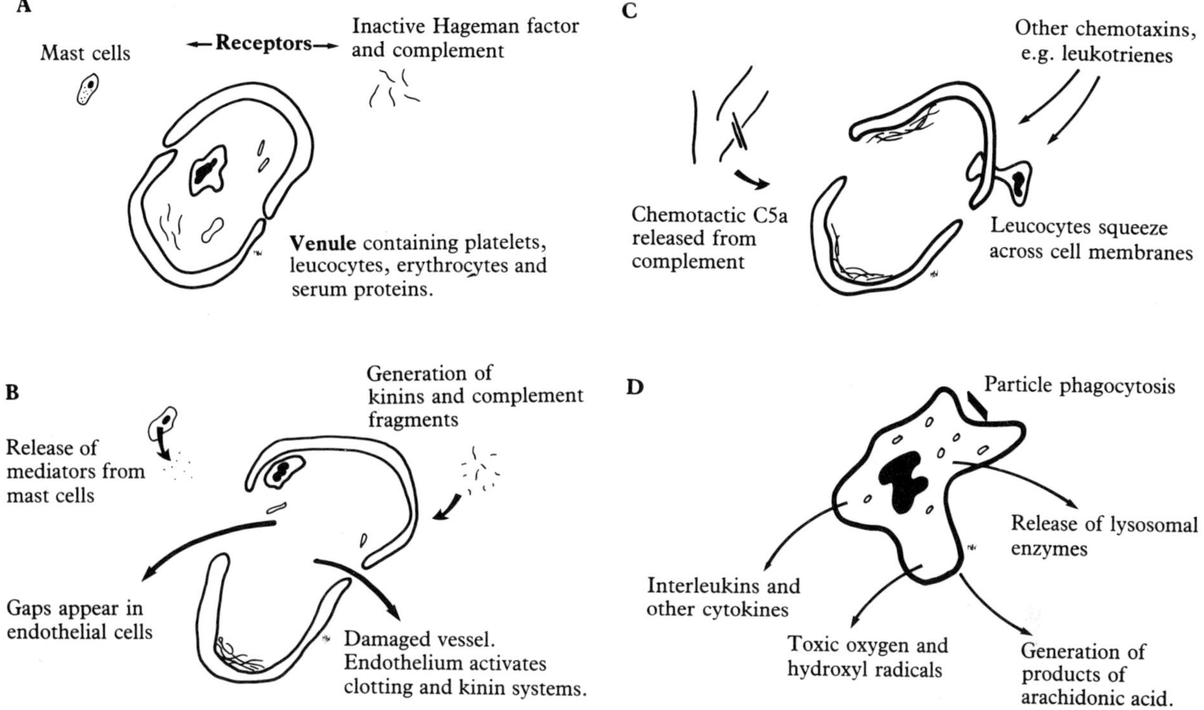

Fig. 1.9 The pathophysiology of inflammation. **A**. Resting state. **B**. Vasodilation. **C**. Chemotaxis. **D**. Phagocytosis and secretion.

inappropriate, and a cause of symptoms and joint damage. Rightly or wrongly, anti-inflammatory therapy is often used.

Pathophysiology of inflammation (Fig. 1.9)

Inflammation is characterised by vasodilatation and the exudation of fluid and cells from the intravascular space into the tissues. Arterioles dilate and gaps appear in the walls of the venules, through which the protein-rich exudate passes. The leucocytes migrate by amoeboid movement across vessel walls. In the early stages polymorphonuclear cells predominate, but macrophages appear in increasing numbers as the process continues. The phagocytic cells remove debris and stimulate the repair process. This has three elements: fibrogenesis, neovascularisation (which forms the granulation tissue) and tissue regeneration.

The main clinical signs of inflammation (as first described by Galen) are due to this vasodilatation and exudation (Table 1.4). Heat, swelling and redness remain important clinical signs in the assessment of activity in joint diseases. Joint pain can have a variety of causes, but if due to inflammation stretching and compressing joint tissue it is usually associated with morning stiffness.

Table 1.4 Relationship between the cardinal signs of inflammation (Celsus, Galen) and the basic pathological changes of inflammation. Heat redness and swelling are caused by acute vasodilation and emigration of fluid and cells into the lesion. Pain results from chemical products such as histamine, kinins and prostaglandins affecting sensory receptors. Fibrosis and new vessel growth are part of the healing process mediated by mononuclear cells. Loss of function can result from physical disruption of the tissue and reflex changes due to pain.

Sign	Pathological change
Heat Redness	Vasodilation
Swelling	Fluid exudate Chemotaxis of phagocytic cells
Pain	Fibrosis
Loss of function	New vessel formation

Table 1.5 The inflammatory cascade

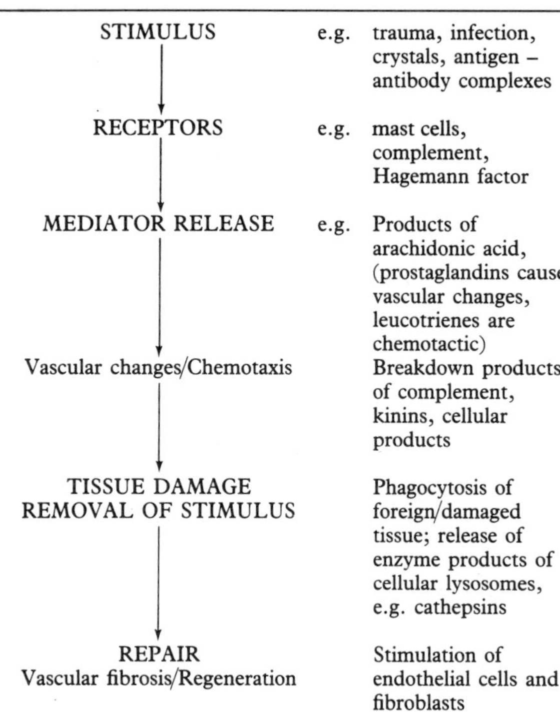

STIMULUS ↓	e.g.	trauma, infection, crystals, antigen – antibody complexes
RECEPTORS ↓	e.g.	mast cells, complement, Hagemann factor
MEDIATOR RELEASE ↓	e.g.	Products of arachidonic acid, (prostaglandins cause vascular changes, leucotrienes are chemotactic)
Vascular changes/Chemotaxis ↓		Breakdown products of complement, kinins, cellular products
TISSUE DAMAGE REMOVAL OF STIMULUS ↓		Phagocytosis of foreign/damaged tissue; release of enzyme products of cellular lysosomes, e.g. cathepsins
REPAIR Vascular fibrosis/Regeneration		Stimulation of endothelial cells and fibroblasts

Mediators of inflammation (Table 1.5)

The main humoral mediators of inflammation include a group of low-molecular-weight substances released from receptors in response to a stimulus. These include packages of preformed histamine and serotonin from mast cells and platelets, and kinins and products of the complement cascade released by cleavage of circulating proteins. As the reaction develops, further mediators are synthesised and secreted from cell membranes and cytoplasm. Products of membrane arachidonic acid have an important role in inflammation and include the vasodilator prostaglandins and the chemotactic leucotrienes (Fig. 1.10). Lysosomal enzymes are important causes of tissue damage, and a variety of the poorly-characterised 'cytokines' (see p 4) are also released. Over the last few years a massive research effort has been centred on the characterisation of these mediators and modulators of inflammation and tissue damage, in an attempt to find pharmacological control of this mechanism of joint disease.

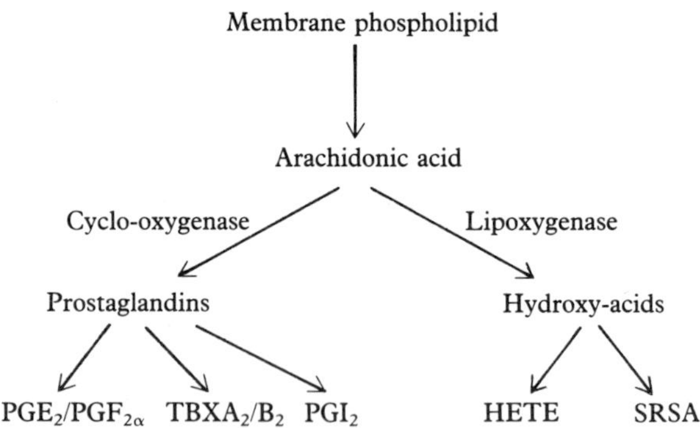

Fig. 1.10 Arachidonic acid cascade. Membrane phospholipids form arachidonic acid, which can be oxygenated into prostaglandins or hydroxyl-acids. Several classes of prostaglandin, with differing actions on inflammation and other tissues, are produced and quickly metabolised. Products of the lipoxygenase pathway include slow-releasing substance A (SRS-A) and hydroxy-acids with chemotactic activity (e.g. HETE).

The systemic response to inflammation (Fig. 1.11):

Local inflammation causes a generalised systemic response which includes fever, malaise, weight-loss, changes in the synthesis of hepatic proteins and changes in the cellular elements of the blood. Many of these effects are probably mediated by the generation of interleukin I from macrophages. These systemic changes may modify local inflammation; in clinical practice they are often used to monitor the activity of a rheumatic disease and its response to therapy.

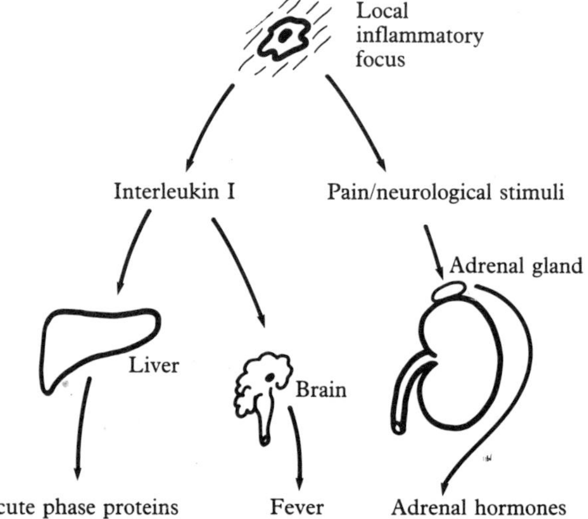

Fig. 1.11 Systemic aspects of inflammation

THE INTEGRITY OF CONNECTIVE TISSUES AND JOINTS

Joints and connective tissues do not 'wear out'. Normal use has been shown to be important in maintaining bone strength and the thickness of articular cartilage and people who pursue demanding physical activity do not develop premature joint disease. It has been estimated that one would have to live for 200 years or more before the subtle age changes in connective tissue led to significant joint damage. The structure and integrative function of each of the connective-tissue elements described are obviously able to withstand many years of repetitive mechanical stress.

The integrity of joints can be disturbed by several different disease mechanisms. Alteration in the ability of the joint to withstand stress may result. Inflammation is a final common pathway in response to most insults to joints. It is one of the body's most important natural defence mechanisms, removing abnormal tissue and initiating repair.

In most people normal joint function is maintained, the defense mechanisms acting as an adequate barrier to disease. The remainder of this book is concerned with the important minority (10–20% of the population, see Chapter 3) who develop significant joint disease.

FURTHER READING

Cruess R L 1982 The musculskeletal system. Embryology, biochemistry and physiology. Churchill Livingstone, Edinburgh

Sokoloff L 1980 The joints and synovial fluid. Academic Press, New York

Panayi G 1982 Scientific basis of rheumatology. Churchill Livingstone, Edinburgh

Gardner D L 1979 Diseases of connective tissue. Journal of Clinical Pathology Suppl 12

Ryan G B, Majno G 1977 Acute inflammation. American Journal of Pathology 86(1): 185–276

Hasselbacher P 1981 The biology of the joint. Clinics in rheumatic diseases 7 (1).

2 Immunopathogenic mechanisms

The identification of rheumatoid factor and the LE cell factor in the 1940s was the first clue that immunological events might be associated with the pathogenesis of certain rheumatic diseases. Since then, the study of immunological abnormalities characterising many of these diseases has gone hand in hand with studies of the immunochemistry and cellular functions of the normal immune system. These have given insights into the cellular, humoral and genetic mechanisms in the immune response, and help to explain associations between various rheumatic diseases and certain histocompatibility antigens and how a particular genetic background might lead to a pathogenic immune response triggered off by an appropriate environmental stimulus. While immunological abnormalities may be secondary to an underlying disorder there is compelling evidence that they may contribute not only to the tissue injury seen in clinical disease but also to the perpetuation of these disorders.

COMPONENTS OF THE IMMUNE SYSTEM

1. The cellular components

The manner in which an antigen stimulates immunity is immensely complex and involves lymphocytes as the specific antigen-recognising cells, and macrophages, mast cells and leucocytes as accessory and effector cells. A multiplicity of effector functions are generated and a fine balance is developed between those which are beneficial and those which are potentially harmful to the host. This control largely depends on subtle cell-to-cell interactions, some of which are genetically determined.

a) Lymphocytes

Lymphocytes have a central role in the immune system since the stimulation of an immune response to both foreign and autoantigens involves activation of specific lymphocytes (Fig. 2.1).

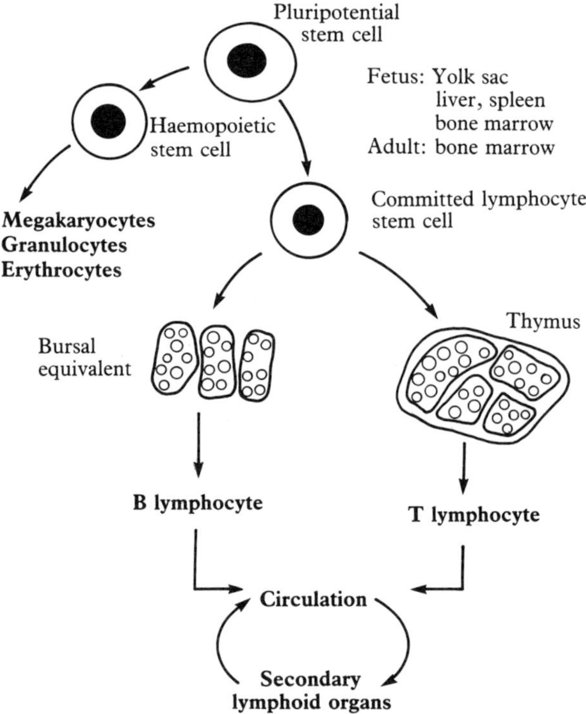

Fig. 2.1 The origin of T and B lymphocytes

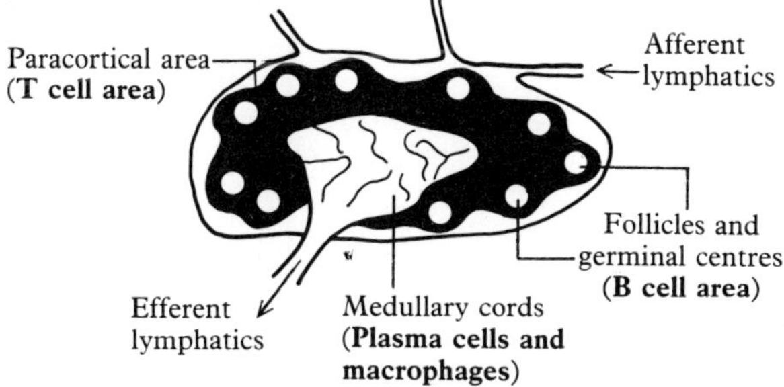

Fig. 2.2 The internal structure of a lymph node

In man, lymphocyte precursors differentiate along two pathways into two major categories, T and B cells. Those that differentiate in the micro-environment of the thymus to become T cells mediate the classical reactions of cellular immunity, which include delayed hypersensitivity, graft rejection and destruction of intracellular pathogens, while those that differentiate in the micro-environment equivalent to the bursa of Fabricius of birds (probably the central lymphoid organs and the lamina propria) to become B cells represent the precursor of antibody-producing plasma cells. T and B cells can be distinguished not only by differences in function and in distribution in peripheral lymphoid tissues but also by cell surface markers (Fig. 2.2 and Table 2.1).

A small proportion of peripheral lymphocytes bear no surface markers for either T cells or B cells. These are termed *null cells* and probably represent a heterogeneous population of cells. A large proportion of null cells bear receptors for the Fc portion of immunoglobulin and are able to kill target cells which are coated with antibody (antibody-dependent cellular cytotoxicity — ADCC) (Fig. 2.3).

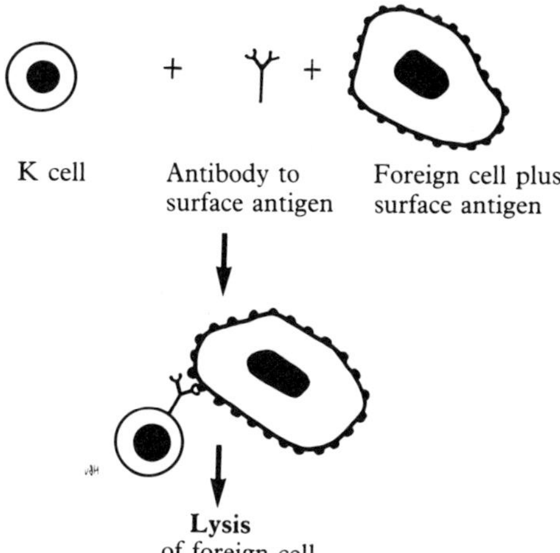

Fig. 2.3 Antibody-dependent cytotoxicity

b) Lymphocytes and the immune response

Immunological effector functions have been classified into two broad categories: (i) *Humoral immunity* — antigen-specific reactions carried out

Table 2.1 Lymphocyte characteristics

	T lymphocyte	B lymphocyte
Function	Delayed hypersensitivity Graft vs host reactions Lymphokine production Killer cells Helper cells Suppressor cells	Antibody production
Anatomical locations		
Blood	70%	20%
Thoracic duct	90%	10%
Lymph nodes	Paracortical areas	Germinal centres and medullary cords
Spleen	Periarteriolar zone	Germinal centres Red pulp
Surface markers	Receptors for sheep RBC Reactive with specific monoclonal antibody, eg. OKT3	Surface immunoglobulin Receptors for C3, EB virus and Fc of immunoglobulin Ia antigens
Functional assessment	Proliferate in response to mitogens: PHA, ConA	Secrete immunoglobulin

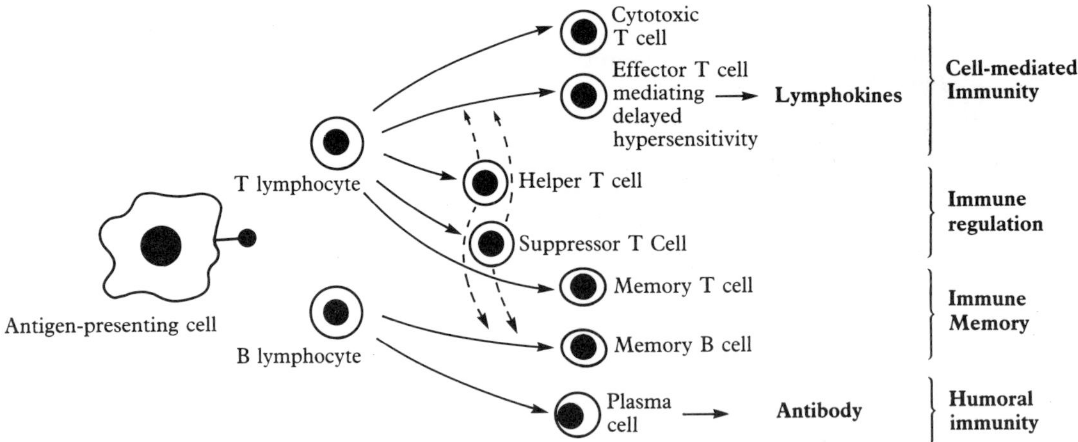

Fig. 2.4 Hypothetical scheme for antigen-induced humoral and cell-mediated immunity

by various classes of immunoglobulin molecules, often associated with amplification systems such as the complement pathway; (*ii*) *Cell mediated-immunity* — antigen-specific reactions carried out by T cells or their products (Fig. 2.4).

(*i*) *Humoral immunity*. In response to an antigenic challenge, B lymphocytes are activated and transform into immunoblasts. Some differentiate further into antibody-producing plasma cells (Fig. 2.5).

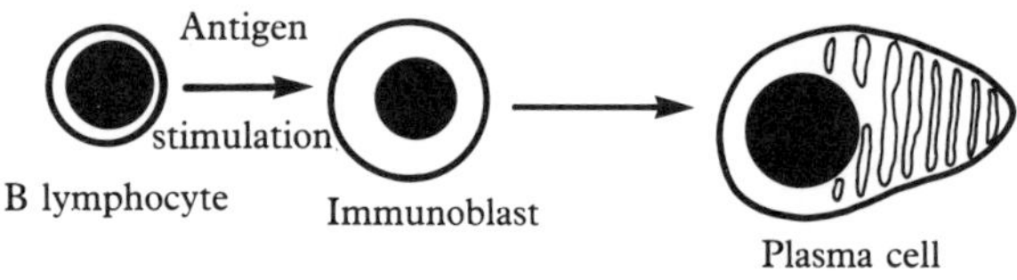

Fig. 2.5 Activation of B lymphocytes by antigen

Subpopulations of B cells are seen which express different classes of surface immunoglobulin. The earliest immunoglobulin-bearing cells generated in the marrow have surface IgM while the majority of mature peripheral B lymphocytes bear both IgM and IgD. It is hypothesised that the type of immunoglobulin receptor determines the result of antigen stimulation: binding of antigen to an IgM receptor leads to tolerance, while antigen binding to IgD leads to immunoglobulin production (Fig. 2.6).

Immunoglobulin in man consists of five distinct groups of proteins: IgG, IgM, IgA, IgE and IgD (Fig. 2.7, table 2.2). Each immunoglobulin class has specific features but they share in common a basic unit composed of a symmetrical structure of four polypeptides: two heavy chains and two light chains that are linked to each other by disulphide

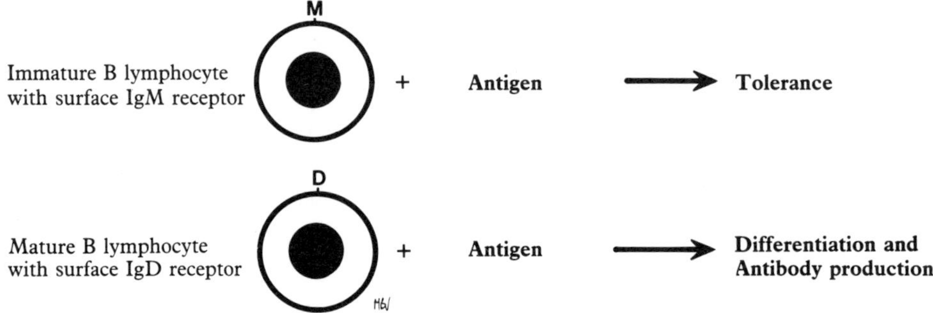

Fig. 2.6 The response of a B lymphocyte to antigen stimulation depends on the type of surface antigen receptor

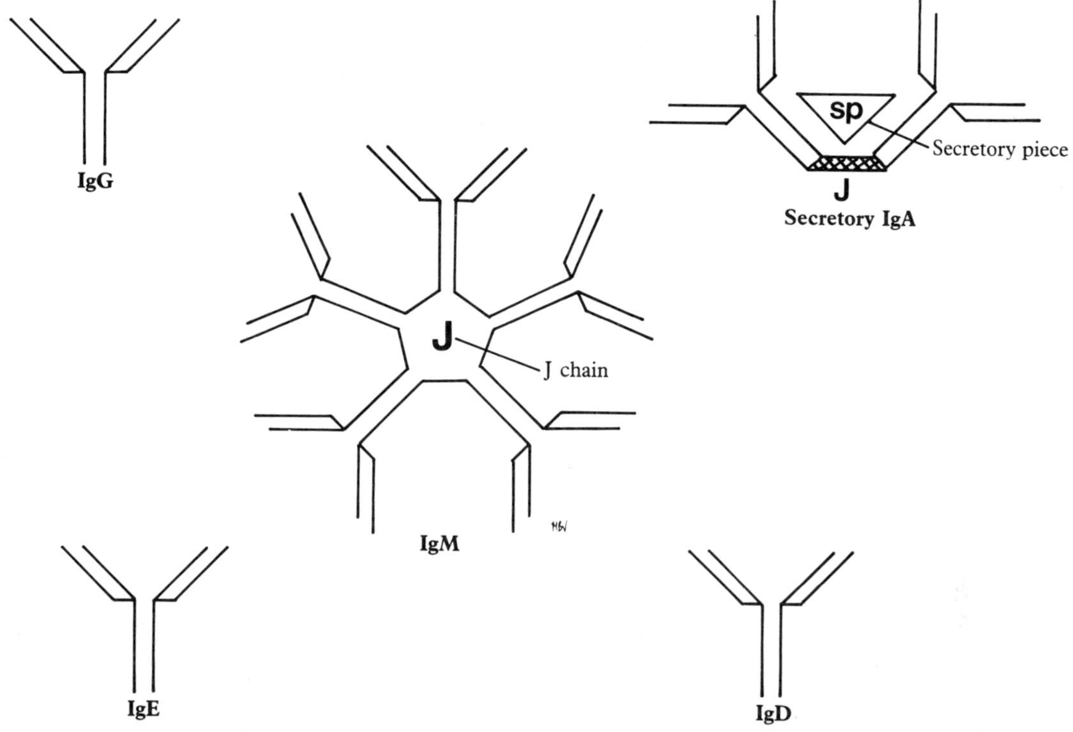

Fig. 2.7 Immunoglobulin classes in man

Table 2.2 Properties of immunoglobulin types

Classes	IgG	IgM	IgA	IgE	IgD
Molecular weight	150 000	900 000	160 000–350 000 (monomer: dimer)	190 000	180 000
Subclasses	1, 2, 3, 4		1, 2		
Presence in secretions	+	+	sIgA	?	?
Concentration in serum (mg/dl)	800–1700 (80% of serum Ig)	50–190	140–420	0.0001–0.0007	0.3–40
Special properties					
Placental passage	+ (1, 3, 4)				
Complement fixation					
— classical	+ (1, 2, 3)	+			
— alternative	+ (4)		+	+	
Binding to macrophages and neutrophils	+ (1, 3)				
Binding to mast cells and basophils				+	
Other properties		Present on lymphocyte membrane	Secretory immune system	Defence against parasites	Present on lymphocyte membrane

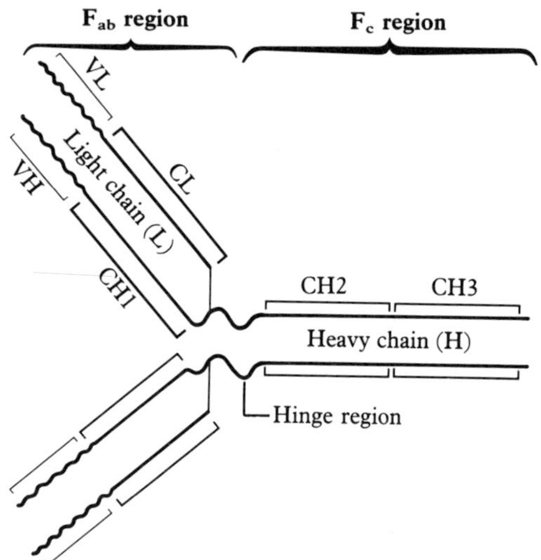

Fig. 2.8 A schematic model for human IgG

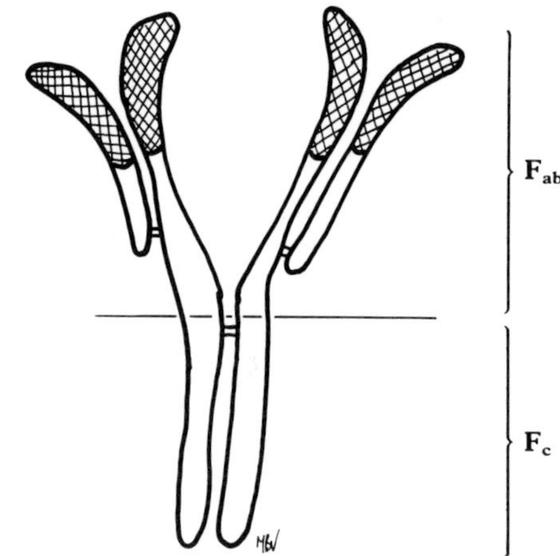

Fig. 2.9 The basic structure of the immunoglobulin molecule showing the F_{ab} and F_c regions. Papain cleaves the immunoglobulin molecule on the amino-terminus side of the inter heavy chain disulphide bridge to yield two identical F_{ab} fragments and the F_c fragment.

bonds (Fig. 2.8). The classes differ in several ways: a) in the aminoacid sequence of their class-specific heavy chains; b) other structural differences, such as the disulphide bridge pattern, number of domains, the type of carbohydrate associated with the protein skeleton and the degree of polymerisation; c) their biological function; d) their distribution in the tissues. IgG and IgA can be further divided into subclasses based on specific antigenic determinants present in the heavy chains. Light chains exist in two different types, kappa (κ) or lambda (λ). They are not class specific and occur in all classes.

In addition to light and heavy chains certain classes of immunoglobin contain other protein components. Polymeric immunoglobulins such as IgM and IgA (which may occur in the serum in monomeric or polymeric form) contain a polypeptide termed the *J chain*. IgA in secretions contains a secretory piece not present in serum IgA.

Each polypeptide chain is built up of small subunit structures, approximately 100 amino acids in length, centred around a disulphide bridge. The variable domain is found at the amino-terminal end of each polypeptide chain. Here there is marked variability in amino-acid residues, and this accounts for antigenic specificity. The variable domains of the light and heavy chains overlap at the aminoterminus of the molecule to provide the antigen-binding region (Fig. 2.9). Even though antibody molecules show remarkable specificity in antigen binding, an antibody will bind any antigen whose structure fits into its antigen-binding region. The better the fit, the tighter the binding, i.e. high-affinity binding (Fig. 2.10). Each antibody, therefore, has its unique spectrum of binding affinities.

The constant domains do not exhibit the same amino-acid variability and are basically equivalent within a given class, although there are allotype differences between individuals. For IgG these allotypes are known as Gm types. At the hinge region of the molecule the arms of the antibody are free to rotate upon binding antigen. The hinge region subdivides the molecule into the Fab portion (the antigen-binding portion of the molecule) and the Fc region, which conveys biological activities to the antibody molecule, including placental transfer, complement activation and binding to receptor sites on cells such as macrophages, polymorphs and mast cells.

(*ii*) *Cell-mediated immunity*. T-cell activity can be divided into three categories: regulation of the immune response, cytotoxicity and production of biologically-active soluble factors (lymphokines). Subpopulations of T cells mediating these different functions can be recognised using

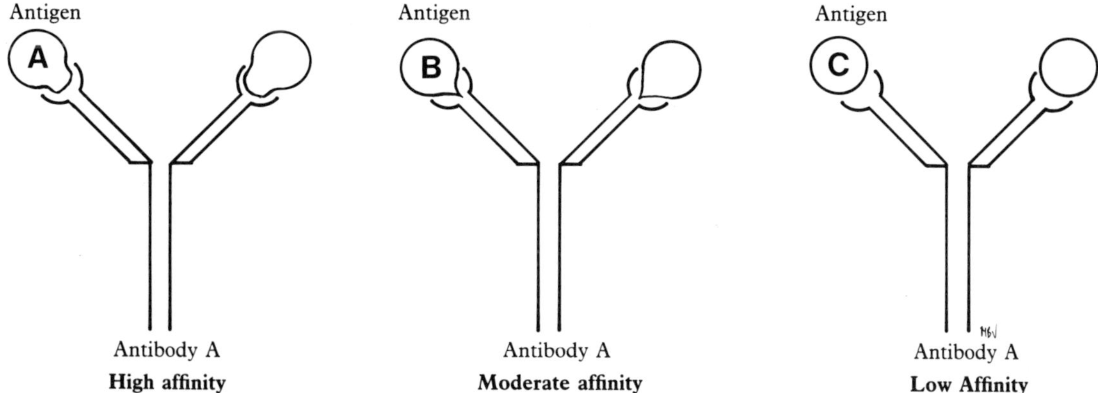

Fig. 2.10 The affinity of binding to an antigen depends upon how well the antigen fits into the antigen-binding site of the antibody

Table 2.3 T-cell subsets defined by monoclonal antibodies (Orthoclone series)

Subset	% peripheral T cells	Function
T4	60%	Helper
T8	20%	Suppressor/Cytotoxic

monoclonal antibodies to cell surface markers (Table 2.3). Cell-mediated immunity has long been identified with elimination of foreign antigen by antigen-specific activation of T-lymphocytes into effector cells with either cytotoxic activity or the ability to produce lymphokines which initiate inflammation and enhance the accumulation and killing ability of macrophages (Table 2.4).

Table 2.4 Example of T-cell lymphokines

Lymphokine	Function
Lymphotoxin	Death of cells
Macrophage inhibition factor	Inhibits macrophage movement
Macrophage activation factor	Localises macrophages in area of antigen–lymphocyte interaction activates macrophages to kill tumour cells and enhances phagocytic potential
Interferon	Blocks viral replication
Interleukin 2	Induces lymphocytes to proliferate

Tissue distribution of the monocyte-macrophage system

1. Blood	Monocyte
2. Connective tissue	Histiocyte; macrophage
3. Brain	Microglial cell
4. Liver	Kupffer cell
5. Bone	Osteoclasts
6. Lung	Alveolar macrophages
7. Synovium	Synovial A cells Multinucleate giant cells
8. Granulomata	Epithelioid cells Multinucleate giant cells
9. Spleen	Macrophages

c) *Macrophages*

Tissue macrophages are derived from the circulating blood monocytes and play a central role in the immune response, both in the initiation and genetic regulation of the immune response and in the effector mechanism as an important source of inflammatory mediators and destructive enzymes. Macrophages mediate at least four distinct but interlinking functions (Fig. 2.11):

(*i*) *Antigen uptake and processing*. Macrophages process antigen in such a way that T-lymphocytes

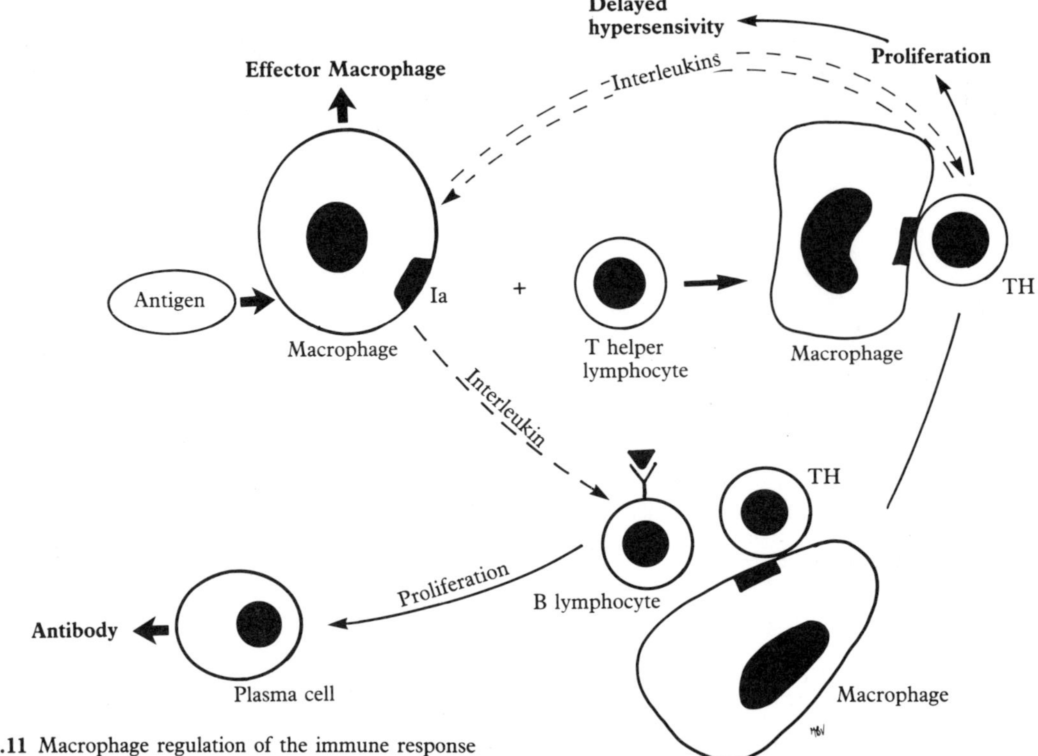

Fig. 2.11 Macrophage regulation of the immune response

which interact with macrophage-bound antigen became immunologically activated. This requires a direct macrophage–lymphocyte interaction and involves recognition of surface alloantigens expressed by genes in the major histocompatibility complex (MHC), as well as the presence of specific antigen.

(*ii*) *Phagocytosis*. Macrophages possess several plasma membrane receptors such as those for the Fc portion of IgG, that augment the killing and phagocytosis of infectious agents.

(*iii*) *Capacity for chemotaxis*. Macrophages can be actively concentrated in the site of an immune response by soluble factors released during the course of an immune response.

(*iv*) *Secretion of soluble factors*. Macrophages and monocytes secrete a wide range of biologically active molecules that influence the development of the afferent limb of the immune response (e.g. interleukin 1) or are directly responsible for many of the major clinical and pathological events of chronic allergic and inflammatory disease. The latter include a wide variety of enzymes which are described further in Chapter 1.

d) *Inflammatory cells*

While the lymphocyte and macrophage are central elements of the immune system there are wide-ranging interactions with other cells involved in inflammation which mediate effector functions of immunity. The immune and inflammatory systems interact via a variety of soluble mediators including immunoglobulins, lymphokines and products of the complement pathway. The cells involved include:

(*i*) *Neutrophil granulocytes*. These constitute the predominant circulating white cell and represent the primary phagocytes of the body. They are capable of chemotaxis and of immune adherence by virtue of Fc and C3b surface receptors. As the result of antigen–antibody interaction and complement activation, polymorphs are attracted in large numbers to the site of an immune reaction where,

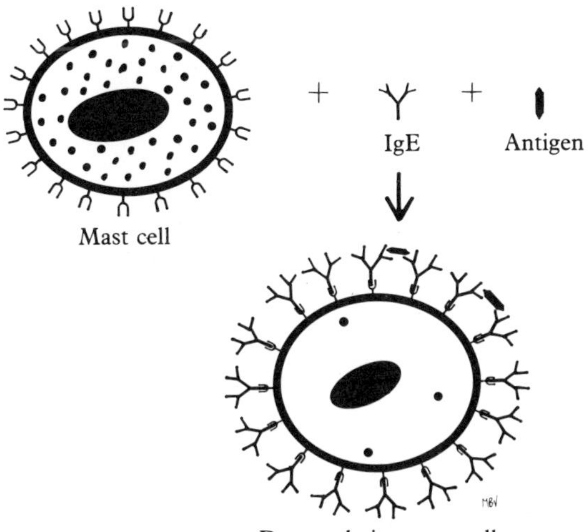

Fig. 2.12 Degranulation of a mast cell following the bridging of two surface-bound IgE molecules by antigen

during the course of phagocytosis, they release large amounts of lysosomal enzymes.

(*ii*) *Basophils and mast cells* (Fig. 2.12). These cells have an important role in immediate hypersensitivity reactions. They bear receptors for the Fc part of IgE and when two of these surface-bound molecules are bridged by binding antigen, basophils and mast cells are activated and degranulate with release of soluble mediators such as histamine, slow-releasing substance of anaphylaxis (SRS-A) and eosinophilic chemotactic factor of anaphylaxis (ECF-A).

(*iii*) *Eosinophils.* Eosinophilia is associated with states of immunity such as allergy, drug reaction and hypersensitivity states. The eosinophil has an important role in mediating immediate hypersensitivity reactions and the host response to tissue-invading parasites. Its role in other immune reactions is still unclear but it is known to be a powerful phagocyte particularly of antigen–antibody complexes.

e) Interactions between lymphocytes and macrophages

The separation of the immune system into two arms is rather misleading, since an optimal immune response to most antigens requires co-operation between macrophages, B cells and T cells. Immune responses are complex and require an intricate interplay of positive as well as negative influences which are mediated by various functional subpopulations of these cells (Fig. 2.13). A large body of evidence indicates that many of these interactions are genetically determined involving genes in the major histocompatibility complex on chromosome 6, which is described later in this chapter.

2. The soluble components

The immune response is closely linked to the process of inflammation through the interaction of humoral systems. In addition to immunoglobulin and lymphokines produced by activated lymphocytes, these include the complement, coagulation, fibrinolytic and kinin systems. These systems are made up of a series of plasma proteins which,

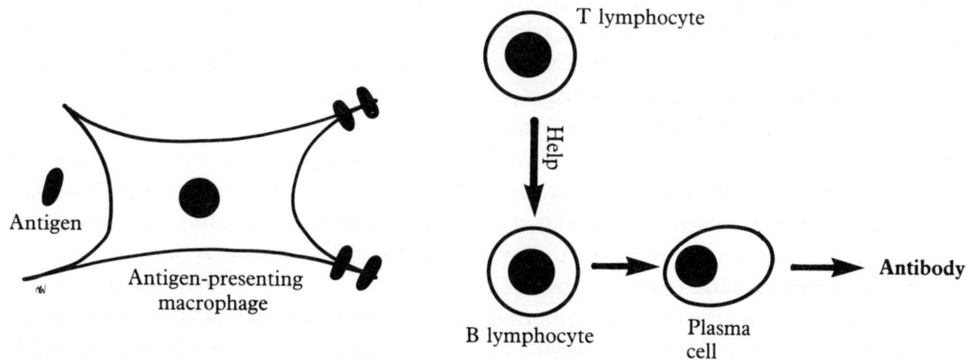

Fig. 2.13 Macrophage – lymphocyte interaction in antibody induction

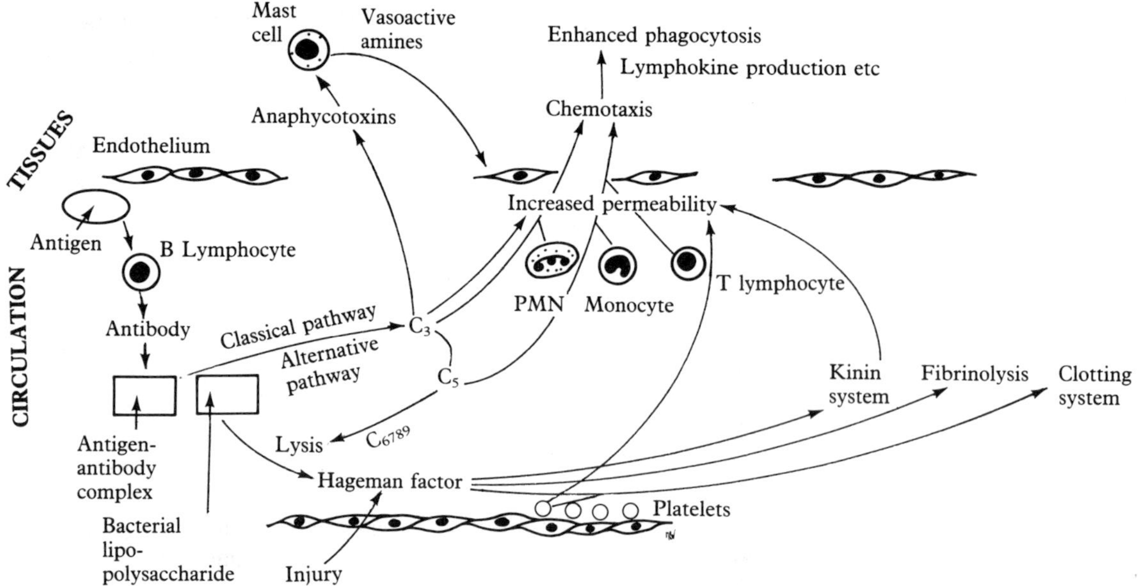

Fig. 2.14 A simplified scheme to show the interaction of complement, coagulation, fibrinolytic and kinin systems in inflammation

when activated, undergo limited proteolytic cleavage to form an active protease which in turn activates the next component in the system, resulting in a cascade of reactions. Figure 2.14 shows a simplified scheme of these interacting systems. Each cascade is controlled by the presence of serum inhibitors, including C_1 esterase inhibitor which regulates each of the four systems.

The complement pathway

The complement pathway is composed of a series of plasma proteins (Table 2.5) which are activated in a set sequence when the system is triggered to result in a cascade of reactions (Fig. 2.15). At each step in the sequence molecules are produced which have important biological activities (Table 2.6) and play a vital role in generating the inflammatory response. Carried to its conclusion, the activated complement sequence leads to holes in the plasma membrane of cells and micro-organisms. The C_{5b}–C_9 complex appears to penetrate the lipid bilayer of the cell membrane to form a channel which allows passage of ions and water. This results in osmotic lysis of the cell. Additional effects of complement activation result from the binding of cleavage products to specific receptors on the surface of cells such as lymphocytes, monocytes and macrophages, neutrophils, mast cells and platelets, and have a role in cellular interactions.

Table 2.5 The complement pathway

Nomenclature	Term	Symbol
Proteins of classical pathway	Component	C eg C_1,C_3 etc.
Proteins of alternative pathway	Factor	B, D, P
Activated proteins		$C_{\bar{1}}$, $C_{\bar{4}}$, $\bar{D}$ etc.
Cleavage fragments		C_{3a}, C_{3b}, Bb etc.
Classical pathway		
Initiation	Immune complexes containing IgG or IgM antibody	
Components	C_1, C_4, C_2, C_3, C_5, C_6, C_7, C_8, C_9 (C_{5-9}: terminal sequence)	
Inhibition	C_1 esterase inhibitor, C_4 binding protein, C_{3b}INA	
Alternative pathway		
Initiation	Bacterial lipopolysaccharide IgA-containing complexes	
Components	B, D, Properdin (P)	
Inhibitors	C_{3b}INA, β1H	

There are two major pathways of complement activation: the 'classical' and the 'alternative' pathways. The classical pathway was discovered first and is triggered by binding of antigen to IgG or

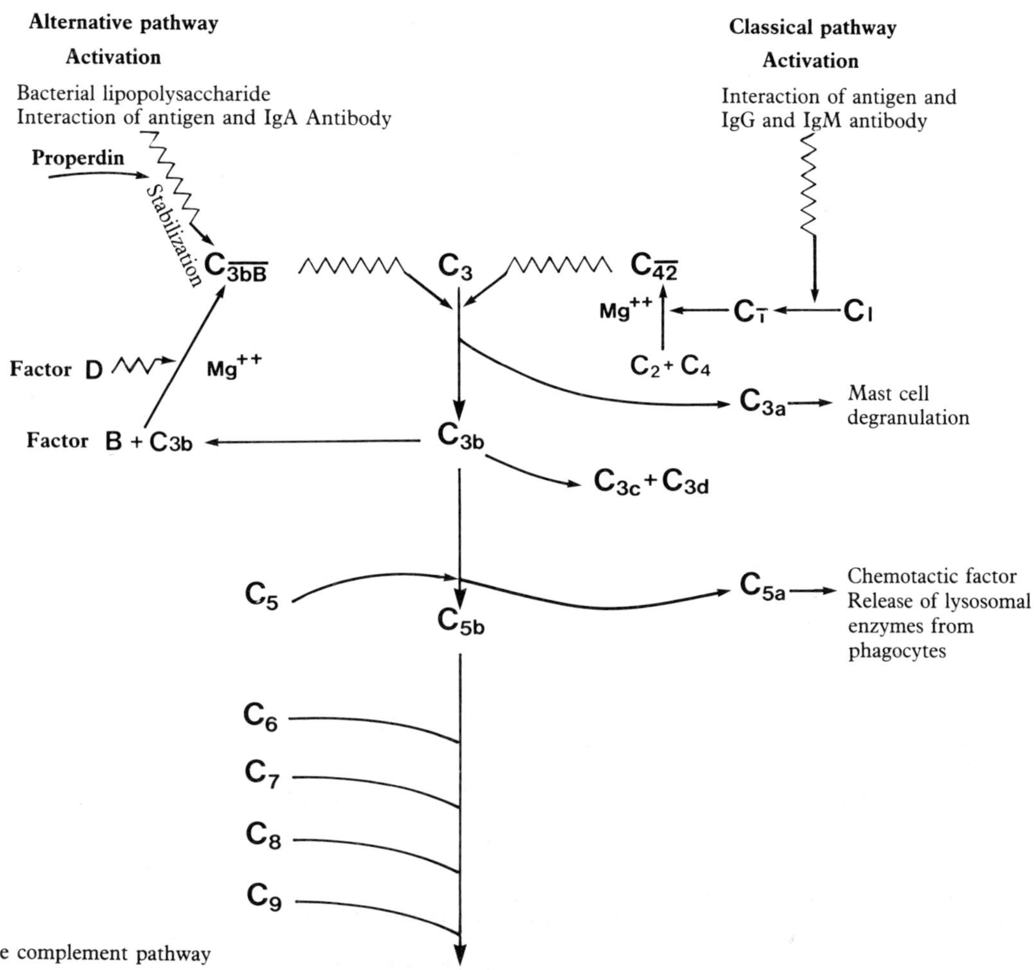

Fig. 2.15 The complement pathway

Table 2.6 Biological activities of complement components

Fragments of C4 and C2	Increases vascular permeability
C4b	Virus neutralisation
C3a	Anaphylotoxin: mast cell degranulation
C3b	Adherence to lymphocyte and phagocyte receptor: promotes phagocytosis; activates B-lymphocytes
C3b and C3d	Binds to monocyte complement receptors
C3bBb	Chemotaxis for polymorphonuclear leukocytes
C5a	Anaphylotoxin: mast cell degranulation Chemotactic factor for polys and monocytes
C567i	Inactive form of C567: chemotactic factor
C5b–9	Membrane lysis

IgM antibody. The alternative pathway is phylogenetically older and can be initiated by direct interaction with substances such as bacterial cell wall lipopolysaccharide and complexes containing IgA, which cannot activate the classical pathway.

The presence of serum inhibitors regulates these pathways. For the classical pathway these include an α-2 neuraminoglycoprotein, C_1 esterase inhibitor, which inhibits activated C_1 and C_4 binding protein and C_{3b} inactivator (C_{3b}INA) which act in concert to control the C_3 convertase (C_{42}) enzyme by degrading C_{4b}. Inhibitors of the alternative pathway are C_{3b}INA and B1H. B1H acts together with C_{3b}INA to degrade C_{3b} and also accelerates the rate of decay of the C_3 convertase (C_{3bBb})

THE HLA SYSTEM

1. Genetics of cellular interactions

The HLA system is the major histocompatibility complex (MHC) of man and is situated on the short arm of chromosome 6. It shows considerable homologies with the MHC of other species, e.g. the H-2 system in mice, and is comprised of closely linked loci containing genes which exert their action on the immune response through cell surface components that appear to be involved in cell-to-cell interactions (Fig. 2.16).

These loci, in the order they are found on the chromosome, are termed HLA-A, HLA-C, HLA-B, HLA-D and DR. Closely adjacent to these loci are others controlling some of the complement components and the Chido (Ch) and Rodgers (Rg) loci coding for red cell antigens. In theory there is space in the MHC for approximately 1000 genes and recently the SB and other loci have been identified but there must be many others as yet undiscovered. Multiple allels are found at each locus: so far nearly 20 alleles of the A locus, 30 of the B locus, at least six of the C locus and 12 in the D locus. However, certain alleles at different loci are found together on the same chromosome more frequently than would be expected by chance (linkage disequilibrium) and distinctive haplotypes are found in certain racial groups, e.g. A1-B8-DR3 and A3-B7-DR2 in Caucasians and AW30, BW42 in Blacks.

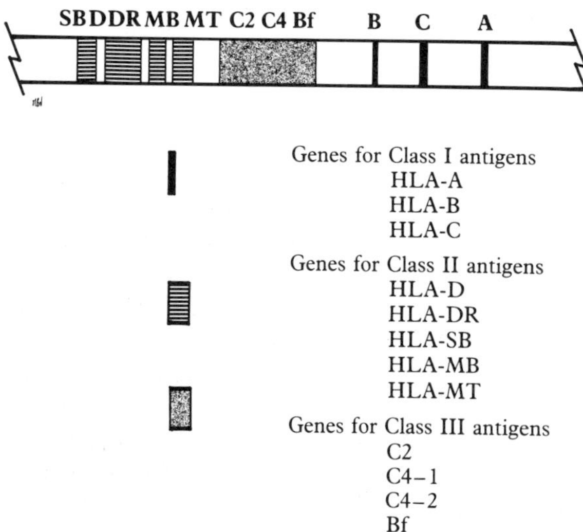

Fig. 2.16 Genetic map of HLA complex on chromosome 6

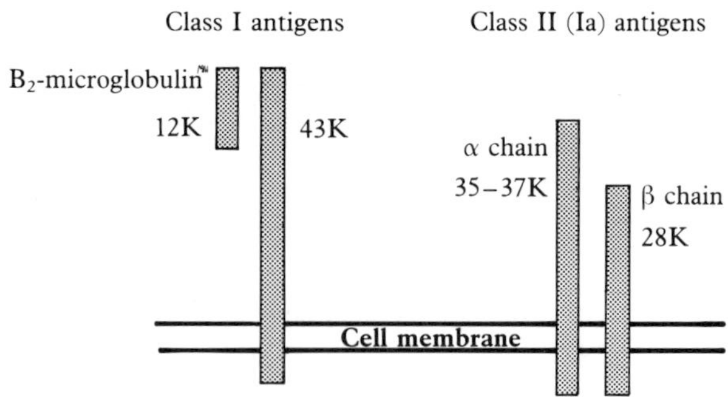

Fig. 2.17 Structure of Class I and Class II (Ia) HLA antigens

Genes in the MHC code for alloantigens on cell membranes (Fig. 2.17). A, B and C locus antigens (the 'classical' HLA antigens) are collectively known as Class 1 antigens, and are present on both T and B lymphocytes and on all other cells except trophoblast cells and mature erythrocytes. The structure of these antigens is known in considerable detail. They are composed of two polypeptide chains: a larger glycoprotein (mol. wt 45 000) carrying the antigenic determinants which is inserted into the cell membrane, and B2 microglobulin (mol. wt 12 000) whose polypeptide sequence is homologous with one of the constant-region domains of human IgG. These antigens function as a recognition site between effector lymphocytes and their target such as virus-infected cells or tumour cells.

A second family of glycoprotein molecules known as Class II antigens are expressed on the surface of B cells (B cell alloantigens), on antigen-presenting macrophages, on stimulated but not resting T cells, and on sperm and vascular endothelial cells but not on other cells. These surface proteins are composed of a bimolecular complex and are coded by genes in the D and DR loci and in related loci such as SB, MB and MT. These antigens show considerable biochemical homology with Ia antigens coded by the immune response genes (IR genes) in mice, and are thus termed Ia-like or Ia antigens. They are involved in antigen presentation by macrophages to T lymphocytes,

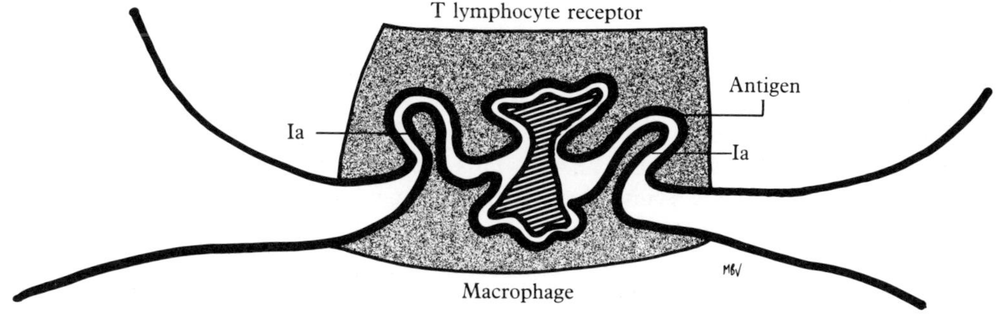

Fig. 2.18 Presentation of antigen to a T lymphocyte by a macrophage in association with Ia receptor

and in interactions between T helper or suppressor cells and B cells. Genes are also present in the MHC complex which code for complement components (class III products) of both the classical pathway (C_2, C_4) and the alternative pathway (Bf).

a) Interactions between macrophage and T lymphocyte (Fig. 2.18)

Antigen-activation of a T lymphocyte requires a double stimulus and needs not only the presence of specific antigen but also recognition of mutual surface alloantigens. Thus the T cell and the macrophage must have the same gene coding for the cell surface Ia receptor.

b) Interactions between T and B lymphocytes (Fig. 2.19)

T helper cell – B cell interactions require a similar double recognition. The antigen-Ia molecular complex presented to the T cell by the macrophage must again be recognised on the B cell surface by the T cell for helper activity to occur. It seems likely that the same is also true for T-suppressor effects on B cells.

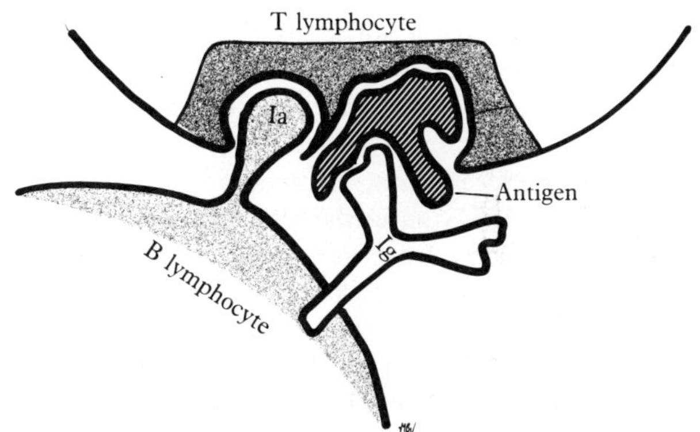

Fig. 2.19 Interaction between T lymphocytes and B lymphocytes also requires recognition of Ia gene product

Table 2.7 HLA and rheumatic disease associations

Disease	HLA antigen	Relative risk
Ankylosing spondylitis	B27	500
Reiter's syndrome *Yersinia, Salmonella, Shigella* arthritis Inflammatory bowel disease with sacro-iliitis Juvenile ankylosing spondylitis	B27	35–50
RA	DW4 DR4	4–10
SLE	DR2 DR3	3–7
Sjögren's syndrome	DR3	3
Systemic sclerosis	DR5	3

2. HLA and rheumatic disease associations

Several rheumatic diseases have been found to have HLA associations (Table 2.7). These fall into two main categories: firstly, the association of the spondyloarthropathy group with B27, and secondly, diseases that have an association with D and DR antigens and only secondarily with HLA-B antigens through linkage disequilibrium. Hypotheses for these observations must explain why the associations are never complete. While a very high proportion of diseased individuals may carry a particular HLA antigen, e.g. B27 in ankylosing spondylitis, not all those with the HLA antigen will develop the disease in question.

Diseases with associations with D and DR antigens frequently manifest auto-immune phenomena. It is hypothesized that this association reflects the presence of genes in the MHC which control immune regulation, resulting either in an abnormal immune response to a particular agent, or to a more generalised impairment of immune regulation not dependent on a specific antigen.

Since ankylosing spondylitis is associated with B27 and not with a particular B cell alloantigen, other hypotheses have been offered emphasising the role of the HLA gene product itself. These include:

1. Molecular mimicry. According to this hypothesis certain HLA antigens bear a structural similarity to certain infectious agents. An immune response to the agents would result in cross-reactivity against the cell surface antigen. There is some evidence that a specific *Klebsiella* serotype cross-reacts with HLA-B27 from cells of patients with ankylosing spondylitis but not controls.

2. Defective cytotoxicity. The association with B27 may implicate the function of B-locus antigens in the recognition phase of cytotoxic effector functions, and reduced efficacy in eliminating certain targets.

ANTIBODIES AS MEDIATORS OF IMMUNOLOGICAL INJURY

The prevalence of auto-antibodies to autologous tissue antigens is a characteristic feature of many of the rheumatic diseases. SLE is the prototype of auto-immune disease in humans and is associated with auto-antibodies to the widest range of tissue antigens. Antinuclear antibodies, and in particular antibodies to DNA, are very characteristic findings. Patients with rheumatoid arthritis also display a wide range of auto-antibodies, especially rheumatoid factors which react with the Fc fragment of human and animal IgG. The stimulus to this auto-antibody response is unknown, but since circulating B cells from normal individuals have the capability to produce anti-DNA and rheumatoid factors, impaired B-cell regulation is thought to be a major factor. Hypotheses to explain this (Figure 2.20) include loss of normal T-cell suppression. This mechanisms has been suggested for SLE, a disease in which functional T-cell suppression is reduced, especially in active phases of disease. Alternatively, abnormal B-cell regulation may occur through bypassing normal T-cell regulation. This might be achieved by modification of self antigens by bacterial or viral antigens or by drugs to render them immunogenic. Clearly, other factors are involved, such as sex hormones and genetic predisposition.

An early observation was that plasma containing high titres of rheumatoid factor did not produce clinical disease in healthy recipients. Similarly, auto-antibodies such as ANA and RF can be found in patients with a variety of non-rheumatic diseases such as tuberculosis and leprosy. It is clear that auto-antibodies do not induce the disease, but under certain circumstances it has been demonstrated that auto-antibodies combining with their specific antigen can lead to tissue-damage and play a role in perpetuating the disease process.

The scope of auto-antibodies in SLE

1. Antibodies to nuclear constituents
   a) Native and denatured DNA
   b) Nucleoprotein
   c) Histone
   d) Soluble nuclear ribonucleoproteins including nRNP, Sm and others
2. Antibodies to cytoplasmic constituents
   a) Ribosomes
   b) Soluble cytoplasmic ribonucleoproteins including Ro(SSA)
3. Antibodies to red cell antigens
4. Antibodies to platelets
5. Antibodies to clotting factors
6. Lymphocyte antibodies
7. Antibodies to RNA
   a) Single-stranded RNA
   b) Double-stranded RNA
8. Antibodies to C-type virus

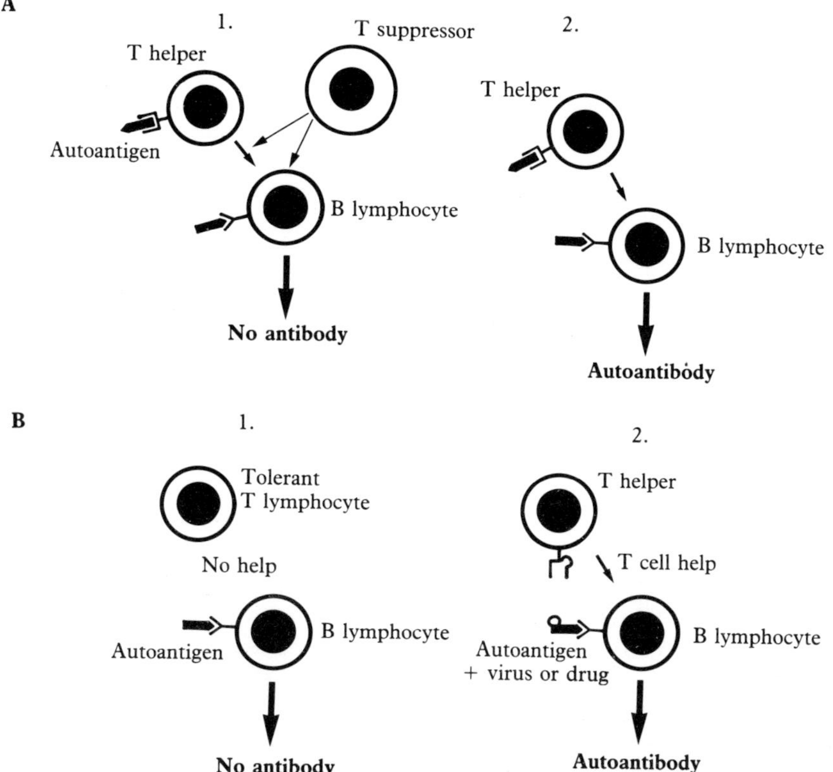

Fig. 2.20 Hypotheses to explain abnormal B lymphocyte regulation. **A**. Removal of T lymphocyte suppression. **B**. Bypassing the T cell block

Antibody-induced tissue-injury can be accomplished directly or indirectly, depending in part on the class of immunoglobin involved, the location of the antigen and the involvement of effector mechanisms. Examples of both can be seen in the rheumatic diseases.

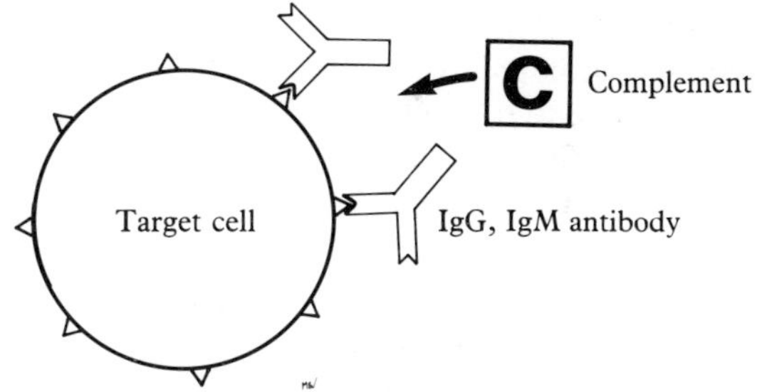

Fig. 2.21 Complement-mediated cytotoxic reaction

1. Cytotoxic reaction

In cytotoxic reactions (Fig. 2.21) immunoglobulin reacts directly with an antigenic site on a tissue or cell surface or to an antigen or hapten intimately associated with the cell membrane. Cell damage is then mediated by complement. Many of the haematological disturbances seen in SLE involve this type of reaction (Table 2.8). Antibodies to membrane antigens on circulating cells are commonly found in SLE and to a lesser extent in RA, especially in patients with Felty's syndrome. Anti-erythrocyte antibodies are found in 18% of

Table 2.8 Cytotoxic antibodies in rheumatic disease

Anti-erythrocyte antibodies	SLE Felty's syndrome
Anti-platelet antibodies	SLE
Anti neutrophil antibodies	SLE Felty's syndrome
Lymphocytotoxic antibodies	SLE RA
Anti-neuronal antibodies	SLE

SLE patients and a third of these develop a haemolytic anaemia. Antibodies to the lymphocyte membrane are a very common feature of SLE, and although under laboratory conditions they are more reactive at 15°C than at body temperature, there is an inverse relationship between the titre of lymphocytotoxic antibodies and the lymphocyte count. All types of lymphocytes are affected but antibodies to T-suppressor cells can be found, and may play a role in impairing immune regulation. Antibodies to lymphocyte antigen also cross-react with other tissues, including brain tissue and the trophoblast, and it is hypothesised that such antibodies have a pathogenic role in the CNS manifestation of SLE and in lupus patients with recurrent abortions.

2. Immune-complex disease

Antibodies are also capable of mediating injury to tissues to which they have no immunological specificity (Fig. 2.22). In this indirect injury the pathogenic agents are soluble macromolecular complexes of antigen and antibody formed in the circulation or in the interstitial tissues.

Studies in laboratory animals demonstrate that under certain circumstances immune complexes deposit in tissues and induce pathological lesions, especially in blood vessels and in the kidney. The classical model for studying the pathogenesis of immune-complex disease is experimental serum sickness. In the acute model (Fig. 2.23), the injection of a large quantity of bovine serum albumin into rabbits induces the production of antibody after several days. As this interacts with antigen, immune complexes can be identified in the circulation, accompanied by a fall in the serum complement level. With increasing antibody concentration, more and larger complexes are formed, and while most are removed from the circulation by cells of the reticulo-endothelial system, some are deposited in the vascular endothelium and renal glomeruli where they interact with the humoral and cellular elements of the host to produce characteristic lesions. In this model it can be demonstrated that tissue-injury is dependent on both complement activation and an influx of neutrophils, and if these factors are abrogated many of the clinical manifestations do not occur. In the glomerular lesions the responsible antigen, host antibody and complement components can be detected in a granular deposition along the glomerular basement membrane. This granular deposition is the hallmark of immune-complex disease.

This model of acute disease can be converted to a chronic model by injecting repeated doses of antigen. If the antigen injections are adjusted according to the immune response of the animal so that an antigen-excess state is maintained, chronic glomerulonephritis is produced, resulting eventually in renal failure.

These, and other models, such as intravenous infusion of preformed complexes into animals, have provided insights into the toxic potential of immune complexes and the pathological events they induce. Since these complexes localise in

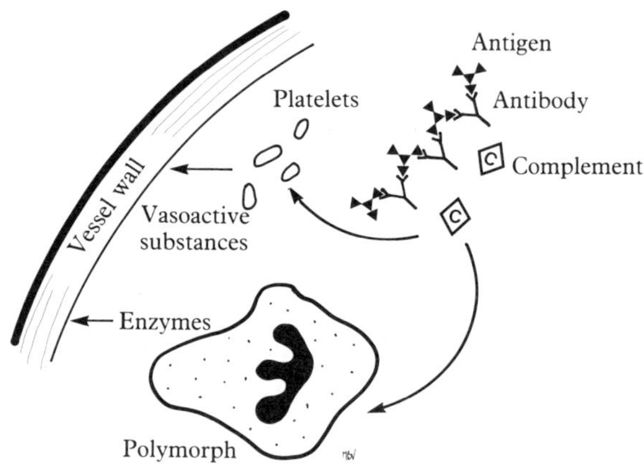

Fig. 2.22 Immune complex-mediated injury

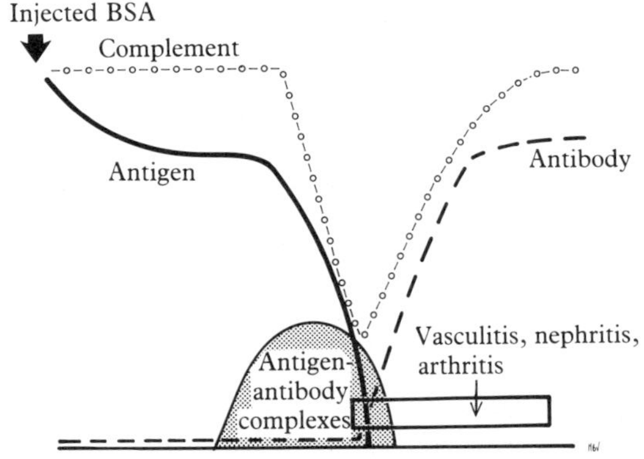

Fig. 2.23 Experimental model of serum sickness

tissues for anatomical and physiological reasons, and not because of any immunological specificity, their physical properties, such as size, solubility, concentration, ability to activate the complement system and the duration of their presence in the circulation, are of great importance. Some of these factors are summarised below:

a) Factors influencing size of immune complex
   (i) Valence of antibody and antigen. Multivalent antigens can be cross-linked by antibody to form a lattice structure.
   (ii) Molar ratio of antigen to antibody. Small soluble complexes are formed in antigen excess.
   (iii) Absolute concentration of antigen to antibody. At a given degree of antigen excess larger complexes are formed if the concentration of the reactants is increased.
   (iv) Affinity of antibody. Low-affinity antibody forms smaller immune complexes than high-affinity antibody.

b) Biological properties of immune complexes
   (i) Activation of the complement system. To produce tissue-lesions, immune complexes must be capable of activating the complement system.
   (ii) Binding to cell surfaces through Fc receptors on neutrophils, monocytes, macrophages, platelets and some lymphcoytes. Large complexes bind more efficiently than small complexes and a sufficient complex size is required for phagocytosis. Large complexes cause platelets to aggregate and release vasoactive substances.

c) Factors affecting clearance of immune complexes by the reticuloendothelial system
   (i) Size of immune complexes. Small soluble immune complexes in antigen-excess are phagocytosed least well.
   (ii) Composition of immune complexes
   (iii) Saturation of the RE system
   (iv) Possible qualitative defects in the RE system. This is proposed for SLE.

d) Factors affecting tissue deposition of immune complexes
   (i) Haemodynamic factors. Sites of turbulence, e.g. branch points of arteries from the aorta, have marked predilection for immune-complex deposition.
   (ii) Size of immune complex. Complexes smaller than 19 S are not nephritogenic in rabbits but larger complexes are trapped in the basement membrane and cause injury.
   (iii) Receptors on endothelial cells of glomerulus or blood vessels. There is evidence for C_{3b} receptors which might bind complement-containing immune complexes.
   (iv) Nature of antigen. Antigens such as DNA bind complement-containing immune membrane, and this may contribute to immune complex localisation.

Certain clinical and pathological events seen during the course of some rheumatic diseases bear a close resemblance to experimental models of immune complex disease. Examples are shown in Table 2.9 and evidence for an immune-complex pathogenesis includes the demonstration of granular deposits of antigen–antibody complexes in the tissue lesions by techniques such as immunofluor-

Table 2.9 Examples of lesions thought to be immune-complex mediated in the rheumatic disease

Tissue-lesion	Proposed antigen	Evidence for immune-complex pathogenesis
Glomerulonephritis in SLE	Autologous tissue antigens esp DNA	Strong (a, b, c, d)
Vasculitis (a) SLE	Autologous tissue antigens esp DNA	Strong (a, b, c)
(b) RA	IgG as antigen for rheumatoid factor	Strong (a, b, c)
(c) PAN	Hepatitis B surface antigen in a minority of cases	Strong in the Hep B cases (a, b, c, d)
(d) Polymyositis	Unknown	Weak (c)
Synovitis in RA	IgG as antigen for rheumatoid factor	Strong (a, b, c)

a = hypocomplementaemia
b = antigen, antibody and complement identified in circulating immune complexes
c = typical IMF and EM appearance of tissue-lesions
d = immunoreactants identified in immune deposits

Table 2.10 Immune complex disease in SLE

Clinical manifestations	Immunopathology
Glomerulonephritis	Complement-fixing antibodies to autoantigens eg DNA
Vasculitis	Hypocomplementaemia
Vasculitis	Circulating immune complexes containing autoantigens, esp DNA
Pleurisy	Antibody and complement
Pericarditis	Granular deposition demonstrated in tissue lesions by IMF and EM containing immunoglobulin and complement
Rash — possibly	DNA and anti DNA demonstrated in immune deposits
Arthritis — possibly	

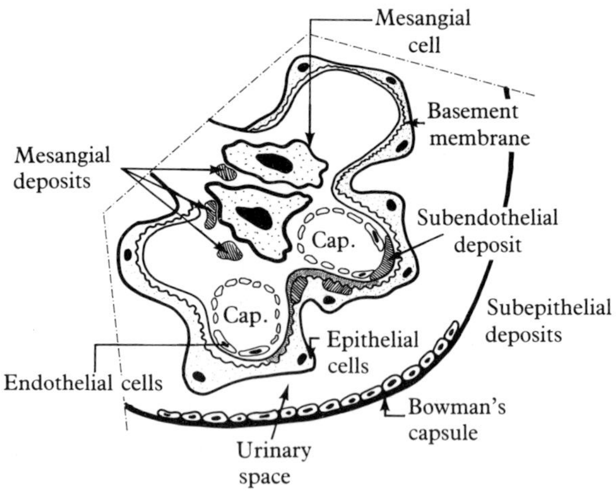

Fig. 2.24 Schematic representation of immune complexes in various areas of the renal glomerulus

escence and electron microscopy, identification of the immunoreactants eluted from the tissue-lesions and the demonstration of circulating immune complexes often accompanied by hypocomplementaemia.

SLE is the best characterised of the human immune-complex diseases (Table 2.10). The development of lesions such as glomerulonephritis and vasculitis is associated with the presence in the serum of complement-fixing antibodies to various auto-antigens, especially DNA, and the presence of circulating immune complexes containing immunoreactants such as DNA, anti-DNA and complement. Immunofluorescence and electron-microscopic studies demonstrate granular deposits in relation to the basement membrane containing immunoglobulin and complement. Evidence that pathogenic complexes are important, particularly in lupus nephritis, has been strengthened further by demonstrating DNA and anti-DNA in these immune deposits. It is hypothesised that such complexes become trapped between the basement membrane and the endothelial or epithelial cells and activate the complement system, and the resulting chemotactic factors attract polymorphs which release lysosomal enzymes to cause splitting and fragmentation of the basement membrane (Fig. 2.24).

There is reason to believe that similar events occur in rheumatoid arthritis (Table 2.11). In this disease pathogenic complexes are composed predominantly of IgG, IgG rheumatoid factor and IgM rheumatoid factor. There is evidence that complexes formed locally within the joint almost certainly contribute to the articular inflammation (Fig. 2.25) and that those formed in the circulation can induce vasculitis.

Table 2.11 Immune-complex disease in RA

Clinical manifestation	Immunopathology
1. Synovitis	Synovial production of immunoglobulin, especially IgG rheumatoid factor Low synovial-fluid complement levels Immune complexes containing immunoglobulin, rheumatoid factor and complement in synovial fluid, within leukocytes, in synovial tissues and in cartilage
2. Vasculitis	High serum levels of IgG and IgM rheumatoid factor Hypocomplementaemia Circulating immune complexes containing immunoglobulin, rheumatoid factor and complement Granular deposits of immunoglobulin and complement in vessel wall demonstrated by IMF and EM

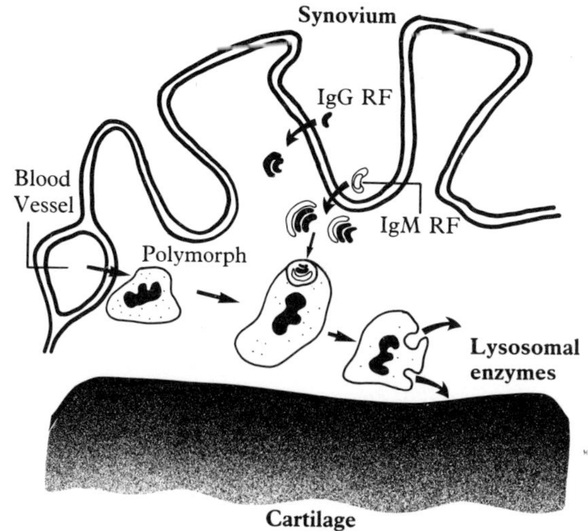

Fig. 2.25 Proposed mechanism whereby immune complexes formed within the joint contribute to inflammation and joint destruction

CELL-MEDIATED IMMUNITY

There is circumstantial evidence that abnormal T-cell function plays an important role in perpetuating RA and other connective-tissue diseases. As a result of a persistent and abnormal immune response, tissue-injury occurs via both arms of the immune system. Evidence for T-cell involvement in these diseases is summarised in Table 2.12 and includes the demonstration of a defective suppressor-cell population, diminished skin tests and abnormal *in vitro* responses of lymphocytes to mitogens and various autoantigens.

Abnormal T-cell suppressor function is particularly marked in SLE, especially during active phases of the disease. This may be an important factor in the production of auto-antibodies but there is not as much evidence for cell-mediated effector mechanisms in this disease as there is in RA and adult polymyositis.

A major role for T cells in RA is suggested firstly by the predominance of T lymphocytes in the rheumatoid synovial membrane, and secondly by the fact that thoracic-duct drainage or total-lymphoid irradiation, which depletes T lymphocytes, often ameliorates the disease. The rheumatoid synovial membrane is characterised by dense collections of lymphocytes, in both a diffuse and a nodular pattern, most of which are T cells. Immunofluorescence studies using monoclonal antibodies to lymphocyte and macrophage surface markers have shown that helper cells predominate greatly over suppressor T cells. In perivascular transitional areas of the synovial membrane between lymphocyte-rich and plasma-cell rich regions, lymphoblasts, plasmablasts and dendritic macrophages are in close association, suggesting that important intercellular interactions are taking place, perhaps triggering not only rheumatoid-factor production but also cell-mediated effector mechanisms (Fig. 2.26). Lymphokines, for example, can be detected in the synovial fluid with the capability of triggering monocyte-mediated inflammation.

Cell-mediated immunity in adult polymyositis is suggested by *in vitro* responses of patients' lymphocytes to muscle antigen. Circulating

Table 2.12 Abnormal T-cell function in rheumatic disease

	Reduced skin tests	Reduced suppressor cells	Abnormal mitogen response	Lymphocyte response to autoantigens	Cell-mediated effector functions
RA	+	+	+	Collagen	Lymphokine in synovial fluid
SLE	+	+	+	DNA	
Systemic Sclerosis		+		Tissue antigens from skin	
Polymyositis				Tissue antigens from muscle	Myocytotoxic lymphocytes

lymphocytes from patients with active disease demonstrate cytotoxicity to foetal muscle cells.

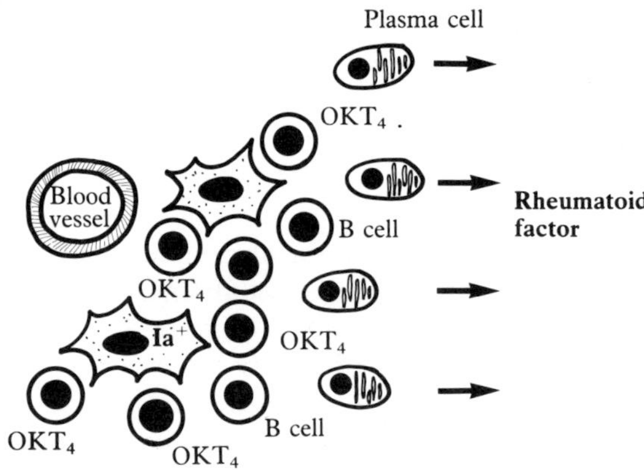

Fig. 2.26 Schematic representation of perivascular region of rheumatoid synovium showing clusters of Ia-positive macrophages (Ia$^+$), T helper lymphocytes (OKT$_4$), B lymphocytes and plasma cells

Clues pointing to cell-mediated immunity in systemic sclerosis inclue the similarity between the vascular lesions of systemic sclerosis and those of chronic homograft rejection, and the observation that a proportion of patients who survive marrow transplantation for more than one year develop Sjogren's syndrome and scleroderma-like skin lesions.

FURTHER READING

Carson Dick W 1981 Immunological aspects of rheumatology. MTP Press, Lancaster

Jasin H E 1982 Scientific overview of systemic lupus erythematosus. Progress in Clinical and Biological Research 106: 65–80

Panayi G F 1982 Scientific basis of rheumatology. Churchill Livingstone, Edinburgh

Schwartz R S 1981 Immunologic and genetic aspects of systemic lupus erythematosus. Kidney International 19: 474–484

3 Epidemiology

The chronic rheumatic diseases are complex disorders and appear to result from the interaction of multiple genetic and environmental factors (Fig. 3.1). Epidemiological studies of the frequency and distribution of disease in populations contribute to our understanding of how these complex inter-relationships determine the expression of a particular disease and its subsequent course. Such studies in rheumatic fever, for example, provided evidence to help establish its streptococcal aetiology.

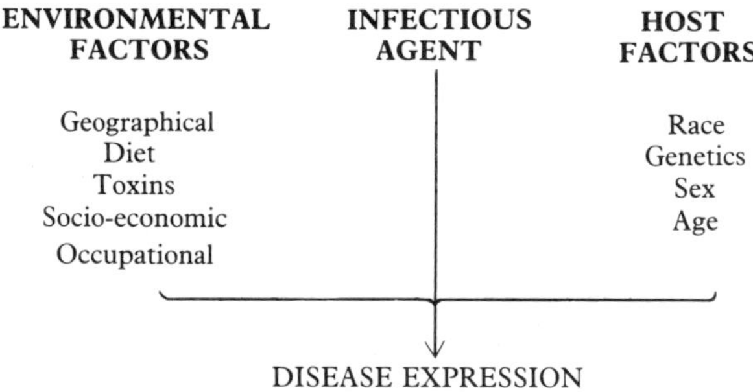

Fig. 3.1 Interaction of environmental and host factors in the development of a rheumatic disease

Incidence and prevalence of disease

The incidence of a disease is the rate at which new cases occur in a defined population during a given period. This reflects factors in the aetiology of the disease, including host predisposition. Prevalence, on the other hand, refers to the number of cases in a given population at a particular point in time or during a specified interval. This reflects not only the risk of developing the disease but also the factors that influence its duration.

Measurement of incidence and prevalence of rheumatic diseases

The incidence and prevalence of rheumatic diseases is difficult to assess because in most cases there is no specific diagnostic test and diagnosis rests on recognising certain patterns of clinical manifestations. To facilitate epidemiological studies, clinical and laboratory criteria have been defined for a number of the rheumatic diseases. Those for rheumatoid arthritis and SLE can be found on pp 46 and 109. Criteria for disease classification are subject to continual updating as previously-recognised entities such as juvenile rheumatoid arthritis are split into clinical subgroups, and as useful laboratory aids to diagnosis become available. The introduction of the technique of indirect immunofluorescence as a sensitive screening test for antinuclear antibodies has been largely responsible for the apparent increased prevalence of SLE during the past two decades (Fig. 3.2). Similarly, the application of immunogenetics to the study of epidemiology has also changed our concepts of incidence and prevalence. This is particularly true for ankylosing spondylitis. Prior to the era of immunogenetics the prevalence of ankylosing spondylitis was estimated to be one case per 2000 of the population. Since the association with HLA-B27 became apparent, and as a result individuals at risk were identified and examined, the

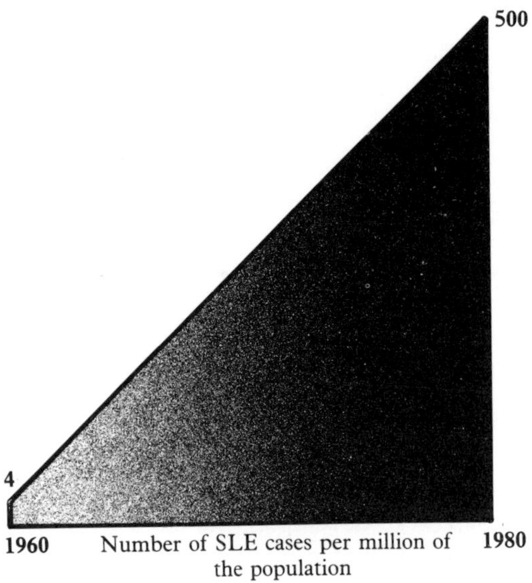

Fig. 3.2 The increasing prevalence of SLE

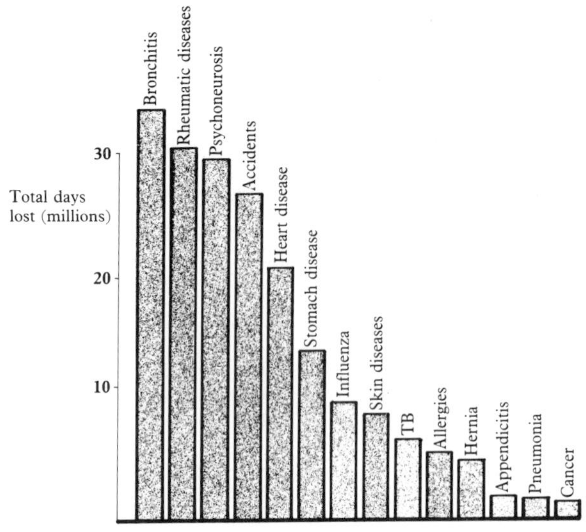

Fig. 3.3 Work days lost through sickness in England and Wales (from National Health Insurance statistics)

prevalence of ankylosing spondylitis is now known to be closer to 1% of the white population.

Other factors which change the incidence and prevalence of rheumatic diseases are: firstly, the changing make-up of the population with, for example, an influx of immigrants with different disease susceptibilities; and secondly, the temporal effect in the expression of a particular disease. In the case of rheumatic fever, for example, there has been a striking reduction in both the number and the severity of cases in North America and Europe. This trend occurred even before the introduction of antibiotics, and probably reflects factors such as changes in social conditions.

Frequency of the rheumatic diseases

The rheumatic diseases are a major cause of incapacity throughout the world. In the UK the number of general-practice consultations due to rheumatic disease is second only to those due to the common cold. These disorders make a major economic impact since they are also a major cause of loss of work. This is revealed by National Health insurance statistics, which show rheumatic diseases second to bronchitis as the most common cause of work-loss due to sickness in England and Wales (Fig. 3.3), where the number of days lost exceeds those lost in industrial action.

The relative prevalence of different rheumatic diseases is shown in Figure 3.4. In many cases the distribution and expression of disease is influenced by geography, by environmental and socioeconomic factors, and by constitutional factors such as genetics, sex and age.

a) Geographic distribution

It is often stated that rheumatoid arthritis is more frequent in temperate rather than in tropical climates. This is not confirmed by epidemiological studies, which show a remarkably constant prevalence of rheumatoid arthritis throughout the world, ranging from 0.3–1.5% with an overall figure of 1%. This suggests that both genetic and environmental factors in the development of this disease are widespread. There are a few pockets of increased prevalence, such as the Yakima Indians in Washington State, and populations with a slightly lower prevalence are found in Japan, Puerto Rica, Jerusalem and Nigeria. In Nigeria and others parts of West Africa, rheumatoid arthritis is generally sero-negative and more benign. Other diseases also thought to have an

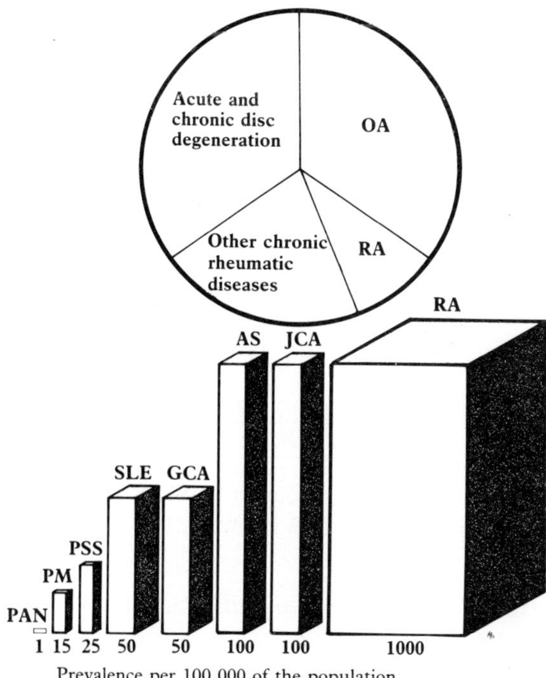

Fig. 3.4 Relative prevalence of different rheumatic diseases (PAN: polyarteritis nodosa; PM: polymyositis; PSS: systemic sclerosis; SLE: systemic lupus erythematosus; GCA: Giant cell arteritis; AS: ankylosing spondylitis; JCA: juvenile chronic arthritis; RA: rheumatoid arthritis)

auto-immune aetiology, such as Hashimoto's disease, are also rare. It has been hypothesised that malaria might have a role in suppressing incipient auto-immune disease, and there is experimental evidence to support this in the adjuvant model of arthritis.

Other rheumatic diseases have a more striking geographic distribution. In some cases this matches the distribution of a particular infectious agent such as epidemic polyarthritis of Australia, Chikungunga, O'Nyong-nyong and Lyme arthritis. The world-wide distribution of ankylosing spondylitis, on the other hand, follows that of the B27 gene (Fig. 3.5). B27, and consequently ankylosing spondylitis, is rare in non-Caucasian populations, such as African Blacks ,Japanese and Australian aborigines. On the other hand, the frequency of B27 is increased in American Indians, especially the Haida Indians (50%), and up to 5% develop ankylosing spondylitis.

Other diseases with a striking geographical and racial distribution are SLE and Behcet's syndrome. The prevalence of SLE is high in Black women in the USA and West Indies and in Chinese women in Asia. While Behcet's is rare in the UK it has a prevalence of 1:1000 in the Japanese population

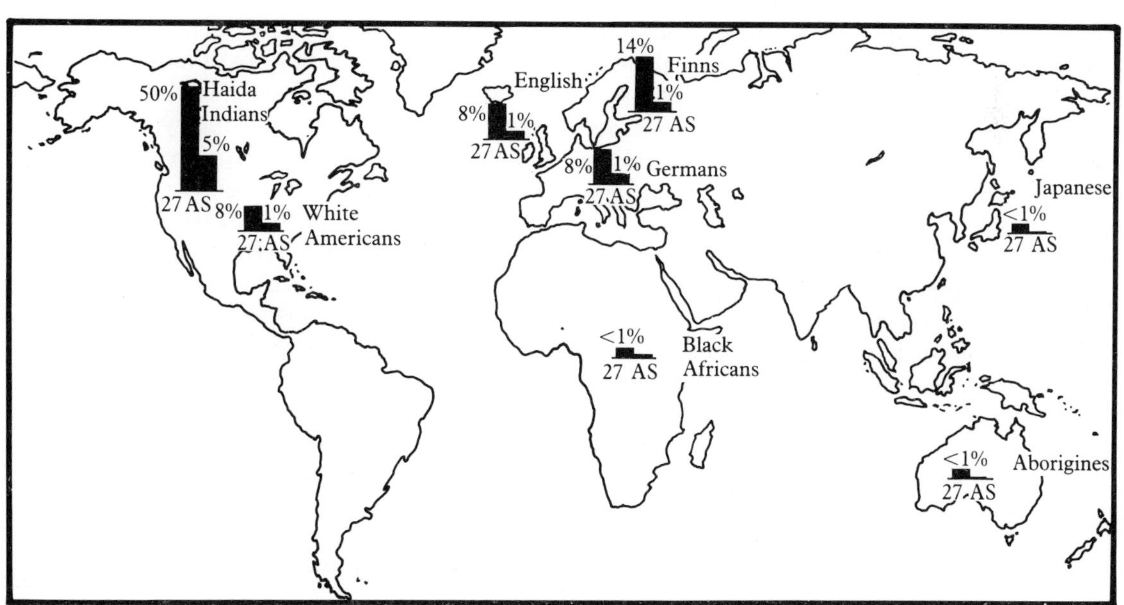

Fig. 3.5 Prevalence of HLA B27 and ankylosing spondylitis in different parts of the world

Table 3.1 Age and sex distribution of some rheumatic diseases

	Male	Female	Both sexes
Children	Juvenile ankylosing spondylitis Haemophilic arthropathy	Juvenile chronic arthritis	Still's disease
Young adults	Ankylosing spondylitis Reiter's syndrome	RA SLE	Reactive arthritis Gonococcal arthritis Enteropathic arthritis
Middle age	Gout	RA Systemic sclerosis Polymyositis	Psoriatic arthritis
Elderly		Pyrophosphate arthropathy PMR GCA	RA

and is one of the major causes of blindness in that country.

b) Environment and distribution of rheumatic diseases

Examples are seen where environmental and constitutional factors appear to interact in influencing the expression of disease. Urban South African Blacks have a higher prevalence of rheumatoid arthritis than those in the rural community, and the high prevalence of SLE in American Blacks contrasts with the low prevalence in West Africa. Another illustration is that hyperuricaemia and increased gout seen in Polynesian populations and in Filipinos living in the USA and Hawaii is the result of a combination of constitutional factors determining purine metabolism and the introduction of Western patterns of life, including dietary habits.

The expression of certain rheumatic diseases is also influenced by socio-economic factors and occupation. The prevalence of rheumatoid arthritis is higher in lower socio-economic levels, and the development of articular erosions is more marked in those with a physical occupation, such as fishermen, builders and farm-labourers. Occupation also affects the joint distribution in OA. For example, the pattern of involvement in the hand can depend on usage, and recurrent minor trauma can predispose to OA at any joint site.

c) Constitutional factors and distribution of rheumatic diseases

1. Genetics. Many rheumatic diseases show an increased prevalence in first-degree relatives, and a high degree of concordance in monozygotic forms. This suggests a genetic predisposition, which is further supported by the identification of association between rheumatic diseases and certain HLA-antigens (Chapter 2).

2. Age and sex (Table 3.1). Many rheumatic diseases show a striking distribution according to age and sex. This demonstrates that host factors have a major influence on the type of rheumatic disease syndrome that is expressed.

Epidemiological studies contribute to our understanding of the rheumatic diseases and, by identifying factors responsible for disease expression, point the way for future research of those responsible for the predisposition, onset and subsequent course of the diseases.

FURTHER READING

Lawrence J S 1977 Rheumatism in populations. Heinemann, London

SECTION TWO

The major rheumatic diseases

4 Rheumatoid arthritis

INTRODUCTION

Rheumatoid arthritis (RA) is the commonest chronic inflammatory disease of joints. Although its major manifestations relate to the musculoskeletal system, it can affect any organ or system in the body so the term *rheumatoid disease* is perhaps more appropriate. Much has been learnt about RA but the cause and cure remain unknown.

The first description of RA was by a French medical student in the early nineteenth century and the present name was given by Sir Alfred Garrod in 1858. It is of interest that a disease with such obvious clinical characteristics should not be mentioned in the Bible or Shakespeare, or be represented in paintings by the great masters. The paucity of erosive disease that might be RA in skeletons retrieved from ancient burial sites further supports the suggestion that RA is a relatively new disease. Rheumatologists who have been in practice for a long time feel that there has been a recent epidemic of RA which now shows signs of abating.

The prevalence of RA in the population is about 3% with three women affected for every one man, but only a proportion have progressive disease and about 2/1000 of the population require sustained treatment. The peak age of onset is around 40 with a spread of 35–50 years. It is a universal disease, the distribution being unaffected by climate or latitude, but its severity varies between countries — more severe, erosive and deforming disease being prevalent in Europe.

AETIOLOGY

The current hypothesis of the aetiology of RA is as follows: a constitutionally susceptible individual encounters a triggering factor which produces joint inflammation. Instead of switching off in the normal way after the acute response, the inflammatory process becomes chronic and self-sustaining long after the initiating factor has disappeared.

Constitutional factors

Age and sex

In the younger age groups female preponderance is striking and may be as high as 6:1, but by the age of 69 the sex distribution is equal. This suggests that hormonal factors may be important and certain other well-established observations support this: onset after delivery is a classic type of presentation; remission of established disease during pregnancy is usual with a flare of activity in the puerperium.

Genetic factors

Many patients feel that RA runs in their families and formal studies show a sixfold increase in siblings and dizygotic twins, with 30% concordance among monozygotic twins. New understanding has come in this area with the discovery that an HLA antigen DR4 is present in 60% of European patients with RA but only 30% of the unaffected population. The presence of DR4 has been calculated to produce a sevenfold risk of developing RA. Much research has now focused on the DR antigens, which play a major role in the regulation of the cellular immune response. Genetic factors in the pathogenesis of RA can be overcome by environmental factors, as was shown in a study of racial groups in South Africa. The Bantu in the homelands have a very low prevalance of RA but members of the same tribe who migrate to the townships near the big cities acquire the same prevalence as the white population.

Potential triggering agents

Infection

Every year or so a new infectious organism is suggested as the cause of RA, but none has ever been regularly isolated from affected tissue and the disease has never been transmitted from one animal to another experimentally. It is postulated that the initiating organism is either eliminated early on before the disease is apparent or persists but is altered in some way so that it is undetecteble by current methods. Such a process has been shown in animals. Erysipelothrix infection in swine causes an RA-like illness. The organism can be recovered in the acute stage but not once the disease has become chronic. It is also interesting that material derived from the bacterial cell wall — peptidoglycans — can cause a polyarthritis in animals.

Current major contenders as likely infecting agents in man are herpes virus, rubella virus, Epstein-Barr virus and mycoplasma. Although these are likely to be superceded in the future, studies with these agents have shown some interesting mechanisms by which organisms can be hidden from the body's normal defence mechanisms and thus persist. For example, mycoplasma are able to absorb host immunoglobulin on to their own surface thereby adopting the guise of self. If the absorbed immunoglobulins were altered in the process, they could become antigenic and act as a stimulus to antibody formation. Such antibodies would, of course, be rheumatoid factors. Genes from a virus may be incorporated into the DNA of a host cell, such as a lymphocyte, as happens with oncogenes in some cancers, and viral antigen may be expressed on the surface of the host cell stimulating antigen and immune complex formation.

Diet

There is growing interest in the role of diet in disease. A very few patients with RA find that disease flares are triggered by certain foods and that they improve on exclusion diets. Certainly in the seronegative spondarthritides, gut-derived antigens may be important.

Psychological factors

Many patients are convinced that their RA was caused by an episode of stress or trauma and these factors also appear to play a role in modulating established disease. It has become less easy to dismiss these claims since it has been shown that severe emotional stress, for example, bereavement, may profoundly surpress the body's immune response.

Perpetuating factors

Auto-immunity

There is overwhelming evidence that the immune system is involved in RA and this has been the dominant area of research in the last two decades. The evidence is as follows:

1. Histologically the synovial tissues in RA show vast accumulation of cells of the immune system including small lymphocytes and plasma cells which are aggregated into lymphoid follicles.

2. These cells are producing, amongst other things, antibodies to IgG which must have been altered in some way so that it is rendered antigenic to the immune surveillance systems. These auto-antibodies are rheumatoid factors and are found in all classes of immunoglobulin, but predominantly in IgM and IgG.

3 Rheumatoid factors can form immune complexes which are taken up by the PMNs and are also thought to activate complement, both mechanisms for generating inflammation.

4. Cell-mediated immunity is abnormal: skin reactivity to antigens such as tuberculin is depressed

in active RA; draining the thoracic duct removes T lymphocytes and ameliorates RA and re-infusing them results in a flare of disease. Total lymphoid irradiation is also often successful in suppressing disease activity.

5. Cytotoxic drugs can be used to induce disease remission and these agents have a profound effect on the immune system.

These facts are generally interpreted to mean that there is an abnormality of both humoral and cellular immunity generating chronic persistent inflammation, but this is not considered to be the actual cause RA.

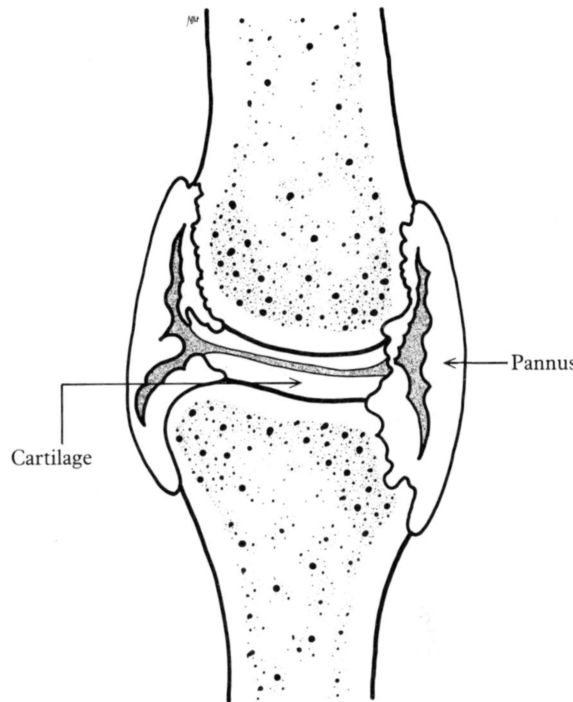

Fig. 4.1 Rheumatoid synovium eroding joint

PATHOLOGY

Synovial pathology

The synovitis of RA affects all joints, tendons and bursae that have a synovial lining. There are two elements in this inflammation: a chronic inflammatory cellular hypertrophy of the synovial tissues and an acute inflammatory exudate of neutrophils into the synovial space.

The earliest changes seen in the synovium are vascular congestion and oedema followed by a marked increase in the numbers of synovial A and B lining cells and fibroblasts; infiltration of cells from the circulation, mainly T lymphocytes and plasma cells; and tissue macrophages derived from circulating monocytes. The lymphocytes and plasma cells aggregate to form recognisable lymphoid follicles and synthesise and secrete rheumatoid factors which react with immunoglobulin to form immune complexes. These activate complement to release leucocyte attractants so that granulocytes accumulate in the synovial fluid. As many as 2 billion have been estimated to exude into the joint space per day. Other inflammation-inducing peptides are also produced by complement activation and the granulocytes themselves are constantly being destroyed, which releases lysosomal enzymes. As the disease becomes established and progresses, the overgrowth of cellular elements causes even more thickening of the synovium and a marked increase in surface area, producing great seaweed-like fronds, hence the name *villous synovitis*. The macrophages in this inflammatory granulation tissue or pannus produce destructive proteases and collagenases which erode demineralised cartilage and bone, starting at the junction between cartilage and subchondral bone at the joint margin and gradually working inwards until the cartilage is totally destroyed (Fig. 4.1). Other major systems are also activated, including the clotting system, resulting in deposition of fibrin over the surface of the cartilage which may interfere with its nutrition by the synovial fluid.

In end-stage RA, the combination of long-standing synovitis and inflammatory joint effusion causes destruction of the joint cartilage, capsule and ligaments with resultant instability, mechanical disarray, subluxation and deformity.

Nodules

An intriguing unsolved mystery of RA pathology is the rheumatoid nodule. These characteristic

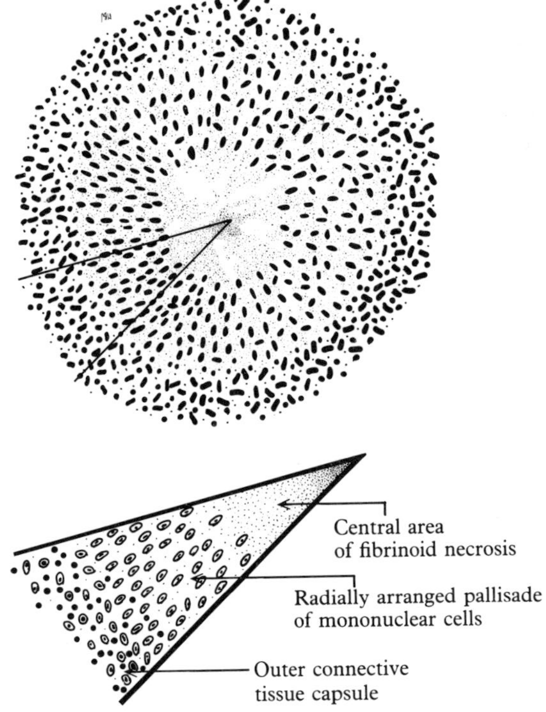

Fig. 4.2 Histology of a rheumatoid nodule

round lumps are found around or far removed from articular structures and may be subcutaneous, intracutaneous, subperiosteal or deep inside organs such as lungs or heart. Histologically, they show an inner necrotic core composed of destroyed collagen, fibrin, cell-fragments and debris; a radially arranged pallisade of mononuclear cells plus the occasional giant cell; and an outer wrapping of chronic inflammatory cells — plasma, cells, lymphocytes, and fibroblasts (Fig. 4.2).

Vascular pathology

Inflammation of blood vessels is a constant early finding in rheumatoid synovium but is also found outside the confines of the joint. Three histological types of vasculitis occur:

1. Obliterative (*non-inflammatory*): intimal thickening leads to thrombosis and occlusion, particularly of small vessels of the hands and is very similar to the vascular changes seen in scleroderma.

2. Subacute inflammatory: the vessels are surrounded by an inflammatory infiltrate. This tends to affect vessels of the skin, muscles and vasa nervorum.

3. Acute necrotizing: this is histologically similar to PAN with fibrinoid necrosis of all layers of the arterial wall. Medium-sized muscular arteries are affected.

Reticulo-endothelial system

This system is persistently overstimulated in RA. Widespread generalised lymphadenopathy and splenomegaly are the rule (p 255).

CLINICAL FEATURES

A classical case of RA is easy to recognise. A youngish women presents with flitting pains in the small joints of the fingers, carpal tunnel syndrome and a sense of general fatigue. After a few months, the MCPJs of the hands start to swell and there is diffuse aching and generalised stiffness in the morning which gradually eases as the day goes on but recurs following a period of inactivity, such as watching television. The feet, knees and shoulders are the next site (Fig. 4.3) of flitting migratory pain which gradually becomes persistent. The symptoms fluctuate widely from day to day, often related to changes in the weather or barometric pressure. Stress and aggravation at work or at home produces flares in activity whereas holidays, rest, domestic harmony, pregnancy and jaundice are associated with improvement. When the disease has become established, depression is common, due to the frustration of not being able to do things and worry about what will happen in the future.

It is important to realise that signs may be absent in the early stages and the patient may have many complaints with very little to show for them. Signs of synovitis: warmth, swelling and tenderness around the joints, appear first in the small peripheral joints; the commonest combination being the MCPJs, PIPJs, wrists and MTPJs with striking symmetry. Tenosynovitis is a prominent feature, particularly in the extensor tendon sheath on the back of the hands and the flexor tendons

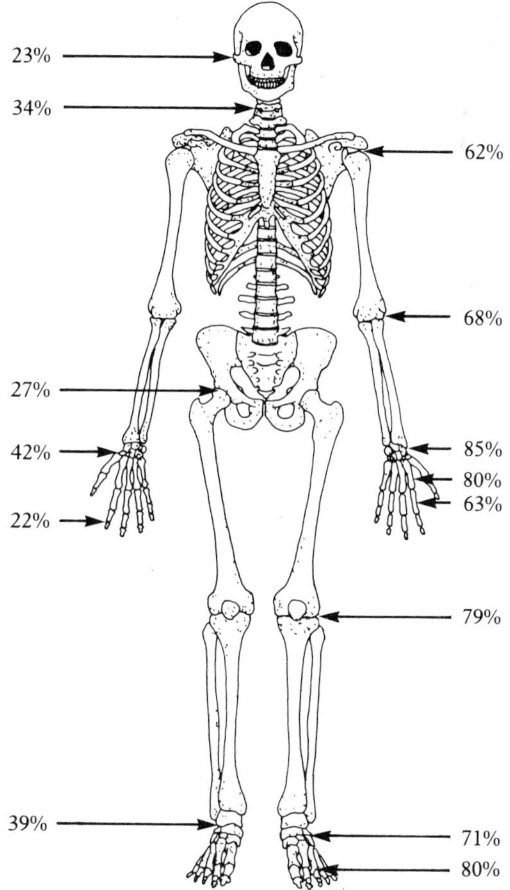

Fig. 4.3 Distribution of joint involvement in rheumatoid arthritis

in the palm, making it difficult to flex the fingers fully and occasionally producing triggering during finger extension.

After several years of persistent synovitis, joint destruction, instability and deformity ensue and systemic features such as vasculitis and sicca syndrome are common. Pain now has more of a mechanical basis and often arises in the large joints, particularly the knees, elbows and shoulders. It is often better after a night's rest, is provoked by joint usage and increases in severity as the day goes on. Deformities are caused by disruption and dislocation of tendons as well as erosion and destruction of cartilage and bone of the joints. Loss of ability to carry out the necessary tasks of daily living and dependence on others are major concerns of the patient at this stage of the disease.

Atypical presentations

Atypical presentations are not uncommon and may cause considerable diagnostic difficulty, particularly in the early stages.

Explosive onset

This often occurs in the older age-groups. The patient may be completely well one day and hardly able to move the next, due to stiffness and pain in the joints and muscles. Slightly less acute forms occur in which the involvement of one joint follows another in rapid succession. Curiously, this form is often associated with a favourable long-term outcome. There are usually high titres of rheumatoid factor in the serum.

Systemic onset

This is particularly common in middle-aged men. Dominant features are non-articular and include fever, anaemia, fatigue, weight loss, myalgia, pleural effusions, pulmonary nodules, neuropathy and cutaneous ulceration. Malignancy and chronic infection such as tuberculosis are obvious differential diagnoses. Arthritis may be a minor component or even be completely absent in the early stages, but high titres of rheumatoid factor and hypocomplementaemia are frequently found.

Palindromic onset

This is characterised by irregular attacks of pain and swelling in one or two joints, often hands, but also knees and shoulders, which last 2–3 days. Afterwards the joints return completely to normal. Periarticular swelling, erythema and transient nodules are often striking features during the acute stage. Rheumatoid factor is often present in the serum and about 50% of patients with this syndrome will progress to RA.

Polymyalgic onset

In the older age-group early RA may be clinically indistinguishable from polymyalgia rheumatica which presents with diffuse stiffness and pain in the shoulders and hips without synovitis. The response to steroids is less dramatic than in true PMR and in time onset of frank joint involvement and presence of rhuematoid factor allow the correct diagnosis to be made.

Mono- and oligoarticular onset

Young women particularly may present with synovitis of one or both knees which may be acute and cyclical or chronic and persistent. ESR and viscosity may be normal and rheumatoid factor absent. Synovial biopsy may be required to exclude other causes of a monoarthritis particularly tuberculosis and PVNS. The course is usually benign, the process often dying out after a few years with no long-term sequelae. It is thought that this may represent a late-onset variant of JCA, though a proportion progress to RA.

DIFFERENTIAL DIAGNOSIS

In the first few weeks, viral diseases (particularly rubella and hepatitis), erythema nodosum, bacterial infection and SLE should be considered. Psychological illness can present with prolonged aching in the joints, often in rather harassed young mothers with small children, who are confined to the home and generally disenchanted with their lot. In the occasional difficult case, a wide range of rare disorders may need to be excluded. Once the disease has become established, the other types of chronic rheumatic disease may need to be considered.

Since so many conditions can resemble early RA and there is no one specific test, a list of criteria has been devised to aid diagnosis.

Early RA — some rare differential diagnoses

1. Gonococcal arthritis
2. Henoch-Schonlein purpura
3. Acne arthritis
4. Oral-contraceptive-associated arthritis
5. Multicentric reticulohistiocytosis
6. Behçet's syndrome
7. Acute leukaemia
8. Familial Mediterranean fever
9. Hyperlipidaemia
10. Polychondritis
11. Amyloid arthropathy
12. Jaccoud's arthritis
13. Sarcoidosis
14. Myxoedema

Rheumatic diseases which may resemble chronic RA

1. Erosive interphalangeal OA
2. Psoriatic arthropathy
3. Chronic pyrophosphate deposition disease
4. Systemic lupus erythematosis
5. Ankylosing spondylitis
6. Reiter's syndrome
7. Chronic tophaceous gout

Criteria for the diagnosis of rheumatoid arthritis

1. Morning stiffness
2. Pain and tenderness in one joint
3. Swelling for 6 weeks in one joint
4. Swelling of one other joint
5. Symmetrical widespread joint involvement
6. Nodules
7. Radiological changes of RA
8. Rheumatoid factor
9. Characteristic synovial histology

7 = classical RA
5 = definite RA
3 = probable RA

SPECIFIC JOINT FEATURES

Hand

In early RA the hand feels stiff, swollen and sore and difficulty is experienced in making a fist, gripping and lifting things. A finger may get stuck in the palm when fully flexed and can sometimes only be released by pulling it out with the other hand (triggering) and symptoms of median-nerve compression such as nocturnal paraesthesiae and numbness in the first three fingers are very common.

Typical signs in early disease are swelling of the second and third MCPJs with loss of the normal valley between the knuckles when making a fist, symmetrical swelling of the PIPJs, guttering between the extensor tendons on the back of the hand due to wasting of the interossei, and prominent swelling on the back of the hand due to tenosynovitis of the extensor tendon sheath (Fig. 4.4).

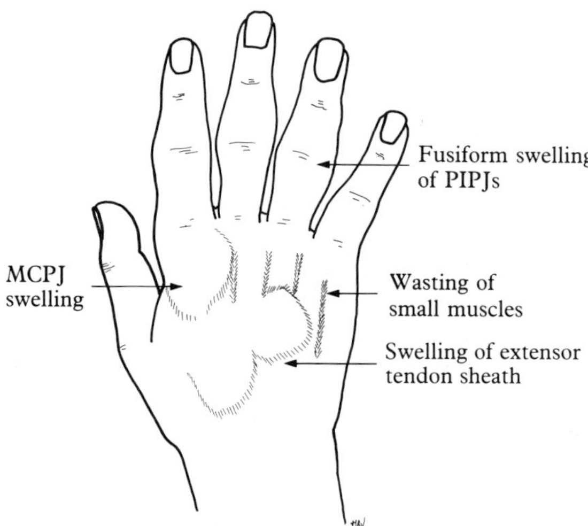

Fig. 4.4 The early rheumatoid hand

In late disease the characteristic rheumatoid deformities develop, including palmar subluxation of the MCPJs with inability to extend the fingers fully, ulnar deviation and boutonnière and swan-neck deformities of the fingers. The patient often has surprisingly few complaints since function may be well-preserved although movements may be executed in an abnormal manner. Swan-neck and boutonnière deformities are the result of tendon dislocations: the former is hyperextension at the PIPJ with flexion of the DIPJ (Fig. 4.5) and the latter is the opposite: flexion of the PIPJ and extension of the DIPJ (Fig. 4.6). The cause of ulnar deviation is not clearly understood but is partly due to to synovitis of the MCPJs causing dislocation of the extensor tendons into the ulnar valleys between the knuckles instead of being attached on the top and partly due to radial divia-

Clinical features of rheumatoid arthritis in the hand

Early

1. Wasting small muscles
2. Extensor tendon sheath swelling
3. Fusiform swelling of PIPJs
4. MCPJ synovitis with filling-in of hollows between knuckles
5. Flexor tendon synovitis
6. Prominent ulnar styloids

Late

1. Deformities
   a) Ulnar deviation
   b) Swan-neck
   c) Boutonnière
   d) Z-thumbs
   e) Subluxation of MCPJs
   f) Dropped fingers
2. Loss of function
   a) Poor grip
   b) Poor opposition

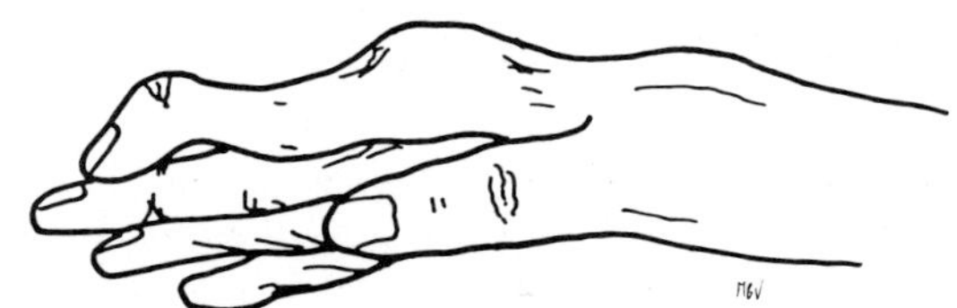

Fig. 4.5 Swan-neck hand deformity

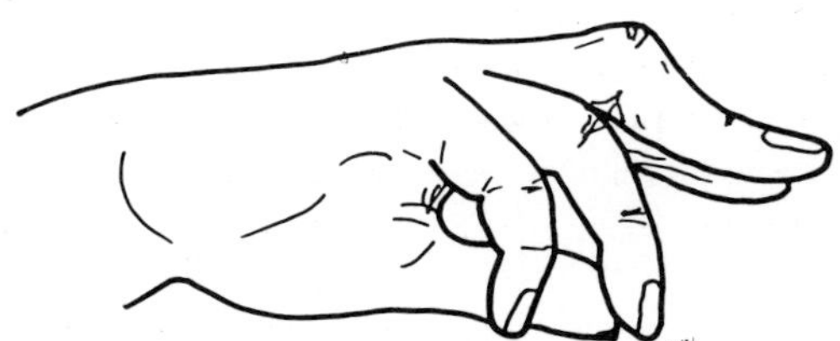

Fig. 4.6 Boutonnière hand deformity

tion of the wrist. Marked resorption of bone of the finger joints can produce shortening and telescoping of the fingers — the 'opera-glass hand' or *main-enlorgnette* — so-called because the fingers can be extended and retracted by pulling on them.

Wrist

In early disease, synovitis of the wrist and inferior radio-ulnar joint causes pain, particularly on lifting heavy objects or performing twisting movements such as unscrewing the tops of bottles or jars. Inflammation in the radio-ulnar joint weakens the normal ligamentous constraints of the ulnar head, which is pulled upwards by the dorsal carpal ligament. This prominence of the ulnar head is very characteristic and is frequently associated with synovitis of the extensor tendons of the fingers which may rupture due to a combination of attrition caused by rubbing over the prominent ulnar head and weakening from active synovitis around the wrist (Fig. 4.7).

Common wrist deformities are dorsal subluxation, producing a 'dinner-fork' deformity, and radial diviation, which may contribute to the ulnar drift of the fingers since in that position the extensor tendons are kept in line with the radius. This is one of the few joints in which fibrous and even bony ankylosis is a fairly frequent occurrence in burnt-out RA.

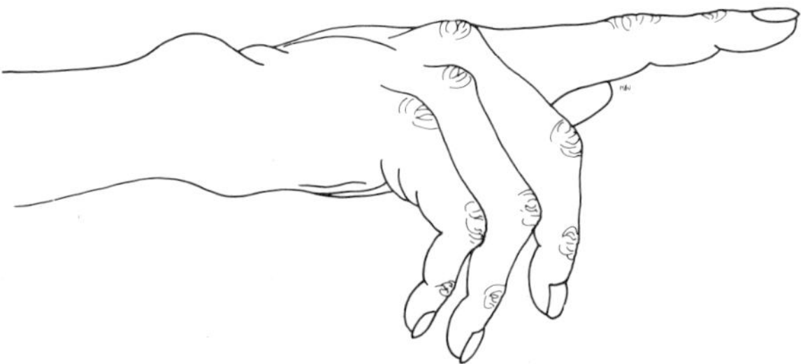

Fig. 4.7 Ruptured extension tendons — 'dropped fingers'

Foot

Foot involvement occurs early but is often asymptomatic even when fairly advanced changes are already present on X-ray. Synovitis of the MTPJs pushes the toes apart — the 'daylight sign' (Fig. 4.8). Occasionally the entire foot is diffusely swollen with pitting oedema. Pain can be elicited by squeezing the sides of the forefoot which compresses the heads of the MTPJs.

Three deformities commonly occur in the forefoot (Fig. 4.9) 1. Metatarsal-head subluxation; 2. Clawing of the toes; 3. Hallux valgus.

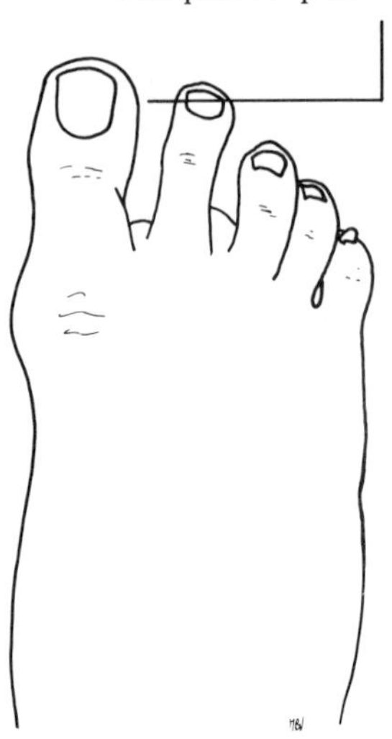

Fig. 4.8 The early rheumatoid foot

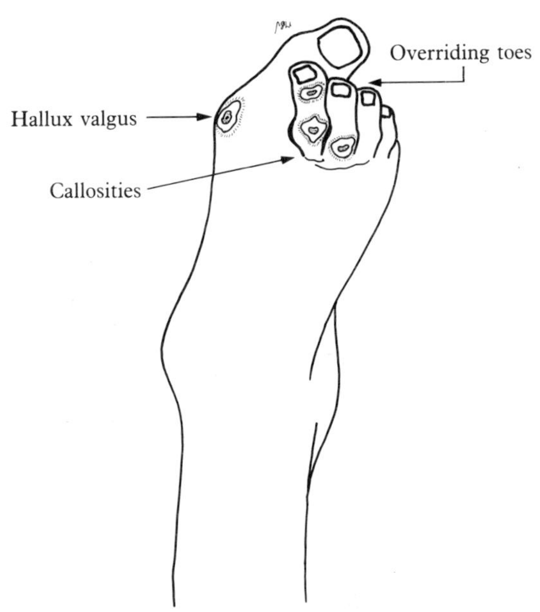

Fig. 4.9 Established rheumatoid foot deformity

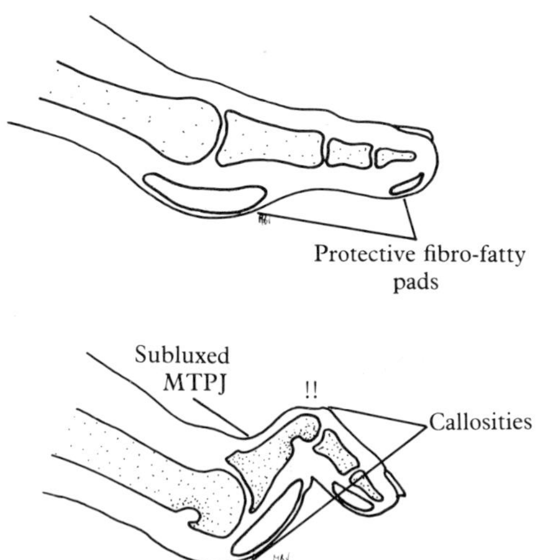

Fig. 4.10 Mechanism of 'cock-up' toe deformity

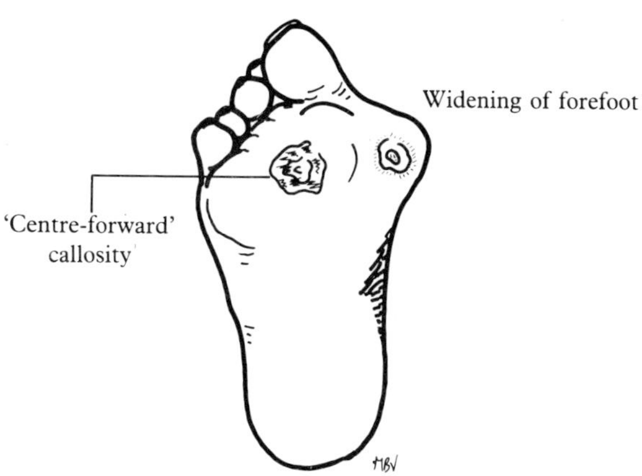

Fig. 4.11 Sole of the rheumatoid foot

The downward subluxation of the metatarsal heads exposes the bare bone to the full weight-bearing on walking without its normal protective padding (Fig. 4.10). This gives the very unpleasant sensation of walking on marbles. Clawed or 'cock-up' toes are the consequence of MTPJ subluxation and result in formation of painful callosities and indolent sores over the PIPJs. Hallux valgus results from lateral drift of the great toes and a large bunion may develop over the first metatarsal head. These deformities make it difficult to find comfortable shoes. Although callosities and bursae develop to protect the bones (Fig. 4.11), these not infrequently become ulcerated and infected, particularly when associated severe knee and hip disease make normal hygiene and nail-cutting difficult.

Midtarsal synovitis causes pain when walking on uneven surfaces and collapse of the longitudinal arch and subluxation of the joints into the sole cause a flat or even 'rocker-bottom' foot.

Ankle and hindfoot

The true ankle joint is infrequently involved in RA, but pain and swelling around the ankle is a common complaint. It can be due to true ankle or subtalar joint synovitis, synovitis of the peroneal tendons or simple oedema.

Early synovitis produces anterior swelling and pain on foot flexion and extension, noticed when 'pushing-off' when walking. Subtalar disease causes pain on inversion and eversion of the foot, noticed by the patient when walking on uneven surfaces. Ankle oedema without synovitis is a characteristic feature of early RA and could be due to disturbance in the lymphatics.

A valgus ankle is the common hindfoot deformity of RA and is probably due to a combination of disease at the ankle and the subtalar joint.

Knees

Knee disease accounts for much lower limb disability, some of which may be preventable. Bilateral, tense boggy swelling of the knee is an early feature caused by a combination of synovial hypertrophy and large effusions, and there is usually a subtle loss of knee extension. Quadriceps muscle wasting and ligamentous laxity may develop rapidly and seriously interfere with the stability of the knee. Walking often pumps the synovial fluid into a bursa in the popliteal fossa which can enlarge to form a popliteal cyst. This can rupture, releasing inflammatory fluid into the calf tissues, producing symptoms and signs indistinguishable from a deep venous thrombosis (p 259).

Persistent synovitis and effusions cause joint and tendon disruption which results in the development of valgus and varus deformities. Disabling fixed-flexion deformities are also common unless steps are taken all along to prevent them developing by the use of exercise and splints. The knee is susceptible to avascular necrosis and infection, particularly in patients on steroids.

Shoulder

This joint has the widest range of movement of any joint in the body, allowing the hand to be used in a wide variety of positions. In RA, inflammation in the gleno-humeral and acromio-clavicular joints and periarticular apparatus is common, and may have disasterous functional effects. Loss of external rotation is the earliest finding, but is usually unnoticed by the patient. Later, elevation, abduction and internal rotation of the arm are imparied so that it is difficult to carry out essential tasks such as combing the hair, dressing or toilet hygiene. Much pain and disability may be due to inflammation in the tendons and bursae around the joint, particularly in the subacromial bursa, and it is important to distinguish these treatable lesions. It is not uncommon in late RA to find the shoulder totally fixed, all movement coming from the scapula. The long head of the biceps tendon runs into the shoulder joint and may rupture, producing a startling lump in the lower forearm on elbow flexion, but this is usually painless and causes surprisingly little disability.

Elbow

This joint may be silently destroyed in the absence of obvious synovitis. Early loss of extension is very common in RA and gradually evolves into fixed-flexion deformity which can seriously interfere with such fundamentally important activities as eating. While the elbow may be relatively pain-free on attempted flexion and extension, pain may be severe on pronation and supination. Olecranon bursitis may be florid but not cause too much discomfort or disability. Nodules are commonly found at the elbow (Fig. 4.12). The ulnar nerve may be compressed behind the medial epicondyle.

Hip

25% of patients with RA develop hip disease.

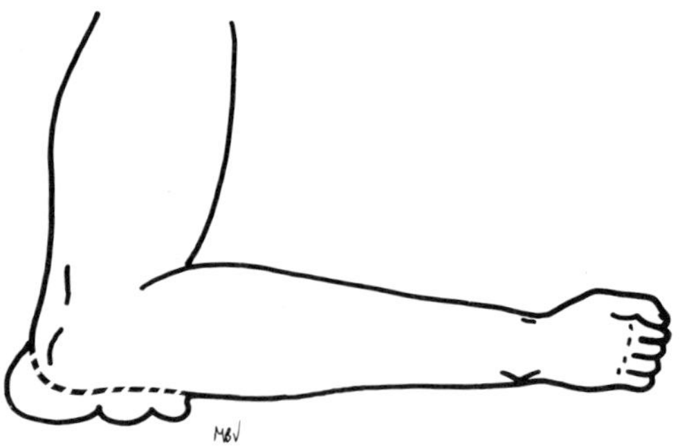

Fig. 4.12 Typical forearm rheumatoid nodules

Synovitis causes pain which is present on weight-bearing and is frequently refered to the knee, a great catch. Inflammation in the trochanteric bursa is common and may erroneously be attributed to hip disease. Signs of inflammation in the hip are minimal because the joint is set deep inside muscles. As pannus destroys the cartilage, there is concentric loss of joint space and the head of the femur migrates upwards, pushing the floor of the acetabulum inwards; this can be seen as protrusio acetabuli on X-ray. Clinically, the hip becomes limited in its range of movement, particularly adduction and external rotation. Extension may be gradually lost and fixed-flexion deformities may develop. Patients on steroids have a high incidence of avascular necrosis of the femoral head, which presents with sudden onset of severe persistent pain with marked reduction of the pre-existing range of movement.

Cervical spine

This is the only part of the axial skeleton significantly involved in RA and the consequences may be dire, leading to quadriplegia and death. It usually occurs in patients with disease of many years duration who have been on steroids. As many as a third of patients have evidence of involvement on X-ray but the incidence of symptoms and neurological consequences is much lower. Changes occur at two sites: the atlanto-axial level and below the second cervical vertebra.

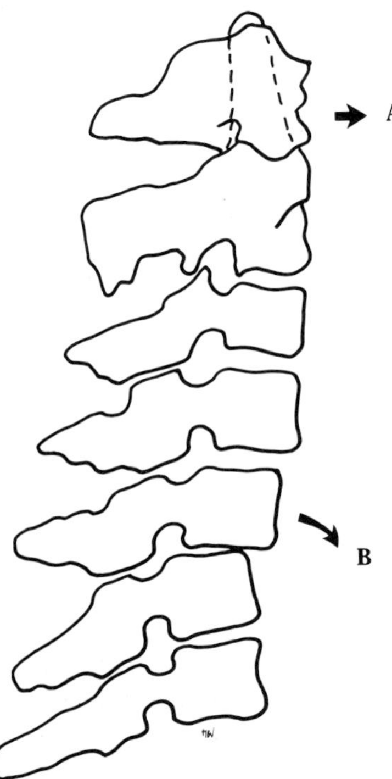

Fig. 4.13 Cervical spine involvement in rheumatoid arthritis. A. Forward slip of the atlas on the axis. B. 'Step-ladder' subluxation, usually most marked around the C5/6 region.

Atlanto-axial changes

Small synovial-lined bursae surround the odontoid peg. Synovitis results in erosion of the peg and weakness and laxity of the transverse ligament. In the normal neck, the distance between the back of the anterior arch of the atlas and the front of the peg is about 3 mm with the neck X-rayed in full flexion, but this distance is very much greater when there is atlanto-axial subluxation (Fig. 4.13). Erosion of the odontoid also leads to instability of the head on the neck. Vertical subluxation may also occur — with the peg rising up into the foramen magnum — detected on lateral X-ray of the skull as encroachment of more than 4 mm above McGregor's line (which joins the back of the hard palate to the occiput).

There is no correlation between the severity of changes on plain X-ray and the patient's symptoms. Pain may be felt in the occipital region due to traction on the second cervical nerve and there may be a history of vertigo and diplopia on rotation of the neck due to pressure on the vertebrobasilar artery. The appearance of neurological signs of cord compression are totally unpredictable, but tend to be a feature of late seropositive disease where corticosteroids have been given. The neurological examination is difficult to perform and assess in RA but the following features should ring alarm bells:

1. Sudden decrease in overall functional ability
2. Lightening pains on neck flexion
3. Upper limb paraesthesiae
4. Segmental sensory impairment
5. Loss of position sense
6. Hyperreflexia
7. Extensor plantar responses
8. Bladder and bowel dysfunction.

The corneal reflex and sensation in the upper part of the face may be diminished, probably due to pressure on the lower fibres of the spinal tract of the fifth cranial nerve which just reaches to the level of the C1–C2 articulation.

Subaxial disease

Involvement below C1–C2 is relatively common both at the synovial apophyseal joints and the non-synovial intervertebral discs and may present with severe pain on neck movement. Subluxation, particularly of C5 or C6, can occasionally cause cord compression.

There are two situations where patients with rheumatoid neck disease are particularly at risk: riding in cars and having anaesthetics. It is usually advisable for the neck to be supported in the first situation with a cervical collar, and for the anaesthetist to be aware of the problem in the second.

Other joints

Inflammation of the crico-arytenoid joints may result in anterior neck pain, difficulty with swallowing, stridor, shortness of breath and hoarseness. Although found in 50% at necropsy, the vast majority are asymptomatic. Very rarely, a tracheostomy is needed and death may result from laryngeal obstruction.

The ossicles in the ear are connected by small synovial joints which may rarely cause conduction deafness.

The sterno-clavicular and manubrio-sternal joints are often affected but rarely cause pain because they are relatively immobile. The sterno-clavicular joint is, however, a favoured site for sepsis and any sudden increase in pain and swelling here should raise this suspicion.

The tempro-mandibular joints are quite frequently involved and cause pain on chewing, accompanied by a 'clunking' sensation and palpable crepitus. Occasionally the patient may suddenly be unable to close the mouth. Severe symptoms can be very debilitating, both psychologically and physically if the intake of food is restricted as a consequence.

EXTRA-ARTICULAR FEATURES OF RA

RA has many features occurring outside the strict confines of the joints. Some are periarticular and result from the inflammatory process impinging on nearby structures — e.g. entrapment neuropathy — others such as eye and lung involvement are remote from joints.

Major extra-articular features of RA

Common

1. Anaemia
2. Lymphadenopathy
3. Oedema
4. Nodules
5. Osteoporosis
6. Muscle wasting
7. Episcleritis
8. Keratoconjunctivitis sicca
9. Entrapment neuropathy
10. Nail-fold vasculitis
11. Peripheral sensory neuropathy

Uncommon

1. Pleural effusion
2. Pulmonary fibrosis
3. Pericarditis
4. Splenomegaly
5. Scleritis
6. Systemic vasculitis
7. Sensorimotor neuropathy

75% of patients with RA have two or more extra-articular features — and generally their presence is associated with sero-positivity, more severe disease and a reduced life-expectancy. Underlying pathogenic mechanisms are not clear but appear to involve immune complexes, antibodies and aberrant cellular immunity.

Nodules

These lumps are a hallmark of RA. They are not usually present at onset but will eventually appear in about 25% of patients. They are firm, round, non-tender and often multiple, with characteristic histological features. *Subcutaneous nodules* favour the elbow, head, sacrum and Achilles tendon. Usually they are mobile but they may, particularly around the elbow, become bound to periosteum. *Intracutaneous nodules* appear around the fingers, particularly in patients who use their hands a lot and tend to come and go quite quickly. *Nodules in tendons* many cause functional disturbance and are often responsible for triggering of fingers when they form inside flexor-tendon sheaths. *Nodules in internal organs*, particularly lung, heart and eye, can cause serious functional impairment and diagnostic confusion.

Nodules may become confluent and grow to a considerable size. Although unsightly, excision is rarely helpful since they nearly always recur. Suppression of the disease by drugs or a spontaneous remission, is often associated with nodules becoming softer, smaller or disappearing altogether. Occasionally, in sites such as the ball of the foot or over the sacrum, nodules break down and discharge — a complication known as *fistulous rheumatism*.

The appearance or increase in size or number of nodules suggests active disease, although there are a small group of patients who develop florid nodules without much synovitis or joint destruction. As a rule they occur only in seropositive patients, except where the disease is being manipulated by therapy and any found in a seronegative patient should be biopsied, since there are several other lumps resembling rheumatoid nodules that can occur in other joint diseases — e.g. gouty tophi, xanthomata and calcific nodules.

Vasculitis

It is accepted that there is a vascular inflammatory element in the pathology of RA thought to be due to the deposition of immune complexes in the walls of arteries and veins but there is considerably controversy regarding frequency, prognosis, association with steroids and management.

Vasculitis tends to be an episodic occurrence but precipitating factors are unknown. Initiation, withdrawal or alteration in the dose of steroids have been implicated. Patients sometimes give a history of intercurrent illness prior to onset. The cutaneous manifestations, like rheumatoid nodules, have a predilection for areas of pressure.

Clinical manifestations of RA vasculitis

1. Nail-fold infarcts
2. Splinter haemorrhages
3. Palpable purpura
4. Cutaneous ulcers
5. Mononeuritis multiplex
6. Scleritis
7. Internal organs
   a) Pulmonary vasculitis
   b) Bowel infarction
   c) Coronary arteritis

In its mildest form, vasculitis presents as small brown periungual and finger-pad lesions or splinter haemorrhages which come and go and are often unnoticed by the patient (Fig. 4.14). These are due to occlusive vasculitis and are certainly not associated with a bad prognosis and require no treatment. When larger vessels are involved, skin ulceration, peripheral neuropathy, mononeuritis multiplex and gangrene of a digit or extremity may occur. Severe necrotising vasculitis presents and behaves much like polyarteritis nodosa and death may result from bowel perforation or myocardial infarction. Patients in the last two categories are often unwell, with low-grade fever, anaemia and weight loss.

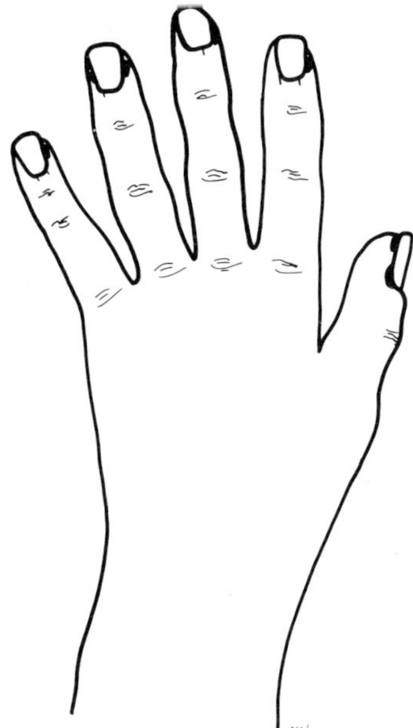

Fig. 4.14 Peri-ungual vasculitic lesions

More severe forms of vasculitis are associated with the presence of nodules, hypocomplementaemia, IgM and IgG rheumatoid factor, cryoglobulinaemia and positive tests for circulating immune complexes such as C1 binding and ACA. Immune complexes may be demonstrated by immunoflourescence around the affected vessels but the significance of this observation is not clear, since they may also be present around vessels in unaffected skin sites in patients with and without vasculitis. Biopsy of rectal mucosa, on the other hand, is often of diagnostic value, since necrotising vasculitis may be detected in the mucosal vessels.

The appearance of systemic vasculitis indicates a bad prognosis. Treatment is indicated (p 62) in the severer forms, which may threaten life.

Anaemia

Anaemia is the rule in active RA and correlates with disease activity. It is usually normochromic and normocytic and results from ineffective erythopoiesis. The iron and iron-binding capacity are both reduced but plenty of sequestered iron can be demonstrated in the marrow, synovium and lymph nodes. The haemoglobin will rise with disease remission and iron therapy is useless.

Common causes of anaemia in RA
1. Active disease
2. Blood loss
3. Marrow suppression by drugs
4. Felty's syndrome

Most patients on anti-inflammatory drugs lose between 5–10 ml of blood a day. This may result in true iron deficiency, which can best be distinguished from the anaemia of chronic disease by the presence of a raised iron-binding capacity. This type of anaemia may respond to iron (p 253). Macrocytosis is five times as common in RA but the incidence of PA is no higher than the general population and may be due to defective folate metabolism. Patients treated with cytotoxic drugs often develop a striking macrocytosis which resolves on withdrawal of the drugs.

Lymphadenopathy

The lymph nodes draining acutely inflamed joints are often enlarged and in about 50% of patients, careful examination reveals a widespread generalised lymphadenopathy. The nodes are soft, mobile and non-tender. Occasionally, one or two become disproportionately enlarged and needle aspiration or excision biopsy may be indicated to exclude a lymphoma. Patients with Sjögren's syndrome may be predisposed to the development of more aggressive lymphoproliferation, with widespread lymphadenopathy, and hepatosplenomegaly with loss of the normal architecture of the lymph node ('pseudolymphoma') but this is very rare.

Osteoporosis

Periarticular osteoporosis is an early X-ray change of RA and indicates significant synovitis. A more generalised osteopenia also develops which cannot always be blamed on steroid therapy and immobilisation may be a contributing factor.

Thin bones are not always due to osteoporosis alone. Osteomalacia is more common in those with RA than the general population, due to a combination of poor diet from a reduced standard of living and confinement to the house by disability. The characteristic X-ray appearances are often not present but multiple fractures are quite common. A bone biopsy may be required.

Oedema

Pitting oedema which is painless is often found round the ankles in early RA, and lymphoedema of the arms has also been described. Both these are probably due to obstructed lymphatic drainage (p 260).

Eye involvement

The eye is frequently involved in RA. 25% of patients have reduced tear secretions due to inflammation and atrophy of the lacrimal glands. Patients are often not aware that the eyes are dry but may complain that they feel gritty and itchy. The cornea sheds its epithelium and superficial ulcers develop on the area of conjunctiva that is exposed when the eye is open (kerato-conjunctivitis sicca). Reduced tear production can be demonstrated using Schirmer test paper but is best confirmed by staining with Rose Bengal and slit lamp examination. Since this potentially serious condition may be asymptomatic, all patients should ideally be screened annually.

Eye involvement in RA
1. Episcleritis
2. Keratoconjunctivitis sicca
3. Scleritis
4. Scleromalacia perforans
5. Marginal corneal ulceration
6. Tenosynovitis of ocular muscles
8. Drug-induced
   a) Steroid cataracts
   b) Chloroquine retinopathy

Mild episcleritis is common, self-limiting and rarely serious. Scleritis is more sinister. Multiple attacks lead to scleral thinning and necrotising scleritis may result in perforation of the eyeball (scleromalacia perforans) and spread to involve the uveal tract.

Inflammation of the tendon of the superior oblique muscle has been reported. There is intermittent diplopia on upward gaze accompanied by a clicking sensation in the orbit.

Lung involvement

The lung is a common site of extra-articular involvement in RA. Middle-aged men with systemic features such as weight loss and fever seem particularly susceptible to develop pleural rubs and effusions which can appear before the onset of arthritis. Effusions can be quite large, cause dyspnoea and require aspiration. The fluid is characteristically high in protein and LDH, low in sugar and C_3 and gives a positive test for rheumatoid factor and immune complexes. It is not blood-stained but appears cloudly due to the presence of numerous white cells and debris. 'Ragocytes' — phagocytic cells containing inclusions — and comet-shaped cells may be identified. A pleural biopsy may show a histological appearance of a flattened rheumatoid nodule.

Lung involvement in RA

1. Pleurisy
2. Pleural effusion
3. Pleural nodules and plaques
4. Parenchymal nodules
5. Interstitial fibrosis
6. Obliterative bronchiolitis
7. Caplan's syndrome

Nodules, solitary and multiple, may occur in the lung parenchyma before or after the onset of arthritis. They seem to have a predilection for the upper lobes where they may cavitate and cause haemophysis and resemble tuberculosis. The presence of a solitary nodule, particularly in a middle-aged man who smokes, may be diagnostically awkward but techniques such as needle and transbronchial biopsy may allow histological material to be obtained without recourse to thoracotomy. Caplan described an interesting phenomenon in miners with pneumoconiosis and RA who developed massive confluent pulmonary nodules.

Classical fibrosing alveolitis with dyspnoea, cyanosis, clubbing, basal rales and honeycomb-shadowing on chest X-ray is uncommon in RA — occurring in about 2% of patients. It is associated with a poor prognosis, death often occuring within 5 years of onset. However, systematic studies have shown that there exists a much milder type of lung fibrosis which is often totally asymptomatic. 40% of consecutive patients with classical RA in one study had an abnormal gas transfer factor although half had completely normal chest X-rays. This type is not associated with an adverse prognosis. It is not clear how RA interstitial lung disease fits into the overall concept of idiopathic fibrosing alveolitis. About 15% of patients who present with advanced lung disease have rheumatoid arthritis and over 50% have elevated rheumatoid factor levels without joint disease.

An extremely rare form of lung disease, obliterative bronchiolitis, has recently been described, distinct from interstitial fibrosis, in which there is rapid and progressive dyspnoea leading to respiratory failure and death within a year, due to widespread small-airways obstruction, often with a normal chest X-ray. Drugs and infection have been implicated in the aetiology.

Heart involvement

Pericarditis is the commonest cardiac manifestation of RA. The usual presenting feature is a painless pericardial rub detected on routine examination. This is usually short-lived but a few patients have a rub which lasts for years. Clinically, pericarditis is present in about 10% of patients but over 30% have significant amounts of pericardial fluid detected on echocardiography. Evidence of present or past pericardial involvement can be found in 40% at post-mortem. Only a few patients show widening

Heart involvement in RA

1. Pericarditis
2. Pericardial effusion
3. Nodules in conducting system
4. Nodules on valves
5. Cardiomyopathy
6. Coronary artery vasculitis
7. Amyloidosis

of the heart shadow on chest X-ray and ECG is often normal or reveals only T-wave flattening or inversion. It can be deduced from these facts that, though common, pericarditis is rarely a problem and no specific treatment is required. Constriction and tamponade are very rare.

Granulomatous lesions with a central necrotic area surrounded by pallisaded histiocytes are present on heart valves in 3% at post-mortem but very rarely cause a problem in life, although aortic incompetence and mitral stenosis are described.

Small nodules in the conducting tissues may cause dysrhythmias and heart block and atrial flutter and fibrillation have been reported during episodes of pericarditis. Many patients at post-mortem have a non-specific inflammatory infiltrate in the cardiac muscle without functional impairment in life. However, there are occasional reports of patients developing cardiomegaly and congestive cardiac failure without any other obvious cause but it is not clear if this is due to a specific rheumatoid cardiomyopathy.

Coronary artery vasculitis may lead to myocardial infarction, and the heart may be involved in amyloidosis (p 318).

Neuromuscular involvement

Many nerves pass through narrow passages near joints and may become compressed by articular and periarticular swelling. The median nerve at the wrist and ulnar nerve at the elbow are particularly vulnerable and are discussed fully on page 281. Median nerve compression is a common and important early feature of RA. In a hand already compromised by joint disease the addition of such a neuropathy may be a functional disaster. Fortunately, entrapment neuropathy is often amenable to treatment either with local steroid injections or by surgical release.

Neuromuscular involvement in RA

1. Muscle wasting
2. Distal sensory neuropathy
3. Entrapment neuropathy
4. Mixed sensorimotor neuropathy
5. Motoneuritis multiplex
6. Radiculopathy
7. Myelopathy
8. Steroid-induced proximal myopathy

Many patients with RA, if examined carefully, show signs of a distal sensory neuropathy which is benign. However, the presence of a mixed sensorimotor neuropathy or mononeuritis multiplex is indicative of vasculitis of the vasa nervosum and has a less favourable outcome.

The radiculopathy and myelopathy associated with cervical spine instability is discussed under that heading.

Most patients develop localised muscle weakness and wasting around inflamed joints thought to be largely due to reflex inhibition secondary to the inflammation. About one-third develop proximal and distal atrophy far removed from joints and this has been attributed to myositis. Muscle biopsy shows a whole range of non-specific abnormalities — often associated with vasculitis. Patients on steroids may develop proximal muscle weakness making it difficult to rise out of chairs and mount stairs, which may be mistaken for increased disability due the arthritis.

Splenomegaly

Splenomegaly may be detected clinically in about 5% of patients and its presence is associated with systemically active disease. Only about 1% of these will eventually go on to develop true Felty's syndrome. In 1924 Felty reported five patients with RA, splenomegaly and leucopenia associated with profound weight-loss, generalised lymphadenopathy and brownish skin discoloration. Ulceration of mouth, legs and cornea were also major features.

The term tends to be applied more loosely nowadays to any patients with RA who develop leucopenia, even in the absence of splenomegaly. The clinical significance of the diagnosis is that there is increased risk of severe infection, particularly of skin, lungs and kidney. The RA has usually been present for 10 or more years with advanced joint deformity and high titres of RF, ANF and cryoglobulins. The WBC varies between 500 and 4500 and infectious episodes do not necess-

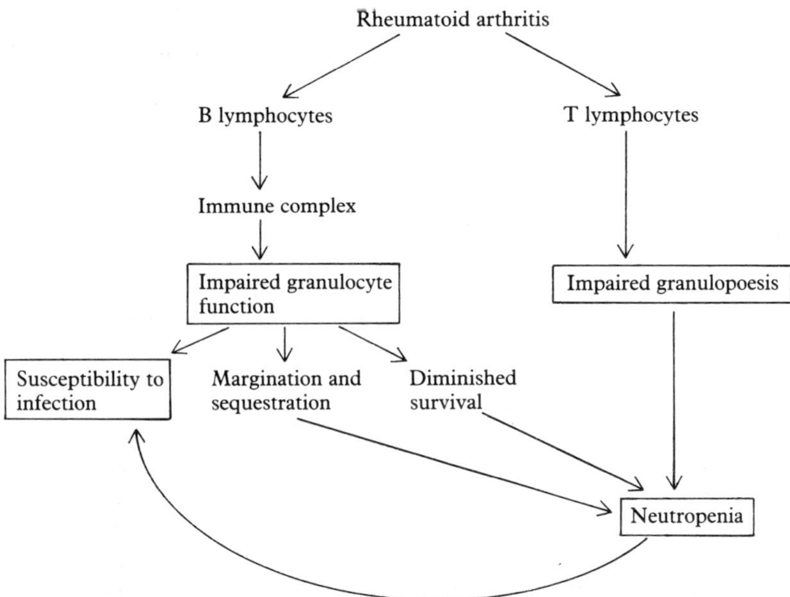

Fig. 4.15 Factors contributing to infection and neutropenia in Felty's syndrome

arily correlate with the degree of neutropenia. The count may also rise during infection making the diagnosis difficult. Platelets can fall, but rarely below 100 000 and purpura and haemorrhage do not occur as a rule. The granuloctyopenia and infection appears to be multifactorial in origin. Decreased production, increased removal, and impaired functions have all been implicated (Fig. 4.15). Splenectomy is recommended for patients with severe recurrent infections, haemolysis, hypersplenism or haemorrhage, but is usually only successful for a few years. Drugs such as lithium carbonate have been tried, with varied success to raise the white count. Gold has been used occasionally with great caution and may be of some benefit.

Renal involvement

Significant renal impairment is not a feature of uncomplicated RA, which is strange in a disease whose many extra-articular manifestations are thought to be due to circulating immune complexes which in other diseases, particularly SLE, target in on the glomerulus. However, post-mortem studies of RA kidneys have shown that many have non-specific interstitial fibrosis. Subtle tests such as urinary NAG excretion and tests of concentrating ability reveal some impairment in life. Amyloidosis may cause nephrotic syndrome and ultimately death from renal failure (p 318). Great rarities are renal tubular acidosis and diabetes insipidus which may develop in patients with Sjögren's syndrome. Analgesic nephropathy is surprisingly uncommon in patients with RA but NSAID drugs may be responsible for some of the subtle decrease in function.

Liver involvement

The existence of 'rheumatoid liver' as a distinct entity is disputed. There is a significantly higher incidence of hepatomegaly in RA patients compared to those with OA and the alkaline phosphatase is more frequently elevated. However, few patients have elevation of the liver transaminases. There is a slightly increased incidence of smooth muscle and antimitochondrial antibodies compared to patients with seronegative polyarthritis. Liver histology during life and at post-mortem reveals no specific structural abnormality except necrotising vasculitis occurring with widespread vasculitis, and nodular regenerative hyperplasia in association with portal hypertension in a few patients with Felty's syndrome. Amyloid deposition may cause striking hepatomegaly. A gold-related hepatocellular necrosis has been described and salicylates may also adversely affect liver function.

INVESTIGATIONS

The diagnosis of RA is essentially clinical and the most useful supporting diagnostic test is radiological examination of affected joints. Blood tests may help to confirm or refute clinically borderline cases and are particularly useful when measured serially as a guide to severity and response to treatment or to watch for adverse reactions to drugs.

Immunological tests

The sera of 75% of patients with RA contain a 19S anti-globulin (IgM rheumatoid factor) which reacts with the Fc portion of autologous IgG. This is often absent at onset, appears as the disease progresses and disappears again in long-standing disease or after treatment with disease-suppressing drugs. Levels fluctuate considerably and are not a reliable guide to disease activity. Persistently high titres are of some prognostic significance and tend to correlate with severe erosive disease and the presence of extra-articular features such as nodules, Felty's syndrome and Sjögren's syndrome. IgM rheumatoid factor is present in about 15% of the elderly population without RA and in 5–10% of patients with other inflammatory connective-tissue diseases. 25% of patients with definite RA never have IgM rheumatoid factor but despite this may have severe erosive disease. Rheumatoid factors also occur in the other classes of immunoglobulins. IgG rheumatoid factor has the characteristic tendency to self-associate to form large immune complexes and high levels may be particularly associated with the development of vasculitis.

Anti-nuclear factors are present in 30% of RA patients and correlate with nodules, Felty's and Sjögren's syndromes, leucopenia and splenomegaly but the DNA antibody level is not raised.

Using highly-sensitive assays such as C1q binding and platelet aggregation, immune complexes can be detected in the sera of most patients with RA at some stage. Tests which detect complement-fixing antibodies, such as the anticomplementary activity (ACA) test, are less sensitive but more significant and the combination of high titres of rheumatoid factor, low complement and ACA correlates with severe systemic disease.

Haematological tests

Normochromic normocytic anaemia is the rule and is discussed further under 'extra-articular' features. The white count is normal in the majority, raised in 25% and may be low in Felty's syndrome (p 57) or as a side-effect of drug treatment. Thrombocytosis is very characteristic of active RA — sometimes counts may exceed one million. Clinical improvement induced by disease-modifying drugs, particularly penicillamine, appears to parallel the fall in the platelet count. The plasma viscosity and ESR are usually raised in active RA but again serial data are more useful that 'spot' measurement.

Biochemical tests

In active disease, the serum alkaline phosphatase of liver origin is often elevated two- to threefold and the serum albumin may be low and revert to normal when the disease goes into remission. Iron and iron-binding capacity may be reduced. The acute-phase proteins, particularly CRP and SAA, are often markedly elevated and serial readings give a good indication of overall activity. Sometimes there is a marked discrepancy between their levels, i.e. one is elevated, the other normal but the significance of this is not yet known.

Radiology

The plain X-ray is helpful in diagnosis of early RA and in assessing the progress of established disease. The early findings reflect the presence of active synovitis and are: symmetrical soft-tissue swelling and juxta-articular osteoporosis, particuularly of the PIPJs and MCPJs of the hands and the MTPJs of the feet. After a variable period of time as the disease progresses erosions appear as small defects with an indistinct margin in the cortex of the bone at the base of the second and third

Common X-ray features in RA

1. Soft-tissue swelling
2. Juxta-articular osteoporosis
3. Marginal erosions
4. Joint space narrowing
5. Geodes
6. Deformities
7. Resorption of distal ends of clavicles
8. C1–C2 subluxation
9. Protrusio acetabuli

metacarpals, the PIPJs, MTPJs and ulnar styloids. These may gradually increase in size and coalesce to form sizeable defects in bone. Erosions also appear at the margins of the large joints but are less easy to visualise radiographically. Continued destruction of the cartilage eventually results in loss of the joint space. Large cysts, or geodes, may form in the subchondral bone where joint fluid is pumped through small defects in the damaged cartilage, particularly in the large weight-bearing joints.

In late disease, juxta-articular osteoporosis and soft-tissue swelling is less pronounced and the long-standing erosions develop a firmer outline. Widespread cartilage destruction, subluxation and deformity are the dominant features and there is occasional ankylosis, particularly in the wrist. New bone formation is not a common radiological feature of RA. In patients with the arthritis mutilans type of disease there is considerable resorption of bone particularly at the MCPJs, and in the phalanges causing shortening of the digits. And many small cysts are seen in patients with the 'typus-robustus' RA in which the hands continue to be used for heavy work despite pain.

Radioisotope scans using technetium-labelled diphosphonate complexes show increased uptake around inflamed joints due to the increased bloodflow but do not offer any great advantage over a plain film in diagnosis and assessment. Techniques employing contrast media are also used. Arthrography will often confirm joint rupture, particularly in the knee and at the wrist. Myelography is essential in the investigation of rheumatoid cervical myelopathy prior to surgery because there may be cord compression at more than one level.

Synovial fluid analysis

Although there are no specific diagnostic features, synovial fluid analysis is useful if only to exclude other condition such as infection in early disease. The fluid in RA is typically a light yellow colour, watery with a negative string test and is cloudy due to a high white-cell count — in the order of 5000–50 000/ml — with 80–90% polymorphs. Rheumatoid factor test may occasionally be positive when the serum is still negative and the complement and glucose are often low. The granulocytes may contain inclusion bodies which represent phagocytosed immune complexes and small fibrinous bodies called rice bodies, may be noted.

Synovial histology

Needle and arthroscopic biopsy of the knee and shoulder joint is technically possible but all other joints must be opened surgically to obtain a satisfactory specimen. The features in RA are nonspecific and may also be seen in other forms of inflammatory polyarthritis, and are: hypertrophy and hyperplasia of the synovial lining cells, an underlying vascular connective tissue infiltrated with large numbers of perivascular lymphocytes and plasma cells, often resembling a lymphoid follicle, many macrophages and some multinucleated giant cells which may contain bone and cartilage debris. Fibrin clot usually covers the synovial surface.

MANAGEMENT

Correct diagnosis is the first step. Although many aspects of management apply equally well to other forms of inflammatory polyarthritis, the label 'rheumatioid arthritis' has prognostic implications and suggests the use of some relatively specific suppressive therapy. It may take some months or even years for the typical clinical, serological and radiological patterns to emerge and it is therefore often important to leave the diagnosis open ('polyarthritis, cause uncertain'), until sure.

The variability of the disease and the different effects of joint damage on different individuals, mean that each patient must be treated individually in the context of his/her life and aspirations. Early tenosynovitis of the fingers, for example, has different implications for the concert pianist and the philosopher and each may require a different approach. However, the assessment and overall aims of therapy are common to all patients.

Treatment depends on the duration, activity and dominant features of the disease and is quite different in early inflammatory polyarthritis and end stage destructive disease.

Assessment and aims of treatment in rheumatoid arthritis

Assessment

1. Duration
2. Activity of disease process
3. Functional impairment
4. Extra-articular features
5. Concurrent diseases and drug therapy
6. Needs and aspirations of the patients

Aims

1. Realistic education to relieve anxiety and allow future plans
2. Relief of symptoms (chiefly pain and stiffness)
3. Prevent disease progression
4. Maintain optimal joint function
5. Modify environment to suit patient needs

Early synovitis

Once the diagnosis of RA has been made the patient and his family should be informed and educated about the disease. Most patients do not become severely disabled or wheelchair-bound, although the majority expect to until reassured. The doctor needs to be honest and to explain clearly what he can and cannot do; many patients need counselling about diet, work, activity, sex and the inheritance of the disease.

Rest and activity

Inflamed joints get better with rest and patients feel generally better, perhaps because products of inflamed synovium contribute to general malaise. Single active joints may benefit from being rested in splints, e.g. wrist and knee, used particularly at night and during inactivity; in generalised polyarthritis a period of strict bed rest for 1–3 weeks, often in hopsital, is helpful and may improve long-term prognosis of the disease as well as the acute inflammation. Careful attention must be paid to posture (Fig. 4.16) and regular passive exercises are needed to maintain a full range of motion. Many patients benefit from taking a rest in the middle of the day and having 8–10 hours sleep a night. A hot bath first thing in the morning is often very helpful in relieving morning stiffness.

Conversely, exercise is important for maintaining the strength of joints and muscles, although the fact that RA is usually worse in the

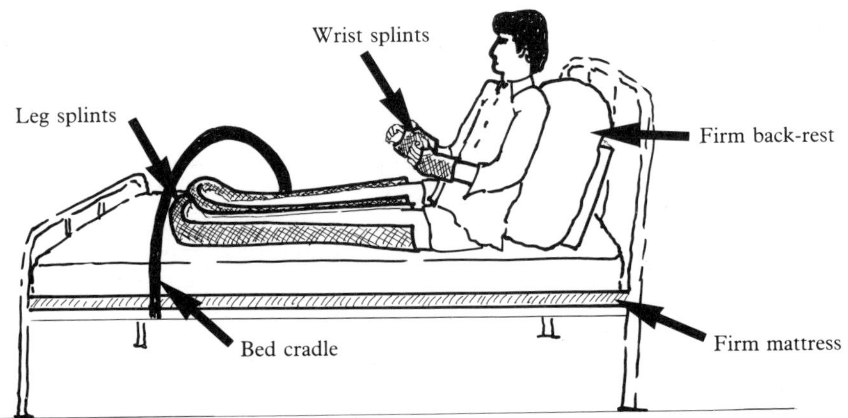

Fig. 4.16 Correct posture during bed-rest

dominant right hand and that it improves in a limb paralysed by polio or a stroke suggests that excessive joint use is not a good thing. It is important to keep a balance between rest and exercise in early disease. Patients should be encouraged to take as much general exercise as they feel they can cope with without causing an increase in pain and stiffness. Swimming is an excellent form of general exercise, particularly if there is a heated pool available. Sets of exercises should be taught which strengthen muscles, preserve movement and prevent deformity. Quadriceps function at the knee is particularly vital. The occupational therapist as well as the physiotherapist can help with these therapeutic and preventative measures which may reduce the risk of progressive joint damage.

Symptomatic relief

Drug therapy is usually helpful in relieving pain and stiffness. In early disease, symptoms are caused by inflammation and respond much better to anti-inflammatory drugs than to analgesics.

Local steroid injections are very helpful in relieving early local pain and pressure from synovitis, tenosynovitis or bursitis. Lasting benefit is particularly likely when long-acting preparations are used in tendon sheaths and the small joints of the hand and in the carpal tunnel. Systemic steroids are hardly ever necessary and are relatively contra-indicated except in the elderly patient with an incapacitating acute onset of RA in whom control can sometimes be achieved with small doses (7.5–10 mg once daily).

The non-steroidal anti-inflammatory drugs are used by most patients; many gain significant symptomatic relief and this leads to functional improvement in many. These drugs need to be tailored to suit the patient (individual variation response is great) and the type and timing of symptoms. Large doses given at night relieve night pain and morning stiffness with a low risk of side effects and provide a particularly useful way of prescribing these drugs in active RA. These drugs have no effect on disease progression.

Prevention of disease progression

In some patients, active symptomatic inflammation persists in spite of the measures mentioned and X-rays show evidence of progressive damage to cartilage and bone. Disease modifying drugs, also called 'second-line' drugs, are available but are toxic. Careful consideration needs to be given before they are used and facilities must be available to monitor their side-effects. Guidelines to general indications and contra-indications and signs of efficacy are listed below.

The drugs used are covered in Chapter 26 and listed below. They all take weeks or months to produce an effect, require careful monitoring, often produce side-effects and have variable response rates. Both doctor and patient must therefore be fully aware of the implications of their

Disease-modifying 'second-line' drugs

Drug	
Gold Penicillamine Hydroxychloroquine	Commonly used
Azathioprine Cyclophosphamide Salazopyrine	Less commonly used
Dapsone Chlorambucil Methotrexate	Reserved for refractory cases

Indications for disease-modifying agents

1. Persistent active inflammatory polyarthritis in spite of optimal general measures and NSAID therapy
2. Progressive joint deformity and functional impairment
3. Progressive radiological changes
4. Severe extra-articular manifestations
5. As steroid-sparing agents

Contra-indications

1. Uncertain diagnosis
2. Disease of less than 6 months duration
3. Inactive disease
4. Lack of adequate facilities to monitor therapy
5. Women of child-bearing age

use. The disease should be monitored clinically, serologically and radiologically so that their effects can be measured.

The remission induced by these drugs is felt as a general improvement in overall well-being as well as just relief of the articular manifestations with a consequent functional improvement and often a reduction in the amount of other therapy.

Features of drug-induced remission
1. Improvement in articular and extra-articular features
2. Reduction in ESR/plasma viscosity
3. Falling titres of rheumatoid factor
4. Slowing of radiological progression

Surgical procedures may also help prevent disease progression. Synovectomy produces only a temporary improvement (usually 2–3 years) but if combined, for example, with removal of the ulnar styloid and dorsal tenosynovectomy at the wrist, can prevent rupture of extensor tendons. Medical synovectomy, using intra-articular radio-active colloids may be useful to interrupt the progression of an individual active joint.

Late disease

In some patients, the disease progresses in spite of all attempts to stop it. The major problems then are mechanical sequelae of damage to the joint and periarticular tissues and/or extra-articular features of the disease and management of these patients is quite different from that used in early synovitis.

Functional problems need to be assessed by doctors, occupational therapists and physiotherapists. Splints may help to support unstable joints and footwear is crucial in the management of joint damage in the lower limb. Shoes to fit deformed forefeet relieve symptoms and prevent pressure areas and support at the ankle may help prevent secondary knee deformity (varus or valgus) as well as relieving pain locally.

Surgery often has a major role at this stage of the disease. Forefoot arthroplasty, arthrodesis of the wrist or ankle and hip or knee replacement are examples of relatively common surgical procedures to help the established rheumatoid arthritis patient.

Some useful operations in rheumatoid arthritis
1. Median nerve decompression
2. Repair of ruptured extensor tendons
3. Hip replacement
4. Excision of subluxed metatarsal heads (Fowler's)
5. Correction of valgus deformity of the great toe (Keller's)
6. Wrist fusion
7. Triple fusion of the hindfoot
8. Synovectomy, particularly of wrist and knee

Pre-operative assessment
1. General health and disease activity
2. Potential sites of infection, e.g. urine, skin, teeth
3. Drugs, particularly steriods
4. Ability to urinate lying down (men)
5. Ability to use crutches (lower-limb surgery)
6. Quality of bone
7. State of cervical spine
8. Condition of other key joints
9. Patient's expectations from surgery

In RA it is more important than in other diseases to assess the patient pre-operatively and to relate a local mechanical problem to the patient's daily activity, his other joint problems, the overall state and treatment of the disease and its likely outcome.

Special problems in late surgery of rheumatoid include the increased risk of infection, thin skin, thin bones, difficulty in mobilisation due to damage to other muscles and joints, drugs and the systemic effects of the disease on the patient and his morale.

For some patients it is more appropriate to modify the environment than the disease. This responsibility may fall partly to the occupational therapist and social worker, as well as the doctor.

Complications

Systemic vasculitis

This can be life-threatening. There are no good controlled trials but several treatments are available. Bed rest and high-dose steroids (e.g. 1 g methylprednisolone) can reduce vascular inflammation; plasma-expanders such as low-molecular-weight dextran may improve blood-flow through damaged vessels; plasmaphoresis may be beneficial by reducing the number of circulating immune complexes and immunosuppressive agents such as cyclophosphamide and azathioprine may dampen down their production. Any or all of these methods can be tried, depending on the clinical situation. Occasionally surgery will be necessary, e.g. amputation of a gangrenous extremity or closure of a perforated bowel.

Cervical cord compression

Immobilisation of the neck in a collar may be protective, particularly with atlanto-axial subluxation, as there is evidence from X-ray screening of the neck that subluxation is not gradual but occurs suddenly at a particular point in neck flexion. Although complete immobilisation is impossible, it may be possible to prevent the critical point being reached. If frank neurological signs are present, surgical fusion may be necessary and is best performed using wires and the new 'superglue' substances which do not involve a long post-operative period in bed on traction, which has a high morbidity in the RA patient. Although some improvement in neurological signs can be expected, this is often incomplete since the neurological damage may be mediated via interference to the blood-supply to the cord. The question of whether cervical myelopathy can be prevented by prophylatic fixation of unstable segments of the spine has not yet been answered.

Ruptured popliteal cyst

Popliteal cyst rupture causes marked inflammation in the calf muscles. The remaining synovial fluid in the knee should be removed and the joint injected with steroid to prevent re-accumulation. The knee and ankle should be splinted in a good position to prevent flexion deformity and foot drop. Quadriceps exercises must be performed regularly to prevent wasting.

Intercurrent illness

Patients with RA who find themselves confined to bed for any length of time, either for medical or surgical reasons, do badly and lose function unless active steps are taken to prevent flexion contractures and muscle-wasting by the methods outlined in the section on general management. Attempts should always be made to get patients back on their feet as soon as possible.

Gastrointestinal bleeding and peptic ulceration

This is a very common occurrence in RA due often to drugs, and is dealt with fully in Chapter 15 VIII. It often poses a great dilemma to the clinician, since ideally all NSAIDs should be stopped but practically this is impossible since it would inflict great suffering on the patient. Often a compromise has to be reached, such as giving H_2 receptor antagonists and continuing the NSAIDs via the rectal route.

Infection

Generally, patients with RA are more susceptible to all types of infection but particularly to septic arthritis because organisms have a predilection for damaged joints and a sudden increase in pain and swelling in an isolated joint should be regarded with suspicion and sepsis should be diligently sought if a patient with RA becomes non-specifically unwell (p 191).

Amyloidosis

RA is one of the commonest cause of reactive systemic amyloidosis, a condition in which there is accumulation in the tissues of a fibrillary protein antigenically indistinguishable from the acute-phase protein SAA and therefore called AA amyloidosis. It presents as a complication of RA in Europe in about 3% of patients, with proteinuria, frank nephrotic syndrome or renal failure. The course is variable but usually progressive and fatal within a year or two of presentation. The diagnosis may be confirmed by demonstrating amyloid in a renal or rectal biopsy. There are no satisfactory treatments but attempts to surpress disease activity and reduce SAA levels are probably sensible (see Chapter 16.VII).

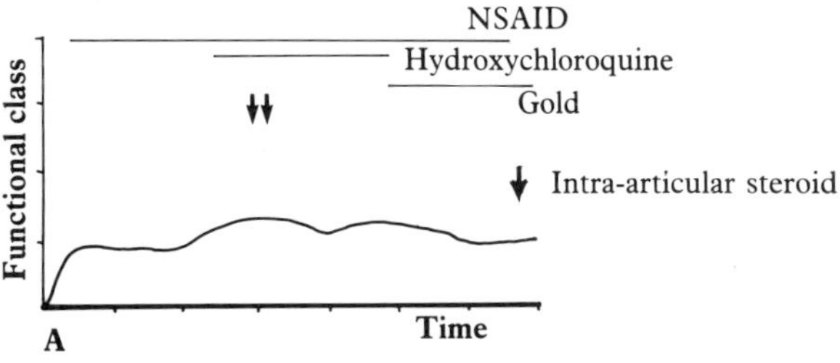

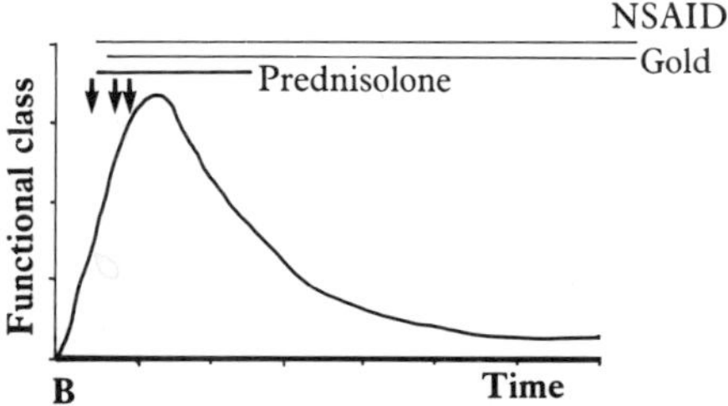

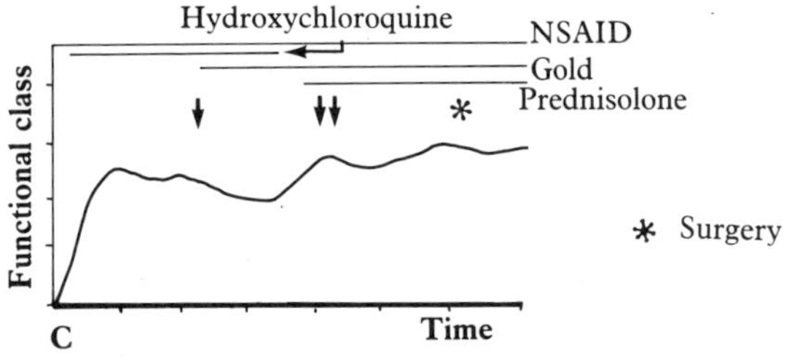

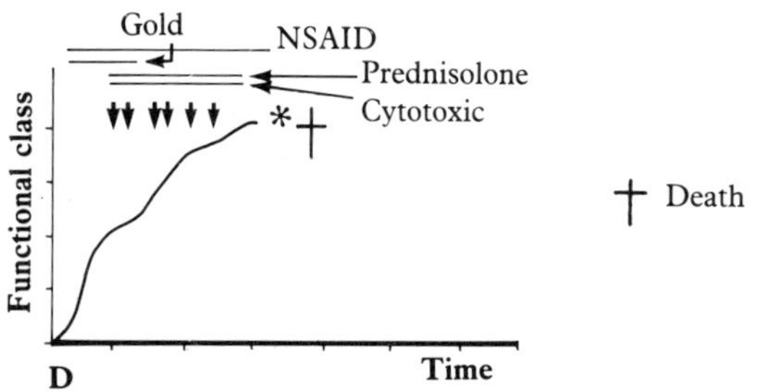

Fig. 4.17 Some typical courses of rheumatoid arthritis. **A**. 'Grumbling'. **B**. Acute remitting. **C**. Acute progressive. **D**. Malignant.

PROGNOSIS

The course of RA is variable and unpredictable for the individual patient in the early stages. Some typical courses are shown in Figure 4.17. Prognosis in terms of functional capacity is reasonably good:

24% remain fit for all normal activities
40% have moderate impairment of function
26% are quite badly disabled
10% are wheelchair-bound cripples

A poor prognosis is indicated by high titres of rheumatoid factor, early appearance of erosions, rheumatoid nodules, systemic manifestations and DR3/DR4 tissue-type. Patients who have remissions generally do better than those with continuous disease. Oddly, an explosive onset is often associated with good outcome.

FURTHER READING

Empire Rheumatism Council 1960 Gold therapy in rheumatoid arthritis. Annals of the Rheumatic Diseases 19: 95
Dumonde D C (ed) 1976 Infection and immunology in the rheumatic diseases. Blackwell Scientific , Oxford
Gardner D L 1972 The pathology of rheumatoid arthritis. Edward Arnold, London
Gifford R H 1975 Corticosteroid therapy for rheumatoid arthritis. In: Azarnoff D L (ed) Steroid therapy. W B Saunders, Philadelphia, pp 78–95
Glick E N 1967 Asymmetrical rheumatoid arthritis after poliomyelitis. British Medical Journal iii: 26
Gordon M H, Ehrlich G E 1974 Penicillamine for treatment of rheumatoid arthritis. Journal of the American Medical Association 229: 1342
Hollingsworth J W 1978 Management of rheumatoid arthritis and its complications. Year Book Medical Publishing, Chicago
Lawrence J S 1977 Rheumatism in populations. Heinemann, London
Mackenzie A H 1970 An appraisal of chloroquine. Arthritis and Rheumatism 13: 280
Masi A T 1967 Population studies in rheumatic diseases. American Review of Medicine 18: 185
Short C L 1974 The antiquitiy of rheumatoid arthritis. Arthritis and Rheumatism 17: 193
Vainio K 1975 Orthopaedic surgery on the treatment of rheumatoid arthritis. Annals of Clinical Research 7: 216

5 Seronegative spondarthritides

I Introduction

DEFINITION AND CHARACTERISATION OF THE GROUP

The demonstration of rheumatoid factors in the 1940s allowed clearer distinction to be made between RA and other forms of polyarthritis, previously considered as 'rheumatoid variants'. As further serological, clinical and radiological differences were recognised, so it became increasingly apparent that several of the 'seronegative polyarthritis' syndromes share certain distinctive features in common that suggest not only a linked interrelationship but also a similar pathogenesis. The term 'seronegative spondarthritides' is applied to this group of diseases which are clinically characterised by the following:

1. Peripheral arthritis — predominantly lower limb and asymmetrical
2. Radiological sacro-iliitis
3. Negative tests for rheumatoid factor
4. Absence of nodules and other extra-articular features of RA
5. Overlapping extra-articular features characteristic of the group
6. Marked tendency to familial aggregation.

The diseases that are accepted as falling within this classification include:

Ankylosing spondylitis (AS) — the prototype of the group
Reiter's disease
Arthropathy of inflammatory bowel disease
Psoriatic arthropathy

Although these are the major conditions characterised in this way, certain childhood cases of arthritis and the arthritis that follows specific gut infections appear to be *formes frustes* of AS and Reiter's disease and demonstrate sufficient typical features to warrant inclusion. Some authors also include Whipple's disease (p 324) and Behçet's syndrome (p 222), but evidence to associate these rare disorders with the other syndromes is tenuous, and they will not be discussed further.

Apart from the clinical similarities listed, the seronegative spondarthritides also share 1. a common pathology and 2. a strong association with the histocompatibility antigen HLA-B27.

Pathology

The pathology of the synovitis that occurs in these conditions is similar in being non-specific and showing only a chronic, mononuclear cell inflammation which, apart from the absence of granulomata, is often indistinguishable from RA.

The major, distinctive histological feature that is common to the group, however, is marked extra-synovial involvement — the major part of the inflammatory process appearing to centre on the enthesis rather than the synovium. A chronic, mononuclear cell infiltrate is seen to affect ligamentous–bony junctions ('entheses'), cartilage, subchondral bone, capsule and periarticular periosteum (Fig. 5.1). Large, central cartilagenous joints

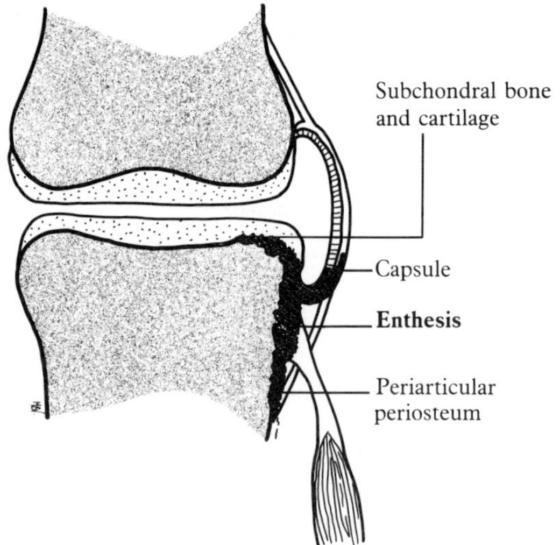

Fig. 5.1 Predominant sites of inflammation in seronegative spondarthritides (note relative sparing of synovium)

(sacro-iliac, intervertebral and sterno-clavicular joints and the symphysis pubis) are particularly involved, but even when synovial joints are also affected (most commonly apophyseal and costo-vertebral joints, hips, knees and shoulders) inflammation of the extrasynovial tissues is still prominant.

Apart from major involvement of the entheses this inflammatory process demonstrates two other characteristic features: 1. Resolution of inflammation by extensive fibrosis; 2. A tendency for the resultant fibrous scar tissue to calcify and ossify.

In the seronegative spondarthritis syndromes, therefore, chronic inflammation, predominantly affecting extrasynovial tissue, may characteristically lead to joint fusion in the relative absence of marked synovitis. Similarly, periarticular osteitis and periostitis may typically result in bony spurs that bridge adjacent vertebral bodies (syndesmophytes) or protrude at sites of ligamentous attachment (e.g. calcaneal spurs).

Association with HLA-B27

Within the seronegative spondarthritides, disease association with HLA-B27 is striking (Table 5.1). Although the mechanism of this association is unclear (p 68) the inheritance of HLA-B27 as an

Table 5.1 Disease association of HLA-B27 in Caucasians

	% positive
Healthy controls	5–14
Ankylosing Spondylitis	90–100
Endemic Reiter's disease	70–90
Shigellosis, salmonellosis or yersiniosis	10
Post-*Shigella* arthropathy (epidemic Reiter's)	80
Salmonella-reactive arthropathy	80–90
Yersinia-reactive arthropathy	80
Inflammatory bowel disease	6
Inflammatory bowel disease + peripheral arthropathy	6
Inflammatory bowel disease + sacro-iliitis	50–60
Seropositive juvenile RA	5–10
JCA without sacro-iliitis	15–25
JCA + sacro-iliitis	40–60
Uveitis	40–50
Balanitis	90

autosomal co-dominant characteristic may at least in part explain two of the clinical observations: 1. The marked familial aggregation so typical of the group; and 2. The observed association between such apparently diverse conditions as sacro-iliitis, uveitis and balanitis, each of which shows independent association with HLA-B27.

PATHOGENESIS OF THE SERONEGATIVE SPONDARTHRITIDES — THE 'REACTIVE' CONCEPT

The combination of shared clinical features, characteristic pathology and a common genetic substrate has led to the suggestion that the seronegative spondarthritides also share a similar pathogenesis. Although the precise pathogenetic mechanism in each of these syndromes is unknown, the clear temporal sequence observed in Reiter's disease supports the view that a 'reactive' response to foreign antigen is the most likely mechanism involved.

The term 'reactive arthropathy' is based on the model of rheumatic fever and describes the situation where an infective insult in a susceptible host provokes an aseptic inflammatory arthritis temporally and anatomically distant from the initial insult. Infection in man, of course, is universal and commonplace and the apparent rarity of post-infectious arthritis implies either special characteristics in the infecting organism and/or individual host susceptibility.

Microbial factors — the triggering agent

It has long been realised that injection of bacterial debris into animals can initiate not only an acute, self-limiting reaction but also a chronic, remittent response depending on: 1. The fragments and vehicle used; 2. The route of exposure; and 3. The strain and species of animal injected.

The ability to produce a chronic response appears to reside particularly in the peptidoglycan polysaccharide (PPS) component of the bacterial envelope (Fig. 5.2), and PPS preparations have been shown capable of producing intermittent granulomatous skin lesions in the rabbit, chronic pericarditis in the mouse and chronic, remittant erosive synovitis in the rat and guinea-pig. PPS heteropolymer is present in the majority of prokaryotes, including all Gram-positive and Gram-negative organisms, and demonstrates remarkable structural similarlity wherever it is found. Cross-reactivity between antibodies raised against PPS from different species is common, and it is of special interest that IgM rheumatoid factors may arise in infective situations, such as infective endocarditis, and may also demonstrate cross-reactivity against PPS. Although the mechanism is obscure, there is increasing evidence that microbial products can modulate the host's immune response (e.g. membrane components of group A streptococci demonstrate immunosuppressive activity in several animal models), and such activity could be of obvious importance in allowing both the development and persistence of inflammation. Adjuvant arthritis in the rat, although used by some as an animal model of RA, in fact closely resembles Reiter's disease.

The route of antigen presentation is important in determining the subsequent inflammatory response in animals, and the same appears to be true in man, e.g. streptococcal infection of the pharyngeal mucosa may give rise to rheumatic fever whereas infection of the skin and subcutaneous tissues (erysipelas) is more likely to provoke glomerulonephritis. The principal portal of entry implicated in reactive syndromes in man is the mucosal surface of the gut (predominantly lower bowel) and urethra. For example:

1. Active inflammatory bowel disease may be associated with peripheral 'enteropathic' arthritis.
2. Exacerbation of AS and acute iritis have been associated, in some studies, with increased colonic colonisation by *Klebsiella* and *Enterobacter*.
3. Reiter's syndrome mav follow sexually-acquired non-specific . urethritis or gut infection by *Shigella*, *Salmonella*, *Yersinia* or *Campylobacter* (all Gram-negative rods).

Elevation of serum IgA, as in psoriatic arthritis, has also been taken as further indication of antigen presentation via mucosal surfaces. Some have even

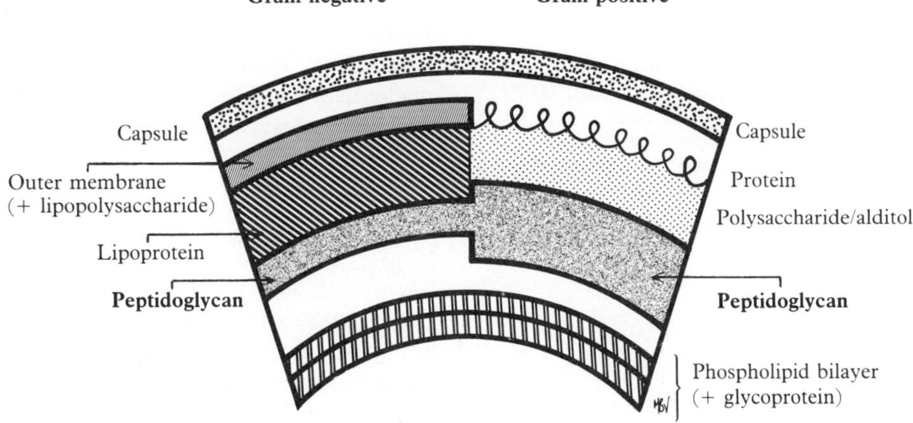

Fig. 5.2 Diagrammatic cross-section of bacterial cell envelope

suggested that the predominance of spinal and sacro-iliac changes in these syndromes results from drainage of infective agents or their products via the prostatic venous plexus or Batson's system, but study of paraplegics with prostatitis (who develop mechanical sacro-iliac joint changes but no sacro-iliitis) does not support this view.

ENTEROPATHIC ARTHRITIS

An interesting human model of 'enteropathic' arthritis is the arthritis that complicates intestinal bypass. Surgical jejuno-colic shunts were first introduced for treatment of morbid obesity in 1956, but the procedure was associated with an unacceptable incidence of metabolic complications, including arthritis in 30%, and was later largely replaced by the metabolically less disturbing procedure of jejuno-ileal bypass. Articular syndromes, however, still occur in up to 40% of such patients, appearing weeks or years after surgery and showing no apparent relationship to other complications or to the degree of weight loss (Table 5.2). Soluble circulating immune complexes occur in those with, but not those without, arthritis and cryoprotein complexes containing immunoglobulin (IgM, IgG and IgA), complement and antibodies to *E. coli* and *B. fragilis* have been identified and shown capable of activating both classical and alternative pathways of complement. These findings, together with the occurrence of Raynaud's, pleurisy and rash, suggest an Arthus-like pathophysiology. This model shows several major differences from the arthritis associated with inflammatory bowel disease or post-dysenteric Reiter's:

1. Joint involvement is more widespread
2. Predilection for lower limb joints is not obvious
3. Sacroiliitis and spondylitis are not associated features
4. There is no relationship to HLA-B27
5. Articular features are inevitably self-limiting, and chronic, recurrent inflammation does not result.

Tetracycline may give relief in some cases but in others steroids may be required. Reconstitution of the bowel inevitably results in prompt remission.

Bacterial debris has also been directly implicated in erythema nodosum leprosum (p 206), and the extra cardiac manifestations of infective endocarditis (p 205). In these situations also, the pathogenesis appears to be an Arthus-like phenomenon and a direct inflammatory action by the debris itself has not been confirmed.

Table 5.2 Rheumatic manifestations associated with intestinal bypass

Arthritis	Acute or insidious onset Usually polyarticular and symmetrical (knees, hips, shoulders, wrists, MCPs, elbows, feet) Remittant course with complete recovery within 12 months
Tenosynovitis	(Hands, wrists)
Raynaud's phenomenon	
Erythema nodosum	
Pleurisy ± effusion ± erythematous, macular rash	

(Other causes of arthralgia in such patients include metabolic bone disease and tuberculosis)

Host susceptibility — the relevance of HLA-B27

Study of the HLA system has provided a ready marker for disease susceptibility in a variety of situations, but in no situation is the association so pronounced as that seen between the seronegative spondarthritides, particularly AS and Reiter's disease, and HLA-B27 (Table 5.1). Although the mechanism of disease association with HLA-B27 remains unclear, two theories of pathogenesis have been suggested:

1. *The linkage disequilibrium hypothesis (two-gene theory)*

This supposes that on chromosome 6, close to the B27 gene, is another putative gene whose product is responsible for disease expression. If both genes are associated by linkage disequilibrium (i.e. the frequency of their phenotypic combination is not equal to the product of their individual frequencies in the population) then B27 may act merely as a marker for the disease susceptibility gene, in the same way that the H2 locus is associated with immune responsiveness in mice.

2. The cross-tolerance hypothesis (one-gene theory)

This suggests that the HLA-B27 gene itself is responsible for disease susceptibility. One way that this might occur is by cross-reactivity between B27 and an external agent, such as a micro-organism. 'Molecular mimicry' is an adaptive response that permits certain parasites to escape immunological detection and destruction, but if only partial cross-reactivity were to occur then an immune response might be elicited and result in antibodies showing high affinity for microbial antigen and low affinity for self antigens. This situation is readily observed in rheumatic fever, the prototype 'reactive' syndrome, where antibody can be demonstrated against both streptococci and cardiac-valve glycoprotein. An alternative mechanism might be that B27 results in an abnormal effector system response.

At present, however, no single theory is entirely satisfactory and several important observations remain unexplained, e.g.

1. Not all individuals with B27 develop disease. In an epidemic of *Shigella* dysentery, for example, only about 20% of B27 positive individuals will develop Reiter's syndrome.

2. Not all patients with AS or other seronegative spondarthritis are B27 positive. A possible explanation for this, which supports the one-gene theory, is the recent report that HLA-B27 negative patients with Reiter's are likely to possess HLA-B7, BW22 or BW42 — all of which may cross-react with HLA-B27.

3. Association between AS and B27 may be marked in Caucasians but is less striking in other populations (Table 5.3).

4. The majority of patients with Reiter's syndrome are B27 positive yet do not develop sacroiliitis.

It therefore seems that other genetic and environmental factors have yet to be determined to account for the 'reactive' response to external triggers. The recent realisation that other rheumatic diseases also display HLA associations (e.g. RA and DR4) has tempted generalisation of the reactive concept and led to renewed interest in microbial agents as aetiological factors in other diseases such as RA (p 41) and SLE (p 99).

Table 5.3 Disease association of HLA-B27 in non-Caucasians

	% positive
American Blacks	
Healthy controls	1–4
Ankylosing spondylitis	50–60
Reiter's disease	50–60
Japanese	
Healthy controls	<1
Ankylosing spondylitis	60
Haida Indians	
Healthy controls (male)	50
Ankylosing spondylitis (male)	100
Pima Indians	
Healthy controls	18
Ankylosing spondylitis (male)	50
Ankylosing spondylitis (female)	10

COMPARISON BETWEEN THE SERONEGATIVE SPONDARTHRITIDES — THE GROUP CONCEPT

Grouping together of the seronegative spondarthritis syndromes serves to emphasise their similarities and appears justified in terms of clinical overlap, common radiological and pathological features, and association with HLA-B27. Clinical similarities, as in overlapping extra-articular features (Table 5.4), are certainly marked (e.g. keratoderma blenorrhagica and pustular psoriasis are indistinguishable both clinically and histologically), but perhaps the most striking argument in favour of grouping together these conditions is their aggregation within families (Fig. 5.3), each syndrome showing an increased familial incidence of other seronegative spondarthritides. With the suggestion that these diseases share a similar 'reactive' pathogenesis, it is tempting to speculate that within a family genetically 'primed' individuals have the potential to develop any of the reac-

Table 5.4 Overlapping extra-articular features of the seronegative spondarthritides

Inflammation of mucosal surfaces
Conjunctivitis
Buccal ulceration
Small- and large-bowel ulceration
Urethritis ± prostatitis
Pustular or heaped-up skin lesions
± nail dystrophy
Uveitis
Aortic root fibrosis
± aortic incompetence
± conduction defects
Erythema nodosum
Pyoderma gangrenosum

tive syndromes, but that the clinical expression depends on which, if any, of the appropriate environmental triggers are encountered. In this respect it is interesting to note that some individuals appear to evolve from one clinical picture to another.

With identification of a common genetic substrate it is perhaps tempting to lump together the various syndroms under the umbrella of 'B27 disease'. However, despite striking similarities, important differences between the syndromes are apparent, suggesting that diagnostic distinction within the group should be retained. For example, peripheral joint involvement is unusual in AS but predominates in Reiter's disease and reactive arthropathy; upper limb involvement is common in psoriasis, occasional in Reiter's, but rare in the others; symmetry characterises AS whereas asymmetry is typical of the other syndromes; 'arthritis mutilans' occurs rarely in psoriasis and Reiter's disease but is not seen in AS. Full clinical comparison between the syndromes is outlined in Table 5.5.

It is increasingly apparent that similarities within the group are more marked between some syndromes than others. Psoriatic arthritis and Reiter's disease, for example, show identical X-ray changes and striking clinical and histological similarity; AS and spondylitis associated with inflammatory bowel disease similarly appear clinically and radiologically identical. These two groups can be distinguished radiologically (Table 5.6) and appear to form separate, distinct subsets. Further elucidation of genetic and environmental factors will hopefully clarify the precise inter-relationship between these syndromes and probably lead to future reclassification of the group.

It is not uncommon to see an asymmetrical oligo- or mono-arthritis predominantly involving knees and ankles in a young seronegative individual who is subsequently found to be HLA-B27-positive. Such patients often give a family history of one of the seronegative spondarthritides and may later develop other features, such as rash or spondylitis, which allow them to be placed into one of the accepted diagnostic categories. Many, however, do not develop such features and remain an apparent *forme fruste* of the seronegative spondarthritis group. The term 'B27 peripheral arthropathy' is a useful diagnostic label in such cases, comparable to 'undifferentiated connective-tissue disease', since it

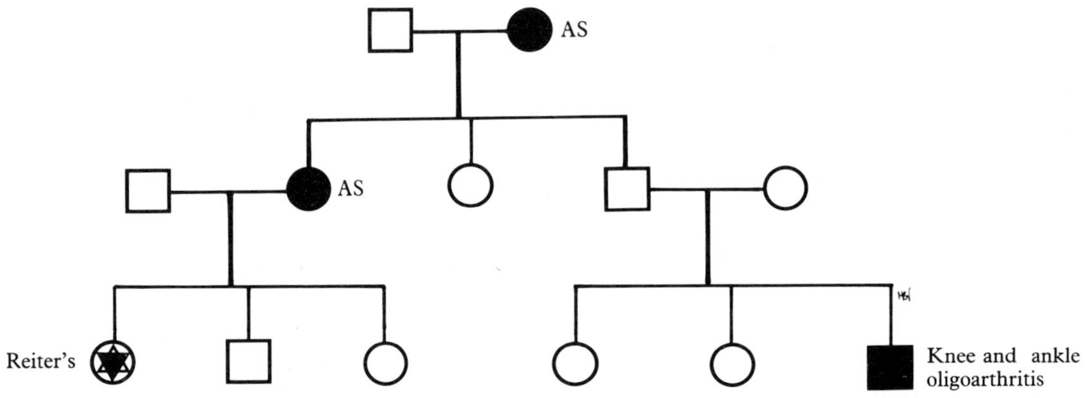

Fig. 5.3 Example of familial aggregation of seronegative spondarthritides

Table 5.5 Comparison between the seronegative spondarthritides

	AS	Reiter's	Intestinal	Psoriasis
Age at presentation	c. 20	c. 20	Any	Any
Sex preponderance	M	M	Equal	F
Onset	Gradual	Acute	(Peripheral — acute) (Axial — gradual)	Variable
Peripheral joints	40%	90%	20%	90%
Predilection	Lower limb	Lower limb	Lower limb	Upper limb
'Sausage digits'	0	+	0	+
Hips, shoulders	+++	+	±	++
Spine	+++	+	±	+
	Symmetrical	Asymmetrical	Symmetrical	Asymmetrical
Sacro-iliitis	100%	20%	Often	20%
	Symmetrical	Asymmetrical	Symmetrical	Asymmetrical
Self-limiting	0	±	+	±
Uveitis	+	++	+	±
Conjunctivitis	+	+++	+	+
Skin involvement	0	+ (restricted)	0	+++(widespread)
Mucous membranes	0	+	±	0
Urethritis	0	+	0	0
Prostatitis	++	++	0	0
Aortic incompetence	+	+	?	0
HLA-B27	>90%	>90%	5% (50% + sacro-iliitis)	20% (50% + sacro-iliitis)

Table 5.6 Comparison between radiological changes of AS/spondylitis associated with inflammatory bowel disease and psoriasis/Reiter's disease

	AS/intestinal spondylitis	Psoriasis/Reiter's
Changes restricted to SIJ/spine	>30%	<10%
Peripheral joint involvement	+	+++
DIP involvement	0	++
SIJ disease	Bilateral, symmetrical	May be unilateral, asymmetrical
Osteitis pubis	+++	+
'Squaring' of vertebrae	+++	+
Syndesmophytes	+++	+
Marginal	+++	+
Non-marginal	−	+++
Symmetrical	++	±
Spread	Progressive ascent	Progress in random fashion
Apophyseal joint involvement	+++	+
Ligamentous ossification	+++	+

broadly categorises the type of process involved and:

1. Implies a generally excellent prognosis
2. Suggests the need for only simple symptomatic treatment and encouragement to full activity
3. Does not preclude future evolution into one of the specific seronegative spondarthritis syndromes

In the following chapters the individual seronegative spondarthritis syndromes will be described, together with the putative trigger agents in each case.

FURTHER READING (INTRODUCTION)

Moll J M H, Haslock I, Macrae I, Wright V 1974 Medicine 53, 343

Moll J M H, Haslock I, Wright V 1978 Seronegative spondarthritides. In: Scott J T (ed) Copeman's Textbook of the Rheumatic Diseases. Churchill Livingstone, Edinburgh

II Ankylosing Spondylitis

This ancient disease represents the prototype of the seronegative spondarthritis syndromes and derives its name from the Greek ankylos (crooked) and spondylos (vertebra). It is a generalised disorder characterised by chronic inflammatory stiffening of the axial skeleton.

INCIDENCE AND DISTRIBUTION

AS was previously considered to be an uncommon disease, almost exclusively affecting men, but with increasing awareness of the condition it appears that the overall incidence in Whites may be as high as 1–2%, with a male:female preponderance of 2:1. Underdiagnosis is certainly commoner in women, due to misconceptions regarding its occurrence in females, clinical differences in presentation (p 76) and reluctance to perform pelvic X-rays. The disease usually manifests about the age of 20. Both the clinical syndrome and X-ray sacroiliitis occur with increased incidence in family members.

The varying frequency of AS in non-Whites largely, though not completely, reflects differences in incidence of HLA-B27 (p 69), being exceptionally rare in Japanese and Black Africans. Haida Indians have a 50% incidence of HLA-B27 and 20% of these show evidence of disease, resulting in a very high prevalence. As discussed in Chapter 5.1, however, other factors apart from B27 influence the incidence of AS in a population.

AETIOLOGY

In common with the other seronegative spondarthritides, individuals with AS demonstrate genetic, constitutional predisposition as evidenced by strong association with HLA-B27 (p 66). There is increasing evidence to suggest that the trigger factor in AS may be an infective agent acting across the bowel mucosa:

1. Correlation has been claimed between disease activity and elevation of serum levels of IgA
2. Increased isolation of *Klebsiella aerogenes* has been obtained from faeces of AS patients with active joint or eye disease
3. Cross-reactivity has been demonstrated between certain *Klebsiella* serotypes and B27-positive cells from AS patients (not controls) and uveal tract tissue, thus strongly supporting the one-gene hypothesis (p 69).

Because of both difficulty in determining disease activity and the normal occurrence of bacteria in the large bowel, the validity of such observations, which have not been confirmed by others, has been questioned. The possibility, however, of lateral transmission of infective agents as a cause of clinical exacerbation is strongly suggested by the finding of T-cell lymphopenia in AS patients during episodes of anterior uveitis and in their household contacts. The male preponderance of AS and the 80% incidence of associated prostatitis have further suggested that urethral, rather than bowel, inflammation may be involved.

The report, as yet unsubstantiated, of reduced PMN phagocytosis in B27-positive AS patients compared to B27-positive controls is of interest in implicating a generalised abnormality of bacterial handling, the gene for which may be in linkage disequilibrium with the B27 gene (the 'two-gene' theory, p 68). The mechanism and distribution of tissue damage remain unexplained, though the typical onset in adolescence and early adult life may be significant since this is the growth period when the entheses are metabolically active, and therefore perhaps more vulnerable to environmental trigger agents.

CLINICAL FEATURES

Articular manifestations

The classical presentation of AS is with an insidious

onset of back-pain and stiffness in a young adult. Early symptoms are deceptive and in most cases aching around the back and buttocks is misdiagnosed initially as sciatica or a chronic mechanical problem. The history of back-pain and stiffness therefore often extends over several years.

Although symptoms may occur anywhere in the spine, including the neck, they are usually maximal in the lumbosacral area. Pain and stiffness are most marked in the morning or after periods of inactivity, and tend to be relieved by exercise: prolonged activity, however, may aggravate symptoms. A patient typically feels worse in the morning and at the end of a working day, but is reasonably comfortable in between. Chronic discomfort frequently disturbs the normal sleep pattern to result in marked fatiguability.

The sacro-iliac joint is usually involved first to produce stiffness and low-back pain which often radiates to one or both buttocks and occasionally into the thighs and down to the back of the knees (Fig. 5.4). Most of the patient's discomfort and disability, however, result from lumbar involvement which makes bending, lifting and turning a formidable chore. The disease tends to ascend the spine and in the thoracic region may cause severe limitation of rotation and a decrease in chest expansion. All axial joints, including the manubriosternal, costovertebral and symphysis pubis, may eventually be affected (Fig. 5.5).

Insertional tendinitis is a common accompaniment that results in aching at many sites, particularly over intercostal muscle insertions ('pleuritic' chest pains), the Achilles tendon and plantar fascia (heel and foot 'sprains').

As the disease progresses over many years there is gradual loss of normal lumbar lordosis followed by an increase in thoracic and cervical kyphosis. Limitation of spinal movement is initially due to pain and stiffness but later results from fibrous and bony ankylosis. Such limitation makes daily tasks such as lifting and driving increasingly difficult and eventually impossible. Pain and stiffness may gradually improve as the spine becomes progressively ankylosed and its mobility is lost.

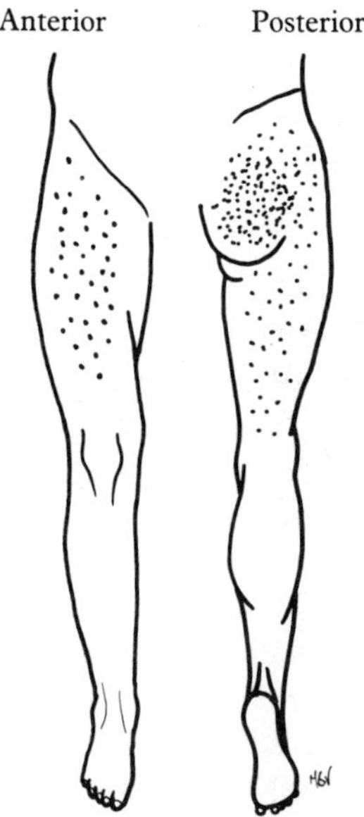

Fig. 5.4 Distribution of sacro-iliac joint pain

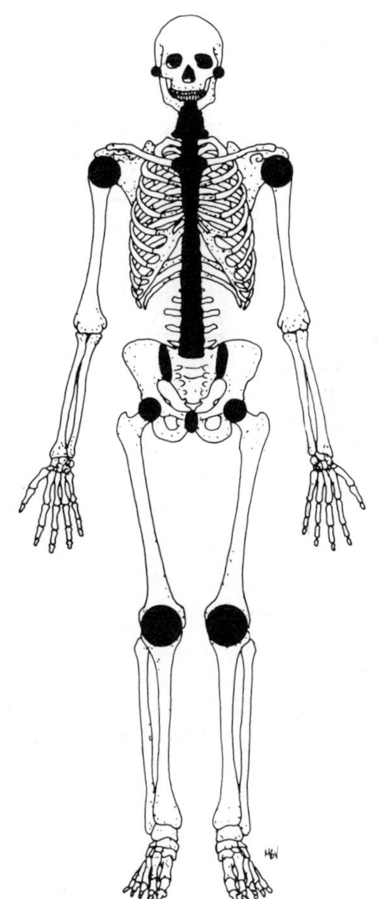

Fig. 5.5 Joint involvement in ankylosing spondylitis

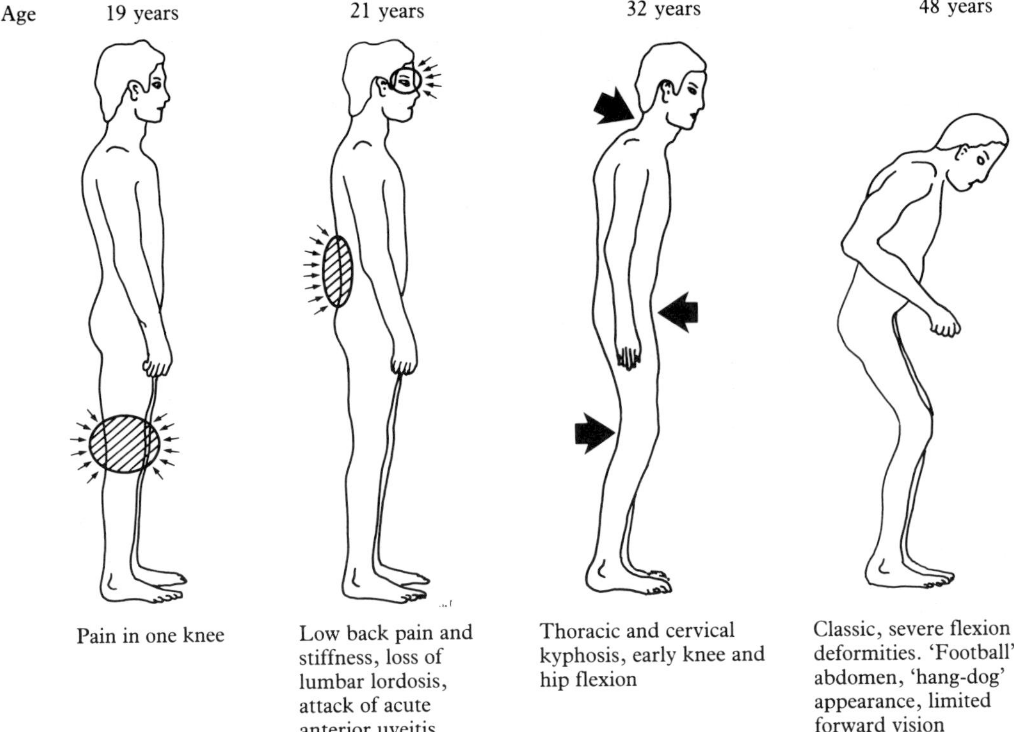

Fig. 5.6 Classic progression of severe ankylosing spondylitis

Up to 40% of patients have extraspinal joint involvement. This is usually asymmetrical at first and results in pain, stiffness and limitation of movement in hips, knees or shoulders. As the disease progresses joint involvement becomes more symmetrical, and fibrous and bony ankylosis may eventually lead to relatively pain-free joint contractures. Flexion contractures of hips and knees, together with progressive angulation of the spine, may produce the late, classic posture of fixed body flexion with subsequent limitation of forward vision, the head held in the 'hang-dog' position and the abdomen taking on the 'football' appearance due to restricted thoracic respiration (Fig. 5.6). Temporo-mandibular involvement with subsequent ankylosis is a further complication in 10%.

As the spine becomes progressively ankylosed, loss of normal righting reflexes, spinal rigidity and secondary osteoporosis strongly predispose to spinal fractures. These present as acute episodes of localised pain which are usually self-limiting over several months. Catastrophic involvement of the spinal cord with paraplegia and death is, fortunately, rare but may particularly occur when muscle protection is reduced during anaesthesia for surgical treatment of intercurrent conditions.

Extra-articular disease

General symptoms of fatigue, weight-loss and low-grade fever are common. A recurrent, non-granulomatous, acute iritis may occur in up to 25% of patients and is apparently unrelated to the severity of the spondylitis, often occurring early in the disease and being more frequent in those with peripheral arthritis. Apart from chronic, asymptomatic prostatitis in 80%, other extra-articular complications usually occur only after many years of active spondylitis and are rare.

Chronic mononuclear cell inflammation of the proximal aortic vasa vasorum may lead to medial necrosis and subsequent fibrosis, resulting in a structurally intact but incompetent aortic valve.

Extra-articular manifestations of AS

1. Uveitis (25%) and conjunctivitis (20%)
2. Prostatitis in 80% of men (asymptomatic)
3. Cardiovascular disease (4%)
   a) Aortic incompetence
   b) Mitral incompetence
   c) Conduction defects
   d) Ventricular dysfunction
   e) Pericarditis
   f) (Aortic root fibrosis is present in 25% of patients at post-mortem)
4. Upper-lobe pulmonary fibrosis (2%)

Extensive subaortic scarring may also lead to permanent conduction defects and involve the base of the anterior mitral leaflet to result in mitral regurgitation. Pericarditis and abnormalities of myocardial contractility are also reported. 'Primary' aortic incompetence, unlike uveitis, is unrelated to HLA-B27.

Chronic infiltrative and fibrotic changes in the upper lobes of the lungs associated with cough, sputum and dyspnoea have been described. Such apical fibrosis may progress to cavitation and be complicated by repeated haemoptysis and secondary infection (especially by *Aspergillus*), thus coming to resemble tuberculosis both clinically and radiologically. Post-inflammatory fusion of thoracic joints may result in a rigid chest wall but ventilation is usually well maintained by the diaphragm. Respiratory disease, however, (particularly pneumonia) occurs with increased incidence in patients with AS.

A low-grade spinal arachnoiditis may occur early in the disease and account for the elevated CSF protein noted in some AS patients. The formation of posterior lumbosacral arachnoid diverticula may lead to a cauda equina syndrome in later life with insidious onset of leg and buttock pain, sphincter disturbance and sensory and motor signs.

DIAGNOSIS

Criteria for diagnosis of ankylosing spondylitis

1. Limited lumbar spine movement in all three planes
2. Pain in thoraco-lumbar or lumbar spine
3. Chest expansion less than 2.5 cm (1″) at the fourth intercostal space

Definite AS: a) Bilateral sacro-iliitis with at least one of the above, or
b) Unilateral sacro-iliitis with either 1, or 2 + 3

Diagnosis in a patient with long-standing AS presents no difficulty, but recognition of early disease requires constant awareness of the condition and a thorough history and examination of the patient. Certain criteria have been proposed for diagnosis and are illustrated above. The most frequent means of satisfying these diagnostic criteria are X-ray demonstration of bilateral sacro-iliitis together with a history of chronic pain.

The usual problem in early diagnosis is differentiation from more common mechanical causes of back pain. Several features, however, in the history and examination should suggest an underlying inflammatory condition (Table 5.7). Examination may reveal the following early signs:

Table 5.7 Differentiating features between back pain of mechanical and inflammatory type

	Mechanical	Inflammatory
Onset	Acute	Insidious
Age	Any age	Usually <35
Effect of exercise	Worse	Better
Morning/inactivity stiffness	±	+++
Pain radiation	Anatomical (L4, 5:S1)	Diffuse
Sensory/motor symptoms	+	–
Other system involvement	–	+
Sleep disturbance	±	+++
Scoliosis	+	–
Decrease in range of movement	Asymmetrical	Symmetrical
Spinal tenderness	Local	Diffuse
Muscle spasm	Local/ asymmetrical	Diffuse/ symmetrical
Sensory/motor signs	+	–
Hip involvement	–	±

1. Loss of lumbar lordosis with tender paraspinal muscle-spasm (diffuse and symmetrical); at first lateral flexion in both directions is affected most severely, but eventually all planes are involved.

2. Symmetrical decrease in spinal mobility: A useful measure of anterior lumbar flexion is the Schober test. With the patient standing, a perpendicular line is drawn from the midpoint between the posterior iliac spines ('dimples of Venus') and a point 10 cm above: an increase of <5 cm on anterior flexion indicates restricted movement (the skin tends to be fixed at the level of the lumbosacral junction). Movement between the lumbar vertebrae can be roughly assessed by placing the examining fingers of one hand over the spinous processes and noting distraction of the fingers during anterior flexion. The ability of the patient to touch their toes is misleading since this is a test more of hip than of spinal flexion.

3. Sacro-iliac joint tenderness. This is elicited by direct palpation or by using various manoeuvres to stress the joint. Clinical tests for sacroiliitis, however, show little correlation with each other and are very insensitive.

4. Tenderness over the pelvic brim, ischial tuberosities and symphysis pubis. Enthesopathy of the numerous ligaments and tendons around the pelvis may reduce the 'intermalleolar straddle' (the distance between the medial malleoli with hips abducted).

Limitation of chest expansion (<2.5 cm at the nipple level), whilst fairly specific for AS, is an insensitive test early in the disease. As the disease progresses, development of thoracic and cervical kyphosis, and manubriosternal, hip and shoulder disease makes the diagnosis increasingly obvious, especially in a patient with a history of iritis.

VARIANTS IN PRESENTATION

Presentation with peripheral arthritis

20% of patients initially present with a peripheral inflammatory arthritis, usually asymmetrical, involving the knee, hip or ankle, several years before the onset of typical back symptoms. This presentation is particularly common in young women and adolescents, particularly boys, but the diagnosis can only be made once other symptoms have developed. Tissue-typing for HLA-B27 may be useful in this situation (B27 peripheral arthropathy, p 70).

Late presentation in the fifth or sixth decades

Such a presentation is unusual and frequently results in the diagnosis not being suspected. Late onset particularly occurs in association with co-existent inflammatory bowel disease.

AS in women

Although both sexes share the same strong association with HLA-B27, in women the disease tends to:

1. More commonly present with peripheral joint involvement
2. Progress more slowly and be associated with less dramatic spinal changes and a more favourable outcome
3. Show more cervical involvement, sometimes with a normal thoraco-lumbar spine
4. Show more osteitis pubis (particularly if parous).

Misdiagnosis is therefore more common, especially with the reluctance to perform pelvic X-rays in a young woman.

INVESTIGATIONS

Laboratory investigations usually reveal non-specific evidence of inflammation e.g. normochromic normocytic anaemia, elevated viscosity, which may be important in alerting one to the possibility of inflammatory rather than mechanical disease. Such abnormalities, however, bear little relationship to clinical disease activity. Tissue typing for HLA-B27 is clinically unhelpful.

X-ray changes, however, often provide the diagnostic evidence of AS. The SIJs usually show the earliest, most marked changes, but such changes may take many years after the onset of symptoms

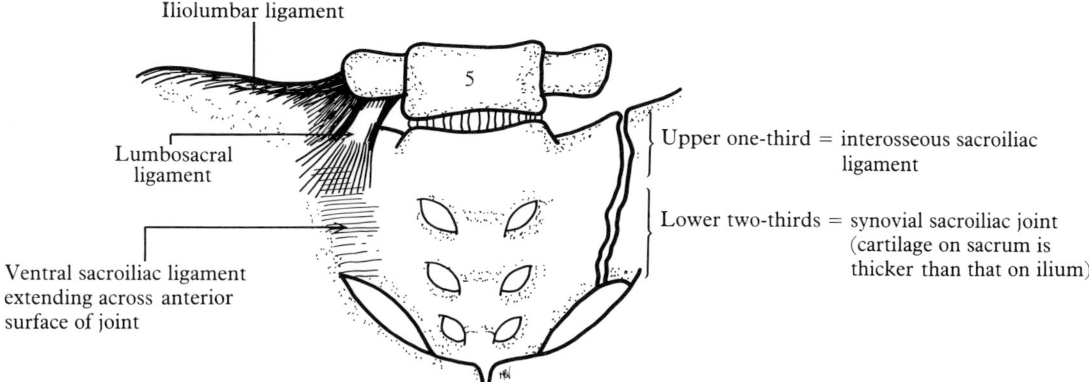

Fig. 5.7 Sacro-iliac joint

to appear. Furthermore, interpretation of sacro-iliac changes is often difficult, especially in adolescents and young adults — just when the diagnosis needs to be made. Other forms of imaging have therefore been tried (e.g. Tc scanning, p 447) in an attempt to demonstrate early sacro-iliitis, but abnormalities with these techniques are often non-specific and difficult to interpret, and plain X-rays remain the investigation of choice.

Each SIJ (Fig. 5.7) consists of a synovially-lined diarthrodial space in the lower two-thirds and a fibrous junction (the interosseous sacro-iliac ligament) in the upper one-third. The joints follow an oblique course and no single X-ray view will look through their entire length: an AP view of the pelvis shows both the anterior and posterior margins of the joints and is sufficient for diagnostic purposes (special views are not indicated). Each joint should show clean margins and a uniform joint-space (2–5 mm wide in young adults). Inflammation in AS produces the changes shown in Figure 5.8.

Various factors, especially age, may confuse radiological interpretation. The 'maturity' of the pelvis is recognised by fusion of the epiphyseal plate along the iliac crest, usually in the late teens, and before this the SIJ may show a wide space and blurred margins. At the other extreme, elderly

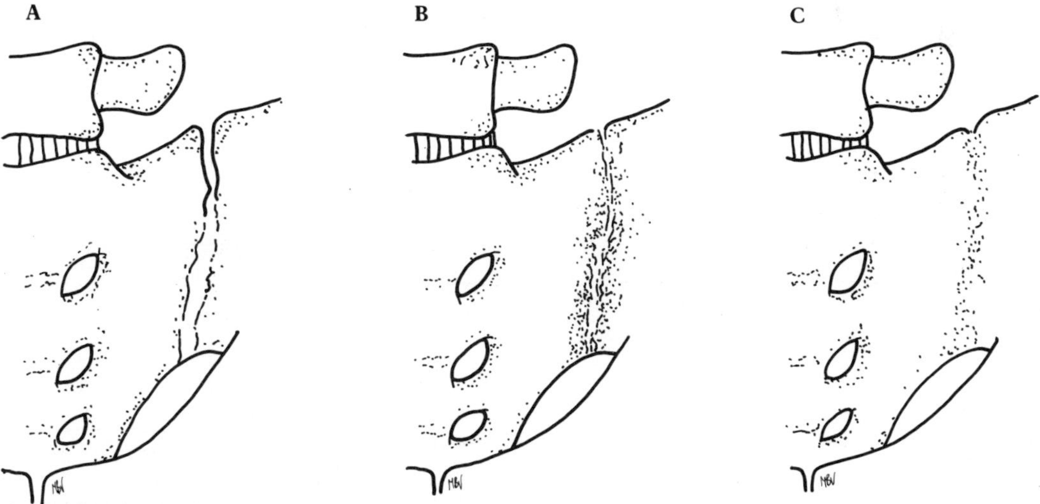

Fig. 5.8 Sacro-iliac joint changes in ankylosing spondylitis (AP view): changes are usually bilateral and symmetrical. **A.** Early: loss of definition of joint space in lower two-thirds of joint, 'pseudowidening' due to cartilage erosion. **B.** Intermediate: progressive joint space narrowing, reactive sclerosis, bony bridging of upper one-third. **C.** Late: Complete fusion across joint with subsequent osteoporosis around it.

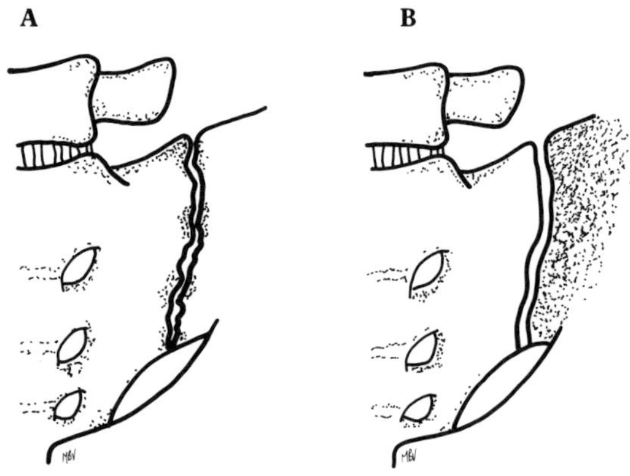

Fig. 5.9 Sacro-iliac joint changes. **A**. Elderly/'degenerative' changes: patchy sclerosis (extends only a few millimetres); irregular joint-space narrowing; margins remain clear. **B**. Osteitis condensans ilii: dense sclerosis in one or both iliac bones.

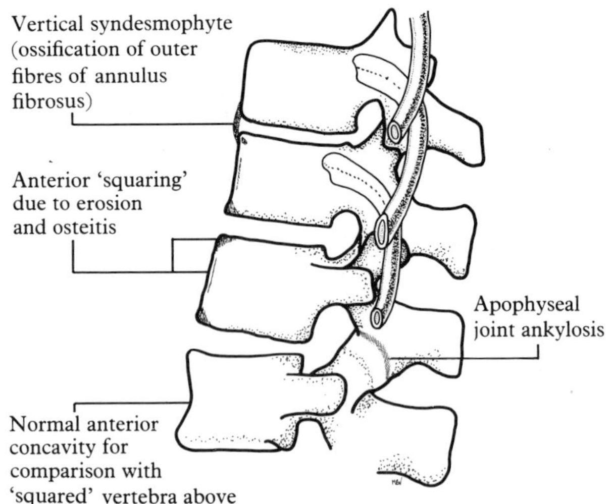

Fig. 5.10 Spinal changes in ankylosing spondylitis

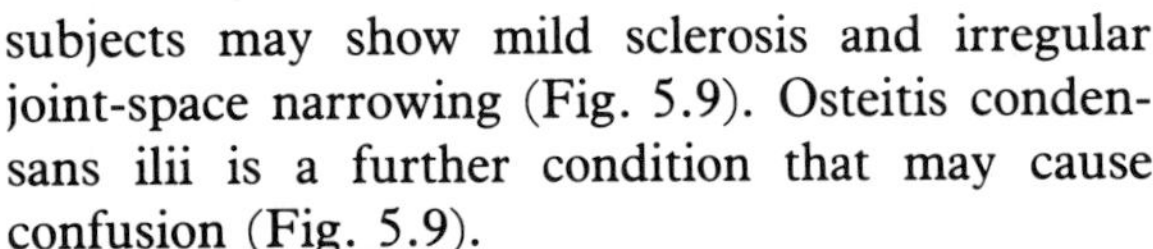

subjects may show mild sclerosis and irregular joint-space narrowing (Fig. 5.9). Osteitis condensans ilii is a further condition that may cause confusion (Fig. 5.9).

Spinal changes in AS are shown in Figure 5.10. Erosion at the insertion of the annulus fibrosus produces scalloping at the anterior corners of the vertebrae ('Romanus lesions') which, together with periostitis of the anterior margin of the body produces 'squaring' and loss of anterior concavity. New bone formation replaces the annulus fibrosis leading to vertical bridging syndesmophytes, with little loss of intervertebral space, and eventually to the classical 'bamboo spine'. Syndesmophytes must be differentiated from osteophytes (Fig. 5.11) and lesions of ankylosing hyperostosis (p 154).

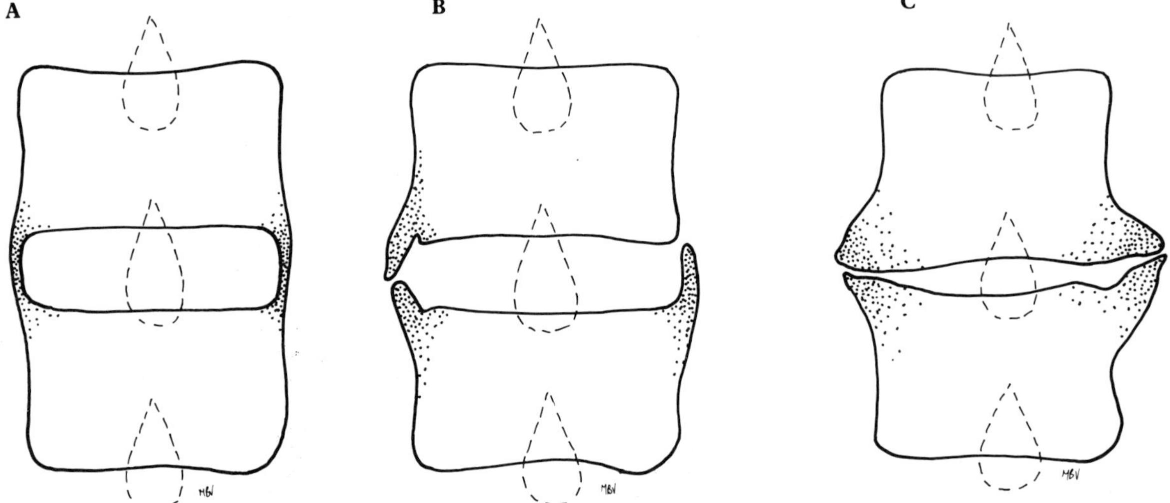

Fig. 5.11 Comparison between syndesmophytes and osteophytes. **A**. Marginal syndesmophytes (AS, spondylitis associated with inflammatory bowel disease). Fine, symmetrical bony bridges occurring from angles of vertebral bodies (i.e. insertion of annulus fibrosus). Disc space perserved. **B**. Non-marginal syndesmophytes (Reiter's disease, psoriatic spondylitis). Coarse, asymmetrical bony bridges originating more from the waist of the vertebral body. Disc space preserved. **C**. Osteophytes. Coarse, horizontal bony outgrowths. Disc space usually narrowed. Asymmetrical.

Occasionally a localised defect in the vertebral end-plate — 'spondylodiscitis' — may be seen in association with acute exacerbation of back symptoms, often following minor trauma. A further late complication is spinal fracture: minor fractures involving pedicle, transverse or articular processes are common but may easily go unnoticed.

Fluffy periostitis leading to exuberant new bone formation may be seen at various enthesis sites, notably along the superior iliac crests, the inferior pubic rami, the calcaneus and at insertions of sacrospinous and sacrotuberous ligaments. The arthropathy of hips and other involved joints is characterised by 'whiskery' marginal and central erosions, proliferative new bone formation and eventual fusion.

MANAGEMENT

Although there is no cure for AS, early and proper management can result in considerable benefit to the patient. Despite chronic discomfort, the overall prognosis is good since few patients progress to total ankylosis and systemic involvement, apart from uveitis, is rare.

The aim of early therapy is to relieve pain and stiffness and to maintain normal posture and mobility. Full explanation of the nature and outlook of the condition is essential if the patient's necessary co-operation is to be obtained. The family also should understand the condition and the necessary modifications to life-style that may have to be made. Education of the patient, and his family, in self-care is the prime object of early management.

Extension exercises are easily taught and should be performed by the patient on a twice daily regime. Steady, regular exercise (e.g. walking, swimming) is actively encouraged, although over strenuous activity (e.g. squash) may result in subsequent exacerbation of symptoms. The posture of the patient during work should be enquired into, and, if unsuitable (e.g. standing crouched forward over a bench for long periods) attempts should be made, where practicable, to alter working conditions or even to change employment. Correct posture and seating at home, with emphasis on maintaining an erect spine, is also important, and patients should be advised to sleep on a firm bed with only one pillow to avoid any tendency towards flexion. Long car journeys, or other activities requiring prolonged inactivity, should be avoided if possible, or else punctuated by brief spells of stretching and walking. Smoking should be abandoned, to avoid respiratory complications, and obesity avoided. Non-steroidal anti-inflammatory drugs are given for symptomatic relief and to allow an adequate exercise programme to be performed. Since symptoms are most marked in the mornings, night-time indomethacin may initially be tried.

If such measures are in general adhered to, the patient may usually lead a full and active life and the chances of developing disabling deformity will be reduced (should the patient's spine eventually become fixed it is far better to be ankylosed with a straight back than in a posture of fixed forward flexion).

Exacerbation of back symptoms due to spondylodiscitis or fracture should be recognised since treatment is then aimed at temporary restriction of spinal movement rather than the exercise programme prescribed for active spondylitis. Spinal X-ray therapy, though symptomatically beneficial, is now no longer used because of the tenfold increased incidence of leukaemia following such treatment.

Management of the later stages of AS may involve aids to daily living and occasionally surgical intervention. Hip and shoulder mobility are obviously vital for an individual with a fixed spine, and hip arthroplasty may be indicated for severe restriction in movement as well as for pain. Re-ankylosis following surgery may occur due to continuing periarticular disease, but the risk of this has probably been overemphasised. Vertebral wedge osteotomy should only be considered as a very last resort to help correct marked flexion deformity where forward vision is severely impaired.

FURTHER READING (ANKYLOSING SPONDYLITIS)

Calin A, Fries J F 1978 Ankylosing spondylitis: discussions in patient management. Hans Huber, Berne

Carette S, Graham D, Little H, Rubenstein J, Rodnan P 1983 The natural disease course of ankylosing spondylitis. Arthritis and Rheumatism 26: 186–190

McEwan C, DiTata D, Lingg C, Porini A, Good A, Rankin T 1971 Ankylosing spondylitis and spondylitis accompanying ulcerative colitis, regional enteritis, psoriasis and Reiter's disease: a comparative study. Arthritis and Rheumatism 14: 291–318

Moll T H M 1980 Ankylosing spondylitis. Churchill Livingstone, Edinburgh

III Reiter's Syndrome

In 1916, Hans Reiter redescribed the symptom complex, previously noted by other observers, of arthritis and conjunctivitis following an outbreak of epidemic dysentery. His name was subsequently linked to this reactive syndrome, which is an important cause of lower-limb arthritis in young adults.

INCIDENCE AND DISTRIBUTION

Reiter's disease is certainly common, many claiming it to be the most frequent cause of an inflammatory oligo-arthritis in a young man. The precise incidence and prevalence of this condition, however, are difficult to assess due to lack of a diagnostic test, presentation to diverse specialities, predilection for a young mobile population, lack of urogenital symptoms in women, a tendency to forget mild enteric features and common presentation as a *forme fruste* of the complete syndrome. Although the majority of patients are aged 16–35 years, rare childhood cases have been reported, usually following diarrhoea. Reiter's disease, particularly the post-venereal form, is diagnosed most commonly in men, with a suggested sex ratio of 15:1. The disease probably occurs worldwide but is apparently more severe in Caucasians: interestingly, the Haida Indians rarely develop this syndrome despite their high population frequency of HLA-B27.

AETIOLOGY

Affected individuals demonstrate the genetic predisposition common to all the seronegative spondarthritis syndromes, as evidenced by strong association with HLA-B27 (p 66) and an increased prevalence of sacro-iliitis, spondylitis and psoriasis in first-and second-degree relatives. Epidemiological studies have clearly shown that 20% of B27-positive individuals who contract *Shigella* or *Salmonella* dysentery will subsequently develop Reiter's syndrome (i.e. 1–3% of all those affected), and that those with the syndrome who are B27-positive will have a more severe and chronic disease than the much smaller number who are B27-negative.

In no other seronegative spondarthritis syndrome is the trigger agent and the time course so clearly established as in post-dysenteric Reiter's syndrome, largely due to ease of documentation. Indeed, it was following the demonstration of HLA-B27 association in Reiter's syndrome that the concept of a 'reactive' arthritis was clearly established (p 66). Post-dysenteric Reiter's may occur 1–3 weeks after infection by several organisms, notably *Shigella flexneri* and *Shigella dysenteriae* (but not, it appears, *Shigella sonnei*), *Salmonella*, *Yersinia enterocolitica* and *Campylobacter jejuni*, the last three commonly giving rise only to the joint manifestations.

There seems little doubt that Reiter's syndrome may also follow infection of the lower genito-urinary tract, and such post-venereal 'endemic' Reiter's is the commonest form seen in England and America (not Europe). Although *Chlamydia* and *Mycoplasma* have been particularly incriminated, such organisms are found with equal frequency in urethritis patients with or without arthritis, and their common role as commensals clouds any clear-cut pathogenetic mechanism. Study is made difficult since patients will usually have eliminated the organism by the time the syndrome develops, and urethritis itself is an integral part of the syndrome.

CLINICAL FEATURES

The acute syndrome

Inflammatory arthritis is the most frequent presenting feature of the triad — conjunctivitis

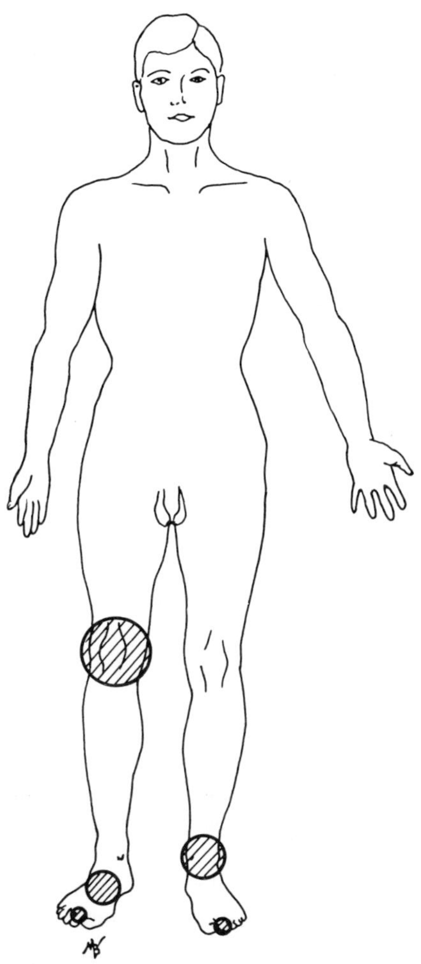

Fig. 5.12 Main joints involved in acute Reiter's syndrome

and urethritis often being so mild as to be missed or not fully appreciated by the patient. The typical presentation is with an acute, asymmetrical oligoarthritis affecting large and small joints in the lower limbs of a young man (Fig. 5.12). Presentation with an acute monoarthritis of knee, ankle, midtarsal joint, MTP joint or interphalangeal joint of the toe is also common, but rarely persistent, and the usual pattern is for three to seven joints to be involved asynchronously over several weeks, with prominent symptoms occurring in only one or two. Inflammation may be quite florid in the most symptomatic joints, with overlying erythema, periarticular and articular tenderness and large, tense effusions. Popliteal rupture may even occur rarely, early in the disease. Although lower-extremity joints are predominantly affected, elbows, wrists and finger joints are occasionally involved in a more widespread polyarthritis.

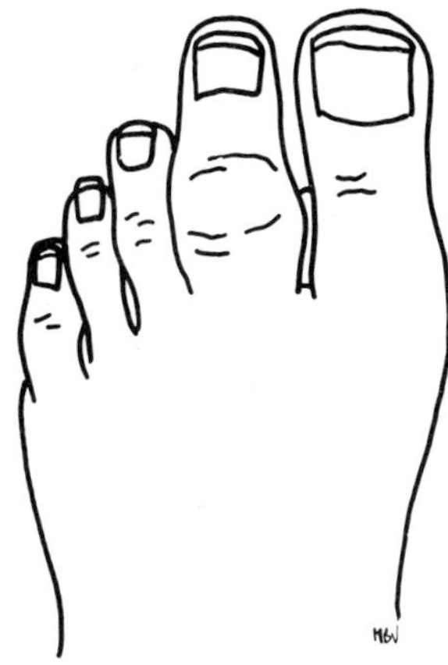

Fig. 5.13 Typical appearance of a 'sausage toe' in Reiter's syndrome (also in psoriasis)

A frequent, characteristic feature is severe but short-lived pains due to inflammatory enthesopathy particularly affecting the Achilles tendon insertion ('lover's heel'), the plantar fascia, the chest wall and lower back. Tenderness of the extensor hallucis longus and 'sausage toes' (Fig. 5.13) are other frequent findings that reflect the enthesopathic nature of the condition.

Conjunctivitis, usually bilateral, occurs in one-third of patients but causes only mild grittiness and scant, sterile discharge which may easily go unnoticed. It is usually self-limiting over 1–4 weeks. Urethritis similarly may produce a mild, non-purulent discharge which is frequently asymptomatic. Cystitis, often the only genito-urinary finding in the female, may also occur in men, and rarely may be haemorrhagic and severe.

Apart from the classic triad of arthritis, conjunctivitis and urethritis, which may develop in any order or occur simultaneously, the following features may also occur 1–3 weeks after the precipitating infection:

1. Keratoderma blenorrhagica (15%) (Fig. 5.14). This appears as discrete, waxy, yellow-brown vesico-papules with desquamating margins, occasionally coalescing to form large crusty plaques.

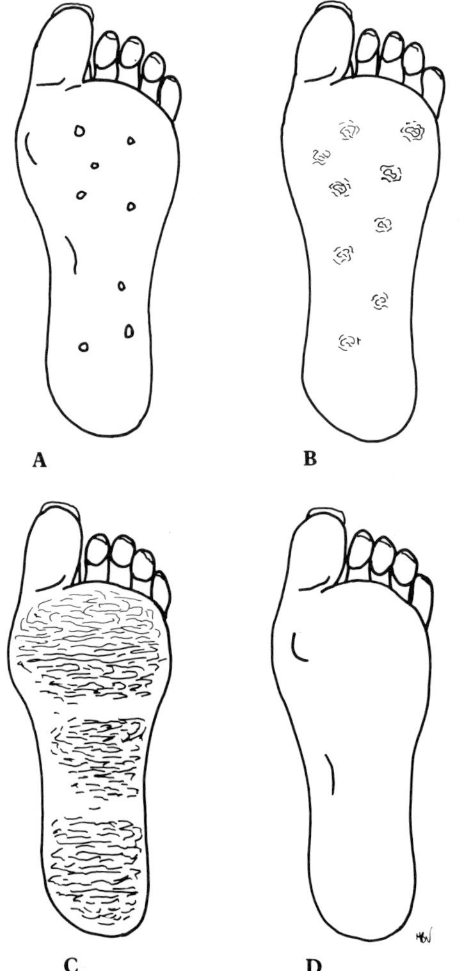

Fig. 5.14 Keratoderma blenorrhagica, showing possible evolution over several months. **A**. Discrete, waxy vesico-papules. **B**. Desquamating margins. **C**. Coalescence resulting in large crusty plaques. **D**. Eventual complete recovery.

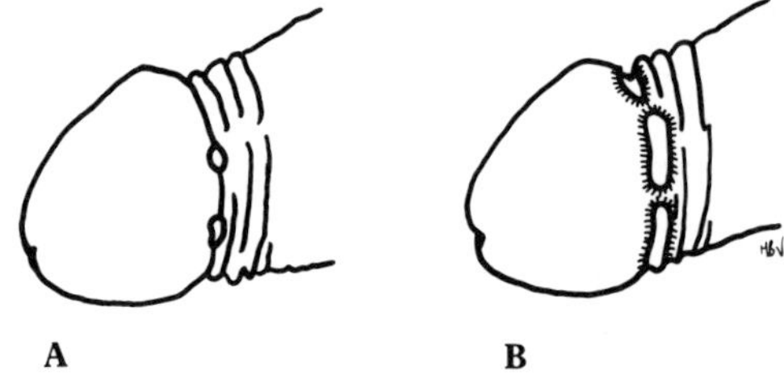

Fig. 5.15 Circinate balanitis. **A**. Early lesion: small vesicles on coronal margin of prepuce and adjacent glans. **B**. Later lesions: Coalescence and rupture to form circinate erosion.

Palms and soles are particularly affected, but spread may occur to involve scrotum, trunk and scalp: in intertriginous areas erosions are more likely than papules. The clinical appearance is indistinguishable from pustular psoriasis. Even the most severe lesions tend to heal completely, without scarring, over several months.

2. Nail dystrophy with subungual hyperkeratosis. This also resembles the gross lesions of psoriasis with subsequent displacement and shedding of brittle, yellow, thickened nails.

3. Circinate balanitis (20–50%) (Fig. 5.15). This is a characteristic feature, appearing first as small vesicles on the coronal margin of the prepuce and adjacent glans and later rupturing to form superficial erosions with minimal surrounding oedema. Some may coalesce to form the circinate pattern. In circumcised individuals the lesions tend to crust and remain discrete; in the uncircumcised they more frequently coalesce and remain moist. Lesions are painless and self-limiting and often escape notice.

4. Buccal erosions (10%). These appear as shallow, shiny red patches on tongue, palate, buccal mucosa and lips. They are painless, rarely deep enough to be called ulcers, and only last a few days.

5. Systemic disturbance. Although general malaise and mild fever are common in patients with Reiter's syndrome, severe systemic disturbance may occasionally dominate the clinical picture and result in an ill patient with acute weight-loss, pyrexia and even toxic confusion. Such a presentation considerably widens the diagnostic possibilities and disseminated infection is invariably suspected, and treated, initially.

Chronic disease

Although the initial syndrome is characteristically self-limiting over several months and leaves no residual disability, recurrent or chronic disease may occur in up to 60% of patients and particularly results in joint and eye complications.

1. Arthritis. Although some patients experience recurrent acute episodes with symptom-free intervals, the majority demonstrate intermittent exacerbations on a background of chronic discomfort.

The relationship between infection and subsequent exacerbation is not as clear-cut as in the initial attack and obvious precipitating 'triggers' are usually absent. It is of considerable interest that episodes of non-specific urethritis or dysentery in a previously affected individual does not invariably provoke a relapse.

As in the acute syndrome ankles, midtarsal joints, MTPs and knees are particularly affected. In addition, other joints including upper limb joints such as elbows and wrists, become increasingly involved (Fig. 5.16). Inflammation is generally less florid than that seen in the initial attack, but repeated exacerbations or chronic disease may lead to eventual joint damage with contractures (predominantly due to periarticular fibrosis) and even bony ankylosis. Disabling deformities are particularly seen to affect the hindfoot and toes.

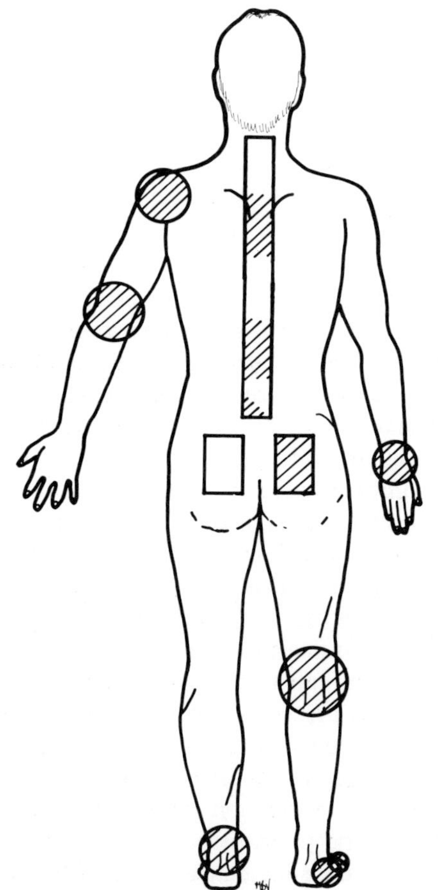

Fig. 5.16 Main joints involved in chronic, recurrent Reiter's syndrome

Sacro-iliitis and spondylitis appear in up to one-third of patients with recurrent disease. Sacro-iliitis is commonly unilateral, and chest expansion is rarely compromised, but otherwise clinical features are indistinguishable from classic AS.

2. *Uveitis*. Usually unilateral, this occurs rarely in the acute syndrome but may affect 30% of patients with chronic disease, especially if sacro-iliitis is also present. Late sequelae include posterior synechiae, glaucoma and persistent subepithelial opacifications.

Apart from joint and eye disease, other late, but rare, features of Reiter's syndrome include:

Aortic regurgitation
Cardiac conduction defects
Pericarditis
Transient pulmonary infiltrates
Peripheral neuropathy (foot-drop, ulnar neuritis)
CNS disease (polyneuritis, seizures, nystagmus, neurophychiatric disturbance)

Diagnosis

The acute syndrome

The diagnosis of Reiter's syndrome should be suspected in any young adult with an acute, asymmetrical oligoarthritis affecting lower-limb joints. A high index of suspicion is required, especially since symptoms of the precipitating infection are usually mild and easily forgotten and *formes frustes* are common, with few patients presenting all the

Suggested criteria for Reiter's disease (acute syndrome)

Typical acute arthritis

1. Seronegative, asymmetrical
2. Predominantly lower-limb
3. ± heel pain, 'sausage' toes

Plus one or more of the following

1. Urethritis
2. Conjunctivitis/iritis
3. Mucocutaneous disease (balanitis, keratoderma, oral ulceration)
4. Preceding dysentery/non-specific urethritis

features of the classical syndrome. Since there are no specific tests the diagnosis is based on clinical features, most of which, apart from asymptomatic urethritis, are evident after a thorough history and examination.

The usual differential diagnosis is between psoriatic arthropathy and acute gonococcal arthritis. Considerable overlap occurs with psoriasis which also may produce asymmetrical oligoarthritis, sausage toes and pustular skin lesions. Circinate balanitis, urethritis, prostatitis and buccal lesions, however, are not features of psoriasis and conjunctivitis is less common. Reiter's syndrome and gonococcal arthritis both occur in the same clinical setting and may co-exist: features that help distinguish the two are outlined on p 199.

Late, chronic disease

The main differentiation in chronic disease is from AS and psoriatic arthropathy. In AS iritis, prostatitis and even urethritis may occur but there is greater tendency for hip and shoulder involvement, sacro-iliitis is always bilateral, 'sausage' digits and foot contractures are not a feature, and X-ray changes are characteristic (p 76). Psoriasis may produce an identical clinical picture to Reiter's disease but shows a greater tendency for upper-limb involvement, severe joint destruction and chronic, widespread skin changes: anterior uveitis is not a usual feature.

Variants in acute presentation

'Reactive arthritis'

Apart from *Shigella*, specific gut infections commonly give rise only to the arthritic component of Reiter's syndrome, thus making diagnosis more difficult and the history of preceding diarrhoea more important. Similarly, non-specific urethritis may give rise to 'sexually-acquired reactive arthritis' (SARA) without the other features of the complete syndrome. The onset and distribution of this 'reactive arthritis' is identical to that seen in Reiter's syndrome, and enthesopathic features such as heel and plantar tenderness are frequently present. Confirmatory evidence of preceding infection may be particularly helpful.

Apart from reactive arthritis, *Salmonella* infection may also give rise to a septic arthritis, particularly in children. This should be suspected when acute, persistent monoarthritis follows *Salmonella* enteritis.

Post-yersinia arthritis.

Yersinia enterocolitica infection, most commonly seen in Scandinavia, may produce additional diagnostic features. Pharyngitis, myocarditis and erythema nodosum may accompany the preceding diarrhoea in adults, whereas infection in children usually results in abdominal symptoms that resemble appendicitis. Iritis and conjunctivitis may occur in B27-positive individuals with reactive arthritis, whereas those who are B27-negative (mainly women) particularly develop erythema nodosum and monarthritis and are less likely to suffer recurrence.

Investigations

The acute syndrome

Routine investigations are generally unhelpful: blood tests (FBC, viscosity, acute phase proteins) demonstrate only the presence of inflammation and seronegativity for rheumatoid factor, and X-rays are usually normal. Confirmation of urethritis or preceding gut infection, however, may be of diagnostic importance:

1. Demonstration of urethritis. Urinalysis may reveal the presence of lower-urinary-tract disease, but the 'two-glass test' is more sensitive, showing mucoid shreds in the first specimen which clear in the second. Examination and culture of urethral smears and fluid obtained by prostatic massage may confirm the presence of mucosal inflammation and also detect any co-existent gonococcal infection (reported in up to 50% of endemic cases). Such rigorous investigation will reveal asymptomatic non-specific prostatitis in 80% of men with Reiter's — a similar incidence to that seen in AS. In practice, examination and culture of urethral smears alone is sufficient.

2. *Confirmation of preceding gut infection.* Except for post-*Salmonella* arthritis, stool cultures are usually negative by the time the arthritis presents. Serum agglutination tests, however, may be of help in confirming previous dysentery.

Chronic, late disease

Haematological investigation may again reveal non-specific evidence of inflammation and a negative rheumatoid factor. X-ray changes, however, may be helpful in diagnosis and become more frequent as further relapses occur: changes may be identical to those seen in psoriatic arthritis (p 89). The main radiological features are outlined below.

Major radiological features in Reiter's syndrome

1. Peripheral joints
   a) Changes usually most marked around ankle, midtarsal, MTPs and interphalangeal joints of toes
   b) Isolated juxta-articular osteopenia
   c) 'Fluffy' periostitis (characteristically producing calcaneal and plantar spurs, showing erosions during active disease)
   d) para-articular erosions
2. Axial joints
   a) Unilateral/asymmetrical sacro-iliitis (p 77)
   b) Large, non-marginal syndesmophytes occurring in 'skip' fashion (p 78)

Anterior uveitis is usually symptomatic and diagnosis is confirmed by slit-lamp examination (p 243).

MANAGEMENT

Early

Since nothing is known to shorten the course of Reiter's syndrome, management of musculoskeletal problems is purely symptomatic and includes initial resting of involved joints, joint aspiration, local steroid injection, simple additional physical therapy and NSAI analgesics. Systemic steroids are anecdotally ineffective in such a predominantly enthesopathic disorder (cf synovitides), but a short course of ACTH or steroids may be considered in the rare patient with predominant systemic features. As a rule, neither the conjunctivitis nor urethritis require treatment.

If non-specific urethritis appears to be the triggering event and urethritis is found at presentation, then some recommend tetracycline 250 mg q.d.s. for 5 days. There is no evidence, however, that antibiotics affect any part of the reactive syndrome and differentiation from reactive urethritis and persistant NSU is impossible. Avoidance of multiple sexual contacts and use of condoms are often both advised, again in the absence of any evidence demonstrating benefit from such measures. Feelings of guilt are common and are certainly not helped by unnecessary courses of antibiotics, talk of 'infection' and advice to modify sexual activities. Such feelings should be elicited and then allayed by adequate explanation of the nature of the disease.

Musculoskeletal symptoms are characteristically self-limiting but usually persist for several months before slowly receding. Residual disability following a first attack is unusual, occurring in <5% but a few patients develop chronic disease that appears to follow directly on from the first attack. Previous views of Reiter's disease as a benign condition are gradually changing with the realisation that up to 60% of patients will develop recurrent or chronic disease. The initial attack should therefore be managed with guarded optimism and a 'treat-and-see' policy adopted, the patient being properly advised on the possibility of a recurrence.

Late

Recurrent joint disease is initially treated along the same general lines as before, utilising joint aspiration and injection, simple physical measures and NSAI drugs. Patients with spondylitis are given the same advice as for those with classical AS (p 79). For the very few patients with severe, relentless joint disease, cytotoxic therapy, especially methotrexate, has been advocated, although confirmation of its efficacy awaits properly controlled trials.

Uveitis is usually controlled by local measures but may occasionally require systemic steroid therapy. Aortic incompetence and heart block are treated surgically or by permanent pacemaker as required.

FURTHER READING (REITER'S SYNDROME)

Calin A 1977 Reiter's syndrome. Medical Clinics of North America 61(2): 365–376

Fox R, Calin A, Gerbo R C, Gibson D 1979 The chronicity of symptoms and disability in Reiter's syndrome: an analysis of 131 consecutive patients. Annals of Internal Medicine 91: 190

Martel W, Braunstein E M, Borlaza G, Good A E, Griffin P E 1979 Radiologic features of Reiter disease. Radiology 132: 1–10

Symposium on Reiter's syndrome 1979 Annals of the rheumatic diseases 38: Suppl 1

IV Psoriatic Arthropathy

Psoriatic arthropathy presents a wide spectrum of axial and peripheral disease. The occurrence of arthritis in patients with psoriasis was previously considered as coincidental association of two common disorders, but 1. epidemiological evidence that arthritis is more common in patients with psoriasis, and 2. the characteristic clinical and radiological features of the arthritis substantiate psoriatic arthritis as a distinct clinical entity and clearly place it within the seronegative spondarthritis group.

INCIDENCE AND DISTRIBUTION

Seronegative arthritis occurs in about 7% of psoriatic patients, representing a six- to tenfold increased incidence over non-psoriatic controls. Since psoriasis affects 1–2% of the population, the prevalence of psoriatic arthropathy may be estimated at 0.1%. An equal sex ratio is seen in both psoriatic arthritis and uncomplicated psoriasis, but the peak age of onset is later for joint disease (fourth and fifth decades) than it is for skin lesions (second and third decades).

AETIOLOGY

Heredity appears to be an important factor in the development of both psoriasis and its associated arthropathy. One third of patients with psoriasis give a positive family history, and although the mode of inheritance remains unclear it is probably multifactorial, thus possibly accounting for the various clinical subgroups described. In common with the other seronegative spondarthritides, the development of arthritis, particularly sacro-iliitis and spondylitis in patients with psoriasis, is clearly associated with the presence of HLA-B27, but HLA haplotypes that are associated with development of psoriatic skin lesions (e.g. HLA-B13 and HLA-B17) occur with equal frequency in those with or without arthritis, and no other marker for joint disease has been discerned.

Evidence for the role of heredity in psoriasis

1. Histocompatibility antigens associated with psoriasis

HLA	Association
B13, B17, Bw38	Increased risk of developing psoriasis
B17	Marker for subgroup with a) early age of onset b) high rate of affected relatives
B12	Marker for subgroup with infrequent family involvement

2. Incidence of HLA-B27 in patients with psoriasis

Psoriasis alone	5–10%
Psoriatic arthritis without sacro-iliitis	20%
Psoriatic arthritis with sacro-iliitis	50–60%

3. Family history of psoriasis present in one-third of patients
4. Increased incidence of sacro-iliitis and other seronegative spondarthritides in relatives of patients with psoriatic arthritis

The pathogenesis of both skin and joint lesions remain unclear, but in psoriatic plaques the observed eightfold increase in epidermal proliferation has been associated with 1. reduced intra cellular cyclic AMP, and 2. a generalised capillary abnormality of meandering vessels, with tight terminal convolutions, showing enhanced reactive hyperaemia.

The Koebner phenomenon, elevated levels of serum IgA and triggering of guttate psoriasis by streptococcal infection, all suggest a strong 'reactive' tendency in individuals who develop psoriatic skin lesions. Support for the supposition that this reactive tendency may extend to development of joint inflammation comes from the demonstration of identical skin lesions (keratoderma blenorrhagica) and indistinguishable joint disease in patients with Reiter's syndrome. The putative trigger agent operating in psoriatic patients, however, awaits identification.

CLINICAL FEATURES

Arthritis

A wide clinical spectrum of joint disease is seen, but five major presentations are recognised:

1. Asymmetrical, oligoarticular type (*c. 70%*). This is the commonest and most characteristic arthropathy. One or a few joints are involved at a time, usually the small distal joints of the hands or feet. A 'sausage' swelling with simultaneous involvement of the DIP, PIP and MCP or MTP of the same finger or toe is typical (Fig. 5.17), much of this appearance being due to accompanying flexor tenosynovitis. Onset is characteristically abrupt, but symptoms are generally mild and systemic features absent. This type may resolve rapidly or persist for several months.

2. Symmetrical polyarthritis (*c. 15%*). Women are predominantly affected by this presentation which, apart from being seronegative and showing more frequent and complete remissions, is often indistinguishable from RA. Onset is commonly acute and may be associated with systemic upset (malaise, weight loss, fever). Although typical rheumatoid complications, such as tendon rupture, may occur, nodules are absent and joint involvement is generally less extensive and more benign than that seen in seropositive RA. Much of the hand deformity appears to result primarily from tenosynovitis and subsequent contractures.

3. Predominant DIP arthritis (*c. 10%*). Although considered by some to be the classic hallmark of psoriatic arthritis, this form is uncommon. Men are particularly affected, involvement varying from one to almost all DIP joints. Symptoms and signs are usually mild, but inflammation is occasionally florid with warmth, swelling and overlying erythema. Psoriatic nail changes are commonly present, and the combination of dystrophic nails and multiple DIP involvement can be striking (Fig. 5.18).

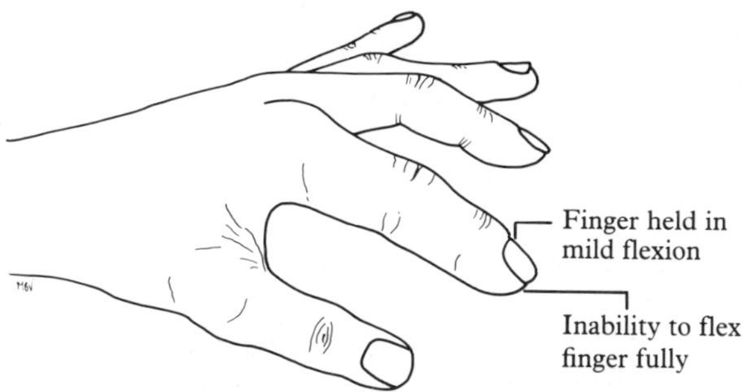

Fig. 5.17 'Sausage finger' — marked swelling of left index finger due to synovitis of DIP, PIP and MCP joints and flexor synovitis

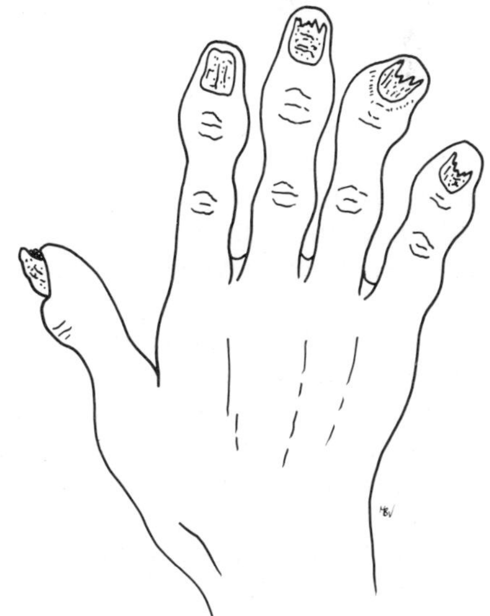

Fig. 5.18 Marked DIPJ arthritis associated with gross nail dystrophy

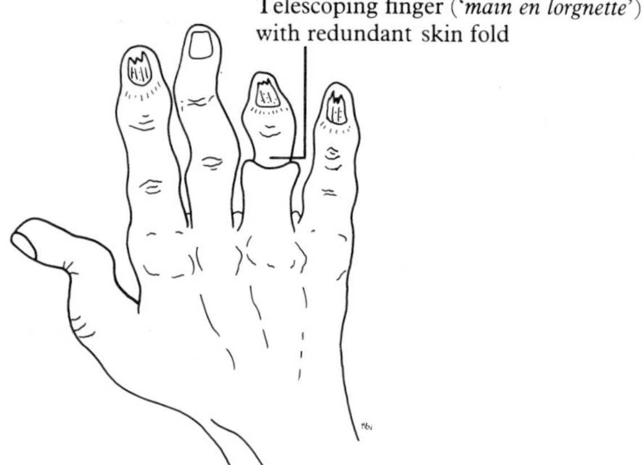

Fig. 5.19 Arthritis mutilans

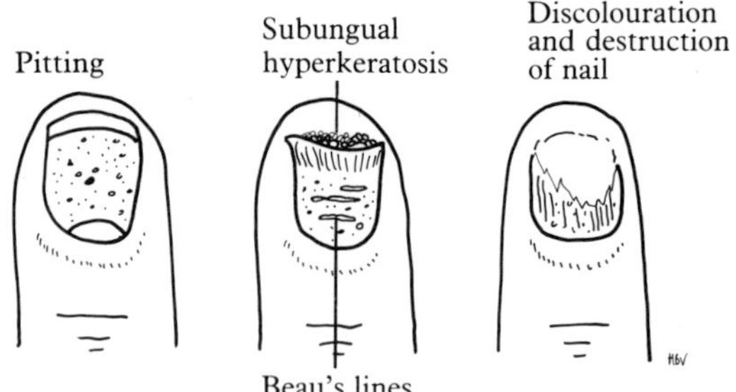

Fig. 5.20 Nail changes in psoriasis (N.B. None are specific and may also be seen in fungal and bacterial infection, lichen planus and Reiter's syndrome)

4. *Predominant axial disease*. Spondylitis may be the major feature in c. 5% of those with psoriatic arthritis, presenting a similar clinical picture to that seen in AS apart from a tendency to less severe symptoms, less widespread spinal disease and less frequent tendinitits.

5. *Deforming erosive arthritis with widespread ankylosis involving multiple small joints of hands and feet, often with sacro-iliitis and spondylitis*. This form may rarely progress to 'arthritis mutilans' with 'opera-glass' hands (Fig. 5.19) and similar deformities of the feet. Often associated with severe skin involvement, this condition has received considerable attention, although occurring in less than 5% of patients.

These clinical groups, however, are not distinct, and many patients show a combination of features as their disease evolves. Presentation in childhood may be with one of the adult onset patterns or may be with a severe systemic syndrome that initially resembles Still's disease (p 93).

The general pattern of psoriatic arthritis is one of intermittent exacerbation followed by varying periods of complete or near-complete remission. Residual disability following each exacerbation, in the majority of patients, is absent or mild.

Nail lesions

Onycholysis, ridging and pitting (more than 20 pits in all the fingernails) are characteristic (Fig. 5.20) and may occur in the absence of skin lesions. Nail changes are more frequent in psoriatic arthritis (85%) than in uncomplicated psoriasis (30%) and correlate more closely than skin changes with the presence of arthritis, appearing with the onset of joint disease in a third of the patients. Although a topographical relationship between involvement of distal joints and affected nails is common, nail changes are in fact more frequent in all patterns of psoriatic arthropathy.

Skin involvement

Of the many clinical patterns of psoriasis recognised, no particular one appears to be associated with the development of arthritis. Some patients may be totally unaware of their psoriasis, particularly if it is confined to the 'hidden areas' of scalp, umbilicus, natal cleft or perineum. Skin lesions usually precede arthritis (75%), but in almost a quarter of cases the arthritis presents first, thus adding to difficulties in diagnosis. An apparently synchronous onset may occur in 5%. In some patients psoriasis and arthritis flare concomitantly, but most exhibit persistent skin disease with intermittent exacerbations of synovitis.

Ocular involvement

Eye lesions are present in up to a third of patients. Conjunctivitis is certainly most common, but anterior uveitis and rarely episcleritis may also occur. Iritis is particularly frequent in HLA-B27 individuals with sacro-iliitis.

DIAGNOSIS

While there are certain presentations which are quite typical of psoriatic arthritis, problems of precise diagnosis may be compounded by minimal, concealed or even absent skin lesions. Despite the wide range of clinical presentations, however, certain features in a patient with a seronegative arthritis should always lead to consideration of the diagnosis.

Features that suggest a diagnosis of psoriatic arthritis in a patient with seronegative arthritis

1. The presence of psoriatic skin lesions
2. The presence of typical nail changes
3. Strong family history of psoriasis
4. Asymmetrical oligoarthritis
5. 'Sausage' swellings of fingers or toes
6. Marked flexor tenosynovitis in relative absence of marked synovitis
7. DIP and PIP involvement with relative sparing of MCPs
8. Spondylitis showing 'skip' involvement and unilateral sacro-iliitis

INVESTIGATIONS

Laboratory investigations are unhelpful apart from confirming seronegativity for rheumatoid factors, and showing non-specific evidence of inflammation (e.g. anaemia, raised viscosity) in patients with active, widespread disease.

X-rays, however, may be important in supporting the diagnosis. Peripheral joints may show erosive changes that superficially resemble RA except that fewer joints appear involved. Features, however, that particularly suggest psoriatic arthritis include:

1. Destructive changes in isolated small peripheral joints
2. Marked asymmetry
3. The combination of marginal erosions and fluffy periostitis — the so-called 'proliferative erosion'. This may produce apparent joint space widening and expansion of adjacent bone, progressing to 'pencil-in-cup' or 'fish-tail' deformities (Fig. 5.21), or even to marked resorption and telescoping of phalanges ('arthritis mutilans').
4. Predilection for DIP and PIP joints with relative sparing of MCP and MTP joints
5. Relative lack of juxta-articular osteopenia
6. Tendency to bony ankylosis
7. Periostitis at enthesis sites (e.g. around calcaneus)

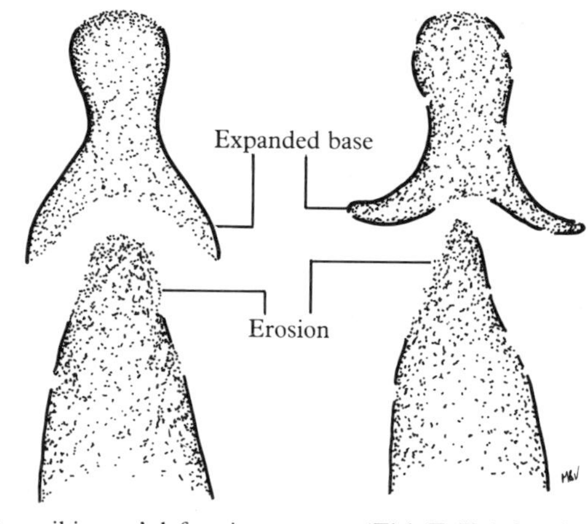

Fig. 5.21 Characteristic 'proliferative' erosions in psoriasis

Radiological changes in the axial skeleton are indistinguishable from those seen in Reiter's disease (pp 77 and 85) and include:

1. Sacro-iliitis — often unilateral or asymmetrical, sacro-iliitis is frequently asymptomatic, being detected in up to 20% of patients with psoriatic arthritis
2. Broad, coarse, asymmetrical syndesmophytes involving ligaments and fibres outside the annulus fibrosus (non-marginal) as well as those of the annulus itself (marginal) (p 78)

MANAGEMENT

Mild disease

In most cases peripheral psoriatic arthritis is a mild condition, patients frequently being bothered more by their skin lesion than their joint symptoms. The commonest oligoarticular form certainly appears usually as more of an intermittent nuisance than a major disability, requiring only symptomatic treatment with NSAI drugs, range-of-motion and muscle-strengthening exercises, and occasional aspiration and local steroid injection (either into joints or into flexor-tendon sheaths). Adequate explanation of the nature of the condition and its generally favourable prognosis should always be given. Patients with spondylitis should be managed in the same way as those with AS, with emphasis on regular, appropriate exercise and maintenance of correct posture (p 79).

Skin lesions are treated according to their severity, preferably under the supervision of a dermatologist. There appears to be no controlled evidence to support repeated claims that improvement in arthritis follows successful treatment of the skin.

Severe disease

In the very few patients (<5%) who develop severe, progressive deforming arthritis, a trial of methotrexate or azathioprine should be considered as an adjunct to the regime of NSAI drugs, local aspiration and injection, simple physical therapy and appropriate exercising. Both drugs may benefit the joint and skin disease, but each is associated with potentially serious side-effects, necessitating careful patient supervision (p 487). If a remission is achieved, attempts at drug withdrawal should be made after 3–4 months, but withdrawal flares are common. Antimalarials should not be tried for fear of provoking exfoliative dermatitis. Gold, also, may produce severe skin reactions, but apparently no more frequently in psoriatics than in patients with RA, and many have claimed to have used this drug with success. Evidence to substantiate the use of these toxic 'second-line' drugs is based largely on uncontrolled trials and reports, the relapsing nature of the arthritis and the wide variation in clinical expression posing considerable problems for controlled treatment studies. At present, however, methotrexate and azathioprine should be tried first.

Prosthetic joint replacement and reconstructive surgery are rarely required, but may considerably benefit patients with severe deformity. The theoretical complications of infection from contaminated plaques and tendency to postoperative fibrosis and ankylosis do not appear to be major problems in practice.

FURTHER READING (PSORIASIS)

Eastwood C J, Wright V 1979 Nail dystrophy in psoriatic arthritis. Annals of the Rheumatic Diseases 38: 226

Kammer G M, Soter N A, Gibson D J, Schur P H 1979 Psoriatic arthritis: a clinical, immunologic and HLA study of 100 patients. Seminars in Arthritis and Rheumatism ix(2): 75–97

Lambert J R, Wright V 1977 Psoriatic spondylitis: a clinical and radiological description of the spine in psoriatic arthritis. Quarterly Journal of Medicine 46: 411

Wright V 1981 Psoriatic arthritis. In: Kelly W N, Harris E D, Ruddy S, Sledge C B (eds) Textbook of rheumatology. W B Saunders, Philadelphia

Wright V, Hall J M H 1976 Seronegative polyarthritis. North-Holland, Amsterdam

V Arthritis Associated with Inflammatory Bowel Disease

Both ulcerative colitis (UC) and Crohn's disease are associated with two distinct forms of arthritis, one peripheral and one axial. Although they behave differently and appear to arise by different pathogenetic mechanisms, both forms of arthritis are included in the seronegative spondarthritis group.

ENTEROPATHIC ARTHRITIS

This term describes a seronegative, inflammatory peripheral arthritis that shows three cardinal characteristics:

1. Joint manifestations occur after the onset of bowel disease
2. Temporal correlation is seen between attacks of arthritis and exacerbation of bowel disease
3. Attacks are followed by complete remission of synovitis

This form of arthritis complicates 20% of patients with Crohn's and c. 12% of those with

UC. The sex incidence is equal and any age may be affected. Attacks tend to predominate in the first few years of bowel disease, and the prevalence of arthritis appears related to:

1. the extent of large bowel involvement — being highest for extensive UC and granulomatous colitis (i.e. Crohn's predominantly localised to colon)
2. the frequency of other extra-intestinal complications — particularly uveitis, aphthous stomatitis, erythema nodosum and pyoderma gangrenosum. Interestingly, the major complications of Crohn's disease — fistula formation and malabsorption — are not particularly associated with joint disease.

Unlike the axial arthritis, enteropathic arthritis shows no association with HLA-B27. Reports of circulating immune complexes showing correlation with active bowel disease, arthritis and liver disease, suggest that the pathogenesis of this condition may resemble the 'bacterial debris' mechanism postulated for the arthritis of jejuno-ileal by-pass (p 68).

Clinical features

Onset of arthritis is characteristically abrupt, reaching a peak within 24–48 hours. Only one to four joints are involved, most commonly the knees and ankles, but occasionally the elbows, interphalangeal joints of the fingers, wrists, shoulders and MCPs (Fig. 5.22). Joint involvement is usually asymmetrical and may show a migratory tendency in the first week. Inflammation is rarely florid and attacks are usually short-lived, the majority showing complete resolution within 2 months. In occasional cases, however, the arthritis may last for 6–12 months, and 10% of patients may have virtually continuous arthritis for several years. Recurrence is unusual and complete recovery is the rule. Correlation between arthritis and activity of bowel disease is less clear-cut in Crohn's disease than in UC.

Concurrent flares of erythema nodosum or uveitis are commonly seen, both occurring with increased frequency in those with bowel disease and arthritis. As with any chronic inflammatory disease, amyloidosis may occasionally occur.

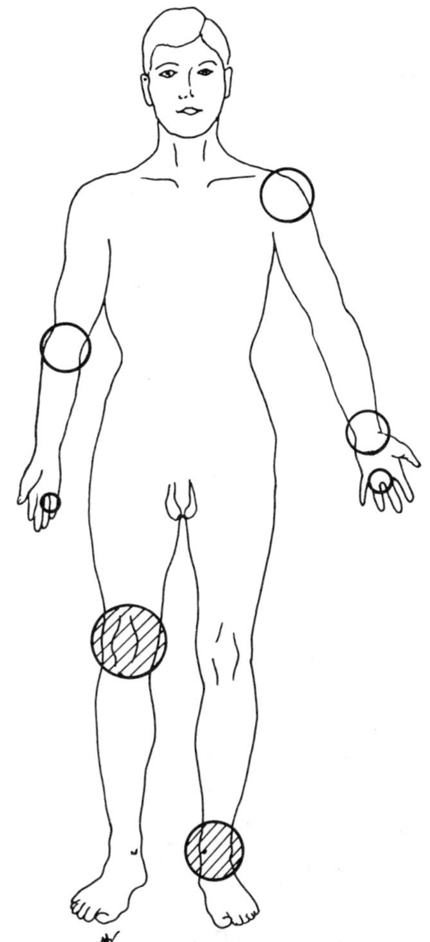

Fig. 5.22 Joint involvement in enteropathic arthritis (involvement of small joints of the hand has particularly been associated, by some, with Crohn's disease). Iritis and erythema nodosum commonly present.

Investigations may reveal anaemia, leukocytosis and elevated viscosity, all principally accounted for by active bowel inflammation. Synovial fluid analysis and synovial biopsy show only non-specific inflammation. X-rays are normal apart from soft-tissue swelling and mild juxta-articular osteopenia: despite repeated attacks joint damage is rare.

Management

Therapy is principally directed towards control of the underlying bowel disease, but may be supplemented by NSAI drugs, joint aspiration and steroid injection. Total proctocolectomy is curative for the joint disease in UC, but resection in Crohn's is less likely to induce remission presumably due to bowel involvement elsewhere.

ANKYLOSING SPONDYLITIS AND SACROILIITIS

Spondylitis, clinically and radiologically identical to idiopathic AS, occurs in c. 4–6% of patients with Crohn's or UC. Several features suggest that the spondylitis and bowel disease are not causally related but are separate diseases occurring in similarly predisposed individuals:

1. Activity of the spondylitis does not parallel that of the bowel disease
2. Spondylitis may predate bowel disease
3. First- and second-degree relatives of patients with bowel disease show an increased incidence of AS and sacro-iliitis

Other features, however, suggest that bowel disease may modify expression of co-existent AS, or even summate with other predisposing factors to precipitate 'secondary' AS in susceptible individuals.

1. Incidence of sacroiliitis in Crohn's and UC is surprisingly high (14–16%), especially in those with severe, chronic disease
2. The usual male preponderance is less marked in AS associated with bowel disease (M:F c. 2:1)
3. The frequency of HLA-B27 in patients with AS and bowel disease is marked (50–70%), but is less than that in idiopathic AS
4. Patients who develop AS after presenting first with bowel disease show later onset of symptoms, more severe bowel disease (with more complications), a lower incidence of HLA-B27 and less frequent uveitis than those in whom AS develops first

The precise interrelationship between bowel and spinal disease, however, remains unclear.

Endoscopic and barium investigation of patients with AS but no bowel symptoms is unrewarding in revealing occult inflammatory bowel disease and should therefore not be performed. Management of spondylitis associated with inflammatory bowel disease is the same as that for classical AS (p 79).

OTHER MUSCULOSKELETAL INVOLVEMENT IN INFLAMMATORY BOWEL DISEASE

Although any joint disease may occur by chance in patients with inflammatory bowel disease, certain conditions appear to be more common in patients with UC or Crohn's, particularly in those with active disease. Such conditions include:

1. Clubbing (p 292) — particularly frequent if a major complication such as fistula is present. Hypertrophic osteoarthropathy, however, is extremely rare.
2. Erythema nodosum (p 317)
3. Septic arthritis of hip — this particularly complicates internal fistula and psoas abscess formation in Crohn's disease (Crohn's now being the commonest cause of psoas abscess)
4. Osteomalacia and osteoporosis (p 333) — caused by malabsorption in Crohn's or by steroid therapy
5. Granulomata in synovium or muscle — these rarely present as a persistent erosive monoarthritis or as an indurated soft-tissue mass

FURTHER READING (INFLAMMATORY BOWEL DISEASE)

Greenstein A J, Janowitz H D, Sachar D B 1976 The extra-intestinal complications of Crohn's disease and ulcerative colitis: a study of 200 patients. Medicine 55: 401

Haslock I, Wright V 1973 The musculoskeletal problems of Crohn's disease. Medicine 52: 217

6 Juvenile chronic arthritis

INTRODUCTION

The term *juvenile chronic arthritis* (JCA) is applied to a group of seronegative chronic inflammatory arthritides of childhood, clinically distinct from rheumatoid arthritis, which are not considered to be just variants of other arthritic conditions whose clinical expression has been altered by the age of the patient. This concept of JCA as a separate disease is supported by the occasional rare case presenting for the first time in adult life. The cause is unknown but potential aetiological features include infection, auto-immunity and heredity. Pathologically, there is villous hypertrophy of synovium with pannus formation. Erosion is uncommon and occurs late due to the increased thickness of young articular cartilage. Deformity and subluxation may develop and there is a tendency to fibrous and bony ankylosis of joints. Extra-articular pathological features include: non-specific inflammation of pleura, peritoneum, pericardium; follicular hyperplasia of lymph nodes; subcutaneous nodules like those of rheumatic fever; and mild vasculitis of cutaneous capillaries and vessels. Since there are no absolute clinical or laboratory diagnostic features of JCA various criteria have been devised. The Taplow criteria are simple and useful but can only be applied retrospectively.

Taplow criteria for juvenile chronic arthritis

1. Onset before 16 years of age
2. Inflammation of four or more joints for at least 3 months
3. If less than four joints, compatible synovial histology
4. Exclusion of other cause of joint disease

CLINICAL FEATURES

Three main forms of JCA are differentiated by their mode of onset and clinical features.

Clinical forms of juvenile chronic arthritis

1. Systemic onset (Still's disease) — 30%
2. Polyarticular onset (more than four joints) — 50%
3. Pauci/monoarticular onset (one to four joints) — 20%

Still's disease

The systemic form of JCA was first described by Sir George Frederick Still in 1897 while a medical registrar at Great Ormond Street Hospital. It occurs mainly in children between the ages of 1 and 4 and is slightly commoner in boys. The child is often acutely and dramatically ill, with severe systemic disturbance. The major clinical features are shown in Figure 6.1.

Many of these features are similar to those seen in an acute infectious illness. The temperature

Major clinical features of Still's disease
1. Pyrexia — 50%
2. Arthritis — 50%
3. Rash — 40%
4. Generalised lymphadenopathy — 35%
5. Splenomegaly — 20%
6. Hepatomegaly — 10%
7. Pericarditis — 10%
8. Subcutaneous nodules — 10%
9. Peritonism (rare)

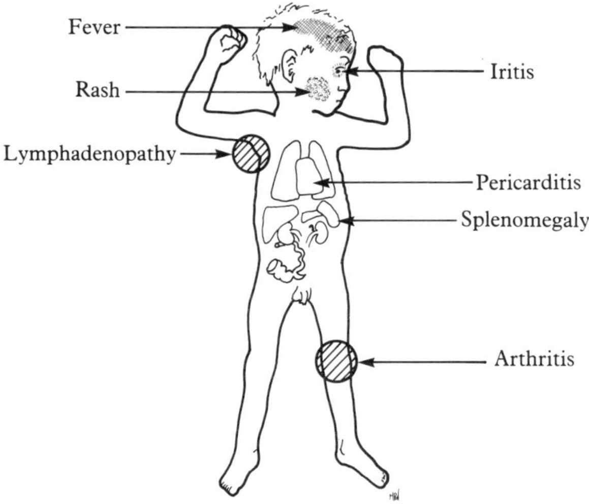

Fig. 6.1 Features of systemic JCA (Still's disease)

often rises to 40°C or more, usually around 6 o'clock in the evening and is accompanied by drenching sweats and rigors. The child may appear extremely ill. After a few hours the fever remits with remarkable improvement in the general condition. This pattern repeats itself over days and weeks, giving a characteristic spiky temperature chart (Fig. 6.2). A pink, evanescent macular rash often appears with the fever or after a hot bath and can sometimes be induced by lightly scratching the skin. Joint involvement may be a minor feature or even completely absent in the early stages. The cervical spine is often affected first and the subsequent joint pattern is variable. About half the children develop an acute generalised polyarthritis which changes with time into a chronic inflammatory arthritis with occasional flares in activity.

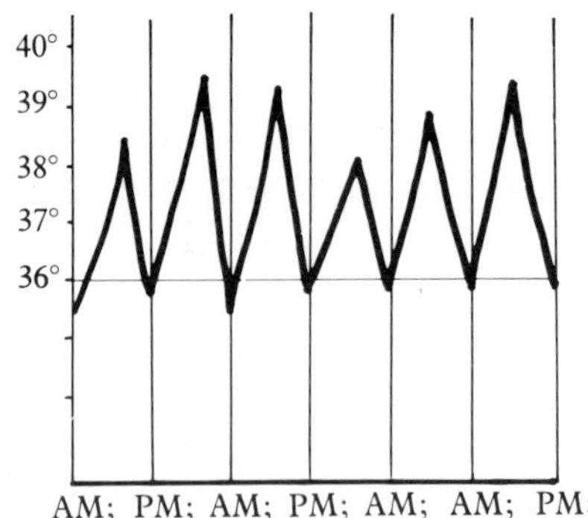

Fig. 6.2 Temperature chart in systemic JCA

The other half have episodic involvement of hips and knees which frequently resolves after a few months. A pericardial friction rub is heard in about 10% but echocardiographic studies reveal evidence of pericardial involvement in over 50%.

Polyarticular onset

Joint symptoms predominate from the onset and systemic upset is mild. It tends to occur at a later age with a peak frequency around 10 and it is commoner in girls. Although virtually all joints can be affected, there is a prediliction for the cervical spine, temporomandibular joints, hips, knees, wrists and ankles. The small joints of the hands and feet are frequently involved, with prominent tenosynovitis but the distribution tends to be asymmetrical and DIPJ synovitis is common. Pain is often disproportionately mild to the degree of inflammation. Growth disturbances are common either from accelerated development or premature closure of epiphyses which results in characteristic deformities (Fig. 6.3).

Growth deformities in juvenile chronic arthritis
1. Short stature
2. Unequal or short fingers and toes
3. Small hands and feet
4. Long or short leg
5. Receding chin
6. Short neck
7. Dental malocclusion

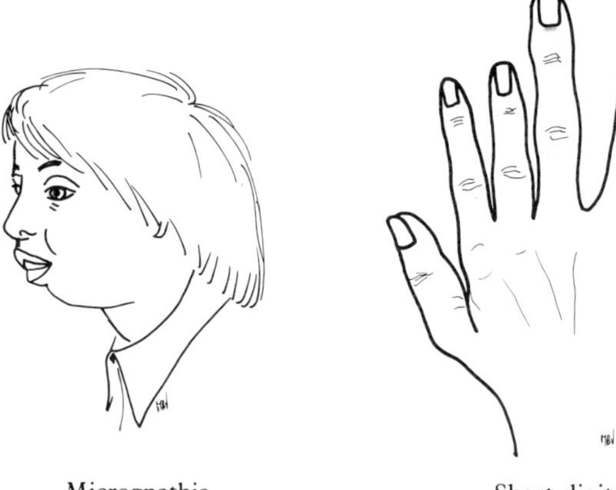

Fig. 6.3 Growth deformities

Pauciarticular onset

There is a gradual onset of arthritis which affects fewer than four joints in the first 6 months. Sometimes only one joint, usually the knee, is involved. It can occur in children of any age but is commoner in girls. Systemic features are mild or absent but there is a high incidence of eye inflammation which may cause blindness. Older boys around the age of 10 with a lower-limb arthritis are prone to acute iridocyclitis which first appears in the middle teens. HLA-B27 is present in a high proportion and often foretells the eventual development of sacro-iliitis or frank ankylosing spondylitis in adult life. Young girls with onset of pauciarticular disease around the age of 4 who are positive for ANF are at great risk of developing a chronic anterior uveitis which is bilateral in two-thirds and causes blindness in one-third if not treated. The insidious inflammation results in posterior syncheiae, cataracts, glaucoma and band keratopathy. Symptoms are minimal and the course prolonged so that regular ophthalmological supervision is mandatory. There is no relationship between the degree of joint activity and eye disease and the role of ANF is unknown.

INVESTIGATIONS

There are no diagnostic tests for JCA. A mild to moderate anaemia is common and reflects disease activity. The white count may be markedly elevated — as high as 60 000 × 10^9/l and the ESR, plasma viscosity and acute-phase proteins are raised in active disease. Rheumatoid factor is negative except in those few children who have classical rheumatoid arthritis starting in childhood. About one quarter of children have ANF. There are no specific radiological features. Erosion of bone is rare; disturbance of growth, premature epiphyseal fusion and ankylosis are common.

DIFFERENTIAL DIAGNOSIS

The seriously ill child with Still's disease without joint involvement is a paediatric emergency. The principal illnesses involved in the differential diagnosis are listed below. Infection, occult malignancy or another connective-tissue disease must be excluded by throat swab, blood, urine and stool culture, ASO titre, Paul-Bunnell, Widal and viral antibody screen. Bone marrow, skeletal survey and urinary VMA exclude leukaemia, metastatic disease and nephroblastoma. High titres of ANF together with raised DNA antibodies suggest SLE and raised muscle enzymes or abnormal EMG suggest dermatomyositis. Often, repeated, careful clinical examination is as useful as investigation — particularly if restriction of neck movement, evanescent rash or pericardial rubs are detected. If there is still uncertainty, a trial of salicylate may help since the fever of JCA usually remits entirely on full doses. If this is inconclusive, a broad-spectrum antibiotic should be tried next and, if fever and malaise improve, a more thorough search for infection is indicated.

Differential diagnosis of systemic juvenile chronic arthritis

1. Bacterial infection
2. Rheumatic fever
3. Leukaemia
4. Nephroblastoma
5. Tuberculosis
6. Glandular fever
7. Other viral infections
8. Systemic lupus erythematosus
9. Dermatomyositis

MANAGEMENT

The aims of treatment are to relieve pain, control disease activity, preserve joint function and prevent or correct deformity while allowing the child to lead as normal a life as possible. Salicylate is the drug of first choice in children given either as soluble aspirin 70 mg/kg/day or as benorylate — a paracetamol/aspirin conjugate — 200 mg/kg/day, aiming to achieve a plasma salicylate concentration of 25–30 mg/dl. If symptoms are not adequately controlled, indomethacin can be tried at a dose of 2–2.5 mg/kg/day. The newer NSAIDs are best avoided in children since experience of them in this age-group is limited. Steroids are indicated in three situations: 1. severe systemic disease uncontrolled by aspirin; 2. chronic uveitis that does not respond to local treatment; and 3. severe inflammatory joint disease uncontrolled by NSAID. Prednisolone can be used in a dose of 1–2 mg/kg given, if possible, on alternate days or as ACTH injections 2–3 times a week. Once activity is controlled, the drug should be gradually withdrawn or reduced to the minimum dose necessary to suppress symptoms. As well as adrenal suppression and risk of sepsis, steroids in children also cause growth retardation. Gold, penicillamine and azathioprine are useful in controlling disease activity in children with chronically active and progressive disease but, particularly with the cytotoxic drugs, there are unanswered questions about the long-term effects on gonadal function and increased risk of malignant disease.

Complete rest will only be needed if there is severe systemic disturbance or many inflamed joints but should be continued for as short a time as necessary. Physiotherapy is the key to maintaining joint function, preventing deformity and preserving muscle power. Working splints for hands and wrists rest the joints without interfering with activities. Swimming and cycling are excellent methods of exercising without full weight-bearing.

Attainment of a good standard of education is vital, since manual work will not be suitable for many of these children. While the majority will still be able to attend their local school, some will fare better at a school for the physically disabled or with home tuition.

Psychosocial problems are frequent in the child and his family and the aid of a social worker or even child psychiatrist may be needed.

PROGNOSIS

The outlook for children with JCA is better than that of adult rheumatoid arthritis but depends on which of the various syndromes the child has. An idea of the overall long-term prognosis can be gained from the following data derived from the work of Dr Barbara Ansell.

40% without limitation of activity
30% slight limitation of activity
7% dead
3% helpless cripples
1% blind

As a general rule, the younger the age at onset the worse the ultimate prognosis. Those with Still's disease and juvenile RA do less well with approximately 30% ending up significantly disabled, whereas those with juvenile AS and monoarticular disease do well. The presence of chronic iridocyclitis also predicts a less favourable outcome with 50% having slight limitation of activity.

Serious stunting of growth is seen in about 0.4%, 15% are left with a receding jaw and 16% have abnormalities of limb growth. Erosions are present on the hand X-rays of about half of the children. 85% of those over school age are either at work or, if female, married and running a home and over a quarter eventually marry although there is an increased risk of divorce.

Death is rare and is due either to infection, usually in those treated with steroids, or to renal failure as the result of amyloidosis which tends to occur in those with the systemic forms of the disease.

FURTHER READING

Ansell B M 1976 Rheumatic disorders in childhood. Clinics in Rheumatic Diseases 2(2)

Ansell B M 1980 Rheumatic diseases in childhood. Butterworth, London

7 Connective-tissue diseases

I Classification

The connective-tissue diseases are a group of chronic inflammatory disorders which predominantly affect women. They involve many different organs and therefore exhibit a wide spectrum of clinical manifestations. Their aetiology is unknown, but it is generally thought to be multifactorial, involving immunological, genetic and environmental, possibly viral, factors.

Diseases included under this category are:

1. Rheumatoid arthritis
2. Systemic lupus erythematosus
3. Systemic sclerosis
4. Poly- and dermatomyositis
5. Polyarteritis nodosa
6. Sjögren's syndrome

The concept of grouping these diseases together was proposed by Klemperer in 1942, who coined the term 'collagen disease'. This was based on pathological features common to these conditions, especially fibrinoid changes in the connective tissue. As a group they must be distinguished from disorders of connective tissue defined by hereditary defects in collagen, such as Marfan's syndrome and Ehlers–Danlos syndrome.

Each connective-tissue disease displays different clinical and pathological features and there is no evidence that they necessarily share a common aetiology or pathogenesis. However, they have enough features in common to be considered as a family of diseases. Common features include: 1. Constitutional factors; 2. Overlapping clinical features; 3. Overlapping pathological features; 4. Prominent immunological abnormalities.

1. Constitutional factors

Host factors such as sex and genetic predisposition appear to have an important role in the pathogenesis and expression of these diseases.

2. Overlapping clinical features

The clinical overlap between these disorders is shown schematically in Figure 7.1. The classification of individual patients depends upon identifying certain clinical and laboratory patterns.

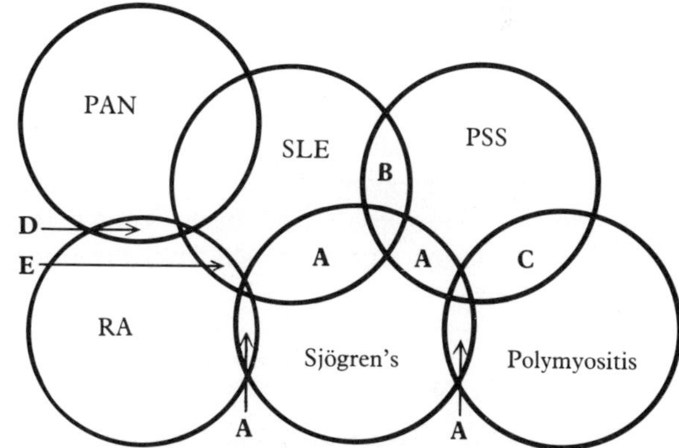

Fig. 7.1 Overlaps between connective-tissue diseases. Common overlaps: **A**) between Sjögren's syndrome and other connective-tissue diseases; **B**) between systemic sclerosis (PSS) and SLE; **C**) between PSS and polymyositis; **D**) between rheumatoid arthritis (RA) and polyarteritis nodosa (PAN); **E**) between RA and SLE.

This is the basis of the American Rheumatism Association (ARA) criteria defining rheumatoid arthritis or systemic lupus erythematosus (SLE), and particular combinations have also been proposed for scleroderma, polymyositis and Sjögren's syndrome. The overlapping between these disorders means that some patients appear to have 'overlap syndromes' and do not fit into traditional diagnostic categories. The term 'overlap syndrome' has been applied to what appears to be a very heterogenous group of disorders including, for example, overlaps between SLE and rheumatoid arthritis, systemic sclerosis and SLE, and systemic sclerosis and polymyositis. The question arises whether or not they represent the co-existence of separate diseases, broad clinical expression of one of the recognised rheumatic diseases, or distinct clinical entities.

In many patients there is difficulty only in the early stages of the disease and the subsequent course resolves the diagnosis. Such patients present with features common to a number of connective-tissue diseases such as arthralgias, Raynaud's phenomenon, hypergammaglobulinaemia and positive tests for antinuclear antibody and rheumatoid factor. They lack the criteria for a single diagnostic category but in time, one pattern gradually emerges.

Less commonly, features of two or more diseases co-exist and the mixed syndrome persists indefinitely. Commonest amongst these are disorders with features of scleroderma combined with those of SLE and/or polymyositis or of rheumatoid arthritis associated with those of SLE. Occasionally, patients sequentially develop two connective-tissue diseases. For example, a patient presenting with typical rheumatoid has been known to develop scleroderma which overshadows the original joint disease.

3. Overlapping pathological features

Blood vessels are a target for involvement in these disorders. Arteries, capillaries or veins of any calibre may be involved and the spectrum of changes ranges from non-inflammatory intimal proliferation to acute necrotising vasculitis.

4. Immunological abnormalities

All of these diseases demonstrate immunological abnormalities and in particular serum auto-antibodies. These not only reflect a basic defect in the immune system but also, in some cases, may have a pathogenetic role. For example, auto-antibodies are implicated in the haemolytic anaemia and immune complex nephritis of SLE, and cell-mediated immunity is implicated in the muscle disease of polymyositis.

The difficulty in classifying patients clinically has prompted the search for serological 'markers' of disease. The identification of antinuclear antibodies (ANA) in SLE was an important step towards this goal and the widely available immunofluorescent test for ANA is the most sensitive screening test for SLE. A positive ANA test, however, is not specific for SLE and ANA are frequently found in other connective-tissue diseases, notably rheumatoid arthritis and PSS. One promising area has been the identification of certain auto-antibodies to individual nuclear and cytoplasmic antigens as listed in Table 7.1. Their clinical significance is still being evaluated but studies suggest that they may be helpful in classifying patients and predicting patterns of disease expression.

Table 7.1 Antibodies characteristic of certain connective-tissue diseases

Antibody	Associated disease
Anti-nDNA	SLE
Anti-Sm	SLE
Anti-nRNP	SLE; MCTD: PSS (rare)
Anti-Ro (SSA)	SLE; Sjögren's
Anti-La (SSB)	SLE; Sjögren's
Anti-centromere	PSS (CREST variant)
Anti-Scl-70	PSS
Anti-Jo-1	Polymyositis
Anti-Mi-1	Polymyositis
Anti-PM-1	Polymyositis–scleroderma overlap
Anti-Ku	Polymyositis–scleroderma overlap

a) Auto-antibodies associated with SLE

The best-studied auto-antibodies are those which react with native or double-stranded DNA. Many reports show that these have a high degree of specificity for SLE. Another serological marker highly specific for SLE is the presence of antibody to a soluble nuclear antigen termed *Sm*, which is detected by precipitation reactions in agarose gels (see p. 465). Antibodies to nRNP, Ro (SSA) and La (SSB) are also characteristically found in SLE sera, but are less specific and occur to some extent in other diseases. Anti-nRNP has been identified, for example, in certain patients with overlap features between SLE, systemic sclerosis and polymyositis. This subgroup constitutes what is known as *mixed connective-tissue disease* (MCTD) and is described in Chapter 7.II. Antibodies to the cytoplasmic protein Ro (SSA) and to La (SSB) are also associated with SLE. Many lupus patients with anti-Ro and anti-La have keratoconjunctivitis sicca, and these antibodies are also found in many patients with sicca syndrome unaccompanied by another connective-tissue disease. This demonstrates that there are serological as well as clinical links between the sicca syndrome and these connective-tissue diseases.

b) Auto-antibodies associated with scleroderma

Auto-antibodies characteristically found in systemic sclerosis but not in other connective-tissue diseases have recently been identified. These include antibody to centromere which is detected by its characteristic pattern of immunofluorescence in the ANA test, and antibodies to a soluble nuclear component, Scl–70. These findings are potentially helpful in classifying PSS patients early in the course of the disease when clinical diagnosis is often difficult. Anti-centromere antibody appears to predict patients who have an indolent course with limited skin involvement and who develop telangiectasia, subcutaneous calcification and oesophageal involvement without prominent involvement of other internal organs; the so-called CREST variant (Chapter 7.III).

c) Auto-antibodies associated with poly- and dermatomyositis

Recently certain autoantibodies have been described in the sera of patients with dermato- or polymyositis. These include antibodies to four soluble cellular antigens, termed *Jo-1*, *Mi-1*, *PM-1* and *Ku*. Antibodies to Jo-1 and Mi-1 are found in polymyositis, while antibodies to PM-1 and Ku occur in patients with overlapping clinical features between polymyositis and scleroderma.

The main interest in these auto-antibody systems is that apparently immune responses to different nuclear and cytoplasmic antigens can be associated with different patterns of disease expression. Research in the future will be directed towards understanding the mechanism for these relationships, thereby leading to a greater understanding of the immunopathogenesis of this group of diseases.

FURTHER READING (INTRODUCTION)

Hughes G R V 1979 Connective tissue diseases. Blackwell Scientific, Oxford

Reichlin M 1981 Current perspectives on serological reactions in SLE patients. Clinical and Experimental Immunology 44: 1–10

II Systemic Lupus Erythematosus

Systemic lupus erythematosus is a chronic inflammatory disorder which predominantly affects young women in their child-bearing years. It involves multiple organ systems and displays a wide range of clinical manifestations accompanied by striking immunological abnormalities. These include serum auto-antibodies to a wide variety of cellular constituents, of which anti-nuclear antibodies (ANA) and in particular anti-DNA are most characteristic. Pathogenetic mechanisms in this disease have been the subject of considerable investigation, and this has tended to highlight SLE out of proportion to its clinical frequency.

Following its description by Kaposi in 1872 SLE became thought of as a frequently fulminating, progressive and fatal disease primarily affecting women in their reproductive years. With the advent of sensitive serological techniques milder cases of SLE are now diagnosed and it is recognised that this disease is more common and displays a broader clinical spectrum than was once thought. This has invalidated previously held concepts of prognosis and treatment. In particular, because different manifestations respond differently to current forms of therapy, treatment needs to be individualised.

INCIDENCE

SLE is uncommon, with an average annual incidence of approximately 70 new cases per million of the population. The incidence appears to be increasing, and this is due to a combination of increased clinical awareness and the availability of sensitive serological tests to aid diagnosis.

Clinical and epidemiological studies have shown that the distribution of SLE is affected by host factors such as age, sex and race. The age of onset and sex distribution is shown in Figure 7.2. The disease occurs predominantly in women and the peak age of onset is between 20 and 30. However, it occurs in childhood and also in the elderly. The ratio of women to men in reported series is at least 9:1.

SLE affects individuals of all races but its prevalence varies from country to country. Its prevalence may be as high as 1:1000 women in some parts of America and even higher in certain racial groups, e.g. Black women in America and the West Indies and Chinese women in Asia. It is thought to be less common in the United Kingdom, but statistics are unavailable.

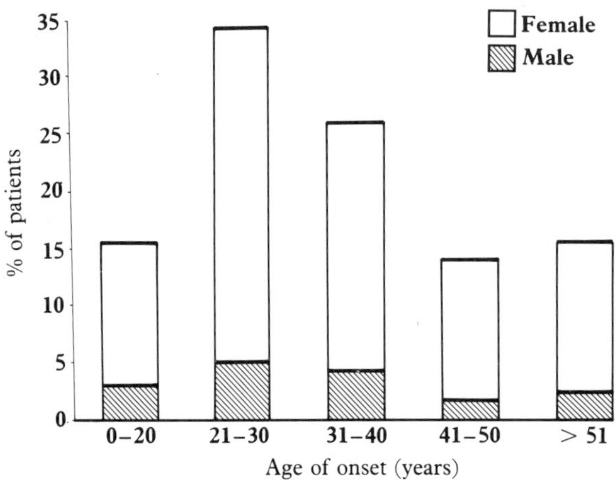

Fig. 7.2 Age of onset and sex distribution of SLE

AETIOLOGY

The aetiology of SLE remains elusive but there is evidence to suggest that a combination of constitutional, environmental and immunological factors are involved (Figure 7.3).

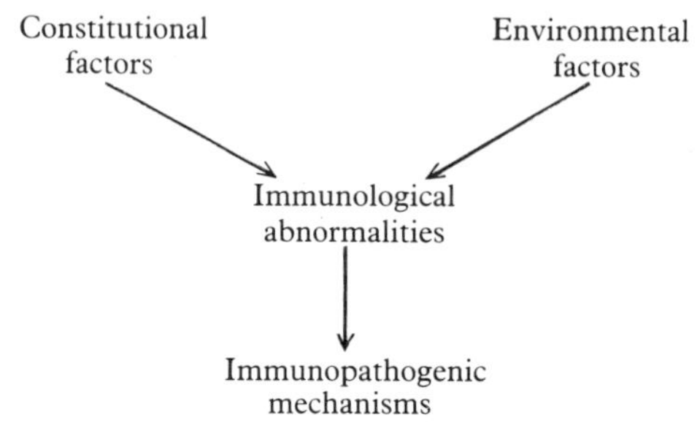

Fig. 7.3 Hypothesis for the aetiology of SLE

1. Constitutional factors

In addition to the striking female preponderance, there is an association between SLE and Klinefelter's syndrome, which is characterised by the XXY phenotype and elevated oestrogen levels. Oestrogens have been shown to accelerate, and testosterone to ameliorate the lupus-like disease that occurs spontaneously in NZB/W hybrid mice.

Genetic factors are also implicated in the development of SLE. The disease occurs in 5% of first-degree relatives of patients and there is a high degree of concordance between identical twins. Recently an association has been shown between SLE and the histocompatibility antigens HLA-DR2 and HLA-DR3. A lupus-like disease has been reported to occur in patients with a hereditary deficiency of early complement components, notably C_2.

There are racial differences in the prevalence of SLE but an important interaction between racial and environmental factors is suggested by the contrast between the high prevalence of this disease in American blacks and the low prevalence in West Africa.

2. Environmental factors

Environmental factors which may be involved include infection, exposure to sunlight and drugs.

Evidence points to a viral aetiology, involving Type C viruses in models of spontaneous lupus occurring in NZB/W mice and dogs. Circumstantial evidence pointing to a viral aetiology is summarised below, but sound documentation is lacking.

Circumstantial evidence for a viral aetiology for SLE

1. Type C viruses implicated in NZB/W mice and dogs
2. Antibodies to double-stranded (?viral) RNA common in human SLE
3. 'Virus-like' structures in organs of SLE patients
4. Isolated reports of components of Type C viruses in SLE kidneys

SLE is exacerbated by exposure to sunlight in 30% of cases. Ultra-violet light is known to cause specific denaturation of DNA with the formation of antigenic thymine dimers.

A variety of drugs may precipitate SLE. Associations are best documented with procainamide and hydralazine, and to a lesser extent with isoniazid and certain anticonvulsants. Anti-nuclear antibodies develop in 50–75% of patients taking procainamide or hydralazine in sufficient doses for 9–12 months. Of these, half develop clinical features. Drug-induced lupus occurs more readily in slow-acetylators, and hydralazine-induced lupus shows a close association with HLA-DR4. It is possible that drugs such as procainamide, hydralazine and isoniazid combine with nuclear macromolecules with the stimulation of an immune response in susceptible individuals. The primary amino group common to these compounds appears to be important, as the acetylated product of procainamide (acetylprocainamide) is much less effective at inducing anti-nuclear antibodies.

A large number of other drugs may on rare occasions cause an SLE-like illness which probably represents an allergic reaction.

Drugs known to precipitate SLE

Frequent association

1. Procainamide
2. Hydralazine
3. Isoniazid
4. Anticonvulsants
5. Chlorpromazine

Rare association

1. Oral contraceptives
2. Chlorthalidone
3. Griseofulvin
4. Levodopa
5. Methyldopa
6. Methylsergide
7. Penicillin
8. Penicillamine
9. Prazosin
10. Propylthiouracil
11. Quinidine
12. Reserpine
13. Streptomycin
14. Sulphonamides
15. Tetracycline

3. Immunological abnormalities

Immunological abnormalities are summarised below.

Abnormal function of B lymphocytes is manifested by generalised B-cell over-activity and the production of antibodies to a wide variety of auto-antigens. There is preferential formation of

Immunological abnormalities in SLE

B-lymphocytes

Abnormal production of auto-antibodies, especially ANA and anti-lymphocytotoxic antibodies

Abnormally high spontaneous immunoglobulin production *in vitro*

T lymphocytes

Abnormal delayed skin tests

Diminished function *in vitro*, notably T-suppressor activity

anti-nuclear antibodies, notably anti-DNA, and anti-lymphocyte antibodies. Abnormal T-cell function has been demonstrated, especially at times of disease activity. A defect in T-suppressor cells has been postulated to account, at least in part, for the abnormal antibody response. The reticulo-endothelial system appears to be less efficient at clearing circulating immune complexes in SLE. Whether or not this is an inherent defect or due to saturation is not known, although evidence points to the former.

4. Immunopathogenetic mechanisms

There is considerable evidence that circulating immune complexes mediate tissue injury, particularly in the kidney. Immune complexes containing DNA and antibodies to DNA have particular importance in this respect but complexes containing other autoantibodies have also been implicated.

An immune complex mechanism may account for tissue injury in other organ systems and may lead to manifestations such as vasculitic skin lesions and pericarditis. However, the pathogenesis of many other features of the disease such as the skin, joint and brain disease, remains to be elucidated.

PATHOLOGY

Pathological findings in many organs are non-specific. A typical change is fibrinoid degeneration, a term which describes homogenous eosinophilic material in the ground substance of small arteries, arterioles and capillaries, and of the connective tissue in synovium and the serosal membranes. Immunofluorescence techniques show this to be composed of immunoglobulin, complement components and other substances such as fibrinogen. A more characteristic, though uncommon, finding is the haematoxylin body, an oval eosinophilic body larger than a nucleus consisting of altered nuclear material and representing the *in vivo* equivalent of the LE cell. Histology of the skin and kidney, however, can point to the diagnosis.

Pathological changes in SLE

General findings

1. Fibrinoid necrosis
2. Haematoxylin bodies
3. Vasculitis of arterioles and capillaries
4. Positive immunofluorescence for immunoglobulin along basement membranes

Skin

1. Liquefaction degeneration of epidermal basal layer
2. Positive immunofluorescence at dermo-epidermal junction

Kidney

1. Mild to diffuse glomerulonephritis
2. Striking immunofluorescence and EM changes

Spleen

'Onion-skin' thickening of arterioles

Heart

Libman-Sachs endocarditis: small verrucous vegetations chiefly on ventricular side of mitral valve

1. Skin

Histological changes typical of lupus in the skin biopsy include epidermal thinning, liquefaction degeneration of the epidermal basal layer, and scattered lymphocytic infiltrates. Granular deposits of immunoglobulin and complement can be detected along the dermal–epidermal junction by immunofluorescence. Similar deposits can be found in clinically-uninvolved sun-exposed skin in two-thirds of SLE patients (lupus band test).

2. Kidney

Various patterns of renal injury can be recognised by light microscopy, immunofluorescence and electron microscopy, although considerable overlap occurs.

a) Minimal lupus nephritis (common)

Here abnormalities are most readily demonstrated

by immunofluorescence and electron microscopy which show granular deposition of immunoglobulin and complement and electron-dense deposits predominantly in the mesangium. These prominent immunofluoresence findings are particularly characteristic of SLE.

b) Mild (focal) lupus nephritis (common)

In this form there is segmental proliferation of some glomerular tufts while others appear normal. Less than half the glomeruli are involved. Immunofluorescence and electron microscopic changes are present in the mesangium of all glomeruli and in the capillary loops mainly at sites of proliferation.

c) Diffuse proliferative nephritis (uncommon)

The tufts of more than 50% of the glomeruli are involved in this form. Active glomerular lesions are more marked than in the previous conditions and include prominent intracapillary cellular proliferation, areas of fibrinoid necrosis, and epithelial crescent formation. This picture is accompanied by striking findings on immunofluorescence and electron microscopy, with granular deposits of immunoglobulin and complement along the peripheral capillary wall and in the mesangium, and electron-dense deposits within the basement membrane and in the subendothelial and subepithelial areas.

A subset of these patients develop progressive glomerular sclerosis.

d) Membranous nephritis (rare)

This form histologically resembles idiopathic membranous nephritis, with diffuse thickening of the glomerular basement membrane, and no proliferative changes. Immunofluorescence reveals immunoglobulin deposited diffusely along all the basement membranes. This form may be complicated by renal vein thrombosis.

CLINICAL FEATURES

1. Presentation

This disease can present in a great variety of ways and the mode of onset varies from insidious to fulminating. The most common presentation is a young woman with marked musculoskeletal symptoms accompanied by constitutional manifestations such as fatigue, malaise, fever and loss of weight with evidence of a mild symmetrical peripheral synovitis. Often there is a history of mild Raynaud's phenomenon. Another common presenting feature is rash. Less common forms of presentation are fever of unknown origin, pleurisy, pericarditis and renal or neuro-psychiatric manifestations. A small proportion present with a 'lupus crisis': extreme weakness and fatigue, severe headaches with chest and abdominal pain and renal or neuropsychiatric involvement. Rarely the presentation may be haematological with 'idiopathic' thrombocytopenic purpura or profound leukopenia.

Presentations in SLE

Common

1. Constitutional symptoms — fatigue, malaise, fever, weight-loss
2. Marked musculoskeletal symptoms
3. Mild peripheral synovitis
4. Rash

Uncommon

1. Fever of unknown origin
2. Pleurisy
3. Pericarditis
4. Renal manifestations
5. Neuropsychiatric manifestations
6. 'Lupus crisis'
7. 'Idiopathic' thrombocytopenic purpura
8. Severe leukopenia

2. Precipitating factors

Precipitating factors can be implicated in the onset or exacerbation of disease in half the cases. These include infection, exposure to sunlight (and, rarely, ultraviolet light in discotheques — 'discolupus'), drugs (see p 101), pregnancy and operations.

3. Course

The course of SLE is unpredictable but the

majority of patients with musculoskeletal and cutaneous manifestations pursue a chronic course dominated by these features, often punctuated by exacerbations and remissions. Some show sequential involvement of other organ systems, though major involvement of kidneys and the neurological system tends to occur early in the course of the disease. A small proportion have a rapidly downhill course with death within 2 years.

4. Involvement of individual organ systems

a) *Joints*

The commonest complaint is joint or muscle pain. Polyarthritis is common and frequently represents the first manifestation of the disease. Pain is often out of proportion to objective signs of inflammation. The arthritis is usually symmetrical, most commonly involving the small joints of the hands, wrists and knees (Fig. 7.4). Occasionally joint deformities develop as a late feature. The hands are most commonly involved with, for example, Z-deformities of the thumb, swan-neck deformities and ulnar deviation of the fingers (Fig. 7.5). Characteristically these occur in the absence of radiological erosions. Rarely a truly erosive arthritis is seen. Another late feature is osteonecrosis of bone especially involving the femoral and humeral heads which occurs in 10% of patients. The diagnosis should be considered in the presence of asymmetrical joint pain, especially in the hip which is otherwise rarely involved in SLE. It is considered

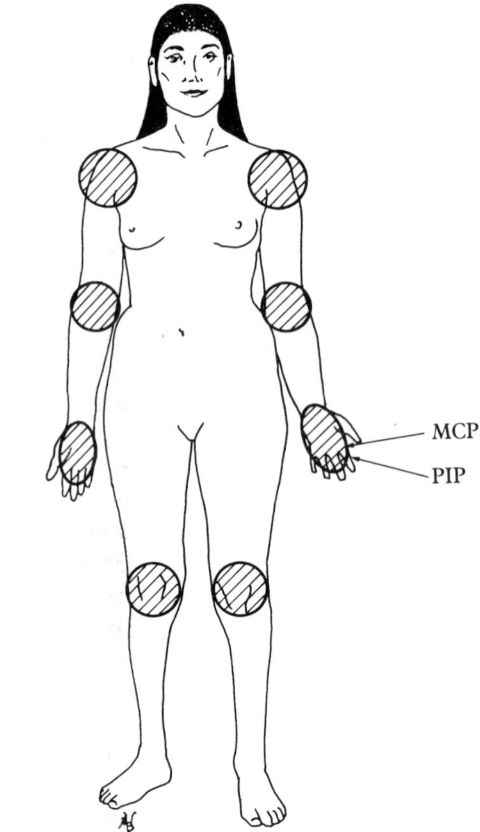

Fig. 7.4 Distribution of arthritis in SLE

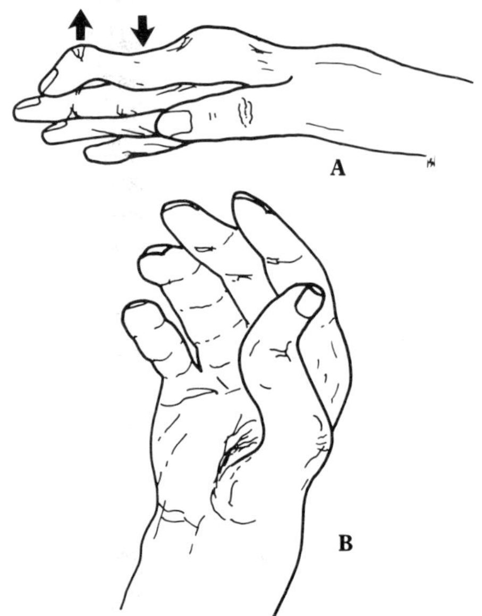

Fig. 7.5 A. Swan-neck deformity. **B.** Z deformity of the thumb in SLE.

Clinical manifestations of SLE

1.	Arthritis	90%
2.	Rashes	80%
3.	Fever	80%
4.	Renal disease	50%
5.	Neuropsychiatric disease	50%
6.	Raynaud's phenomenon	40%
7.	Pleurisy	40%
8.	Lymphadenopathy	40%
9.	Alopecia	30%
10.	Pericarditis	30%
11.	Mouth ulcers	30%

to be a complication of long-term steroid administration but tends to occur in young patients with a history of severe disease.

b) Muscles

Myalgias are very common and occasionally the typical clinical picture of polymyositis develops (Chapter 7.IV). In the elderly a polymyalgia rheumatica-like presentation may occur.

c) Skin and appendages

Mucocutaneous involvement occurs at some time during the course of the disease in the majority. The erythematous butterfly rash is the most well-known feature, and occurs in half the cases. Widespread maculopapular eruptions are common, and characteristically involve the dorsal surface of the fingers between the joints. Discoid lupus lesions occur in 10% (Chapter 15.I). Skin lesions have a predilection for sun exposed areas and photosensitivity is marked in approximately one-third. Urticaria, bullous lesions, purpura and ulcers occur less commonly.

Mucocutaneous manifestations of SLE

Skin

1. Non-specific maculopapular rash
2. 'Butterfly' erythema
3. Discoid lupus
4. Photosensitivity
5. Cutaneous vasculitis
   a) Urticaria
   b) Purpura
   c) Ulcers
   d) Bullae
   e) Livedo reticularis
6. Thrombocytopenic purpura
7. Raynaud's phenomenon
8. Lupus profundus
9. 'Rheumatoid' nodules

Mucous membranes

Ulceration

Hair

1. Alopecia
2. 'Lupus hair'

Nails

1. Pitting
2. Onycholysis

Abnormality of the hair, mucous membranes and nails are also common. Alopecia may be focal and associated with scarring of the scalp or diffuse when it is often associated with a clinical exacerbation. A characteristic feature is fragmentation of the frontal hairs leading to a receding hairline with shortened, broken off hair, known as 'lupus hair'.

Ulceration of the oral mucosa is common during clinical exacerbations. Often it is painful, but asymptomatic ulceration of the hard palate is a very frequent finding.

Nail-lesions occur and include pitting and onycholysis (separation of the nail from underlying nail-bed).

Lupus profundus is an uncommon manifestation and refers to panniculitis causing tender indurated nodules on the face generally associated with an overlying discoid rash. In rare cases more severe panniculitis, resembling Weber-Christian disease, occurs particularly on the buttocks and upper arms and resolves leaving a depressed scar.

d) Blood vessels

Raynaud's phenomenon is common, usually mild, and may precede other manifestations by many years.

Periungual erythema may be marked and dilated nail-fold capillaries are common (p. 261).

Recurrent deep venous thrombosis, sometimes complicated by pulmonary embolism occurs in a few.

A late feature is premature atherosclerosis which has been linked to prolonged corticosteroid therapy. This may cause myocardial infarction or, rarely, intermittent claudication.

e) Lungs

Pleurisy occurs most commonly causing pain and a small effusion. Large effusions are uncommon.

Other pulmonary manifestations are less common although pulmonary function tests are

Lung involvement in SLE

Common
1. Pleurisy
2. Asymptomatic diffusion defects

Uncommon
1. Pulmonary infiltrates
2. High diaphragm on X-ray
3. 'Disappearing lung syndrome'

frequently abnormal, even in the asymptomatic patient, with reduced carbon monoxide diffusion.

Marked pulmonary symptoms including dyspnoea, cough and haemoptysis may accompany a severe generalised exacerbation of SLE. Clinical findings include râles and the chest X-ray shows patchy infiltrates or areas of plate-like atelectasis. This is lupus pneumonitis which must be distinguished from infection.

A raised diaphragm is another radiological finding; the result of the combination of repeated episodes of pleurisy, atelectasis and abnormal diaphragmatic function. In severe cases this can be associated with marked restriction defects in lung function: 'the disappearing lung syndrome'.

Pulmonary hypertension is a rare and late feature of SLE.

f) The heart

Pericarditis is the commonest cardiac manifestation and is usually transient and mild. Tamponade and constrictive pericarditis are very rare.

Myocarditis leading to heart failure is uncommon and clinically significant endocarditis is very rare.

Isolated cases of myocardial infarction due to coronary vasculitis have occurred. However, ischaemic heart disease secondary to accelerated coronary atherosclerosis appears to be a major hazard of long-term corticosteroid treatment.

g) The kidney

Clinical evidence of renal disease occurs in half of the patients, usually early in the course of the disease. The most common manifestation is mild to moderate proteinuria, sometimes accompanied by microscopic haematuria and casts, which fluctuates with disease activity. Renal insufficiency and nephrotic syndrome occur less frequently. Anuria is a rare complication due to severe interstitial nephritis.

A minority of patients have progressive renal failure leading to hypertension and 'end-stage' kidney.

Kidney involvement in SLE

Common
1. Proteinuria (0.5–2 g/24 h)
2. Microscopic haematuria
3. Casts

Less common
1. Renal insufficiency
2. Nephrotic syndrome

Uncommon
Progressive renal failure

Rare
1. Renal vein thrombosis
2. Anuria due to interstitial nephritis

h) The neurological system

Neuropsychiatric manifestations occur in 50% and include a wide range of neurological and psychiatric features which are usually transient and do not result in a residual organic defect.

Headaches are common and sometimes have the features of migraine. Psychiatric manifestations are also common, but often it is difficult to determine what is due to disease, due to treatment and due to reaction to a chronic disease.

The most serious manifestations are seizures which are usually grand mal, organic brain syndromes and strokes. These manifestations usually accompany active disease of other organ systems. Peripheral neuropathy is uncommon and takes the form of a mononeuritis multiplex or a sensory neuropathy. Rare manifestations are Guillain-Barré syndrome and transverse myelitis of the spinal cord.

Visual impairment is rare but fundal examination often shows cotton wool exudates (cytoid

Neurological involvement in SLE

Common
1. Headaches
2. Psychiatric disturbance

Less common
1. Seizures
2. Strokes
3. Cranial-nerve lesions
4. Organic brain syndrome

Uncommon
Mononeuritis multiplex

Rare
1. Cerebellar ataxia
2. Chorea
3. Guillain-Barré syndrome
4. Transverse myelitis

bodies) and haemorrhages during exacerbations of disease activity.

Diagnosis rests on clinical suspicion since conventional neurological investigations are of limited value. Abnormalities of the CSF are seen in two-thirds, usually a raised CSF protein with or without pleocytosis. Depression of CSF levels of the complement component C4 sometimes occurs, but samples have to be analysed immediately since C4 activity in CSF spontaneously disappears. The EEG is frequently abnormal, often showing diffuse slow wave activity. This may be helpful when psychiatric manifestations predominate. Brain scans and computed tomography are abnormal in some cases but not others.

i) Miscellaneous manifestations

Generalised lymphadenopathy and hepatosplenomegaly are common. Mild elevation of serum liver enzyme levels is also seen but clinically significant liver disease is rare. Mesenteric arteritis occasionally leads to ileal and colonic ulcers which may perforate. Rarely a protein-losing enteropathy occurs.

Ocular involvement includes keratoconjunctivitis sicca with or without other features of Sjögren's syndrome, and, less commonly, episcleritis.

j) Infection in SLE

Infection is a serious complication and fever should be attributed to infection unless proved otherwise, particularly in a patient on steroids or immunosuppressive agents. It is the most common cause for pulmonary infiltrations in SLE, sometimes with opportunistic organisms such as TB and pneumocystis. Diagnosis often requires bronchoscopy and lung biopsy.

5. Clinical subgroups

a) Characterised by cutaneous manifestations

(i) *Discoid LE*. Chronic discoid cutaneous lupus (DLE) is the term used when chronic scarring cutaneous lesions are the predominant manifestation and there are few or no systemic signs and symptoms. The discoid lupus lesion starts as a circumscribed indurated erythematous plaque which develops a central area of hyperkeratosis, follicular plugging and atrophy. Plaques generally occur on the face, behind the ears and on the scalp, but may be widespread. Most patients with DLE have a low incidence of systemic complications and ANA (5–10%), and auto-antibodies characteristic of SLE, especially antibodies to native DNA, are absent. Most physicians, however, view DLE as part of the spectrum of lupus erythematosus and approximately 10% subsequently develop features of SLE.

(ii) *Subacute cutaneous lupus erythematosus (SCLE)*. Subacute cutaneous lupus erythematosus identifies a subset of lupus patients with a characteristic non-scarring dermatitis. These patients exhibit a wide distribution of photosensitive lesions, with the face, arms and trunk being frequently affected and they often present first to a dermatologist. Most have a mild systemic illness and the majority have positive tests for ANA. Serious organ involvement, however, is less frequent than in 'classical' SLE and patients with SCLE have a low incidence of renal disease.

b) SLE in childhood

Clinical manifestations and prognosis are similar to the adult disease. Previous reports that prognosis was worse in children was based on studies of more 'classical' and severe disease and the previous failure to recognise milder cases of SLE.

c) SLE in the elderly

Patients in whom disease onset occurs after the age of 55 comprise 10–15% of the total lupus population. Age modifies the disease: mode of onset tends to be more insidious and pattern of organ involvement is different with more interstitial lung disease and less arthritis, Raynaud's, alopecia and lymphadenopathy.

d) SLE in pregnancy

It is now agreed that pregnancy is safe for most patients with SLE. It is best undertaken during remission but pregnancy apparently has little effect on the disease process. Post-partum exacerbation may occur though in practice it is rarely seen in well-controlled patients There is an increased risk of abortion, especially if SLE is active. A number of mechanisms have been postulated, including decidual arteriolitis with interference of decidual placental perfusion and the presence of lymphocytotoxic antibodies which are known to cross-react with the trophoblast. Otherwise, the newborn are generally unaffected, although occasionally transient lupus rashes are seen and babies with heart block have been reported. These manifestations have been associated with the passage of maternal antibodies to the Ro(SSA) antigen across the placenta.

e) Drug-induced SLE

Drug-induced lupus occurs more often in the elderly, and the clinical picture is very similar to idiopathic lupus in this age group, with prominent cutaneous, joint, pericaridal, pleural and pulmonary manifestations but rarely renal involvement.

ANA are present in high titre. These can be shown to react predominantly with histones, especially the H_2 fraction. Antibodies characteristic of idiopathic lupus such as anti-native DNA are only rarely present and serum complement levels usually remain normal.

Features of drug-induced lupus

Common

1. DRUGS: procainamide; hydralazine, sufficient cumulative dose required
2. RISK FACTORS: slow acetylator status; HLA-DR4 (for hydralazine)
3. Older age-group; female preponderance
4. Polyarthritis
5. Rash
6. Pleurisy and/or pericarditis
7. Pulmonary infiltrates
8. ANA in high titre (mainly to histones)
9. Resolution after discontinuing drug

Rare

1. Renal and neuropsychiatric disease
2. Anti-native DNA antibodies
3. Low serum complement levels

Discontinuation of the offending drug usually results in rapid resolution of the symptoms, although antinuclear antibodies may persist for several months.

f) SLE associated with C2 deficiency

A lupus-like disease has been reported to occur in patients with an inherited deficiency of the complement component C2. The disease is characterised by the predominance of cutaneous manifestations, particularly discoid skin lesions, a lower incidence of renal disease and a low prevalence of antibodies to nDNA. It is of interest that, unlike typical DLE, the presence of immunoglobulin and complement is frequently lacking in the skin lesions of these patients.

6. Disease associations with SLE

Associations have been noted between SLE and myasthenia gravis, porphyria cutania tarda, hereditary complement deficiency states especially of early complement components such as C2 and hereditary deficiency of Cl-esterase inhibitor (hereditary angio-neurotic oedema).

LABORATORY FINDINGS

1. Acute-phase reactants

The erythrocyte sedimentation rate (ESR) is usually elevated in active disease. In contrast the level of C-reactive protein is often normal even when SLE is active, although it usually rises in the presence of infection.

2. Haematology

A mild to moderate normochromic normocytic anaemia is common and the haemoglobin often reflects disease activity. A haemolytic anaemia occurs in a few patients.

Haematological findings in SLE

Common
1. Normochromic normocytic anaemia
2. Leukopenia (WBC less than 3×10^3)
3. Lymphopenia (with active disease)
4. Thrombocytopenia

Uncommon
1. Circulating anticoagulant
2. Haemolytic anaemia
3. Severe thrombocytopenia

Leukopenia is a very common finding, and lymphopaenia in particular reflects disease activity.

Mild thrombocytopenia is common but only in the minority is it severe and accompanied by purpura.

A circulating anti-coagulant is seen in some patients but is rarely significant clinically.

3. Serological findings

SLE is characterised by the presence of antibodies to a wide variety of auto-antigens. ANA detected by immunofluorescence and antibodies that react with double-stranded (native) DNA are particularly characteristic and aid diagnosis (Chapter 24.v.).

Antibodies to DNA are found in most patients with SLE. They can be detected to a number of different antigenic determinants on the DNA molecule but can be subdivided into two broad categories: those that react with native (double-stranded) DNA and those that react preferentially with denatured (single-stranded) DNA. Antibodies to ssDNA are found in at least 80% of patients with active SLE but are also found in a variety of other disorders (Chapter 24.V.). Antibodies to nDNA, on the other hand, are found in two thirds of patients with active, untreated disease and are highly specific for SLE. Titres of anti-DNA (ss and n) often fluctuate with disease activity and can be used in conjunction with complement levels to help assess disease activity.

Common serological findings in SLE

1. Hypergammaglobulinaemia	80%
2. Anti-nuclear antibodies	95%
a) to DNA	70%
b) to nucleoprotein	70%
c) to soluble ribonucleoptoteins (including nRNP, Sm, Ro, La)	70%
3. Rheumatoid factor	40%
4. Positive Coomb's test	30%
5. False-positive VDRL	20%

4. Serum complement

Hypocomplementaemia may occur in association with clinical exacerbations. Profound falls in complement almost always indicate the presence of active renal disease.

DIAGNOSIS

The diagnosis of SLE depends on recognising a characteristic pattern of clinical and laboratory abnormalities.

The criteria for SLE revised by the American Rheumatism Association in 1982 are as follows:

1. Malar rash
2. Discoid rash
3. Photosensitivity

4. Oral ulcers
5. Nonerosive arthritis
6. Pleurisy or pericarditis
7. Renal disorder:
   a) persistent proteinuria (>0.5 g per day)
   or
   b) cellular casts
8. Neurological disorder:
   seizures or psychosis
9. Haematological disorder:
   a) haemolytic anaemia
   or
   b) leukopenia (<4000 mm^3) on two occasions
   or
   c) lymphopenia (<1500 mm^3) on two occasions
   or
   d) thrombocytopenia (<100 000 mm^3)
10. Immunological disorder:
   a) positive LE cells
   or
   b) anti DNA
   or
   c) anti Sm
   or
   d) false-positive VDRL
11. ANA
   4 or more criteria required for the diagnosis of SLE

These were designed for classification for use in clinical and therapeutic studies rather than for bedside diagnosis. Indeed, using these criteria mild cases will be missed. It is in this situation that serological tests are helpful.

Serological tests for SLE
1. ANA by immunofluorescence
2. Antibodies to DNA
3. Antibodies to nRNP, Sm, Ro(SSA) or La(SSB)
4. Positive lupus band test

The immunofluorescence test for ANA is a valuable screening test and has replaced the LE cell test in most laboratories. It is not a specific test, however, and ANA are frequently found in other connective tissue diseases, in other autoimmune diseases and in approximately 5% of the normal population (Chapter 24.V). Antibodies to native DNA are present in two thirds of patients and are rarely found in other conditions. Antibodies to certain ribonucleoproteins of the nucleus and cytoplasm (nRNP, Sm, Ro (SSA) and La (SSB)) are also common findings, and may support the diagnosis of SLE when anti-DNA is absent.

Lupus band test

Granular deposits of immunoglobuin and complement can be detected by immunofluorescence in clinically uninvolved skin from the extensor surface of the upper third of the forearm in two thirds of SLE patients and only very rarely in patients with other conditions. This may be used as an aid to diagnosis.

Useful pointers to the diagnosis of SLE are shown below.

Diagnosis of SLE

1. *Pointers to diagnosis*
   a) Young women (<40)
   b) Arthritis but no joint erosions after 2 years
   c) Alopecia
   d) Neuropsychiatric manifestations
   e) Lymphopenia
   f) Positive ANA
   g) High titres of anti-DNA
   h) Positive lupus band test
2. *Differential diagnosis* includes
   RA; SBE; lymphoma; sarcoidosis; ITP; TTP; gonococcal septicaemia

SEROLOGICAL SUBSETS INCLUDING MIXED CONNECTIVE-TISSUE DISEASE

The technique of immunodiffusion has been used to identify antibodies to certain soluble nuclear and cytoplasmic ribonucleoproteins (Table 7.2). Their major importance is that they identify certain patterns of disease expression, rather than being diagnostic tools.

Table 7.2

Antibody	Frequency in SLE	Present in other CTD	Associated clinical pattern
anti-nRNP	30%	PSS RA	Raynaud's Overlap features (MCTD)
anti-Sm	10%	–	CNS lupus
anti-Ro (SSA)	40%	Sjögren's	Photosensitive rashes SCLE Sjögren's 'ANA-negative' SLE
anti-La (SSB)	10%		

1. Antibodies to nRNP

These antibodies identify patients who rarely develop nephritis but who often have severe Raynaud's phenomenon and may develop overlapping features of scleroderma and polymyosis. This overlap has been called *mixed connective-tissue disease*.

Mixed connective tissue disease (MCTD)

Clinical features commonly described in MCTD are shown in Table 7.3.

Most reported cases are women with a mean age of onset in the fourth decade. It occurs in children but the childhood disease appears to be more severe with more renal, cardiac and haematological complications.

Table 7.3 Clinical and laboratory features of MCTD

Common features	Rare features
Raynauds	Severe lupus nephritis
Polyarthritis	Severe CNS disease
Fever	Diffuse scleroderma
Malar rash	Malignant hypertension
Pleurisy/pericarditis	Scleroderma kidney
Swollen hands	Pulmonary hypertension
Sclerodactyly	Widespread sclerosis of GI tract
Abnormal oesophageal motility	Myocarditis
pulmonary fibrosis	
Myositis	
Hypergammaglobulinaemia	
Positive ANA (often speckled pattern)	

The clinical picture is variable, especially at the start. Usually patients present with an 'SLE-like' picture in which non-deforming arthritis, erythematous rashes, serositis, fever and leukopenia are present though at times there is a 'scleroderma-like' appearance in which Raynaud's phenomenon, puffy hands, sclerodactyly and abnormal oesophageal motility dominate the clinical picture. Proximal muscle weakness at the onset may suggest polymyositis and some patients are initially considered to have rheumatoid arthritis.

Raynaud's phenomenon is prominent, sometimes producing severe morbidity and it frequently precedes other manifestations by months or years. Skin manifestations of SLE are frequently seen and sclerodermatous features such as swollen fingers or sclerodactyly also occur. Abnormal oesophageal motility is common, but serious systemic complications of PSS affecting the intestinal tract, lungs and kidneys occur only rarely. Non-deforming polyarthritis is common, but in some cases the joint disease suggests rheumatoid arthritis with radiological erosions, subcutaneous nodules and positive tests for rheumatoid factor. Clinical renal disease is rare and so is neuropsychiatric disease, although several cases of trigeminal sensory neuropathy have occurred.

Laboratory characteristics include an ANA test positive in high titres, often with a speckled pattern of fluorescence, the predominance of antibodies to nRNP and the relative absence of antibodies to other nuclear antigens such as DNA, typical of SLE. The serum complement levels usually remain normal.

2. Antibodies to Sm

Anti-Sm occurs almost exclusively in SLE. Some consider that patients with anti-Sm constitute a distinct clinical subset. Although these patients develop nephritis it is reported to be mild and follows a benign course. It had also been observed that antibodies to Sm are associated with the development of central nervous system disease particularly when it occurs as an isolated clinical manifestation.

3. Antibodies to Ro (SSA) and La (SSB)

SLE patients with these antibodies tend to have a high frequency of photosensitive skin rashes. Patients classified as SCLE (page 107) nearly always have anti-Ro antibody. These antibodies also identify lupus patients who develop clinical features of Sjögren's syndrome.

A small proportion of lupus patients with anti-Ro have persistently negative immunofluorescence tests for ANA and have been designated 'ANA-negative SLE'.

TREATMENT

Since there is no known cure, treatment of SLE is based on symptomatic relief and suppression of inflammation.

1. General measures

Patient education is needed because it is still a popular concept that this is invariably a fatal disease. General treatment measures include adequate rest during phases of active disease, avoidance of sun exposure by those who demonstrate a photosensitive element, and early identification of complicating infection.

2. Symptomatic measures

Many patients do not require systemic corticosteroids since they never develop major organ involvement. Topical steroids are valuable when relatively small areas of skin are involved. Musculoskeletal symptoms can usually be controlled with non-steroidal antinflammatory agents, and symptoms due to pleurisy and pericarditis usually respond also. Aspirin has been largely superseded by newer anti-inflammatory agents, such as proprionic acid derivatives, which are better tolerated. It should be remembered that high doses of aspirin may be hepatotoxic in SLE and non-steroidal anti-inflammatory drugs occasionally cause a reduction in creatinine clearance, particularly in patients with renal impairment.

3. Suppression of severe disease

a) Antimalarials

Antimalarial drugs, particularly hydroxychloroquine, are useful to suppress troublesome arthritis and skin rashes not responsive to other conservative therapy.

Retinal toxicity is not a major problem if smaller doses are used (200–400 mg a day) although 6 monthly opthalmological examinations are recommended during treatment (See Chapter 27).

b) Systemic corticosteroids (Table 7.4).

It may be necessary to resort to using corticosteroids for manifestations such as arthritis, rash, serositis and constitutional features such as fever if they are unresponsive to other measures and are causing major morbidity. These manifesations are usually suppressed by prednisolone in a dose of 0.5 mg/kg body-weight/day.

Table 7.4 Indications for corticosteroids in SLE

Indication	Initial dose
Severe nephritis Seizures, coma or other severe CNS disease Severe thrombocytopenia Vasculitis involving major organs or peripheral nerves	1 mg/kg/body-weight
Arthritis, Rashes and other non-life threatening disease organs not responsive to other measures and causing severe morbidity	0.5 mg/kg/body-weight

Otherwise, the use of steroids should be restricted to more serious manifestations such as severe nephritis with renal impairment and severe neurological disease. For these complications prednisolone in a dose of 1 mg/kg body weight should be used, though on rare occasions higher doses may be required. Pulse intravenous therapy with megadoses (1 gram) of methylprednisolone has been used with success in treating some cases of severe SLE, especially those with deteriorating renal function.

When clinical response has been achieved the steroid dosage is tapered to the smallest possible daily dose or preferably alternate day therapy.

c) Immunosuppressive drugs

Immunosuppressive agents in the treatment of SLE are still controversial. Several investigators, however, advocate the combination of azathioprine and corticosteroids in severe lupus nephritis. Azathioprine appears to have an important steroid sparing effect in this situation and improved survival associated with a low infection rate has been reported.

d) Experimental forms of treatment

Experimental forms of therapy include plasmapheresis. Early results suggest that this may supplement treatment in patients with active and severe disease who are resistent to corticosteroids and cytotoxic drugs alone.

e) Which drugs to avoid?

There is no evidence that any drug should be avoided in all patients. Drugs able to exacerbate SLE should only be used under careful supervision. These includes penicillin, sulphonamides and oral contraceptives. On the other hand, there is no evidence that drugs known to precipitate drug-induced lupus exacerbate idiopathic SLE. Anticonvulsants may be required to control seizure activity and can be used with safety. Similarly, there is no contra-indication to immunisations, although common sense suggests that they should be performed whenever possible when the patient is not taking large doses of steroids or immunosuppressive drugs and when the disease is not very active.

f) Late complications

A small proportion of patients with end-stage renal failure require chronic haemodialysis. Renal transplantation is not contra-indicated in SLE *per se*.

Prosthetic surgery is sometimes required for avascular necrosis of the hip.

g) Laboratory parameters to monitor treatment

DNA antibody titres and serial estimations of serum complement are helpful in conjuction with clinical assessment in assessing disease activity and monitoring treatment. Abnormal laboratory values in the absence of clinical disease are not, however, an indication for treatment.

PROGNOSIS

Prognosis in SLE has improved dramatically from a 2-year 90% mortality before the Second World War to the current 10-year survival rates of 90%. This apparent improvement is in part due to increased clinical awareness and the widespread use of sensitive serological tests to diagnose milder cases and in part due to the introduction of antibiotics for infectious complications and improved methods of treating renal failure. Active glomerular lesions appear to respond to corticosteroid and immunosuppressive therapy and early treatment with these agents may be partly responsible for the great improvement seen in the prognosis of patients with severe renal disease.

FURTHER READING (SLE)

Hughes G R V 1979 Systemic lupus erythematosus. In: Connective tissue diseases. Blackwell Scientific Publications

Hughes G R V 1982 Systemic lupus erythematosus. Clinics in Rheumatic Diseases, April 8:1

Rothfield N 1981 Clinical features of systemic lupus erythematosus. In: Kelley W M, Harris E D, Ruddy S, Sledge C B (eds) Textbook of rheumatology. W B Saunders, Philadelphia

III Progressive Systemic Sclerosis

Progressive systemic sclerosis (PSS) is a generalised disorder of connective tissue, predominantly affecting women in the fourth to fifth decade. It results in diffuse fibrosis of the dermis (sclero-

Classification of scleroderma

1. *Progressive systemic sclerosis (PSS)*
   a) 'Classic disease'. Diffuse skin involvement and early appearance of systemic disease
   b) Limited skin involvement (fingers and face) with late systemic involvement and prominent calcinosis, Raynaud's, oesophageal dysfunction, sclerodactyly and telangiectasia (CREST variant)
2. *Localised scleroderma*
   Including — Morphea
   — Linear localised scleroderma

Terms used in the description of scleroderma

1. *Sclerodactyly*
   Sclerodermatous changes limited to the digits distal to the MCP and/or MTP joints
2. *Acrosclerosis*
   Sclerodermatous changes limited to the fingers, hands and to a lesser extent the distal parts of the forearms and face
3. *Diffuse scleroderma*
   Skin involvement of proximal extremities and/or trunk with acrosclerosis
4. *Calcinosis*
   Radiological evidence of soft-tissue calcification
5. *Telangiectasia*
   Visible macular dilatation of a superficial blood vessel which empties upon pressure and fills slowly when the pressure is released. It is distinguished from a rapidly-filling spider angioma with a central arteriole and from dilated linear superficial vessels.
6. *Raynaud's phenomenon*
   Episodic pallor and/or cyanosis of part or whole of one or more digits in response to cold exposure or emotion

derma), subdermal tissues and certain internal organs, notably the gastro-intestinal tract, heart, lung and kidney. Raynaud's phenomenon is a regular and frequently early symptom and other vascular abnormalities, affecting chiefly the microcirculation, constitute a common feature of the disease.

Scleroderma, meaning tightness, tethering and induration of the skin, is the hallmark of PSS, but this term is also applied to a heterogenous group of conditions designated collectively as localised scleroderma. This includes morphea and linear localised scleroderma.

The expression of systemic sclerosis is very variable and the spectrum ranges from generalised cutaneous involvement with rapidly progressive and fatal visceral involvement to an indolent form with restricted skin involvement (fingers and face). In some patients skin involvement is absent (scleroderma sine scleroderma).

INCIDENCE

It is an uncommon disease which affects all races and occurs in all parts of the world. It occurs in females four times more commonly than in men, and the peak onset is in the fourth and fifth decade. Although it occurs at any age, it is uncommon in children.

AETIOLOGY

The aetiology of this disease is unknown. Fibrosis of the skin and internal organs, however, result from overproduction of collagen. In rapidly-progressive stages of scleroderma skin collagen contains newly formed labile cross-links consistent with new collagen formation but its composition is identical to normal collagen. In addition to increased synthesis there have been some reports of reduced collagenase activity in involved skin, which may result in decreased degradation.

The cause of collagen overproduction remains a mystery. It has been postulated, however, that a derangement of tryptophan and serotonin metabolism may be responsible. Indirect evidence for such a hypothesis includes: 1. Scleroderma of the trunk and extremities in some children with phenylketonuria; 2. Scleroderma-like changes in some patients with carcinoid; 3. Retroperitoneal fibrosis, sometimes produced by the antiserotonin agent methysergide. No direct evidence for such a disorder exists however.

Endothelial-cell injury is considered by some to be the primary event in this disease. Suggested pathogenetic mechanisms for such injury include 1. immunological mechanisms and 2. a serum component, as yet undefined, selectively cytotoxic to endothelial cells which has been detected in patients with scleroderma.

Immunological mechanisms

Immunological mechanisms may play a role in the pathogenesis. Antinuclear antibodies, often producing a speckled or nucleolar pattern of immunofluorescence are found in virtually all patients. Peripheral lymphocytes from scleroderma patients have been shown to respond *in vitro* to partially-characterised constituents of skin extracts. Other evidence linking scleroderma to immunological events includes: 1. the similarity between the vascular lesions seen in scleroderma with the vascular lesions characterizing chronic homograft rejection; and 2. the observation that a substantial proportion of patients develop scleroderma-like skin lesions 12–18 months after bone marrow transplantation.

PATHOLOGY

The earliest pathological change appears to be vascular, with intimal proliferation, adventitial fibrosis and sometimes fibrinoid degeneration affecting small arteries and arterioles throughout the body. The other characteristic change is progressive fibrosis of the dermis and internal organs.

In the skin, for example, the earliest change is oedema accompanied by perivascular infiltration of interstitial subcutaneous tissues with mononuclear

Organ changes in PSS

General

1. Changes in small arteries and arterioles: intimal proliferation; adventitial fibrosis; fibrinoid degeneration
2. Progressive fibrosis

Skin

1. Early
   Oedema and mononuclear cell infiltrate
2. Later
   Dermal fibrosis; atrophy of epidermis and appendages

Heart

1. Pericarditis
2. Diffuse myocardial fibrosis
3. Intimal proliferation of intramural coronary arteries and 'contraction band' necrosis

Lungs

1. Interstitial fibrosis
2. Bronchiolectasia
3. Involvement of pulmonary arteries and arterioles

Gut

1. Smooth muscle replaced by fibrosis
2. Wide-mouthed colonic diverticula an uncommon but specific finding

Kidney

1. Involvement of small arteries and arterioles and fibrinoid degeneration in glomerular capillary loops
2. Cortical infarcts
3. Small granular kidneys

Muscles

1. Common: extensive perimysial and epimysial fibrosis with muscle-fibre degeneration
2. Uncommon: typical polymyositis

Joints

1. Fibrin covering synovial surfaces
2. Synovial infiltration with mononuclear and plasma cells

cells. Subsequently there is an increase in dermal collagen and late changes include atrophy of the epidermis and appendages. EM and biochemical studies indicate that the collagen is predominantly immature.

CLINICAL FEATURES

1. Presentation

A 'typical' patient is a woman in her 40s who presents with puffiness and stiffness of her fingers, often accompanied by arthralgias, and a history of severe Raynaud's phenomenon for months or years. Less common modes of presentation are polyarthritis, proximal muscle weakness with features typical of polymyositis, or accelerated hypertension. A rare presentation is malabsorbtion in the absence of skin changes (*scleroderma sine scleroderma*).

Clinical presentations of progressive systemic sclerosis

Common
1. Raynaud's
2. Puffiness and stiffness of fingers
3. Arthralgias

Less common
1. Polyarthritis
2. Polymyositis
3. Accelerated hypertension

Rare
1. Malabsorbtion

There are no obvious precipitating factors, though renal involvement has followed operations, dehydration and the administration of corticosteroids and ACTH.

2. Course

The course is unpredictable, but in the majority (60%) diffuse involvement occurs gradually with progression of skin changes from the fingers to the hands, forearms, portions of the lower extremities, face and trunk. The disease follows an indolent course over the next two to three decades. Later in the course symptoms result from progressive visceral involvement, although the hide-bound skin tends to soften after 10–15 years.

In a smaller proportion (20%) skin involvement remains limited to the finger (sclerodactyly) or distal extremities and face (acrosclerosis). In the minority (10%) there is a rapid progression to diffuse scleroderma with early visceral involvement.

3. Involvement of individual organ systems

Systemic manifestations of systemic sclerosis are listed below.

Systemic manifestations of systemic sclerosis

1. Raynaud's	95%
2. Skin	95%
3. Oesophagus	90%
4. Lung	80%
5. Heart	60%
6. Kidney	50%
7. Intestine	30%
8. Joints	25%
9. Muscle	20%

a) Blood vessels

Raynaud's phenomenon affecting the hands and usually the feet is practically universal and may antedate cutaneous changes by several years. Small areas of ischaemic necrosis leaving pitted fingertip scars are common. Abnormalities of the nail-fold capillaries including dilated and distorted capillary loops (p. 261) can be observed with a magnifying glass as one of the earliest findings. A less common occurrence is gangrene of the extremities.

b) Skin

Skin changes occur in 95% and are the hallmark of PSS. Puffy or taut fingers are often the earliest sign of skin involvement and inability to retract the lower eyelid is the earliest indication of facial involvement. As the scleroderma progresses, the

Skin involvement in systemic sclerosis

Early

1. Oedema
2. Thickening and tightening
3. Pruritis

Late

1. Dermal atrophy
2. Loss of hair and dermal appendages
3. Telangiectasia
4. Pulp atrophy of fingertips
5. Ulceration
6. Subcutaneous calcification

skin becomes increasingly taut, shiny, indurated and bound down to underlying structures. There is decreased mobility of the hands, with flexion deformities of the fingers, and the face assumes a pinched look, with radial furrows around the mouth and a reduced mouth aperture. Late features include:

(i) telangiectasia, mainly on the fingers and palms of the hands, the face, lips and tongue
(ii) loss of the pulp of the fingertips
(iii) ulceration of the skin over bony prominences such as the knuckles and medial malleoli
(iv) subcutaneous calcification (calcinosis circumscripta), chiefly affecting the volar aspect of the terminal phalanges and extensor surfaces, e.g. the forearm. The association between subcutaneous calcification and scleroderma was previously recognised as the Thibierge–Weissenbach syndrome.

c) *Oesophagus*

The oesophagus is the most common site of systemic involvement. Hypomotility of the lower two-thirds of the oesophagus occurs in 90% of patients, and in half of these the loss of peristalsis results in symptoms such as heartburn or dysphagia.

d) *Gastrointestinal tract*

Involvement of the gastrointestinal tract may be diffuse, and barium studies have demonstrated dilatation and prolongation of transit time throughout the small and large bowel. Fibrosis of the small bowel with lymphatic obstruction and diminished arterial blood supply may result in malabsorption, abdominal fullness and cramps. Alteration of the bowel flora may add to the problems of malabsorption.

e) *Lungs*

Diffuse interstitial lung disease is the most common pulmonary involvement in systemic sclerosis. Its onset is insidious and initially patients are usually asymptomatic, although some degree of restrictive lung disease or impairment of gas exchange can be detected by pulmonary function tests in most patients. Progressive fibrosis of the lungs occurs in a proportion of patients, leading to cough and dyspnoea after months or years accompanied by basal crepitations and abnormal chest radiographs.

Extensive sclerosis of small pulmonary arteries may occur with or without pulmonary interstitial fibrosis leading to pulmonary hypertension and subsequently cor pulmonale.

Pleurisy causing pain accompanied by a friction rub is uncommon and occurs early in the disease. Silent effusions are more common. A rare late complication is alveolar cell or bronchiolar carcinoma.

f) *Heart*

Diffuse myocardial fibrosis may result in dysrhythmias, including complete heart block and ventricular failure. These tend to be late complications of PSS. Acute asymptomatic pericarditis is a rare manifestation which occurs early in the course of the disease. Small silent effusions are frequently detected by echocardiography.

g) *Kidneys*

Clinical renal disease usually takes the form of highly-malignant arterial hypertension, leading to rapidly-progressive and irreversible renal failure. This is most often seen in patients with diffuse scleroderma within 3 years of onset. Although hypertension and high plasma renin levels are the rule, renal failure occasionally occurs with normal blood pressure.

h) Joints

A true inflammatory polyarthritis may occur, usually early in the course of the disease and predominantly involves small joints (Fig. 7.6). Joint limitation and stiffness in advanced cases of PSS with skin involvement is related to hardening of the skin and underlying tissues. Joint erosions are occasionally seen radiographically and bone changes are predominantly confined to the distal phalanges. These usually consist of osteolysis (Fig. 7.7) which may occasionally be seen elsewhere (mandible and ribs). In many patients characteristic coarse crepitus may be felt over tendons, e.g. the flexor and extensor tendons at the wrist. This has been related to fibrinous deposits on the surfaces of tendon sheaths and overlying fascia.

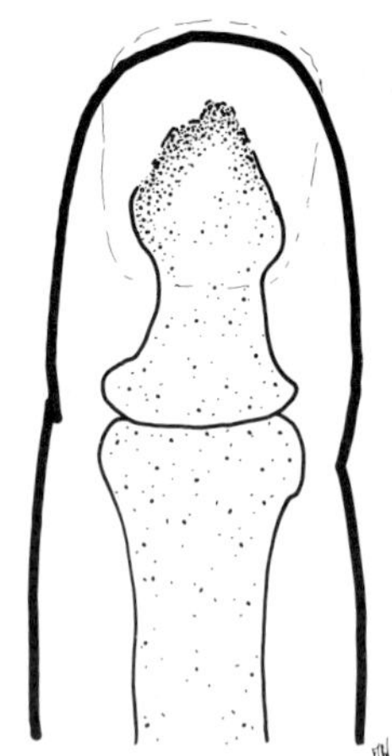

Fig. 7.7 Osteolysis of the distal phalanx

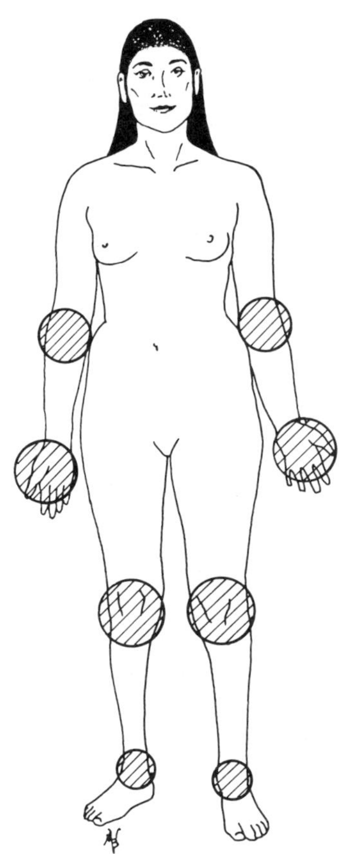

Fig. 7.6 Distribution of arthritis in systemic sclerosis

i) Other features

An inflammatory myositis indistinguishable from polymyositis may accomapny PSS. Dry eyes and dry mouth may result from fibrosis of lacrimal and salivary glands, but a true Sjögren's syndrome may develop, with lymphocytic infiltration of these organs.

LABORATORY ABNORMALITIES

The ESR and specific acute-phase reactants such as CRP are often normal. A micro-angiopathic haemolytic anaemia often accompanies renal disease. Otherwise, anaemia usually reflects visceral involvement and its complications such as malabsorption and renal failure. The white cell count and differential are usually unremarkable and the presence of eosinophilia points to the diagnosis of eosinophilic fasciitis.

Serological findings are common. These include antibodies which are characteristically found in PSS but not in other connective-tissue diseases, such as anti-centromere antibody and antibody to a soluble nuclear antigen, Scl-70.

Serological findings in systemic sclerosis

1. Hyperglobulinaemia	50%
2. ANA	90%
3. Anti-centromere antibodies	30%
4. Anti-Scl-70 antibodies	20%

DIAGNOSIS

The diagnosis is simple when advanced fibrotic changes are present in the skin and visceral organs. Early in the course of the disease, however, diagnosis may be very difficult. Helpful pointers to an early diagnosis are shown below.

Aids to early diagnosis of PSS

Clinical

1. Scleroderma proximal to MCPs
2. Skin biopsy
3. Abnormal pulmonary function tests
4. Abnormal oesophageal motility

Serological

1. High titres of anti-nucleolar antibody
2. Anti-centromere antibody
3. Anti-Scl-70 antibodies

The presence of sclerosis of the skin proximal to the MCPs is highly suggestive of scleroderma. Biopsy of early skin lesions shows characteristic changes. Asymptomatic involvement of internal organs, especially the lungs and oesophagus, is very common in early stages of the disease. Oesophageal dysmotility can be demonstrated by barium swallow performed with the patient in a recumbant position, or oesophageal manometery, in virtually all patients. Serological findings may be helpful. High titres of antibodies to the nucleolus detected by immunofluorescence are rarely found other than in systemic sclerosis and antibodies highly specific for scleroderma such as anti-centromere antibody and anti-Scl-70 can be found in half the cases.

VARIANTS AND DIFFERENTIAL DIAGNOSIS

1. Crest syndrome

C = *c*alcinosis
R = *R*aynaud's
E = o*e*sophageal dysfunction
S = *s*clerodactyly
T = *t*elangiectasia

The CREST syndrome denotes patients in whom scleroderma is limited to sclerodactyly and is accompanied by prominent Raynaud's phenomenon, calcinosis and telangectasia. Raynaud's phenomenon accompanied by puffy fingers is the initial manifestation and it may be decades before other features become apparent. Attention was given to this form because of its indolent course and better prognosis. Except for oesophageal dysfunction, systemic involvement is not prominent for many years, but it is now known that pulmonary hypertension leading rapidly to cor pulmonale can be a devastating late complication in this subgroup.

Anticentromere antibody is found in two thirds of these patients but is found only rarely in patients with diffuse scleroderma.

Primary biliary cirrhosis can be associated with the CREST variant.

2. Diffuse eosinophilic fasciitis

Diffuse eosinophilic fasciitis, described by Shulman in 1975, is now considered to be a variant of scleroderma. It predominantly affects young adult males, when induration of the skin of the extremities and trunk, accompanied by pain, swelling and tenderness, occurs sometimes after a history of recent heavy exertion. There may be marked eosinophilia (up to 50% of the granulocytes) and hypergammaglobulinaemia. The diagnosis is made by a deep wedge biopsy including skin, fascia and muscle which shows infiltration of the subcutaneous space with mononuclear cells with or without eosinophils and dense fibrosis of the deep fascia. These patients do not develop Raynaud's phenomenon or systemic features of PSS. However, carpal tunnel syndrome may occur with a synovitis and/or tenosynovitis and occasionally the subsequent occurence of aplastic anaemia has been reported. It responds to corticosteroids but may resolve spontaneously.

3. Drug-induced scleroderma-like conditions

Some workers exposed to vinyl chloride have developed Raynaud's phenomenon, localised scleroderma-like changes on the dorsum of the hands, fingers and forearms and osteolysis of the distal phalanges accompanied by hepatic portal fibrosis, splenomegaly and pulmonary fibrosis. The antimitotic agent bleomycin may also cause scleroderma-like changes and pulmonary fibrosis.

A proportion of patients who developed Spanish oil disease in 1981 after ingesting contaminated rapeseed oil (p 330) showed chronic progression with the development of scleroderma-like changes affecting the face and limbs. They also developed pulmonary fibrosis and pulmonary hypertension, with widespread vascular changes demonstrated histologically. The precise nature of the toxic agent is not known, but hypotheses include acetanilide contamination of the oil which reacted with fatty acids to produce toxic oleoani lides, and vinyl chloride contamination from the plastic containers.

4. Localised scleroderma

In morphea, well-circumscribed indurated plaques of varying size occur at any site and become sclerotic with ivory-coloured centres and violaceous borders. This occurs at any age but most commonly in children and young adults.

Linear localised scleroderma also starts most commonly in childhood with linear streaks of sclerosis involving the skin and underlying muscle and bone, usually involving an upper or lower extremity or the fronto-parietal area of the forehead and scalp (*coup de sabre* lesion).

These conditions may be associated with arthralgias, but there is no convincing evidence of transformation of localised scleroderma to PSS with visceral involvement.

Certain rare conditions which produce scleroderma-like changes are listed above. These lack the visceral component of PSS and display their own characteristic diagnostic features. Scleroedema is a rare self-limiting condition, which occurs mainly in children but also in adults, in which symmetrical oedematous induration of the skin of the face, scalp, neck, trunk and proximal portion of the extremities follows an infection, particularly a streptococcal throat infection. This condition resolves spontaneously in 6–12 months.

Variants and differential diagnosis of PSS

Variants of scleroderma

1. CREST syndrome
2. Eosinophilic fasciitis
3. Drug-induced conditions
   a) Polyvinyl chloride disease
   b) Bleomycin-induced fibrosis
   c) Spanish oil disease

Localised scleroderma

1. Morphea
2. Linear localised scleroderma

Conditions producing 'scleroderma-like' changes

1. Scleroedema
2. Scleromyxoedema
3. Phenylketonuria
4. Carcinoid syndrome
5. Porphyria cutanea tarda
6. Cutaneous amyloidosis
7. Werner's syndrome
8. Progeria
9. Diabetic cheiroarthropathy

TREATMENT

The number and variety of therapies attempted in PSS testifies to the failure to find adequate treatment for the underlying pathological process in this disease.

To date the most effective management is aimed at symptomatic relief. In addition to avoiding exposure of the hands to the cold, the mainstay of treating Raynaud's phenomenon has been the use of agents which block sympathetic vasoconstriction. These generally give disappointing results, but measures such as intravenous reserpine, infusions of low-molecular-weight dextran and infusions of prostaglandin E_1 can help to heal indolent ulcers. Fibrinolytic agents such as stanozolol, calcium-channel blocking drugs such as nifedipine and antagonists of serotonin such as ketanserin are currently under review for Raynaud's phenomenon. Metoclopramide helps oesophageal dysfunction in some patients by stimulating oesophageal peristaltic activity and increasing low oesophageal sphincter pressure. Broad spectrum antibiotics have proved helpful in some cases of malabsorption. Non-steroidal antiinflammatory agents are helpful in the symptomatic control of articular symptoms.

Hypertension should be vigorously treated to protect renal function. Potent new anti-hypertensive beta-blockers are effective agents and drugs that specifically block renin such as captopril also show great promise. Occasionally, bilateral nephrectomy has been life-saving. Once renal failure has occurred haemodialysis is required. Kidney transplantation has not generally been successful.

No drug has been shown to reduce fibrosis of the skin or other organs in adequately controlled trials and this is true for D-penicillamine and colchicine, agents which have received attention in recent years. There is evidence, however, from retrospective studies that penicillamine might retard progression of the disease and improve patient survival. Corticosteroids should generally be avoided but may be required in cases with associated myositis. The use of immunosuppressive drugs and forms of treatment such as plasmapheresis are still in the investigative stage.

PROGNOSIS

The prognosis of this disease is very variable and depends entirely on the degree of visceral involvement. The overall 5-year survival is 70% and the commonest causes of death are due to kidney and lung involvement. Pulmonary hypertension leading to cor pulmonale is liable to occur as a late feature in patients with the CREST variant.

The prognosis is worst in those who develop the disease under the age of 50 and in those who develop clinical involvement of the heart, lungs and kidney early in the course of the disease. Malignant hypertension followed by oliguric renal failure was previously uniformly fatal but this outcome has been modified by the availability of new and potent antihypertensive agents and of improved haemodialysis procedures.

FURTHER READING (Progressive systemic sclerosis)

Rodnan G P 1978 Progressive systemic sclerosis. In: Samter M(ed) Immunological Diseases. Little Brown and Co., Boston, p 1109–1141

LeRoy E C 1981 Scleroderma. In: Kelley W M, Harris E D, Ruddy S, Sledge C B (eds) Textbook of rheumatology. W B Saunders, Philadelphia, pp 1211–1277

IV Polymyositis and Dermatomyositis

INTRODUCTION

Polymyositis is an uncommon clinical syndrome, chiefly occurring in the middle-aged, in which weakness is accompanied by inflammatory changes within muscles. In the presence of a characteristic skin rash the term *dermatomyositis* is applied. Polymyositis or dermatomyositis may occur alone or may be associated with underlying malignancy or with another connective-tissue disease.

Classification of polymyositis and dermatomyositis

1. Adult polymyositis	33%
2. Adult dermatomyositis	33%
3. Myositis associated with malignancy	8%
4. Childhood poly- or dermatomyositis	6%
5. Myositis accompanying other connective tissue diseases	20%

Several different ways of classifying this group of disorders have been suggested. While no method is completely satisfactory, the simple classification given (on p 121) has much to recommend it. Classifications such as this do not suggest that each of the groups is a distinct entity, since it must be emphasised that there is considerable overlap between these groupings, but are proposed in order to focus on some of the characteristic features of each group.

INCIDENCE

These uncommon conditions can occur at any age and have been reported in children of 2 and in old people in their ninth decade. Most cases occur between the fifth and sixth decades and the overall sex incidence is in favour of women 2:1. The precise incidence is unknown but in England approximates 3 per million annually. Of the primary myopathies affecting proximal muscles, polymyositis is more common than muscular dystrophy in adults but much less common in children.

AETIOLOGY

The cause and pathogenesis of these disorders are not known. Multiple factors may be involved. However, viruses and immunological abnormalities are promising areas for further research.

Viral aetiology

Support for a viral theory comes from the observation of possible myxovirus or picornavirus-like particles in involved muscle, and the clinical association of certain infections with a myositis. Isolation of coxsackievirus from involved muscle has been reported in a few isolated and rather unusual cases of polymyositis. This has not been achieved in typical cases of polymyositis or dermatomyositis. Since some species of coxsackievirus have affinity for muscles resulting in myocarditis or epidemic pleurodynia this connection requires further investigation.

Infections associated with myositis

1. *Bacterial*
   a) *Cl. welchii*: gas gangrene
   b) *Cl. tetani*: tetanus
   c) Staphylococci: septic myositis
   d) *M. leprae*: leprous myositis
2. *Viral*
   a) Rubella
   b) Epidemic pleurodynia
   c) Post-influenza
   d) Infectious mononucleosis
3. *Parasites*
   a) *Trichinella spiralis*
   b) Cysticercosis
   c) Toxoplasmosis
   d) Schistosomiasis
   e) Sarcosporidiosis

Other organisms have been implicated and an association between some cases and toxoplasma has been suggested by the finding of raised toxoplasma antibodies in a large proportion of one series of patients with poly or dermatomyositis.

Immunological factors

Auto-antibodies are commonly found in the sera of patients. Some, such as antimyosin antibody, are nonspecific while others such as antibodies to a soluble nuclear constituent termed Jo-1 (see later), are very disease-specific. Vascular deposits of immunoglobulin and complement have been reported in biopsies of muscle and other involved organs in cases of childhood polymyositis and this raises the possibility of humoral mechanisms in pathogenesis. There is even scantier evidence for humoral mechanisms in adult disease, either immune-complex-mediated or organ-specific. Evidence points, however, to an important role for cell-mediated immunity. Several investigators have shown that peripheral mononuclear cells from patients proliferate in response to muscle antigens and that the degree of response is directly proportional to the degree of disease activity. Peripheral blood lymphocytes are also shown to be myotoxic *in vitro*. The model of experimental allergic myositis adds support to the role of lymphocytes in the pathogenesis of polymyositis. In this model, animals develop myositis after immunisation with skeletal muscle antigens and adjuvant. Lymphocytes from immunised animals are shown to be cytotoxic.

Immunogenetic studies have shown associations with the B-cell alloantigen HLA DR3. An association with C3 deficiency has also been reported.

PATHOLOGY

Changes of inflammation and regeneration are seen in skeletal muscle. Widespread atrophy and degeneration of types 1 and 2 muscle fibres are seen, together with hyalinization, swelling, vacuolation and disruption of muscle cells. Simultaneously, some muscle-cell regeneration occurs, reflected by basophilia, large vesicular nuclei and prominent nucleoli. An inflammatory cell infiltrate is also seen, most prominent around vessels but also, to a lesser extent, between muscle fibres. Lymphocytes predominate with a moderate mixture of histiocytes and occasional plasma cells, polymorphs and eosinophils.

In the skin the picture is very similar to SLE, with epidermal atrophy, liquefaction degeneration of the basal layer of the epidermis, and infiltration of the dermis with mononuclear cells.

CLINICAL FEATURES

Muscle weakness is the principal manifestation and the most common presentation is symmetrical weakness of proximal muscles and anterior neck flexors which may progress over weeks or months with or without dysphagia or respiratory muscle involvement.

Presenting clinical features are summarised below. Rash distinguishes patients with dermatomyositis; otherwise the spectrum of muscle disease is similar in each disease subgroup.

Presenting clinical features of polymyositis

Common
1. Proximal muscle weakness
2. Rash
3. Myalgias
4. Arthralgias

Uncommon
1. Dysphagia
2. Raynaud's
3. Sclerodactyly

Adult polymyositis

In typical cases of adult polymyositis, muscle weakness begins insidiously either in the lower (most common) or upper limbs, chiefly affecting the proximal muscle groups. Rare cases develop acutely, with myoglobinuria, but most occur over weeks or months. Very occasionally the onset is insidious developing over 5–10 years, making the differential diagnosis from muscular dystrophy very difficult. However, the specific pattern of muscle weakness seen in muscular dystrophy is not seen. Early symptoms include difficulty in climbing stairs and arising from a chair, clumsy gait and difficulty in raising arms and combing the hair. In approximately half the cases weakness is accompanied by pain and tenderness. The distribution of weakness is usually symmetrical and diffuse and shows a considerable range of severity. Weakness of the neck flexors occurs in 30%, 4% have significant respiratory embarrassment and 4% have significant bulbar weakness producing dysphagia and dysphonia. The pattern of muscle involvement is seen in Table 7.5. Ocular muscles are virtually never involved. Advanced cases may show atrophy and sometimes there is widespread subcutaneous calcification (calcinosis universalis).

General malaise and loss of weight are common. Features such as Raynaud's, polyarthralgias and symmetrical polyarthritis occur in approximately 20% and sometimes it is difficult to differentiate such involvement in polymyositis from a co-existent connective tissue disease. ECG abnormalities occur in 50%, usually non-specific T-wave changes or S-T segment abnormalities. Heart involvement is occasionally symptomatic, resulting in dysrhythmias and heart failure. Pulmonary fibrosis some-

Table 7.5 Pattern of muscle involvement in polymyositis (after DeVere et al)

Site of weakness		% of patients
Upper limbs:	proximal	86
	proximal and distal	39
Lower limbs:	proximal	92
	proximal and distal	32
Neck:	flexors	47
	extensors	14
Respiratory muscle weakness		4
Bulbar		6
Facial		4
Muscle tenderness		43
Muscle atrophy		40
Contractures		11

times occurs and on rare occasions dominates the clinical picture.

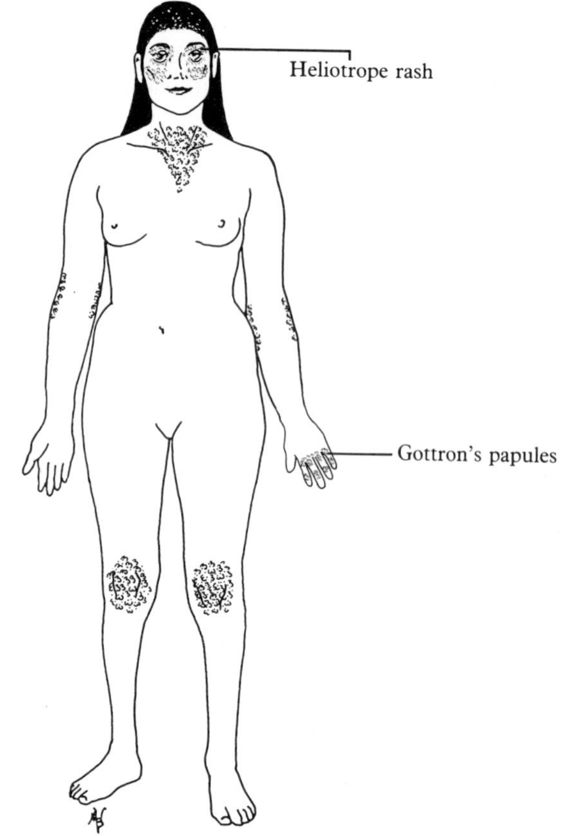

Fig. 7.8 Distribution of rash in dermatomyositis

Dermatomyositis (Fig. 7.8)

Dermatomyositis is a recognisable syndrome characterised by rash, especially a purplish dusky rash on the eyelids (heliotrope), cheeks and other light exposed areas, with periorbital oedema. A scaly erythematous dermatitis may also be seen on the extensor surfaces of the knuckles, elbows and knees and on the medial malleoli. Slightly elevated plaques (Gottron's papules) may develop over the knuckles, and linear streaks may occur on the back of the hands and fingers. Hyperaemia of the nailfold is very characteristic. During active phases of the disease plaques often become tender and elevated, while in quiescent periods they become whitened and atrophic.

Malignancy

Polymyositis is associated with an underlying malignancy in about 8% of cases. This association occurs mainly in the middle aged (representing approximately a tenfold greater frequency of malignancy than in the general population), and is highest in men over the age of 50 with dermatomyositis when the frequency of associated malignancy may be as high as two-thirds. In practice, investigations for occult malignancy should be performed in those patients over the age of 50.

Carcinoma of the lungs, ovary and breast are the tumours most commonly found in association, but a variety of other neoplasms have been reported including lymphoma, Hodgkin's disease and both benign and malignant thymomas. Muscle weakness usually antedates the appearance of the tumour by 1–2 years. Skin changes occur more commonly than not; otherwise there are no distinguishing clinical features between those with and those without malignancy. Not surprisingly, the prognosis is worse in this group due to the effects of malignancy, not the underlying muscle condition. There are the occasionaly reports of remission of the myositis following tumour removal.

Childhood poly- and dermatomyositis

These disorders occur most commonly in children between the ages of 4 and 10. In most cases there is little difference between the childhood and adult form of the disease. Extensive subcutaneous and muscular calcification, however, is seen more commonly in the childhood disease. There is a smaller subgroup of childhood myositis, with a more severe disease characterised by rapidly-progressive weakness accompanied by vasculitis which may result in fatal gastrointestinal complications such as haemorrhage or perforation.

Overlap syndromes

Systemic sclerosis is the most common connective tissue disease to be associated with myositis (50% have myositis) with SLE next (10%) and rheumatoid arthritis, Sjogren's syndrome and polyarteritis nodosa less commonly.

VARIANTS OF POLYMYOSITIS

Occasionally typical skin lesions occur without evidence of myositis (amyopathic dermatomyositis). On rare occasions poly- or dermatomyositis is dominated by the clinical features of diffuse interstitial fibrosis.

Focal nodular myositis

Focal nodular myositis is an uncommon variation of polymyositis when it presents as focal nodules which require differentiation from skeletal muscle tumours. This condition may remain localised although cases showing evolution to more typical diffuse polymyositis have been reported.

LABORATORY FINDINGS

The erythrocyte sedimentation rate and serum gammaglobulin levels are inconsistently elevated. Rheumatoid factor, anti-nuclear antibodies and false positive tests for syphilis are occasionally seen but offer no help diagnostically.

Antibodies to myosin can be demonstrated in 75% but this is a non-specific finding also found in other forms of muscle disease. Recently auto-antibodies to partially characterised cellular antigens including Jo-1, Mi-1 and PM-1 have been identified in the sera of about half the patients and are reported to be specific for polymyositis or overlap syndromes between polymyositis and systemic sclerosis (Table 7.6).

Table 7.6 Auto-antibodies characteristic of polymyositis

Antibody	disease
Anti-Jo-1	Polymyositis
Anti-Mi	Polymyositis
Anti-Ku	Polymyositis–PSS overlap
Anti-PM1	Polymyositis–PSS overlap

Serum muscle enzymes

Elevation of serum levels of muscle enzymes including creatine phosphokinase (CPK), aldolase and transaminases is valuable both for diagnosis and for following clinical activity and response to treatment. CPK is an especially sensitive indicator of muscle fibre damage. During treatment a decrease in CPK levels may precede clinical improvement by three to four weeks. Likewise, relapses may be heralded by elevated levels, sometimes as much as six weeks before the clinical deterioration is detected. Enzyme levels are not infallible guidelines, however. Sometimes they remain within normal levels despite active myositis. This is particularly true in long standing cases where muscle atrophy is extensive.

When available, measurements of urinary excretion of creatine and serum levels of myoglobin using sensitive techniques such as radioimmunoassay may be helpful in monitoring disease activity. Both represent nonspecific indicators of muscle damage.

Electromyography

The triad of 1. polyphasic short small motor-unit potentials, 2. spontaneous fibrillation, and positive sharp waves with increased insertional irritability and 3. bizarre, high-frequency repetitive discharges is particularly suggestive of polymyositis and dermatomyositis. In 10–15% of cases these changes cannot be elicited from proximal muscles. In such cases it is important to check the paraspinal muscles.

Muscle biopsy

The muscle to be biopsied, preferably the quadriceps or deltoid muscle, should be clinically involved but not too atrophic. Since involvement is symmetrical, a clinically-abnormal muscle can be confirmed by EMG and the same muscle on the opposite side used for biopsy to avoid artefactual changes produced by the electrode. Frequent findings are shown below. Involvement is often patchy and this may account for a negative biopsy in 20%. Because of this, open biopsy is usually used but needle biopsy is less traumatic and has been claimed to yield very good results. In a recent study needle biopsy of the vastus lateralis muscle proved to be a sensitive diagnostic procedure and if histological changes were added to morphometric changes the two parameters gave more than 90% positivity.

Common findings at muscle biopsy in polymyositis

1. Degeneration of muscle fibres	83%
2. Mononuclear cell infiltrate	75%
3. Variation in cross-sectional diameter	73%
4. Necrosis of muscle fibres	59%
5. Regeneration	44%
6. Fibrosis	21%
7. Phagocytosis	19%

DIAGNOSIS

The criteria for diagnosis of these disorders are shown below. In the absence of generally-accepted criteria for diagnosis, Bohan and Peter proposed the following:

Criteria for diagnosis of polymyositis

1. Proximal muscle weakness
2. Typical muscle biopsy changes
3. The triad of EMG abnormalities
4. Elevated serum levels of muscle enzymes
5. Characteristic rash

1. Definite dermatomyositis, at least three criteria plus the rash
   Definite polymyositis, four criteria (without the rash)
2. Probable dermatomyositis, two criteria plus the rash
   Probable polymyositis, three criteria (without the rash)
3. Possible dermatomyositis, one criterion plus the rash
   Possible polymyositis, two criteria (without the rash)

Differential diagnosis

Polymyositis must be differentiated from any disease that affects skeletal muscle.

Acute and subacute myositis can be precipitated by a variety of known infectious agents, listed on p 122. Bacteria cause an acute focal suppurative myositis while viruses and parasites may cause a diffuse myositis which may resemble polymyositis clinically and pathologically.

The major causes of weakness which must be differentiated from polymyositis are disorders of the peripheral and central nervous system, and muscular dystrophy. Polymyositis is not accompanied by neurological abnormalities and the former can be excluded by careful examination and the results of laboratory investigations.

The distinction from muscular dystrophy may be much more difficult. A familial history and slow insidious onset suggests muscular dystrophy while global weakness including the neck flexors and the presence of systemic disease suggests polymyositis. The EMG and biopsy findings can be identical, however, and in some cases it is impossible to distinguish between these conditions and a trial of steroids may be needed.

Differential diagnosis of polymyositis

1. *Disorders of peripheral and central nervous system*, including:
   a) Denervating condition e.g. motor neurone disease
   b) Peripheral neuropathies
   c) Carcinomatous neuromyopathy
   d) Disorders of neuromuscular function, e.g. myasthenia gravis
2. *Muscular dystrophies*
3. *Drug-induced myopathy*, including:
   a) Corticosteroids
   b) Chloroquine
   c) Penicillamine
4. Endocrine myopathies, including:
   a) Hypo- and hyperthyroidism
   b) Acromegaly
   c) Cushing's disease
   d) Addisons's disease
   e) Hypo- and hyperparathyroidism
   f) Osteomalacia
   g) Hypokalaemia
   h) Hypocalcaemia
5. Polymyalgia rheumatica
6. Infections of muscle

Corticosteroids, especially fluorinated compounds, may cause a proximal myopathy. It should be remembered that corticosteroid myopathy can occur in patients receiving high doses of prednisolone therapy for dermato- or polymyositis. This should be considered if a patient on long-term treatment begins to weaken without concomitant increase in the CPK level. A muscle biopsy will show type 2 fibre atrophy rather than inflammatory changes.

Endocrine myopathies, for example chronic thyroid myopathy, are rare causes of muscle weakness but closely mimic the distribution of weakness seen with polymyositis.

Polymyalgia rheumatica causes pain and stiffness of the proximal muscles but can be distinguished from polymyositis by the absence of weakness, absence of muscle enzyme changes or changes on muscle biopsy.

TREATMENT

The aims of treatment are to suppress the muscle inflammation, to support vital functions, especially respiration, in severe cases, and to counteract the effects of muscle disease such as weakness and flexion deformities.

Supportive measures

In most cases prolonged management and long-term follow-up are necessary. In the early stages of disease respiratory function, especially vital capacity, should be monitored serially. In some cases assisted ventilation is required. Measures should be taken to avoid aspiration in patients with pharyngeal muscle weakness. During the early stages passive range-of-motion is carried out to prevent contracture of limbs and an active range-of-motion exercise programme is continued by the patient when the disease is suppressed.

Suppression of muscle inflammation

Most cases respond to corticosteroid and/or immunosuppressive agents. This statement is based on clinical observation since there is a lack of control trials of these agents in these conditions.

Corticosteroids

Corticosteroids are considered by many to be the drugs of choice. An initial dose of 1 mg/kg body weight results in improvement in the majority. This dose should be continued for 4–6 weeks followed by gradual reduction to maintenance levels. Alternate-day steroids are often effective in maintaining remission.

Immunosuppressives

Immunosuppressive agents have been shown to be useful adjuvants to prednisolone, especially in those resistant to treatment. A number of studies have shown that intermittent parenteral methotrexate had an important steroid-sparing effect. Azathioprine, cyclophosphamide and chlorambucil have been reported to have similar steroid-sparing effects. These agents have generally been added to prednisolone when the latter has been found to produce an inadequate response after 2–4 months. There have been reports, however, of remissions being induced by methotrexate alone. Control trials are required in the future, since there is one recent report of a double-blind control trial of azathioprine in patients stabilised on prednisolone which failed to show a difference between azathioprine and placebo in reducing the amount of steroid.

Other measures

Isolated cases of patients resistant to other forms of therapy have been improved by plasmapheresis or whole-body irradiation. In some cases associated with malignancy, resection of the primary tumour has resulted in remission of the myositis.

PROGNOSIS

The prognosis has apparently improved with the introduction of steroids. The overall prognosis in recent large studies is 72% survival after 6 years compared with less than 50% before the steroid era. Patients treated early in the course of their illness are expected to improve more than those in whom extensive muscle atrophy has occurred. The highest proportion of deaths occur within the first 2 years after diagnosis; treatment should, therefore, be concentrated on this high risk period.

Prognosis is less good in the elderly and the mortality rate has been shown to be directly proportional to the age of onset of the disease. This is, in part, due to the increased association with malignancy which has particularly ominous prognostic implications.

FURTHER READING (POLYMYOSITIS AND DERMATOMYOSITIS)

Bohan A, Peter J B, Bowman R L, Pearson C M 1977 A computer-assisted analysis of 153 patients with polymyositis and dermatomyositis. Medicine 56: 255

Bradley W G 1981 Inflammatory diseases of muscle. In: Kelley W M, Harris E D, Ruddy S, Sledge C B (eds) Textbook of rheumatology. W B Saunders, Philadelphia pp 1255–1276

V Systemic Vasculitis

Systemic vasculitis is a descriptive term for diseases characterised by inflammation and frequently necrosis of blood vessel walls. It may occur as a separate condition, or may be associated with other diseases, especially connective tissue disorders. A simple classification of these disorders is shown below. While distinct clinicopathological entities such as Wegener's granulomatosis can be recognised it must be emphasised that there is considerable overlap of both clinical and pathological features between the subgroups shown in the table and this method of classification reflects the inadequacy of our knowledge of underlying pathogenic mechanisms.

Vasculitis may involve vessels of different types, sizes and locations (Fig. 7.9) and this results in the broad spectrum of clinical manifestations seen in these disorders.

The aetiology in most cases is not known. The prevailing theory is that these vasculitic syndromes

Classification of systemic vasculitis

1. *Polyarteritis nodosa group*
   a) 'Classical' PAN
   b) Churg–Strauss vasculitis
   c) Wegener's granulomatosis
   d) Cutaneous PAN
2. *Vasculitis associated with connective-tissue diseases*, including
   a) Rheumatoid arthritis
   b) Systemic lupus erythematosus
   c) Systemic sclerosis
   d) Polymyositis
3. *Leukocytoclastic allergic vasculitis*
4. *Large-vessel vasculitis*
   a) Giant cell arteritis
   b) Takayasu's arteritis

are caused by immunopathogenic mechanisms. It is thought that many of these vasculitic syndromes are caused by deposition of immune complexes in blood vessel walls. Indirect evidence that this plays a role includes similarities between these conditions and experimental serum sickness, the presence of hypocomplementaemia and circulating immune complexes and the identification of immunoglobulin and complement in vessel walls in the human disease. There is direct evidence in some cases of PAN associated with hepatitis-B surface antigen (HBAg). HBAg has been reported in the sera in circulating immune complexes and in affected vessel walls in some patients with PAN.

The histopathology of certain types of vasculitis suggest that other types of immunopathogenic mechanisms may be involved in vascular damage besides classical immune-complex mediated injury. For example, cell-mediated immune reactivity may be involved in forms of vasculitis, such as Wegener's, characterised by extra-vascular granulomata.

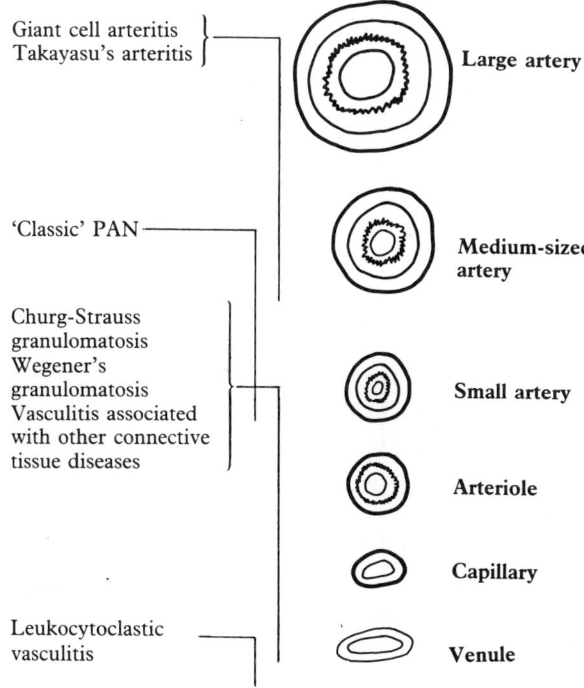

Fig. 7.9 Spectrum of vessels involved in systemic vasculitis

POLYARTERITIS NODOSA GROUP

Included in this category are conditions characterised by widespread vasculitis often with aneurysm (nodosa) formation. Churg-Strauss granulomatosis and especially Wegener's granulomatosis can be recognised as clinicopathological entities distinct from classical PAN. However, many similarities in clinical manifestations, pathology and therapeutic response suggests that they are part of the same disease spectrum.

1. CLASSICAL POLYARTERITIS NODOSA

In 1866 Kussmaul and Maier described the first case of necrotising vasculitis in a patient with widespread inflammation of medium-sized and small arteries and named it *periarteritis nodosa*. In some areas inflammation of the vessel had caused nodules along the course of the artery.

Clinico-pathological features of 'classical' PAN are summarised overleaf.

Incidence

This is a rare disorder: one study in New York City described an incidence of 0.2 cases per 100 000 of the population per year. All age groups are involved but most cases occur between 40 and 60 with males affected twice as commonly as females.

Aetiology

The prevailing theory is that PAN is caused by deposition of immune complexes in blood vessel walls. In a proportion of cases there is good evidence that immune complexes containing hepatitis-B surface antigen (HBAg) are involved. The incidence varies widely in different series from high frequencies (up to 80%) in some parts of the USA, France, Hungary and South America to less than 10% in the UK, Canada and other parts of the USA. It is apparent that other mechanisms are involved. PAN has been described in patients with acute serous otitis media, in association with polychondritis, hairy-cell leukaemia, intravenous

Typical clinico-pathological features of 'classical' PAN

Common features

1. Necrotising vasculitis of small and medium-sized muscular arteries
2. Multisystem disease affecting skin, renal, cardiac, pulmonary, gastrointestinal and peripheral nervous systems
3. Peak age of onset 40–60; Male:Female 2:1
4. Renal involvement
   a) 70% vasculitis; glomerulitis
   b) 10% develop acute renal failure
5. Peripheral neuropathy (60%) mononeuritis multiplex
6. CNS (30%) hemiplegia; seizures
7. Gastro-intestinal (70%) infarction of viscera
8. Hepatic:
   Clinical abnormality in association with HBAg (10–54%); Asymptomatic vasculitis in 50%
9. Hypertension (60%)
10. Coronary arteritis: especially in infants
11. Testicular pain

Uncommon

Allergic history; eosinophilia; granulomata

Differential diagnosis

Other connective tissue diseases; SBE; malignancy: left atrial myxoma

methamphetamine abuse and following hyposensitisation. These conditions may provide clues for identification of further antigens associated with this disease.

Pathology

The cardinal feature is inflammation affecting small and medium sized arteries with a predilection for the site of vessel bifurcation. Fibrinoid necrosis is common and the cellular infiltrate (polymorphonuclear leucocytes in early lesions and later mononuclear cells) involves all three layers of the vessel. The arterial involvement may be segmental, sometimes proceeding to aneurysm formation, or circumferential with massive inflammation leading to occlusion. The major clinical manifestations result from infarction and haemorrhage due to aneurysmal rupture.

Figure 7.10 shows the frequency of different organ involvement in autopsy studies. Renal involvement is very common. In one-third, inflammation of interlobar arteries and arterioles is accompanied by glomerulonephritis. The most typical picture is a necrotising proliferative glomerulonephritis with epithelial crescent formation. Immunoglobulin and complement detected by immunofluorescence is usually absent in contrast to the nephritis of systemic lupus erythematosus.

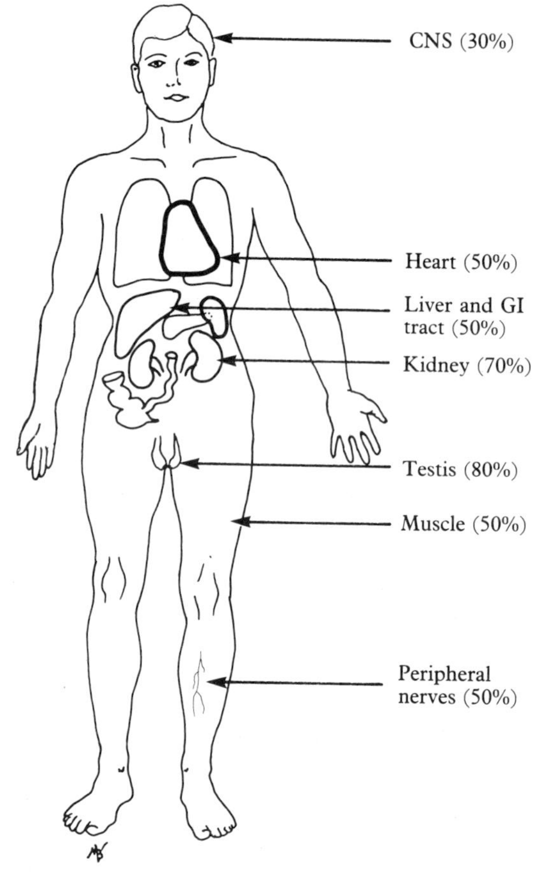

Fig. 7.10 Distribution of organ involvement at post mortem in PAN

Clinical features

1. Presentation

The typical patient is a middle-age man, and the most common presentation is a combination of systemic features such as fever, malaise and loss of weight, together with involvement of one or more of the following systems: skin; kidney; heart; gastrointestinal tract; peripheral nervous system. Initial manifestations, for example, include acute abdomen and mononeuritis multiplex. The subsequent course varies from indolent to fulminating.

Presenting features of systemic vasculitis
1. PUO and weight-loss
2. Nephritis
3. Rapidly-developing hypertension
4. Acute abdomen
5. Myocardial infarction
6. Muscle pain, tenderness and wasting
7. Peripheral neuropathy (predominantly motor)

2. Involvement of individual organ systems (Fig. 7.11)

a) Skin. Cutaneous manifestations include livedo reticularis, cutaneous ulcers and infarcts. Cutaneous nodules originally described by Kussmaul and Maier are rare. A cutaneous form of PAN without visceral manifestations is associated with a good prognosis.

b) Joints. A symmetrical polyarthritis affecting small peripheral joints is common, especially early in the course of the disease. Progression to joint deformity does not generally occur.

c) Gastrointestinal tract. Abdominal pain is common and patients may present as surgical emergencies. Intestinal perforation or infarction are uncommon but usually fatal complications of PAN.

d) Central and peripheral nervous system. Neurological involvement is common, particularly mononeuritis multiplex which is often painful and sudden at its onset and is one of the hallmarks of PAN. Cerebral arteritis and a variety of neuropsychiatric manifestations may also occur.

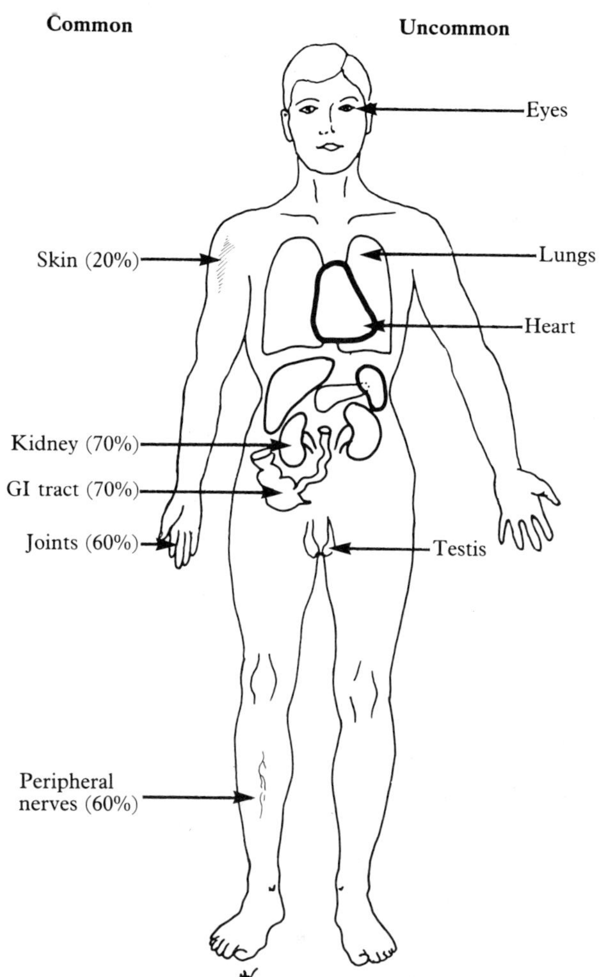

Fig. 7.11 Distribution of clinical organ involvement in PAN

e) Kidneys. Haematuria and proteinura are the commonest manifestation of renal involvement. However, a large proportion develop progressive renal failure, often accompanied by hypertension, which is the commonest cause of death. In 10% renal failure is acute and fulminant.

f) Less common organ involvement. Although the heart is frequently found to be involved at autopsy, clinical involvement including pericarditis, myocardial infarction and dysrhythmias occur less often. Lung involvement characterised by asthma and transient radiographic shadows is relatively rare in classical PAN. Other clinical features include testicular pain, which may affect up to 18% of patients with classical PAN. Vascular involvement of the eye results in visual loss, uveitis, scleritis and conjunctivitis.

Laboratory findings

Laboratory findings are non-specific and reflect the systemic nature of the disease. Normochromic normocytic anaemia an elevated ESR and a polymorphonuclear leucocytosis are present in the majority. Anti-nuclear antibodies and low titres of rheumatoid factors occur in some patients. Hypocomplementaemia is rare except in patients with hepatitis-B-related vasculitis

Diagnosis

The diagnosis of PAN is based on a combination of clinical features and finding necrotising arteritis on biopsy or arterial aneurysms on visceral angiography. Aneurysms are seen in up to 60% of patients with classical PAN.

Clinically involved sites such as the kidney, muscle, testis, skin or sural nerve should be biopsied although visceral angiography prior to renal biopsy has been recommended because of the danger of aneurysmal rupture.

If a clinically-involved organ is not available for biopsy, the following sites may be biopsied "blind' based on their frequent involvement in autopsy studies: kidney (positive in 60%); rectum (positive in 40%); muscle (positive in 30%); liver (positive in 30%); testis (positive in 20%).

Treatment

Vigorous treatment to suppress the disease is required since untreated the prognosis is very poor.

Prednisolone is required in a dose of 1 mg per kg body-weight and, in patients who respond, resolution of aneurysms has been seen on angiography.

Recent reports suggest that cytotoxic drugs, particularly cyclophosphamide should be used in combination with corticosteroid. Plasma exchange may be useful as adjunctive therapy in acute episodes of disease.

Prognosis

Corticosteroids have improved the 5-year survival from 15% (with no treatment) to 50%.

A poor prognosis is associated with severe renal disease, old age at onset and intestinal infarction. Most deaths occur within 3 months. Late deaths may be due to active vasculitis or complications such as chronic renal failure, cerebrovascular disease, cardiac failure and sepsis.

2. CHURG-STRAUSS GRANULOMATOSIS

In 1951 Churg and Strauss described patients with systemic vasculitis who differed from those with 'classical' PAN in features such as a prominent allergic history, particularly asthma, blood eosinophilia and the presence of extra-vascular granulomata, and suggested the term *allergic angiitis and granulomatosis*.

It is rare and predominantly affects middle-aged males.

Typical clinico-pathological features of Churg–Strauss vasculitis

Common features

1. Extravascular granulomata; involvement of capillaries and veins as well as small and medium-sized arteries
2. Peak age of onset 50–60; Male:Female 2:1
3. Allergic history, especially asthma (mean duration prior to vasculitis 8 years)
4. Lung involvement
5. Peripheral eosinophilia ($>1500/mm^3$)
6. Raised IgE in some
7. Otherwise similar to 'classical' PAN

Differential diagnosis

Broncho-pulmonary aspergillosis

Pathology

This condition is characterised by extravascular granulomata and small vessel involvement including capillaries and veins as well as small and medium sized arteries which is unusual in classical PAN.

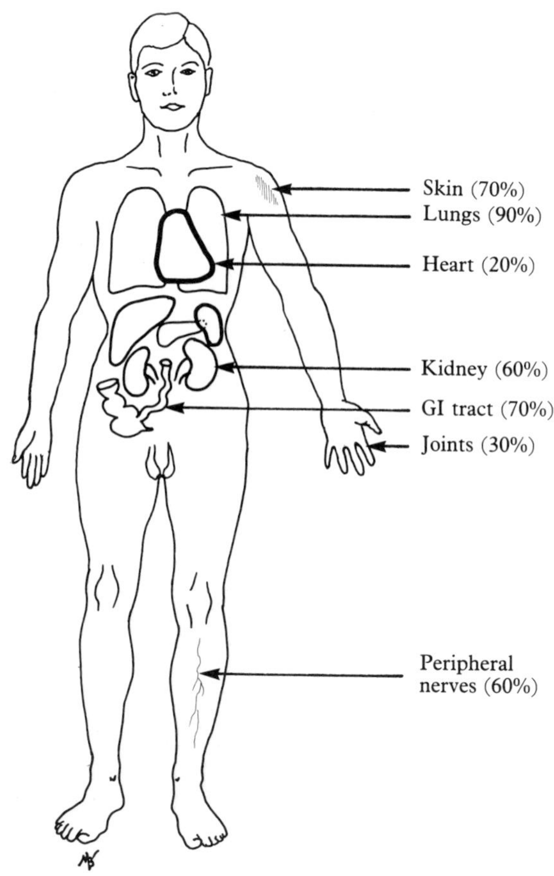

Fig. 7.12 Distribution of clinical organ involvement in Churg–Strauss granulomatosis

Clinical features (Fig. 7.12)

It is the prominence of respiratory tract involvement which distinguishes this condition from classical PAN. Respiratory symptoms are usually the earliest feature, with a history of asthma or, less commonly, allergic rhinitis, preceding the development of systemic vasculitis, often by many years.

The clinical presentation of systemic vasculitis and the pattern of organ involvement is similar to classical PAN. However, chest X-ray abnormalities such as patchy, shifting infiltrates or bilateral nodular densities, are seen in over 50% and renal involvement is less prominent.

Laboratory findings

Eosinophilia is a characteristic finding and absolute eosinophil counts may be as high as 20 000 mm^3. In some patients there is an elevation of IgE levels.

Diagnosis

The clinical diagnosis is based on the combination of systemic vasculitis with an allergic history, non cavitating pulmonary infiltrates and blood eosinophilia. Confirmation of systemic vasculitis is achieved as for PAN.

Treatment

Most patients respond to corticosteroids. Prednisolone is required initially in a dose of 1 mg per kg body-weight. The efficacy of cytotoxic drugs in this condition is not known.

Prognosis

The prognosis of this condition is generally thought to be better than classical PAN with a 5-year survival exceeding 70%. Patients with a short interval between the onset of asthma to the appearance of vasculitis appear to have a worse prognosis.

3. WEGENER'S GRANULOMATOSIS

Wegener's granulomatosis is more easily recognised as a distinct clinical entity. The respiratory tract is always involved, usually without an allergic history, and necrotising granulomata are seen in the nasopharynx, paranasal sinuses and lungs together with a necrotising arteritis of small and medium sized arteries and a segmental necrotising glomerulonephritis.

Clinical features (Fig. 7.13)

The most common presentation is with symptoms referrable to the respiratory tract, especially acute or chronic sinusitis, chronic rhinitis or nasal mucosal ulceration in a combination with consti-

Typical clinico-pathological features of Wegener's granulomatosis

Common

1. Necrotising granulomata in respiratory tract; arteritis of small and medium-sized arteries; glomerulonephritis
2. Mean age of onset 45; Male:Female 2:1
3. Paranasal sinuses: 90% rhinorrhoea and sinus pain
4. Nasopharynx: 75% mucosal ulcers; saddle-nose deformity
5. Lungs: 95% cough; chest pain; haemoptysis; multiple nodular infiltrates, sometimes cavitating
6. Kidney: 90% focal, segmental glomerulitis; necrotising glomerulonephritis
7. Joints: 50% arthralgias
8. Skin: 40%
9. Eyes: 40% keratoconjunctivitis; granulomatous sclero-uveitis
10. Nervous system: 25% mononeuritis multiplex

Uncommon

History of allergy; eosinophilia

Differential diagnosis

Midline granuloma; lymphomatoid granulomatosis

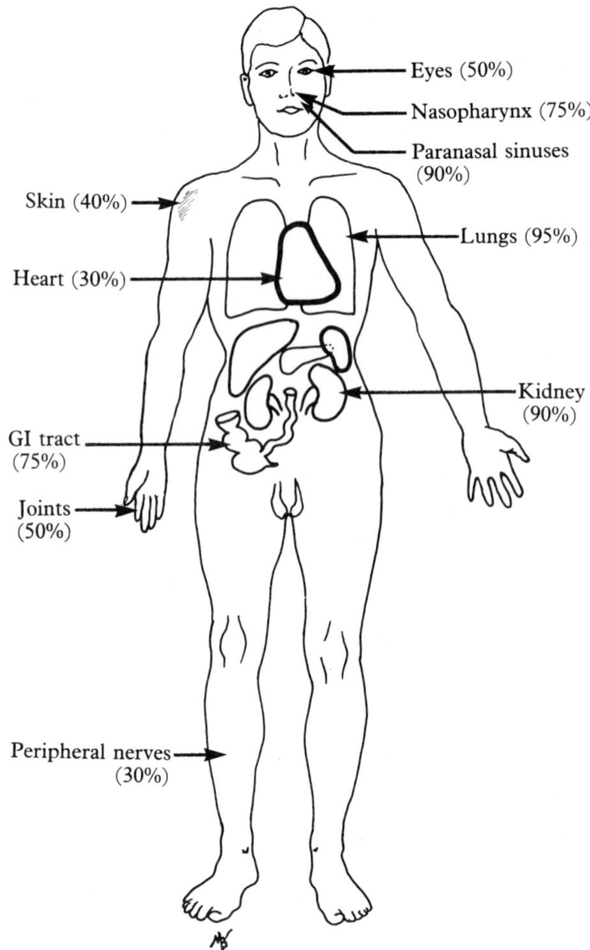

Fig. 7.13 Distribution of clinical organ involvement in Wegener's granulomatosis

tutional features such as fever, malaise and loss of weight. Subsequently lower respiratory tract and renal involvement occur in virtually all patients and often there are features of systemic vasculitis affecting the skin, joints, gastrointestinal tract and neurological system identical to PAN.

a) *Upper and lower respiratory tracts*

Upper respiratory tract involvement occurs in virtually all patients and early symptoms include rhinorrhoea, nasal mucosal ulceration and symptoms of sinusitis. These are accompanied by ulceration of the nasal mucosa and radiological evidence of sinusitis: mucosal thickening and subsequent destruction of bony walls. Lung involvement is nearly always seen in Wegener's granulomatosis and is characterised by symptoms such as cough, haemoptysis, dyspnoea and occasionally pleuritic pain, and pulmonary infiltrates which are usually visualised on the X-ray as multiple nodular opacities which may cavitate.

b) *Kidney*

Clinical renal involvement is not usually an initial manifestation but eventually develops in the majority, with proteinuria and haematuria accompanied by progressive renal failure. Deterioration of renal function is often rapid, but hypertension is not common.

c) Other organ involvement

Systemic vasculitis produces manifestations similar to PAN. Local granulomatous lesions may occur in the orbit of the eye causing proptosis, uveitis or keratitis.

Laboratory findings

Laboratory findings are similar to PAN. Eosinophilia is not a feature as in Churg-Strauss granulomatosis.

Diagnosis

The clinical diagnosis is based on the combination of characteristic clinical features and typical histological findings: necrotising granulomata and vasculitis. Nasal biopsy may be useful for the diagnosis but open lung biopsy may occasionally be necessary.

Treatment and prognosis

Wegener's granulomatosis was almost uniformly fatal, due to renal involvement, before 1960. Corticosteroids were reported to improve some cases but the overall mortality was not affected. Cyclophosphamide (given orally in a dose of 1–2 mg per kg body-weight) has now been shown to be effective and is the treatment of choice in this disease. Many patients benefit from additional short-term corticosteroids for severe skin vasculitis, eye involvement or pericarditis. The dose of cyclophosphamide may be tapered once the patient has been asymptomatic for one year. Total and long lasting remission in this disease has now been reported.

OTHER CLINICAL VARIANTS OF THE PAN GROUPS

1. Localised forms

Necrotising vasculitis of medium-sized arteries has been seen in isolated organs in the absence of systemic disease. Involved organs have included the appendix, gall bladder, uterus and testis. A localised form of cutaneous PAN is reported to have a good prognosis.

Carrington and Liebow described a limited form of Wegener's granulomatosis with pulmonary involvement but no renal complications.

2. PAN associated with HBAg

The clinical features of HBAg-associated PAN are similar to other forms of PAN except for the presence of a variable degree of hepatic dysfunction. There is no constant relationship between the onset of PAN and liver disease.

3. Infantile PAN and Kawasaki's disease (mucocutaneous lymph node syndrome)

PAN is rare in children but when it occurs there is a predisposition towards involvement of the coronary arteries which may result in sudden death.

In 1967 Kawasaki described a well-defined entity, mucocutaneous lymph node syndrome, which is closely associated with infantile PAN. Cases were described in Japan and subsequently in Europe and North America, usually between 6 and 18 months of age, who developed a febrile illness with a macular exanthema accompanied by conjunctivitis, cervical lymphadenopathy, erythema of the mucous membranes of the lips and tongue (strawberry tongue) and subsequent desquamation of the skin of the fingertips. In most cases recovery occurs in 3–4 weeks but 2% die suddenly. Autopsy findings indicate a necrotising vasculitis of the coronary arteries, indistinguishable from infantile PAN.

In some survivors, however, ECG evidence of myocarditis and aneurysms or stenosis of the coronary vessels have been demonstrated.

VASCULITIS ASSOCIATED WITH OTHER CONNECTIVE TISSUE DISEASES

Vasculitis may occur in association with other systemic rheumatic diseases, especially rheumatoid arthritis and SLE.

Systemic vasculitis is a common but well-recognised feature of rheumatoid arthritis. It is usually seen in patients with long-standing nodular and seropositive RA but with a relatively inactive synovitis. The average age of onset is 60 years and men and women are equally affected.

Blood-vessels of all sizes may be affected, particularly small arteries such as the vasa nervorum and the digital arteries. The extent of involvement ranges from small nail-fold, nail-edge, or digital infarcts occurring alone, representing the most common and relatively benign form, to systemic vasculitis resembling PAN.

In the most severe form vasculitic features occur such as cutaneous ulceration, peripheral gangrene and neuropathy. Vasculitic ulcers are deep, painful, punched out, develop suddenly and often affect unusual sites such as the calf and dorsum of the foot. The most common neuropathy is a peripheral sensory neuropathy but mononeuritis multiplex indicates more serious disease and if widespread is associated with a poor prognosis.

Rarer manifestations of vasculitis include coronary arteritis, cerebral vasculitis and intestinal infarction and renal involvement with lesions identical to those of PAN.

Laboratory findings

Most patients have high titres of rheumatoid factor and circulating immune complexes and immunoglobulin and complement have been identified in the walls of the affected blood vessels. Laboratory markers of active vasculitis are IgG rheumatoid factor, anti-complementary activity in the serum and hypocomplementaemia.

Diagnosis

A diagnosis of vasculitis is confirmed by biopsy. The traditional biopsy sites are muscle, sural nerve and skin. Rectal biopsy may be used as a blind biopsy site and evidence of arteritis has been found in 40% of patients with clinical vasculitis.

Treatment

Treatments used in severe rheumatoid vasculitis such as systemic steroids, gold, D-penicillamine and cytotoxic drugs have not given satisfactory results. Experimental forms of treatment including intermittent bolus doses of cyclophosphamide and methylprednisolone given intravenously with or without plasma exchange have given encouraging results and are still being evaluated.

Prognosis

Patients in whom RA is complicated by vasculitis have an increased mortality. Motor neuropathy, severe weight-loss and a positive rectal biopsy are associated with a poor prognosis.

LEUCOCYTOCLASTIC ALLERGIC VASCULITIS (Hypersensitivity vasculitis)

This term refers to a heterogeneous group of clinical syndromes in which vasculitis predominantly involves smaller vessels, especially the post-capillary venule. The characteristic histological feature is infiltration of necrotic vessel walls with polymorphonuclear leucocytes and scattered nuclear debris ('nuclear dust'), hence the term *leucocytoclasis*. A variety of aetiological factors have been implicated, including drug hypersensitivity (sulphonamides, penicillin, thiazides, phenylbutazone), infection (streptococci) and malignancy. The skin is the most common organ involved and often there is no systemic involvement. Cutaneous lesions are usually purpuric, mainly on the lower extremities, buttocks, forearms and hands. The purpura is usually palpable. A variety of other rashes may be seen including papules, nodules, vesicles, bullae, ulcers or urticaria. The condition is usually self-limiting and benign, though occasionally recurrent and chronic.

Leucocytoclastic allergic vasculitis may be associated with the various systemic diseases shown opposite. In addition three clinical syndromes with systemic involvement are characterized by leucocytoclastic vasculitis.

1. Henoch Schonlein Purpura (anaphylactoid purpura) (Fig. 7.14)

This occurs most commonly between the ages of 4–11 but may occur at any age, including the

Conditions associated with leukocytoclastic vasculitis

1. Drugs: incl.	sulphonamides penicillin phenylbutazone thiazides allopurinol phenytoin vaccines animal serum gold barbiturates
2. Infections: incl.	Group A Strep *Staph. aureus* Neisseria Hepatitis B virus CMV
3. CTD: incl.	RA Sjögren's PSS PAN SLE
4. Malignancy: incl.	carcinoma lymphoma Waldenstrom's macroglobulinaemia
5. Miscellaneous: incl.	chronic active hepatitis primary biliary cirrhosis bacterial endocarditis intestinal bypass syndrome

elderly. It is characterised by a combination of purpura, arthritis, glomerulonephritis and abdominal pain.

The majority of cases are thought to be due to hypersensitivity or food allergy and have a good prognosis.

A characteristic pathological finding is the deposition of IgA in the glomerular and cutaneous lesions and IgA containing immune complexes may be detected in the serum.

5–10% have a relapsing and chronic course and a minority may develop severe and permanent renal damage. Steroids have little effect on the renal disease but are reported to improve abdominal symptoms.

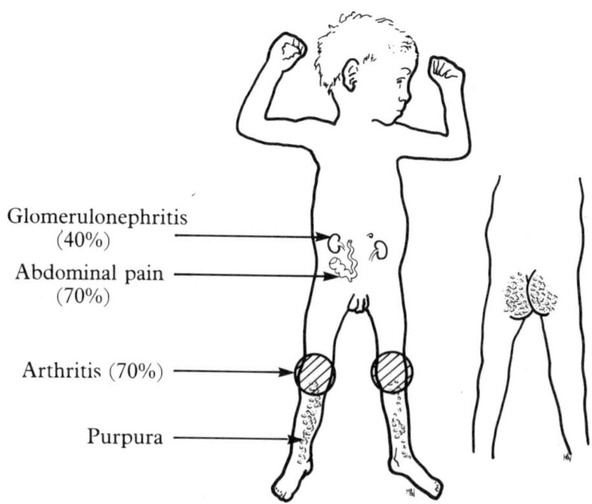

Fig. 7.14 Distribution of clinical organ involvement in Henoch–Schönlein purpura

2. Essential mixed cryoglobulinaemia
(Meltzer–Franklin syndrome)

This uncommon condition occurs predominantly in middle-aged females and shows varying degrees of severity from idolent and mild to fatal (renal failure). The major clinical manifestations are purpura, arthralgia, anaemia, splenomegaly, lymphadenopathy and progressive glomerulonephritis.

The hallmark of this disease is the presence of cryoglobulins containing IgM with rheumatoid factor activity and IgG.

This is considered to be an immune complex disease, and in addition to cryoglobulinaemia there are low complement levels, and immunoglobulin and complement have been demonstrated in the affected vessel walls and glomerular basement membrane.

This is another syndrome associated with hepatitis-B surface antigen, since there are reports that HBAg or antibody to HBAg have been detected in the serum or cryoglobulins in two-thirds of the patients.

Patients who develop severe glomerulonephritis have a poor prognosis and this disease is reported to progress despite corticosteroids or cytotoxic treatment.

3. Hypocomplementaemic vasculitis

In 1973 McDuffie described a rare syndrome in young women characterised by chronic urticaria affecting the face, upper extremities and trunk accompanied by arthralgias and mild renal involvement. Laboratory abnormalities include hypocomplementaemia and C1q binding material in the serum. Renal biopsy shows mild to moderate membranoproliferative glomerulonephritis and immunoglobulin and complement have been demonstrated in the basement membrane.

LARGE VESSEL VASCULITIS

GIANT CELL ARTERITIS

Giant cell arteritis is recognised as an entity with an onset over the age of 55 which classically results in a clinical picture comprising typical headache, constitutional symptoms and fever accompanied by anaemia and high ESR. The vascular lesion predominantly involves the cranial branches of arteries originating from the arch of the aorta. It is now recognised that it may also involve medium-sized and larger arteries throughout the body. There is a strong association with polymyalgia rheumatica (Chapter 12): some suggest that PMR is a manifestation of GCA while others view them as separate entities tending to occur together.

Incidence

The mean age of onset is 70 years and women are affected more than men. The prevalence of giant cell arteritis in the population over the age of 50 is approximately 0.2% and the annual yearly incidence is 10 cases per 100 000 of the population.

Pathology

There is a pan-arteritis which tends to be segmental. In early lesions a mononuclear cell infiltrate occurs in the region of the internal or external elastic lamina or adventitia accompanied by intimal thickening. In more advanced lesions there is necrosis of portions of the artery wall with fragmentation of the elastic lamina and granulomata containing giant cells. Electron microscopy shows giant cells in close proximity to fragments of the elastic lamina.

Clinical features

1. Presentation

The typical presentation is an elderly women who develops a headache in association with systemic features such as fever, malaise, and loss of weight. Symptoms usually develop over weeks but the onset may be abrupt. Sometimes the onset is identical to polymyalgia rheumatica (Chapter 12) and less commonly the initial symptom is blindness. Other forms of presentation are PUO and anaemia.

2. Local manifestations

Local clinical manifestations depend on the artery involved. Headache occurs in two-thirds and is usually severe and often localised to the region of the inflamed artery, though it may be diffuse. Scalp tenderness is common, especially over the temporal artery, and occasionally over the occipital artery. Rarely there is gangrene of the scalp.

Ocular involvement leading to sudden blindness is the most serious complication. This occurs in approximately 20% and although it may be the initial symptom it usually follows other symptoms by several weeks or months and is frequently preceded by transient visual symptoms.

Intermittent claudication of the muscles of mastication on chewing is a pathognomonic feature.

Clinical evidence of large artery involvement elsewhere is found in 15% and includes claudication of the extremities, bruits and diminished pulses in the neck and limbs, carotid sinus sensitivity, and CNS involvement such as hemiparesis and organic brain syndromes. In rare cases, coronary artery involvement causes myocardial infarction.

3. Systemic manifestations

Fever and loss of weight are common. Features of polymyalgia rheumatica occur in half the cases.

Typical features of giant cell arteritis

1. Disease of the elderly; Female:Male 2:1
2. Involves branches of carotid, especially superficial temporal artery, vertebral artery, ophthalmic artery, posterior ciliary artery, but also any medium or large-sized artery
3. Pan-arteritis: giant cells in granulomata; fragmentation of elastic lamina
4. *Clinical features*
   a) Headache associated with classical complex of fever, anaemia, raised ESR
   b) Systemic
      (i) Fever (50%), sometimes PUO
      (ii) Anaemia
      (iii) Reduced weight
      (iv) Abnormal liver-function tests (50%), usually raised alkaline phosphatase
      (v) Polymyalgia rheumatica (40–60%)
   c) Local — depending on arteries involved
      (i) Headache; temporal or occipital
      (ii) Scalp tenderness; rarely necrosis
      (iii) Jaw claudication — pathognomic
      (iv) Sudden blindness
      (v) Aortic arch syndrome
      (vi) Carotid sinus sensitivity
5. *Diagnosis*: temporal artery biopsy — multiple sections as lesions often segmental
6. *Treatment*: steroid-responsive

Laboratory findings

The ESR is almost invariably raised, although there are rare biopsy-proven cases with a normal ESR. A mild to moderate normochromic, normocytic anaemia is common and liver function tests, especially a raised alkaline phosphatase, are abnormal in 50%.

Diagnosis

The diagnosis must be considered in any patient over the age of 50 with a new headache, transient or slight loss of vision, polymyalgia rheumatica, fever, anaemia or an elevated ESR.

Temporal artery biopsy may confirm the diagnosis. It is important to choose a symptomatic or clinically abnormal segment, several centimetres long, and to examine multiple sections. This is because of the segmental involvement. Superficial temporal angiography had been advocated to locate arteritis in a vessel normal to palpation. However, both false positive and false negatives are common in this procedure.

Treatment

Since sudden irreversible blindness can occur, immediate institution of therapy is essential.

This condition is generally steroid responsive. Prednisolone 1 mg per kg body weight is given initially and continued for 2–4 weeks until there is resolution of the symptoms and a fall in the ESR. Subsequently the dose is gradually reduced by no more than 10% of the total every 2 weeks as gauged by the symptoms and ESR. This allows identification of the minimum suppressive dose. In the few patients who are steroid-resistant, the disease can usually be controlled by adding an immunosuppressive agent such as azathioprine. GCA generally follows a self-limited course over several months to several years and steroids can be withdrawn in the majority.

TAKAYASU's ARTERITIS (PULSELESS DISEASE)

Takayasu's arteritis is also a pan-arteritis characterized by inflammation of medium sized and large arteries. However, there are clear-cut differences to GCA in age range, distribution of involved vessels, associated clinical features and response to treatment.

This is a rare disease which predominantly affects females most commonly between the ages of 10 and 30. After its description in Japan cases have been reported from all over the world.

Pathology

There is a predilection for the aortic arch and its branches but it may involve large and medium arteries anywhere, including the pulmonary artery. There is a pan-arteritis with fragmentation of the elastic lamina. A mononuclear cell infiltrate is seen with occasional giant cells. The intima is thickened often with overlying thrombosis and there may be obliteration of the arterial lumen.

Clinical features

This disease tends to have a chronic indolent course. Early or non-specific systemic symptoms such as malaise, arthralgia and weight-loss predominate but later there are features of vascular insufficiency. Important manifestations are tenderness and bruits over the affected arteries (especially brachial, subclavian and carotid) and reduced peripheral pulses. Subsequently there may be claudication of affected extremities and atrophic changes with ischaemic ulcers. Hypertension is common and involvement of the pulmonary artery may result in pulmonary hypertension. Vertigo, syncope, seizures and dementia may develop as a result of reduced cerebral blood-flow. Similarly, features or mesenteric and coronary artery stenosis and occlusion may develop. The diagnosis is confirmed by arteriography. Typical arteriograms show vascular segments with smooth-walled, tapered, focal or prolonged narrowing. These changes are usually most pronounced in the region of the aortic arch and its primary branches.

Treatment

Corcitosteroids are said to suppress the symptoms and reverse arterial stenosis in the early stages of the disease. In later stages, however, arterial surgery may be required. The disease follows an indolent course and in one study the five year survival rate was 85%.

FURTHER READING (PAN)

Alarcon-Segovia D 1980 The necrotizing vasculitides. Clinics in Rheumatic Diseases August 6:2

VI Sjogren's syndrome

INTRODUCTION

Sjogren's syndrome is characterised by the infiltration of the exocrine glands and other organs with lymphocytes and plasma cells leading to destruction and glandular insufficiency. The cardinal features are dryness of the eyes and mouth (the Sicca complex).

The Sicca syndrome may occur alone (primary Sjogren's syndrome) but approximately 50% of cases are accompanied by rheumatoid arthritis (secondary Sjogren's syndrome) and a few have other connective tissue diseases such as SLE and scleroderma.

Classification of Sjogren's syndrome

Primary Sjogren's syndrome — Sjögren's syndrome occurring alone

Secondary Sjögren's syndrome — associated with other diseases, e.g.

1. Rheumatoid arthritis
2. SLE
3. Systemic sclerosis
4. Primary biliary cirrhosis
5. Chronic active hepatitis
6. Polymyositis
7. Thyroiditis

INCIDENCE

Sjogren's syndrome occurs predominantly in women and the highest incidence is between the ages of 40 and 60 years. Its frequency in RA is 20% and therefore Sjogren's syndrome is most commonly seen in this context. Primary Sjogren's syndrome and Sjögren's associated with other conditions occur less commonly.

AETIOLOGY

The aetiology of Sjögren's syndrome is unknown but may involve constitutional and immunological factors.

1. Constitutional factors

Sjogren's syndrome occurs predominantly in women and is one of several auto-immune diseases with an association with the histocompatibility antigen HLA DR3.

2. Immunological factors

Immunological abnormalities include a marked hyperactivity of B-lymphocytes with hyperglobulinaemia and serum autoantibodies, some organ specific such as antibodies to salivary duct epithelium and others non-specific such as antinuclear-antibodies and rheumatoid factor. Impaired cellular immunity with defective suppressor T-cell function has been reported in some patients but not in others.

Both T lymphocytes and B lymphocytes have been identified in the tissue lesions and local synthesis of immunoglobulins have been demonstrated. Since the lymphocyte infiltration has been demonstrated to be initially periductular in location lymphocyte cytotoxicity directed against antigens on salivary gland duct cells has been postulated.

PATHOLOGY

Typical histological findings in the major salivary glands include lymphoid infiltration, acinar atrophy, hypertrophy of ductal, epithelial and myoepithelial cells resulting in what is known as epimyo-epithelial islands. Focal lymphocyte infiltrates with acinar destruction also occurs in minor salivary glands enabling labial biopsies to be used for diagnostic purposes.

In addition to the major and minor salivary glands and the lacrimal glands this disease may affect a variety of other organs and the characteristic lymphoid infiltration also occurs in the nasal cavity, pharynx, trachea, bronchi, sweat glands, vagina and, in severe cases, may involve the lungs, kidney and skeletal muscle resulting in functional abnormalities of these organs.

In some patients lymphoid infiltration is more invasive, leading to pseudolymphoma or even frank lymphoid malignancy.

CLINICAL FEATURES

1. Presentation

The typical case is a middle-aged woman in whom sicca symptoms develop insidiously. Less commonly it presents with parotid swelling or with constitutional symptoms such as malaise and arthralgias. Rarely the presenting feature is cutaneous vasculitis, a cranial neuropathy usually involving the trigeminal nerve, a peripheral neuropathy, or the hyperviscosity syndrome. Sicca symptoms tend to develop more rapidly in primary Sjogren's syndrome, when episodic parotitis and involvement of other organs is more common.

Presenting features in Sjögren's syndrome

Common

Insidious development of Sicca symptoms

Uncommon

1. Parotid swelling
2. Constitutional symptoms: malaise, arthralgias
3. Cutaneous vasculitis
4. Cranial or peripheral neuropathy
5. Hyperviscosity syndrome

2. Involvement of exocrine glands (Fig. 7.15)

Ocular symptoms due to reduced lacrimal secretion and dessication of the cornea and conjunctiva (keratoconjunctivitis sicca) include a gritty or sandy sensation, reduced tearing, photophobia and the presence of a ropey discharge, particularly at the inner canthus. Recurrent infections are also common. In advanced cases the cornea may be severely damaged and complications include corneal ulceration and occasionally perforation.

Decreased saliva results in dryness of the mouth (xerostomia) which leads to dysphagia, abnormalities of taste and adherence of food to the buccal surface.

Widespread involvement of mucosal glands elsewhere may result in dryness of the nose, posterior pharynx, trachea, bronchial tree, skin and vagina. Involvement of the respiratory tract leads to an

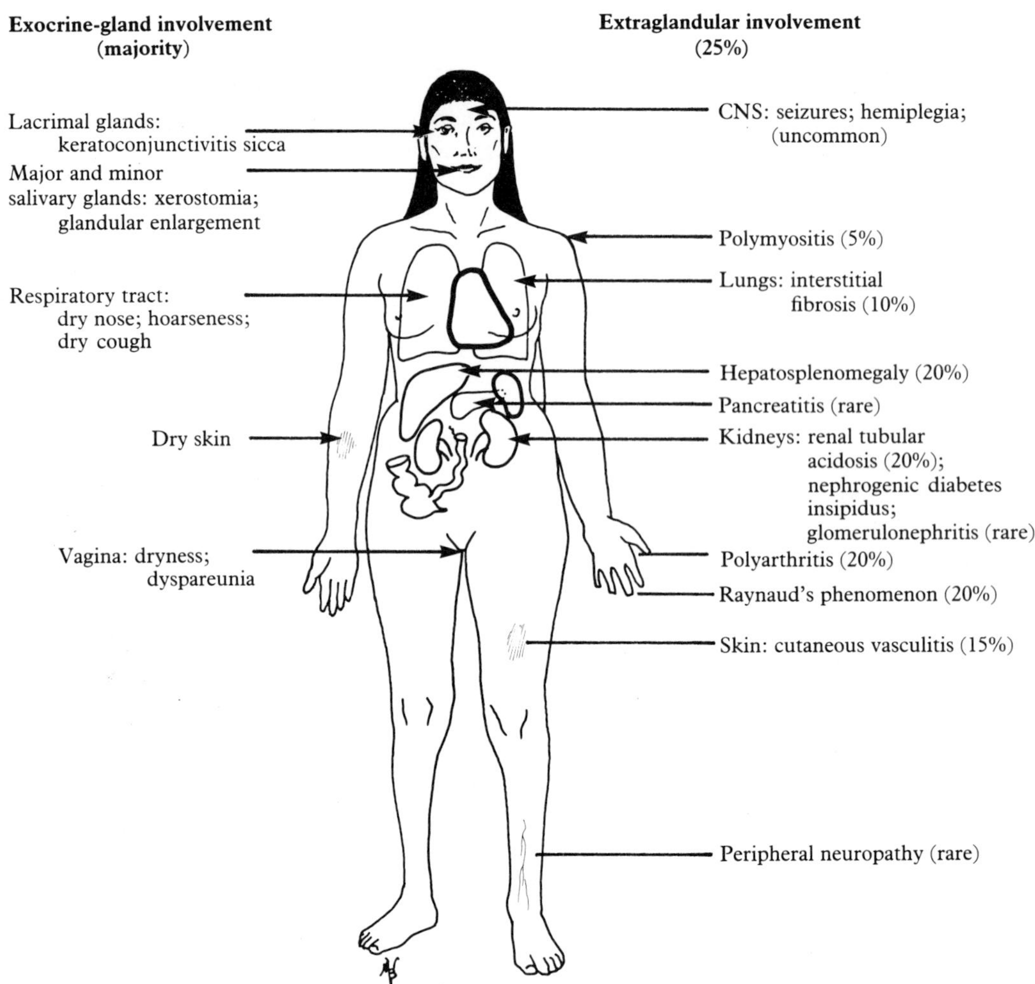

Fig. 7.15 Distribution of clinical organ involvement in Sjögren's syndrome

increased frequency of upper and lower respiratory tract infections and otitis media.

There is parotid gland enlargement in 50% of cases (80% in primary Sjögren's) sometimes accompanied by pain and fever.

3. Extraglandular involvement (Fig. 7.15)

Extraglandular lymphoproliferation occurs in 25% of primary Sjögren's syndrome, and involves the reticuloendothelial system, kidney, muscle and lungs. Systemic manifestations are varied and include diffuse interstitial pneumonitis, renal tubular abnormalities, peripheral and cranial neuropathy, non-thrombocytopenic purpura and the development of pseudomalignant and malignant lymphoid proliferation.

Malignant lymphoma occurs more often than can be explained by chance alone, and Sjögren's syndrome has often been considered to be a link in the spectrum between auto-immune disorders and lymphoproliferative disorders.

LABORATORY ABNORMALITIES (Table 7.7)

Auto-antibodies to salivary duct, gastric parietal

Table 7.7 Serological findings in Sjögren's syndrome

	Primary Sjögren's (%)	Sjögren's with RA (%)
Rheumatoid factor	90	100
ANA	80	70
Anti-Ro (SSA)	70	5
Anti-La (SSB)	50	5
Salivary duct antibody	10	70
Gastric parietal cell antibody	30	30
Thyroglobulin antibody	30	20

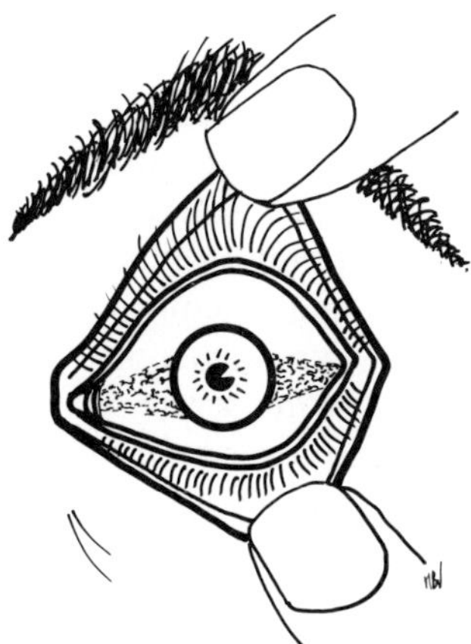

Fig. 7.16 Appearance of cornea after Rose Bengal staining

cells, thyroglobulin, mitochondria and smooth muscle are frequently present. Rheumatoid factor is found in over 90% and anti-nuclear antibodies in approximately 70%. Serum antibodies to two partially-characterised cellular antigens Ro (SSA) and La (SSB) are commonly found in primary Sjögren's syndrome.

DIAGNOSIS

The Schirmer's test is a simple test for dry eyes in which tear production is estimated by placing filter paper strips under the eyelids (less than 5 mm of wetting in 5 minutes indicates dry eyes). The frequency of false-negative and false-positive tests, however, is high. The characteristic signs of keratoconjunctivitis sicca are best seen using a slit lamp after Rose Bengal staining to detect punctate corneal ulceration and attached filaments of corneal epithelium. (Fig. 7.16) Definite KCS can be identified in approximately two-thirds of patients with Sjögren's syndrome.

Lip biopsy of the minor salivary glands is a sensitive diagnostic procedure. Lymphocytic infiltration in the labial glands is similar to that in the major salivary glands and not only appears to be specific to Sjögren's syndrome but also the degree of infiltration correlates with the severity of the disease.

Other methods used to examine the salivary glands include parotid flow measurements, salivary scintigraphy and sialography. Parotid flow measurements and scintigraphy measure salivary gland function. Parotid flow rates are assessed under conditions of maximal gland stimulation with lemon juice. Levels of less than 0.5 ml min are virtually diagnostic of sicca syndrome. Scintigraphy using technetium pertechnetate ($^{99m}TcO_4^-$) is a sensitive technique to demonstrate reduced uptake, concentration and excretion of the radioisotope. Serial scans can be used to assess progression of disease. The technique of sialography involves injecting a radio-opaque contrast medium into the parotid duct to demonstrate the gross distortion of the normal intrasalivary duct system. In Sjögren's syndrome there is marked dilatation of the ductules (sialectasis). This technique is used less often now that simpler methods such as lip biopsy are available.

TREATMENT

Sjögren's syndrome is generally a benign disorder and management is aimed at symptomatic relief and preventing damage due to dry eyes.

Eye symptoms are best treated with the frequent instillation of artificial tears containing methylcellulose. Some recommend the use of soft contact lenses to protect the cornea in severe cases.

Symptoms due to xerostomia are notoriously difficult to treat and simply increasing fluid intake is the most effective way. Careful brushing of the teeth is essential and regular dental supervision may prevent or delay the rampant dental caries which frequently complicates xerostomia.

Severe systemic manifestations occasionally warrant corticosteroid or immunosuppressive therapy. Painful parotid swelling often responds to corticosteroids, and immunosuppressives have been used to treat extra-glandular lymphoid infiltrates associated with severe renal and lung disease. Hyperviscosity syndrome is a complication which may require plasmaphoresis.

The management of associated conditions such as rheumatoid arthritis is not affected by the presence of Sjogren's syndrome, although there may be an increase in drug side-effects in this group of patients.

FURTHER READING (SJÖGREN'S SYNDROME)

Shearn M A 1971 Sjogren's syndrome. Major problems in internal medicine. W B Saunders, Philadelphia

Moutsopoulos H M 1980 Sjogren's syndrome (sicca syndrome). Current issues. Annals of Internal Medicine 92: 212–226

8 Osteoarthritis

Osteoarthritis is one of a number of terms used to describe a condition characterised by: 1. destruction of hyaline articular cartilage and 2. increased activity of subchondral bone.

Synonyms include *osteoarthrosis, degenerative joint disease, arthrosis* and *hypertrophic arthritis*.

The condition is best thought of as 'joint failure' (synonymous with heart failure), and does not described a single disease entity. Thus, although osteoarthritis can be recognised by certain clinical, radiological and pathological features, several different joint conditions can result in these changes.

Classification of osteoarthritis

1. Primary (no known cause)
   e.g. 'generalised' or 'nodal' osteoarthritis
2. Secondary (identifiable predisposition(s) to joint failure)
   a) Predominant local mechanical cause
      e.g. Post-traumatic
      Post-meniscectomy
      Post slipped femoral epiphysis
   b) Predominant metabolic or systemic predisposition
      e.g. Ochronosis
      Haemachromatosis
      Generalised hypermobility
      Familial chondrocalcinosis
      Familial premature OA
   c) Secondary to pre-existing inflammatory rheumatic disease
      e.g. Gout
      Rheumatoid arthritis

CLASSIFICATION OF OSTEOARTHRITIS (OA)

The traditional division of OA is into primary (no known cause) or secondary (obvious predisposing factor) cases. Alternative divisions might be made according to the pattern of disease or the apparent causative factors.

Metabolic diseases, inflammatory joint disease and structural abnormalities can all predispose to OA. Thus severe joint destruction can result from the isolated abnormality of amino-acid metabolism seen in ochronosis; monoarticular OA may follow meniscectomy or a slipped epiphysis; and inflammatory joint disease can result in changes indistinguishable from those of 'primary' OA.

Cases of primary OA occasionally have a strong familial history (as in some cases of premature disease of the hip, or in epiphyseal dysplasias presenting as OA); others may cluster in geographical areas, suggesting an important environmental factor. However, the commonest form of 'primary OA' seen in the UK is the so-called generalised nodal OA of middle aged women (synonyms 'menopausal arthritis', primary GOA, inflammatory GOA). This is a destructive condition which may have a relatively acute onset and prominent inflammatory component causing confusion with rheumatoid arthritis. The joint involvement (DIPs and knees especially) is characteristic, and as the disease progresses typical OA changes of weight-bearing joints may develop.

As our knowledge and understanding of OA advances and as the concept of 'joint failure' gains ground, the primary or secondary classification becomes less useful. OA is obviously an end-stage condition of multi-factorial origin. Different patterns of disease can be distinguished and in some a clear metabolic, inflammatory or mechanical factor dominates the condition (Fig. 8.1). As in other areas of rheumatology, pattern recognition and a search for possible associated factors (see below) is more important to the clinician than any rigid classification.

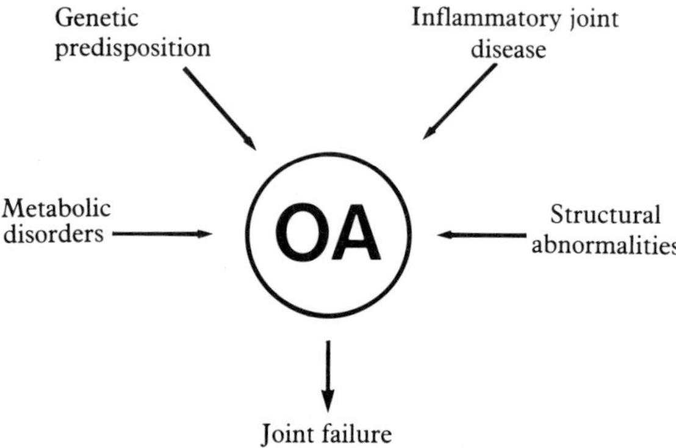

Fig. 8.1 Osteoarthritis can be regarded as 'joint failure'. The pathogenesis is multifactorial, although genetic, inflammatory, metabolic or mechanical (structural) factors may dominate in individual cases.

EPIDEMIOLOGY

Osteoarthritis (OA), is a very common, age-related phenomenon. Radiographic evidence of the condition rises with age and is slightly more common in women than in men, so that over half the population over the age of 60 and nearly everyone over the age of 75 have changes of OA. Fortunately, clinical expression of the condition does not occur in all those with X-ray changes; nevertheless, it is estimated that over five million people in the UK alone suffer significant pain and disability from OA.

Epidemiological studies have shown that racial, geographical and occupational factors affect the incidence and pattern of the disease. For example, OA of the knee is rare in Chinese, whereas OA of the hip is common in working men in the North of England; Pima Indians have a high incidence of Heberden's nodes, and generalised disease is commonest in White women. Thus, although OA is known to affect many races, and has been common throughout man's history, genetic make-up and joint usage are clearly important in its expression.

THE PATHOLOGY OF OSTEOARTHRITIS

OA affects all parts of a synovial joint. The most striking changes are those seen in the load-bearing cartilage and subchondral bone (Fig. 8.2). The tissues involved are very active, with an increase in cellular numbers and metabolism; this is interpreted by some as attempted regeneration in the face of tissue destruction.

Articular cartilage

Cartilage is composed of a small number of cells (chondrocytes), confined to the middle and lower zones; a network of collagen fibres (10%); large aggregates of proteoglycans (15%); and water (70%), which is attracted to the hydrophilic proteoglycan (see also Chapter 1).

In early OA the water content increases (perhaps due to disruption of the collagen network allowing the matrix to swell); cells increase in number and activity and form clumps; the proteoglycans are depleted, altered in composition and aggregate less easily; and there is an increase in the concentration of degradative enzymes. In advanced OA there is a marked disruption of the collagen network and matrix, especially in the superficial layers and the deeper layers become vascularised and may mineralise.

The morphological changes seen as the disease progresses are shown in Figure 8.2. Early disease is characterised by surface fibrillation (which can be shown up by Indian ink staining) and loss of metachromatic staining (due to proteoglycan depletion). Not all areas of surface fibrillation progress to OA, but in those which do tangential splits appear in the surface and this leads into loss

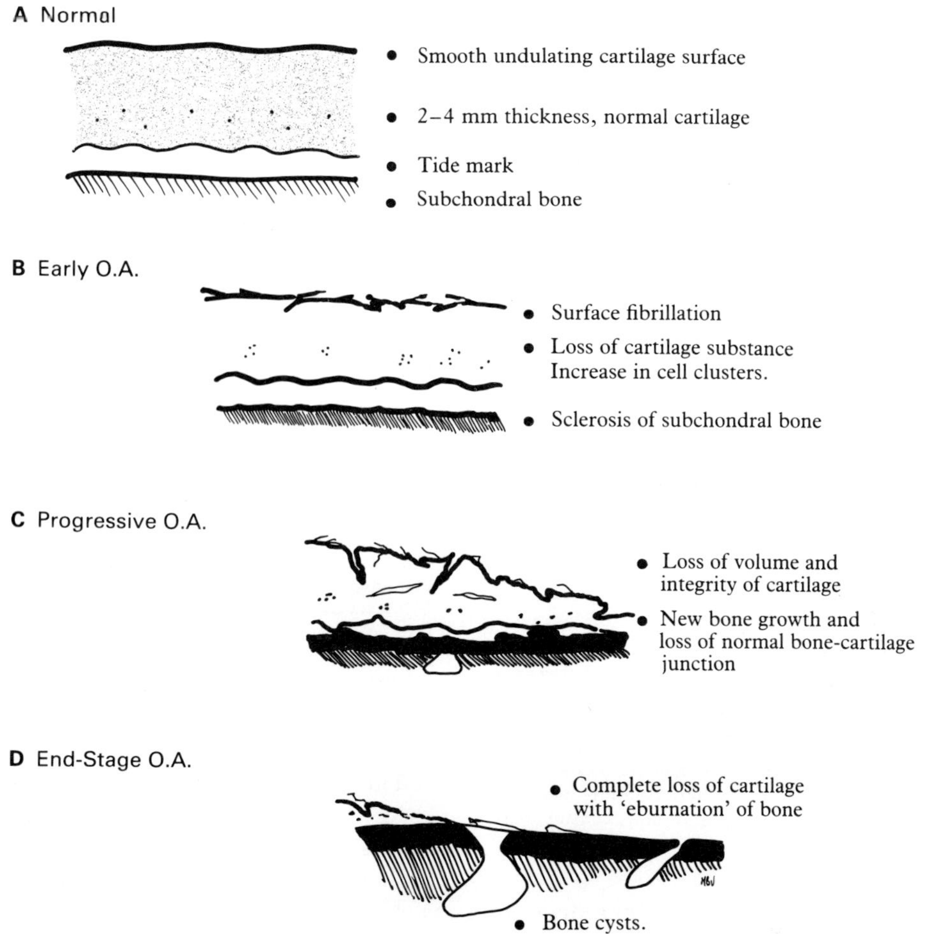

Fig. 8.2 Progressive changes seen in the cartilage and subchondral bone in osteoarthritis (OA).

of cartilage volume. The realisation that cartilage fibrillation can be progressive or non-progressive is important, and implies multiple aetiological factors. In the deeper layers the nests of cells are apparent and the tide-mark separating bone and cartilage becomes indistinct due to invasion with new vessels and partial mineralisation.

Subchondral bone

There is abnormal activity of subchondral bone, with the cells, vascular component and density of the tissue all increasing. Dense bone is interrupted by the development of cysts, which may communicate with the joint space, and which contain degenerate connective tissue. At the margin of the joint new bone forms the 'osteophytes' covered by fibrocartilage.

This intense activity produces a line of dense, hard, resilient bone just below the cartilage, tending to extend into it. In addition, it causes remodelling of the joint, and a change in the contour and congruity of the weight-bearing surface which may result in new areas of the cartilage taking the load (Fig. 8.3).

Soft tissues

The synovium shows mild, variable, patchy inflammatory changes. The predominantly mononuclear cell infiltrate may contain plasma cells, lymphocytes and giant cells. Fragments of carti-

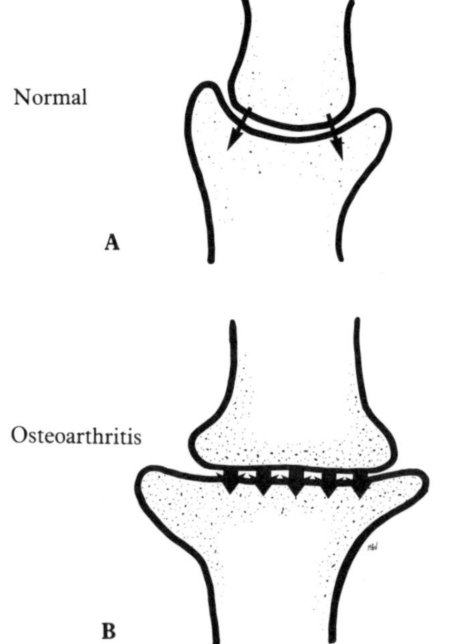

Fig. 8.3 Normal joint contours and congruity are altered in osteoarthritis, leading to changes in the area of weight-bearing in a joint. **A**. Normal — normal joints are non-congruous. Weight-bearing is on limited areas of cartilage at joint margin. **B**. Osteoarthritis — remodelling of subchondral bone and osteophytic growth alters bony contour, increases congruity and changes weight-bearing to new, central areas.

lage and bone and areas of new mineral deposition may also be seen. In advanced cases the synovial changes are sometimes bad enough to mimic those of rheumatoid disease.

The joint capsule is often thickened and gross fibrosis may occur, helping, along with the osteophytes, to 'splint' the joint.

Periarticular soft-tissue cysts may also develop. These are most obvious at the distal interphalangeal joint; if needled, thick, clear jelly is extruded, consisting principally of hyaluronic acid. Synovial extensions (Baker's cysts) can form in OA as in other, more overtly inflammatory conditions, and they may rupture.

Synovial fluid

A modest increase in the amount of synovial fluid is usual in OA joints, and it is qualitatively, as well as quantitatively, abnormal. It is viscous and contains predominantly mononuclear cells, in counts ranging from about 500 to 5000/dl. Fragments of cartilage and bone may be seen, and crystals of hydroxyapatite are often present. This inflammatory exudate is quite different from that of rheumatoid arthritis and allied conditons, in which polymorphonuclear cells, rather than monocytes, dominate the reaction.

RADIOGRAPHIC FEATURES OF OSTEOARTHRITIS

The radiographic changes are a direct consequence of the pathology described above (Table 8.1).

Table 8.1 Relationship between the main pathological and radiological features of osteoarthritis

Pathology	Radiology
Loss of articular cartilage	Joint space narrowing
Increased activity of subchondral bone	Subchondral sclerosis Cysts Osteophytes

The characteristic features are loss of joint space, subchondral bone sclerosis and cysts, osteophytes, and sometimes mild soft-tissue swelling or areas of visible mineral deposition (Fig. 8.4).

The pathological changes need to be fairly well advanced to cause radiographic changes, and an accurate assessment of the disease may necessitate special views and weight-bearing films to help outline the bone changes and cartilage loss.

CLINICAL FEATURES OF OSTEOARTHRITIS

Clinical osteoarthritis is difficult to define, and no established criteria exist. The diagnosis is usually based on: 1. Signs and symptoms in affected joints; 2. The distribution and pattern of involved joints; and 3. The time course of the disease.

Signs and symptoms

Pain is the main symptom; it is usually worst on joint usage and at the end of the day; it is relieved

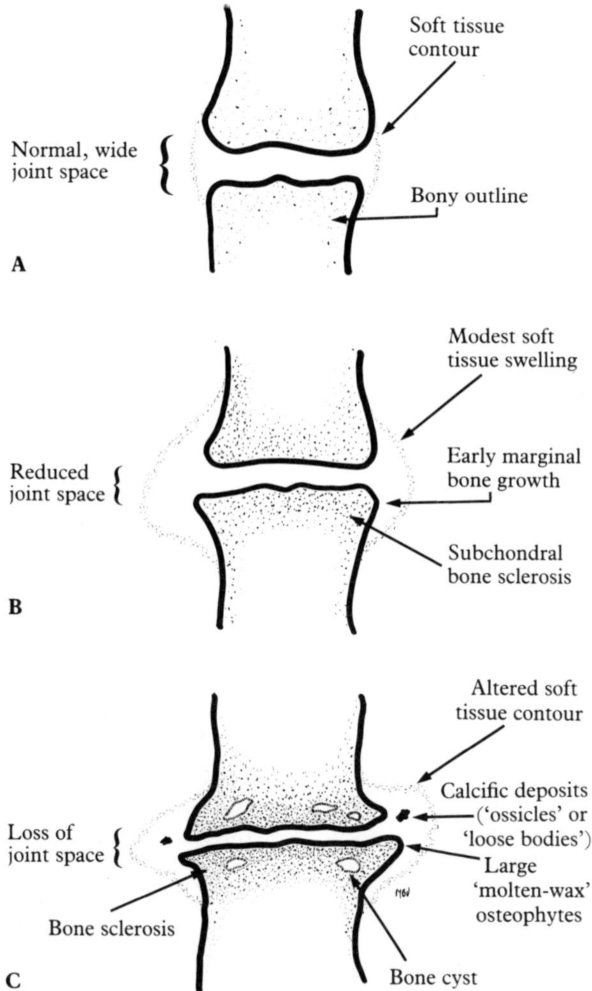

Fig. 8.4 Radiological changes in osteoarthritis (OA). **A**. Normal. **B**. Early OA. **C**. Advanced OA.

Main Clinical Features of Osteoarthritis

Symptoms

1. Pain
   a) With joint use
   b) Worst at end of day
2. Stiffness
   a) Severe, short-lasting stiffness after inactivity
   b) Mild early-morning stiffness

Signs

1. Painful limitation of joint movement
2. Crepitus
3. Modest soft-tissue changes
4. Bony swelling and tenderness at joint margin

by rest, and at night. Mild, short-lasting early-morning stiffness and more severe 'gelling' of the joints after a period of inactivity are also characteristic. On examination the joints have a limited range of movement accompanied by pain and crepitus, mild effusions, warmth, or soft-tissue swelling, and tenderness over the joint line. Periarticular areas, such as the capsular and ligament insertions, are often an important cause of localised pain and tenderness around the joint.

In early disease soft-tissue changes may dominate the clinical features, but in late OA severe deformity and destructive changes may result in gross mechanical abnormalities dominating the clinical presentation.

Distribution

The joints commonly affected by OA are shown in Figure 8.5. Monoarticular disease sometimes occurs, especially in the hip, but involvement at two, three or four different sites is usual. Polyarticular disease, with prominent changes in the distal interphalangeal joints and carpo-metacarpal joints of the thumb is common in middle-aged women; whereas hip disease, with or without spinal involvement, is commoner in men.

Time course

The onset of clinical features can occur at any time from early adult life, but peaks in the sixth decade; OA affects women more than men (F:M ratio approximately 2.5: 1). The onset is usually insidious, and the spread from one joint site to another is slow (mean interval approximately 1 year). The condition is usually slowly progressive, its course being interrupted by variable exacerbations and remissions of symptoms, although spontaneous recovery can rarely occur. Relatively little is known about the natural history of the disease.

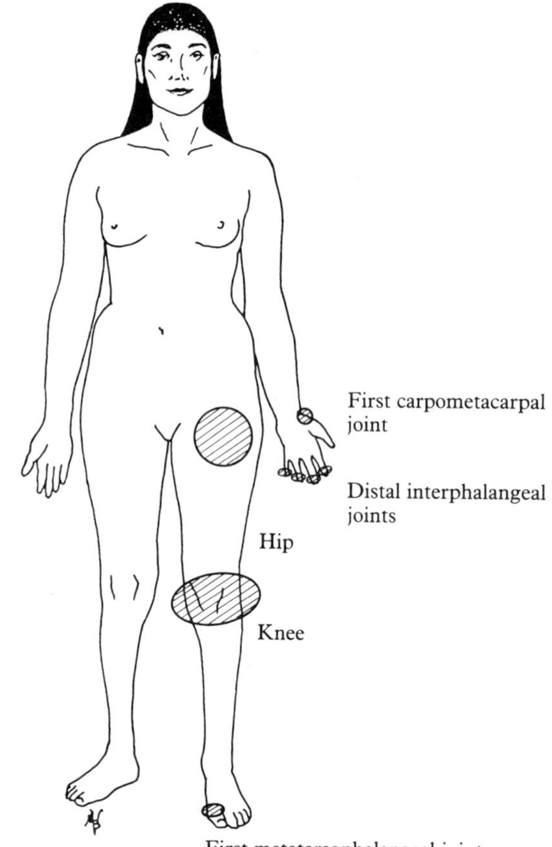

Fig. 8.5 Distribution of peripheral osteoarthritis

PRESENTATIONS

The majority of patients with OA present in one of three ways:

1. The insidious development of pain related to activity, and of stiffness after rest, in one or more large joints is the commonest mode of onset. In men the hip joint is often the major site, but the classical case would be a woman in her 50s or 60s with pain in one or both knees. The differential diagnosis is wide-ranging, but exclusion of a periarticular or referred cause of pain, or of another major rheumatic disease, is the main problem.

2. Pain, swelling and stiffness in the fingers of a middle-aged woman, developing over a few months shortly after the menopause, is another presentation. Examination reveals mild inflammatory arthritis of the interphalangeal joints which in the course of a few years develop the classical nodes. There may be mild OA of other joints. This polyarticular presentation is often misdiagnosed as RA.

3. Exacerbation of pain and/or swelling in a hip or knee following trauma (often mild) is the third classical presentation. The patient has usually been aware of intermittent mild joint discomfort and stiffness for some years, but only presents when trauma causes a marked local increase in symptoms. Such exacerbations usually subside over a few weeks, and in many patients OA runs a very variable course punctuated by these episodic 'flare-ups'. At presentation the differential diagnosis may include any cause of acute arthritis, especially pseudogout.

OA is a variable condition differing according to the major predisposing factors (see p. 145) and the main joint sites involved. It can therefore present in many other guises, and diagnosis is largely made by exclusion (see below).

OSTEOARTHRITIS AT DIFFERENT JOINT SITES

Special clinical and radiographic features accompany involvement of different joints. The commonest sites are the hands, feet, hips, knees and spine (Fig. 8.5).

The hip

Pain in the groin or thigh and stiffness of the hip, are frequent early symptoms. In about 20% of cases most hip pain is referred to the knee; this can cause confusion but rotation of the hip with the knee fixed, will elicit true hip pain.

The earliest sign is loss of internal rotation with pain exacerbated by extremes of movement and on weight-bearing. In advanced disease an antalgic gait is present (Fig. 8.6; the pelvis lurches down on the affected side), and shortening of the leg, muscle wasting and gross restriction of movement develops.

Conditions that can cause pain around the hip, mimicking OA, are listed opposite. Pagetic pain may be particularly difficult to distinguish from OA, although a constant, deep, bony pain, unrelated to activity, suggests bony pathology.

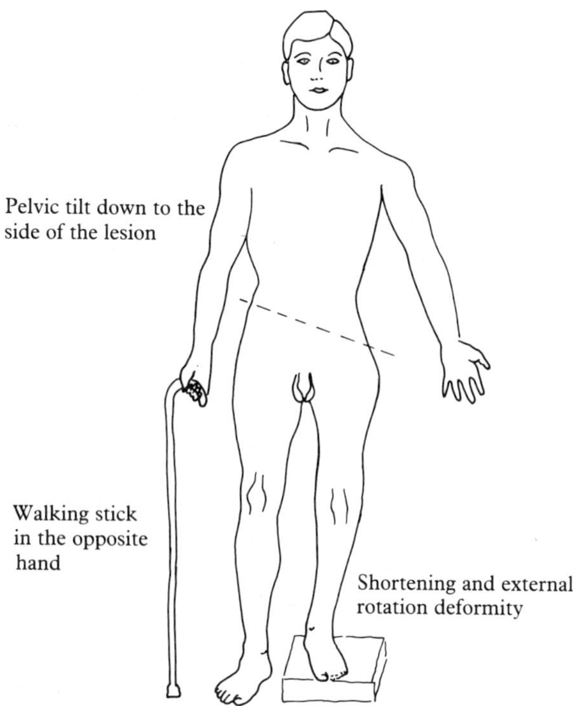

Fig. 8.6 Deformities due to osteoarthritis of the hip

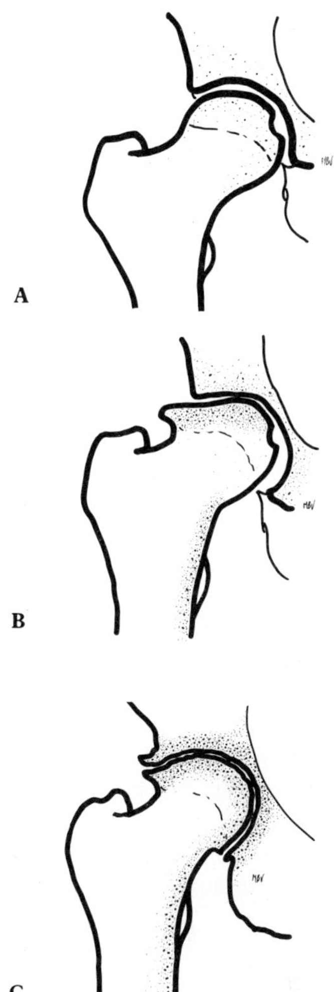

Fig. 8.7 Radiological patterns of hip osteoarthritis. **A**. Normal. **B**. Superior pole (associated with back disease, poor prognosis). Superior loss of joint space and lateral migration of femoral head. **C**. Concentric (associated with hand and knee disease, good prognosis). Concentric loss of joint space and 'jet-stream' marginal osteophytes.

Conditions which may be confused with OA of the hip

1. Trochanteric bursitis
2. Adductor tendinitis
3. L3 root compression
4. Entrapment of lateral cutaneous nerve of the thigh
5. Paget's disease
6. Fractured neck of femur
7. Other forms of arthritis
8. Secondary bone deposits from neoplasia

Radiological assessment is very important. Many cases of OA hip are secondary to a pre-existing anatomical abnormality such as old dislocation, slipped epiphyses, Perthes disease, or minor tilt abnormalities of the femoral head. In addition the distribution of the changes in the hip varies: monoarticular cases often affect the superio-lateral aspect, causing the head of the femur to migrate up and out (especially common in men), whereas polyarticular disease will usually be associated with concentric changes all round the hip joint (more common in women) (Fig. 8.7). The radiograph also allows assessment of the severity of disease, and the presence of any complications such as avascular necrosis.

The knee

Pain on use is the most important symptom. Stiffness also occurs, and, as with the hip, may result in 'gelling' after inactivity, and in difficulty getting out of chairs. Early on in the disease symptoms vary, periarticular tenderness may be prominent, and the patient may notice episodic effusions; in advanced cases deformity may develop causing severe disability and more persistent severe pain.

On examination there is often restriction of movement, joint crepitus, a small effusion and articular or periarticular tender spots; muscle wasting (especially of the vastus medialis) is always present, and instability and deformity may develop. It is important to establish the source of pain, which may arise from any one of the three compartments of the joint (lateral, medial and patello-femoral) or periarticular tissues such as ligament insertions or bursae (commonly the inferior attachment of the medial collateral ligament). Patello-femoral disease causes severe symptoms on coming down stairs, and signs include pain and crepitus on palpation of the patella. Medial or lateral joint-line tenderness and instability of collateral ligaments are indicative of tibio-femoral disease.

The radiographs (like the clinical examination) should include a weight-bearing view. AP and lateral views will allow visualisation of the three compartments and show the severity of cartilage loss, bone changes and the soft-tissue response.

Hands

The distal interphalangeal joints (especially of the index finger) and carpometacarpal joint of the thumb are commonly involved; proximal interphalangeal joint disease is less frequent, and the wrist and other CMC joints are rarely affected (Fig. 8.8).

Symptoms may be absent, but disease at the base of the thumb can cause a good deal of difficulty with pinch grip, or with other activity such as wringing out clothes, and the interphalangeal joints may be stiff, painful and tender. In severe disease hand function may be severely limited.

Joint swelling is usual and the firm, superior-lateral swellings over interphalangeal joints are called Heberden's (distal) or Bouchard's (proximal) nodes. The joints may be tender and in about 10% redness (due to periarticular inflammation) is present. Cysts over the PIPs occur in a minority.

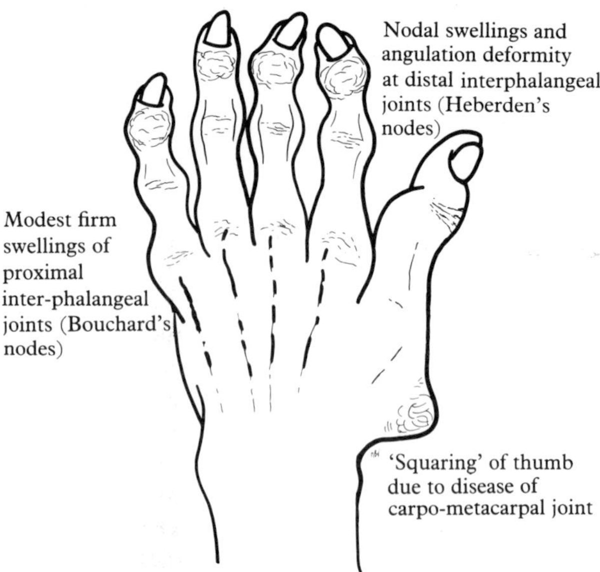

Fig. 8.8 The hand in generalised osteoarthritis

Feet

The first metatarso-phalangeal joint is commonly affected, resulting in stiffness (hallux rigidus) or deformity (hallux valgus) (Fig. 8.9). Other MTPs are sometimes involved but OA of other joints in the foot is uncommon. Metatarsalgia can occur but symptoms are often secondary to pressure

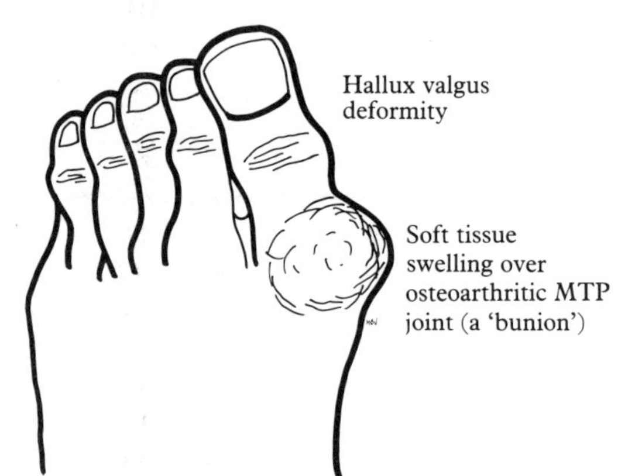

Fig. 8.9 The foot in osteoarthritis

areas from footwear causing periarticular inflammation over deformed joints (e.g. the 'bunion' of hallux valgus, sometimes called 'poor-man's gout').

The spine

The posterior apophyseal joints (the facet joints) of the spine are synovial and they commonly acquire changes of osteoarthritis. Functionally these joints are inextricably linked with the fibrous inter-vertebral joints, and disease of both types of articulation commonly coexist. The apophyseal joints may give rise to back pain which can be referred to the relevent dermatome and aggravated by motion. However, it is often difficult to differentiate the anatomical source of back pain, and the relationship between pathological, radiological and clinical changes in these joints is particularly weak. The differential diagnosis of back pain is considered further in Chapter 22.

CORRELATION BETWEEN CLINICAL, RADIOGRAPHIC AND PATHOLOGICAL CHANGES

A brief description of the features of OA implies that pathological changes inevitably cause both a radiographic abnormality and symptoms. This is not the case. The changes in bone and cartilage must be both advanced and extensive to be seen on the X-ray; if there is only an isolated area of cartilage ulceration for example, no joint-space narrowing will be seen on the radiograph. Similarly, pathological or radiological changes do not always cause clinical signs or symptoms.

In many joint sites (especially the spine) the discrepancy between the X-ray and the clinical status can be striking. Thus, although in general the most severely-damaged joint is the most symptomatic, some advanced X-ray changes are seen in asymptomatic patients, and severe symptoms may accompany minor radiographic changes.

The cause of symptoms in OA remains unknown. One may speculate that clinical OA is a dual condition: requiring both OA pathology plus 'factor X' which allows its symptomatic expression. OA has been defined as a condition characterised by destruction of articular cartilage and activity of underlying bone; nerve endings are absent from the cartilage and sparse in the bone. Raised intra-osseous pressure may explain some symptoms, and may also account for the symptomatic relief caused by osteotomy. Capsular stretching and disease of other innervated periarticular structures may also give rise to OA pain. However, the severely damaged but asymptomatic joint remains a common clinical paradox.

ASSOCIATED CONDITIONS

Several conditions with pathological, radiological and clinical features of OA but other distinguishing factors have been described. These include: 1. Chondromalacia patellae; 2. Inflammatory (erosive) OA; 3. Diffuse idiopathic skeletal hyperostosis; 4. Neuropathic joints; 5. Calcium phosphate crystal deposition disease.

Chondromalacia patellae

This condition principally affects young women; it presents as knee pain exacerbated by walking down stairs, or on sitting with flexed knees. Compression of the patella, which is often especially mobile and tender on its margin, reproduces the pain. Radiographs may show some narrowing of the patello-femoral joint space, and arthrography or arthroscopy shows fibrillation of the patello-femoral articular cartilage. Histology shows softening and fibrillation of the cartilage. The condition is often self-limiting, but may progress to patello-femoral OA. However, relatively little is know about either the aetiology or natural history of this condition, and its relationship to OA remains controversial.

Inflammatory (erosive) osteoarthritis

The tendency for middle-aged white women to acquire a disease of their interphalangeal joints has already been mentioned. In some the articular and periarticular inflammatory features are particularly striking, and radiological erosions may be seen

Conditions affecting the distal interphalangeal joint
1. Generalised osteoarthritis
2. (Possible further subset of 'erosive'/inflammatory OA)
3. Rheumatoid arthritis (usually mild)
4. Psoriatic arthropathy
5. Juvenile chronic polyarthritis
6. Sarcoidosis

(although it is difficult to distinguish erosions from collapsed subchondral bone cysts). Some cases seem to develop into rheumatoid disease and in others it is difficult to distinguish between OA and, for example, psoriatic arthropathy. Many authors describe the inflammatory form of OA as a distinct subset, others regard it as an exaggerated form of generalised nodal OA. As yet, no obvious distinguishing factor has emerged to help unravel this problem.

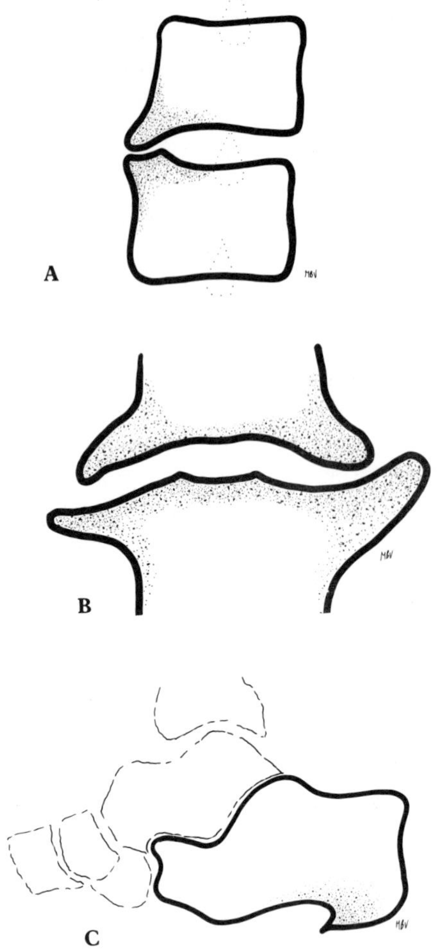

Fig. 8.10 Features of diffuse idiopathic skeletal hyperostosis (DISH). **A**. Large, right-sided antero-lateral osteophytes of four or more disc spaces with normal preservation of disc spaces. The osteophytes may fuse. **B**. Large, flowing, molten-wax osteophytes in association with peripheral OA. **C**. Calcification of tendon insertions, e.g. heel spur on the calcaneus.

Diffuse idiopathic skeletal hyperostosis (DISH)

Large antero-lateral osteophytes around four or more normal disc spaces in the thoraco-lumbar spine is the agreed definition of spinal hyperostosis or *Forrestier's disease*. It is now recognised that this radiological finding in the spine, which is common in middle-aged or elderly people, is often associated with peripheral joint changes. Large osteophytes and ossification of tendon and ligament insertion points occurs, and if OA is present massive bony overgrowth can occur, justifying the old term 'hypertrophic arthritis' (Fig. 8.10). Severe OA in conjunction with DISH and extensive bony overgrowth is therefore regarded as a distinct OA subset by some authorities.

Neuropathic (Charcot) joints

Grossly disorganised, destroyed joints associated with bony debris and soft-tissue calcification, occasionally occur in patients with neurological disease. The usual co-existing conditions are neurosyphilis, syringomyelia, diabetic neuropathy or pain insensitivity (Fig. 8.11). Many aspects of the pathology or radiology are similar to that of severe OA, particularly if associated with crystal deposition. (Chapter 9)

Calcium phosphate crystal deposition

Evidence of mineral deposition in the cartilage, soft tissues or synovial fluid is common in OA joints. The usual salts are hydroxyapatite (bone

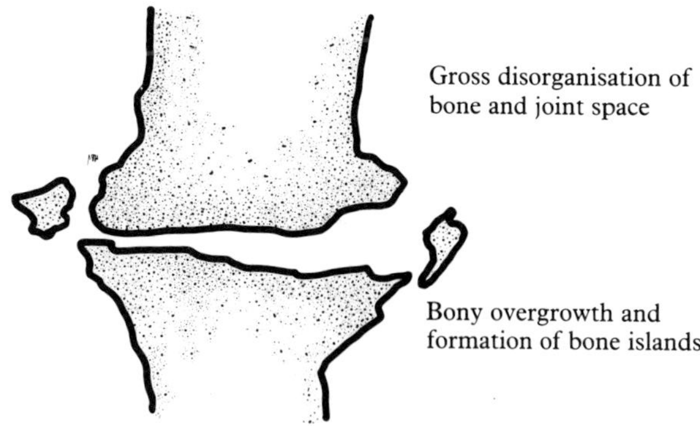

Fig. 8.11 Charcot joint. Common associations are: neurosyphilis, syringomelia, diabetes, pain insensitivity.

mineral, $Ca_{10}(PO_4)_6.OH$) or calcium pyrophosphate dihydrate ($Ca_2P_2O_7.2H_2O$). Pyrophosphate deposition is sometimes associated with a severe, characteristic form of destructive OA centred on knees and wrists (see Chapter 9.III); and hydroxyapatite crystals tends to be found in the more severely-damaged joints (see Chapter 9.III). It appears that mineral deposition can both result from, and add to, joint damage, providing an accelerator pathway to joint damage in OA; an 'amplification loop' mechanism (Chapter 9.1.).

DIAGNOSIS AND ASSESSMENT OF OSTEOARTHRITIS

OA tends to present in an older population. It is a diagnosis made on clinical and radiological grounds, but without strict criteria or any available diagnostic test. Furthermore, radiological changes of OA are almost invariable in the elderly, but often asymptomatic.

The problem is therefore one of deciding whether the OA is the cause of the problem (usually pain, stiffness or difficulty with daily tasks), rather than deciding if it is present.

A careful history and clinical and radiological examination should elucidate the extent of the problem and the source of the pain. Further tests are generally unnecessary, and should only be used to exclude other possible causes of symptoms such as polymyalgia rheumatica or hypothyroidism.

There is a statistical association of OA with obesity, hypertension and hyperuricaemia; but there are no other clear disease associations unless the OA is secondary to some other joint condition (see p. 145), and no search for associations is either warranted or fruitful.

The more important consideration is the possible existence of some other condition (elderly people frequently have more than one disease) which may be complicating the clinical picture. Symptoms of OA may be exaggerated by co-existing depression, pain-amplification or Parkinsonism, for example and disability may be made far worse by the presence of some other problem such as visual handicap or a tremor.

Mistakes can be made by assuming that symptoms can all be explained by a radiographic report saying 'OA present'.

TREATMENT

No specific disease-modifying therapy is available. Treatment is therefore symptomatic, and in view of the chronicity of the disease should be kept as safe and simple as possible.

The reassurance that the diagnosis is OA and not, for example, rheumatoid disease, may be the only therapy needed. Present evidence suggests that patients should also be advised to keep active, and to continue to use their joints (the advice most are looking for). The use of a stick to reduce

Treatment of OA
1. A positive attitude
2. Education and reassurance
3. Advice to keep active
4. Avoidance of abnormal loading of affected joint
5. Maintain muscle bulk
6. Intermittent use of analgesic or anti-inflammatory drugs
7. Occasional periarticular or intra-articular steroids
8. Surgery for end-stage disease

weight-bearing on an OA hip or knee, aids in the home, or simply weight-reduction, may all reduce symptoms considerably and obviate the need for any drugs. Physiotherapy to maintain muscle power and movement is especially important in hip and knee disease, and local heat may provide temporary relief of symptoms.

Drugs or surgery are therefore frequently unnecessary. However, many patients continue to be severely disabled or in considerable pain in spite of the measures outlined above. Simple 'on demand' analgesics help some; non-steroidal anti-inflammatory drugs are more effective and can be used for short periods. Long-term use of drugs should probably be avoided, but is necessary for some patients. There is no place for steroids (either locally or systematically) except in cases where a single periarticular tender spot can be identified, or in a few cases of carpo-metacarpal joint disease or knees with raised intra-articular pressure; local injections of depot-steroid and anasthetic can then be useful. Severely-damaged joints may benefit from splints or require prosthetic surgery: hip replacement has revolutionised the lives of many of the more advanced cases of hip OA.

Sensible management of OA patients requires first and foremost a careful assessment of the precise local or general factors contributing to the disability: the simple, non-invasive measure is often the best. Management should however be positive; much can be done for most patients: the attitude that 'it is just OA — nothing can be done' is as damaging as over-treatment.

SPECULATION ON THE AETIOLOGY AND PATHOGENESIS OF OA

This chapter has tried to keep to a fairly factual description of the known features of this condition. Surprisingly little is known for certain of its aetiology and pathogenesis. There are, however, a number of observations that can be made:

1. Normal use of joints, however heavy, does not apparently increase the risk of OA but can affect its distribution.
2. Instability, or a major mechanical abnormality of a joint, increases the risk markedly but does not invariably cause OA.
3. Racial and familial predisposition to OA is apparent, especially in polyarticular disease and nodal GOA.
4. Inflammatory features are common and often occur early in the disease; all tissues of the joint are involved.
5. A variety of quite different stimuli can lead to OA; these include ochronosis, dietary factors as in Kashin-Beck disease, crystal deposition diseases, epiphyseal dysplasis and inflammatory arthropathies.
6. Although normal cartilage ageing has some features in common with OA, ageing alone is an insufficient explanation for the destructive and regenerative changes seen.
7. Epidemiological data suggests that several subsets of OA can be identified; hip disease, for example, has a quite different distribution, age-sex incidence and relationship to other joint OA from knee disease.
8. Most radiological, pathological, biochemical or clinical studies have been on advanced OA of the hip.

These observations suggest that OA is neither a single disease entity nor has any simple aetiology. The difficulty in unravelling this group of conditions is the relative lack of markers of subsets, or of known key pathogenic mechanisms. One can, however, say with confidence that OA is not a 'wear-and-tear' disease and that many of the other long-held views are misconceptions. Osteoarthritis and related disorders provide an exciting new area of challenge for both doctors and basic scientists interested in joint disease.

FURTHER READING

Ali S Y 1978 New knowledge of osteoarthritis. Journal of Clinical Pathology 31(Suppl 12): 191–199

Nuki G 1981 The aetiopathogenesis of osteoarthritis. Pitman Medical, London

Radin E L 1973 The physiology and degeneration of joints. Seminars in Arthritis and Rheumatism 2: 245–257

Wright V 1976 Osteoarthrosis. Clinics in Rheumatic Diseases 2,3.

9 Crystal deposition diseases

I Introduction

A crystal deposition disease can be defined as a pathological condition associated with the presence of crystals and one in which the crystals contribute to tissue damage. The joints of the body are one of three systems particularly susceptible to both deposition of crystals and crystal-induced damage. Other organs affected include the lungs, susceptible to inhaled particles, and the excretory ducts of the liver and kidney in which the concentration of many sparingly soluble salts is high (Fig. 9.1).

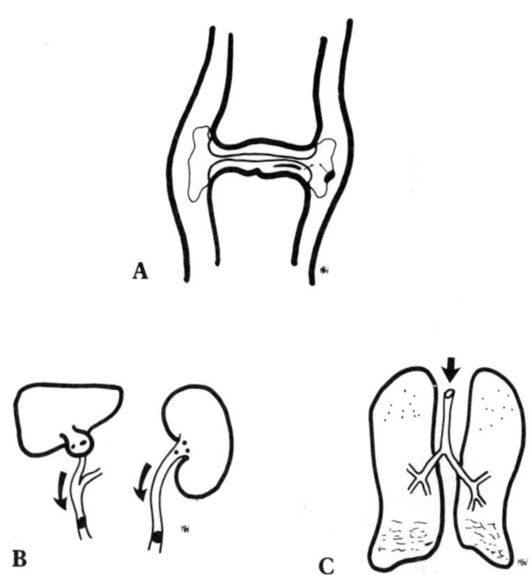

Fig. 9.1 The different systems commonly affected by crystal deposition diseases. **A.** Joints — crystals deposited in cartilage and soft tissues can cause direct local damage, and may be shed into the synovial space, causing an inflammatory reaction. **B.** Liver and kidney — the concentration of sparingly soluble salts is deliberately raised to aid excretion. Crystal deposits (stones) can form in the collecting ducts. **C.** Lungs — inhaled particles and crystals lodge in the small airways and alveoli, and cause an inflammatory reaction leading to fibrosis of the lung (e.g. asbestosis).

PARTICLES IN JOINTS

Crystals and other particles found in joints are of three types: 1. those deposited in the tissue as part of a pathological change, e.g. urate and calcium crystals; 2. particles derived from normal joint tissue, e.g. fragments of cartilage or subchondral bone; and 3. particles entering the joint percutaneously, e.g. corticosteroid crystals injected for therapeutic reasons, or thorns penetrating the skin. (Fig. 9.1). The most important of these are the monosodium urate monohydrate, calcium pyrophosphate dihydrate and hydroxyapatite crystals which grow in the articular cartilage, synovium and periarticular tissues. Cholesterol, calcium oxalate and a variety of other calcium-containing crystals occasionally form at the same sites.

THE GROWTH AND DISSOLUTION OF CRYSTALS IN JOINTS

The human body has to be able to form and maintain the crystalline mineral of bones and teeth (calcium phosphates), but prevent crystallisation

Classification of joint particles

1. Crystals deposited from solutes in body fluids
   a) MONOSODIUM URATE MONOHYDRATE
   b) CALCIUM PYROPHOSPHATE DIHYDRATE
   c) HYDROXYAPATITE
   d) Cholesterol
   e) Other lipid crystals
   f) Calcium oxalate
   g) Dicalcium phosphate dihydrate
   h) Calcium carbonate
   i) Other calcium salts
2. Particles derived from the joint itself
   a) Fragments of bone and cartilage
   b) 'Rice bodies'
3. Extrinsic particle entering the joint from the outside
   a) Steroid crystal injected for therapy
   b) Other therapeutic or diagnostic agents
   c) Plant thorns
   d) Other foreign bodies

Classification of crystal deposition diseases

Dystrophic crystal deposition

Local deposition at a site of tissue injury
Usually hydroxyapatite (dystrophic calcification)
Examples
a) Calcified haematomas
b) Calcified tuberculous focus
c) Skin and muscle calcification in connective-tissue diseases

Ectopic crystal deposition

Deposition at multiple sites due to raised solute levels in body fluids
Examples
a) Hyperuricaemia causing gout and urate tophi
b) Hyperparathyroidism causing calcification in the eye, joints etc
c) Calcific periarthritis in patients on renal dialysis

Mixed ectopic and dystrophic deposition

In many cases a combination of metabolic predisposition (raised solute) and local tissue factors dictate the presence and distribution of crystal deposits

of solids elsewhere. The concentration of calcium and phosphate therefore has to be fairly high, and the body is also saturated with respect to calcium carbonate. Special mechanisms exist in bones and teeth to activate the formation of crystals from these solutes, whereas other tissues contain chemical inhibitors of crystal growth.

Crystals form outside the skeleton if the concentration of solute rises, and/or there is loss of the normal tissue inhibitors. Thus many organs calcify at a site of local damage (e.g. calcification of tuberculous and traumatic lesions) and widespread calcification can also result from hypercalcaemia or hyperphosphataemia.

The joints and periarticular tissues are particularly susceptible to crystal deposition, especially when damaged. This presumably reflects a relative lack of inhibitors. Thus hyperuricaemia is more likely to result in crystals growing in joints, hence gout, than it is to cause urate crystallisation anywhere else. Similarly the joints often calcify in hyperparathyroidism, and the periarticular tissues in the hyperphosphataemia induced by renal dialysis. Increasing age and joint trauma enhance the susceptibility of local tissues; in most cases of calcium crystal formation these factors are more important than any generalised metabolic abnormality.

Crystals form by a process of nucleation, followed by a phase of crystal growth (Fig. 9.2). Nucleation requires a high concentration of the solute to form in a small area, and is often an active, energy-dependent step. Growth, in the case of most crystals relevant to joint disease, is a very slow process that can only continue if the solute concentration of the surrounding medium remains above the saturation point. It usually takes months or years to form sizable deposits in the tissue.

Dissolution can be a much faster process, and will inevitably occur if the solute concentration

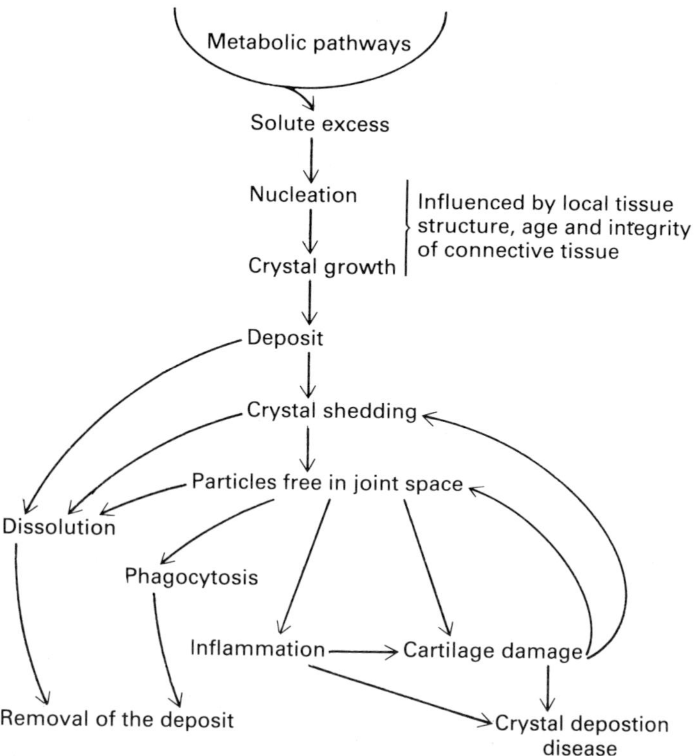

Fig. 9.2 A simplified diagram of some of the pathways involved in the crystal deposition diseases

drops below the solubility line. Crystal deposits can also be disrupted, shedding their contents into nearby tissue spaces such as the synovial cavity. The individual particles may then be dispersed by lymphatics or phagocytosis, or dissolve because they are in a less saturated environment (Fig. 9.2). Most crystal deposits found in and around the joints have a slow natural turnover, with alternating phases of overall growth or dissolution.

THE IDENTIFICATION OF CRYSTALS

Large deposits can be identified by clinical examination, radiography or gross inspection of pathology samples; individual crystals can only be found by microscopic examination of joint tissue or synovial fluid.

1. Clinical examination: finding tophi

Prolonged hyperuricaemia or hyperlipidaemia can result in the formation of subcutaneous deposits of urate or cholesterol crystals respectively. Subcutaneous deposits of hydroxyapatite sometimes form in the extremities in the connective tissue diseases (especially scleroderma), and occasionally develop spontaneously. The distribution of tophi of urates, lipids and calcium salts is similar to that of rheumatoid nodules, favoured sites including the extensor surface of the elbow, the tendons in the hand, front of the knee and Achilles tendons (Fig. 9.3). Urate tophi have a greater predilection for the helix of the ear and big toe than other rheumatological nodules.

2. Radiology

Urate and lipid deposits are radiolucent, although their presence can sometimes be inferred from the distribution of soft-tissue swellings or associated changes in bones and joints. Deposits of calcium pyrophosphate, hydroxyapatite or other calcium salts will show up on the radiograph, as long as

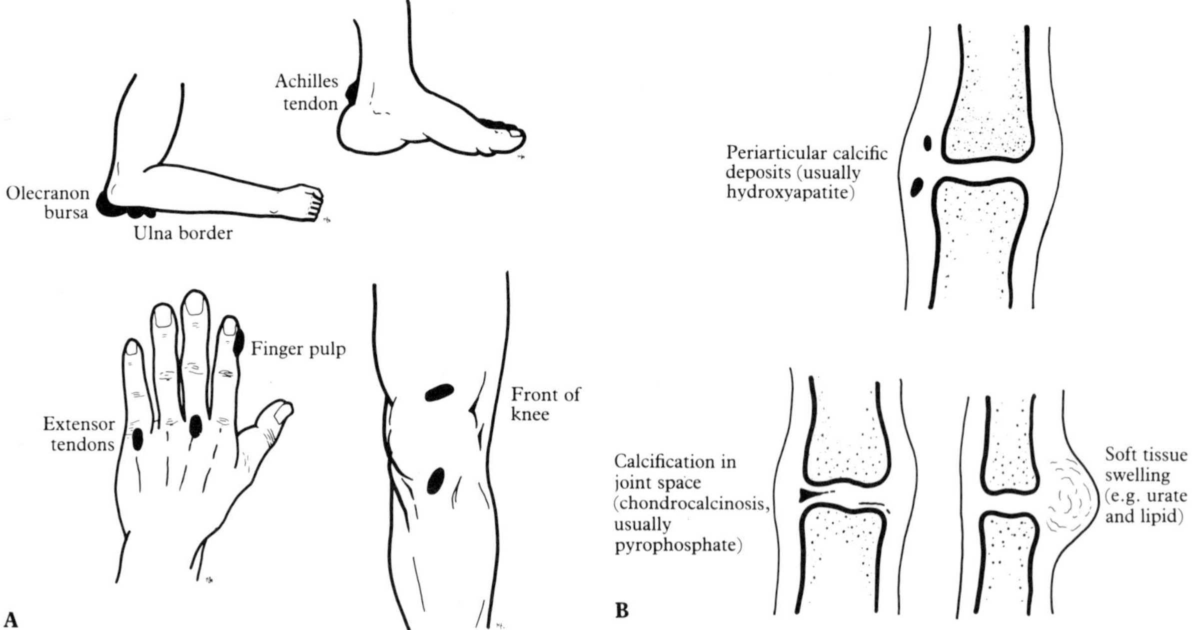

Fig. 9.3 Clinical and radiological recognition of crystal deposits. **A**. Common sites of rheumatological nodules. **B**. Radiological identification of tophi.

they are big enough. Pyrophosphate tends to be deposited in the mid-zone of cartilage, giving rise to the typical linear shadow of chondrocalcinosis, whereas hydroxyapatite deposits tend to be rounded (Fig. 9.3). However, apatite in joints cannot usually be seen because the individual crystal clumps are far too small.

3. Microscopy of tissues and joint fluids

Joint puncture (Chapter 24) allows easy access to synovial fluids for crystal identification, and tissue is sometimes available at operation to aid diagnosis. Crystals of urate, pyrophosphate or lipids usually grow to a sufficient size to be seen by light microscopy, although polarised light is needed to visualise them properly. Using this technique the different crystals can be identified by their different morphology and sign of polarisation (Fig. 9.4).

Plane polarised light is split into two emergent rays by birefringent crystals, with an effective change in the vector and wavelength. The polarised light microscope utilises this property. The change in vector of the light allows the crystals to be seen against a dark background if the stage is placed between crossed polars (Fig. 9.4), and the wavelength change can be seen as a colour shift if a suitable filter (compensator) is inserted into the light path. Fortunately for rheumatologists, urate and pyrophosphate crystals have opposite signs of birefringence, negative and positive respectively. This means that using the conventional system, with a first-order red compensator, urate crystals appear yellow and pyrophosphate blue when aligned with their long axis on the optical axis of the compensator (Fig. 9.4).

A careful search of a drop of synovial fluid or suitably-prepared tissue sample, in a polarised light microscope, allows positive identification of crystals in the majority of cases. The routine examination of synovial fluid is discussed further in Chapter 24.

Hydroxyapatite crystals are too small to be seen in the light microscope, although staining tissues or fluids with calcium stains such as alizarin red will allow the larger clumps to be seen. Electron microscopy is needed to visualise individual apatite particles and a number of sophisticated analytical attachments can be used to aid identification.

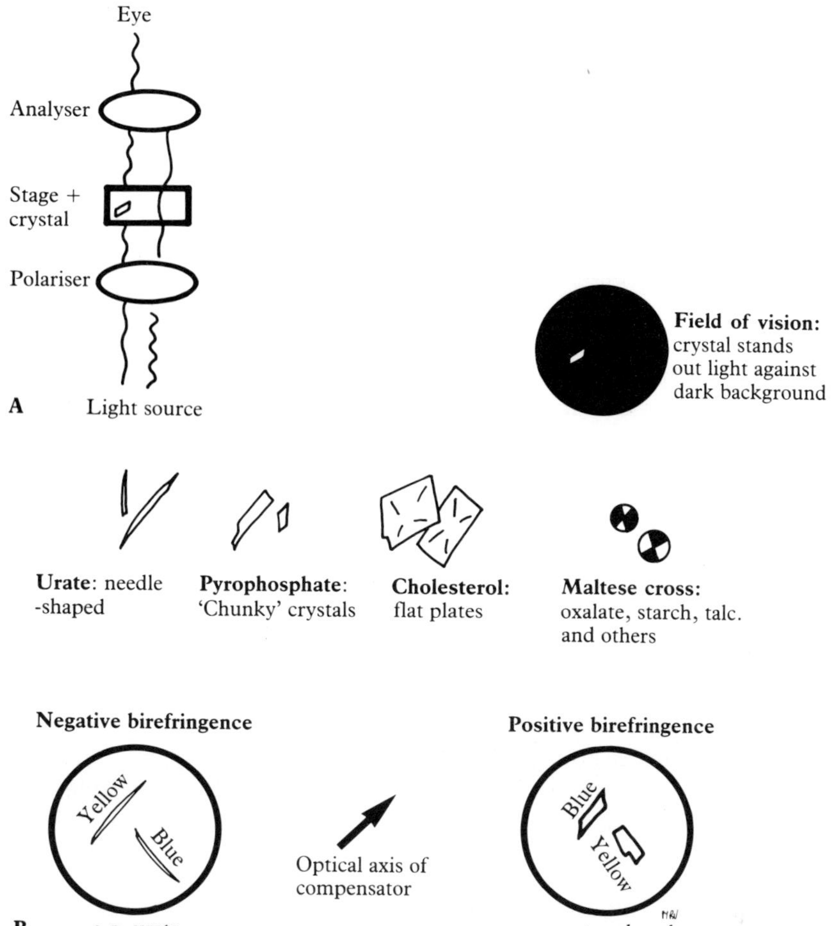

Fig. 9.4 Identification of joint crystals by polarised light microscopy. **A**. The polarised light microscope. The polariser only allows light of one vector to the stage. Crystals alter the vector, allowing light through the analyser. **B**. Morphology and signs of birefringence.

4. Other methods

Further information about visible crystal deposits can be obtained by using specific solvents such as uricase for urate or alcohol for lipids. Deposits can also be obtained for X-ray diffraction or infra-red spectrophotometry if further identification is needed.

CRYSTAL-INDUCED TISSUE-DAMAGE

Deposits of crystals in and around joints often remain asymptomatic. However, they can also cause two types of arthritis: 1. acute self-limiting attacks of inflammation and 2. chronic destructive joint disease.

The three most important crystals — urate, pyrophosphate and hydroxyapatite, are each associated with both types of pathological reaction (Table 9.1).

1. Crystal-induced inflammation

The biological properties of crystals depend on their having internal symmetry and relatively large surfaces. The surface of the crystal has repeating units throughout, which apparently bind to and

Table 9.1 The three major crystal deposition diseases of joints

Crystal	Distribution of deposits	Acute inflammatory disorder	Chronic destructive disease
Monosodium urate monohydrate	Peripheral (feet, hands)	Acute gout	Chronic tophaceous gout
Calcium pyrophosphate dihydrate	Intermediate (knees, wrists, elbows, hips, shoulders, hands)	'Pseudogout'	Chronic destructive 'pyrophosphate arthropathy'
Hydroxyapatite	Central (shoulders, hips, spine, knees)	Acute calcific periarthritis	Some forms of osteoarthritis

may alter proteins and cell membranes. Not all crystals cause inflammation, those that do have a charged, atomically 'rough' surface and it is the interaction of this surface with proteins and cells that activates inflammatory mediator systems (Fig. 9.5).

The two most important extracellular mediators are Hageman factor (Factor XII of the clotting system) and complement. Both can be activated directly by crystal surfaces, although prior coating of crystals with other plasma proteins such as IgG may enhance or alter this ability. Hageman-factor activation can trigger generation of kinins and the clotting cascade; complement activation releases chemotactic, vasoactive and membranolytic factors.

Phagocytic cells are also important in crystal-induced inflammation, cell depletion resulting in a marked reduction in response. Phagocytosis may be enhanced by protein coating, but can occur in its absence. A large number of inflammatory mediators are released during phagocytosis, including toxic free radicals, lysosomal enzymes and, in the case of urate, a specific polymorphonuclear chemotactic factor. Simple attachment of the crystal surface to cell membranes can also cause mediator release without phagocytosis, and macrophages and platelets are activated by crystals as well as polymorphonuclear cells.

Calcium-containing crystals interact with macrophages and synovial lining cells in other ways and

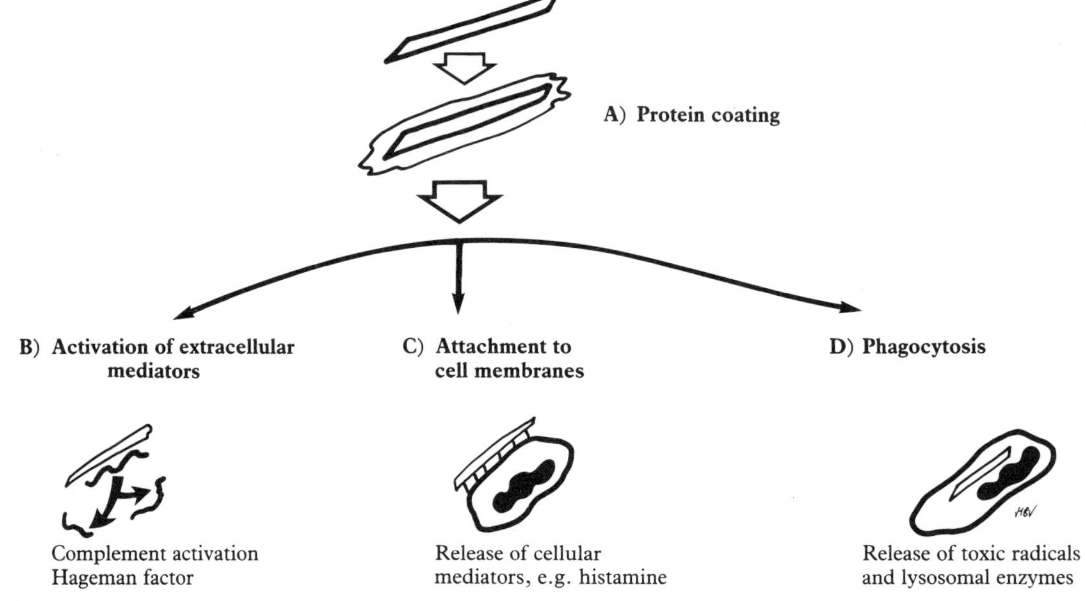

Fig. 9.5 Some of the pathways involved in crystal-induced inflammation

appear to enhance release of collagenase, prostaglandins and possibly cytokines, as well as being mitogenic.

Crystals can therefore activate cellular and extracellular inflammatory mediators. In the case of urate the acute, polymorphonuclear cell response is dominant, whereas calcium containing crystals activate the chronic macrophage dependent response to a greater degree. All reactions are dependent on the dose, size, surface area and protein coating of the particles. Most acute reactions are also self-limiting, although it is not clear what stops the inflammatory reaction once it has started.

2. Joint destruction

A small proportion of those with crystal deposits in their joints develop progressive destructive changes resulting in attrition of cartilage and underlying bone. The mechanisms involved are not clear. Deposits may cause mechanical disruption of cartilage, and surface wear (like sandpaper), but the frequent chance radiological finding of large deposits in an otherwise normal joint argues for other factors being involved.

Low-grade inflammation, or release of destructive factors from synovial lining cells without acute inflammatory mediator activation, are also possible. It has been suggested that crystal deposits can lead to a cycle of destruction involving shedding of particles, release of collagenase and other mediators, further cartilage and bone damage, and thus more particles released. This may explain the relatively sudden development of severe disease in the few people who shed sufficient crystals from preformed deposits.

SUMMARY AND CONCLUSIONS

Joint tissues are susceptible to deposition of crystals of a variety of chemical types. Increasing age and joint damage as well as metabolic abnormalities enhance this predisposition. Once a deposit is formed it may cause no problem, some crystals going through cycles of growth and dissolution without causing joint damage. However, shedding of crystals into the joint space can result in an attack of severe but self-limiting inflammation, and in a few people joint destruction occurs. In any patient with unexplained acute attacks of arthritis or chronic joint damage a clinical and radiological screen for crystal deposits should be supplemented by synovial fluid examination under polarised light to see if crystals can be identified which might be contributing to the disease.

FURTHER READING

Dieppe P A, Calvert P 1983 Crystals and joint disease. Chapman & Hall, London

Dieppe P A, Doherty M, Macfarlane D G 1983 Crystal-related arthropathies. Annals of the Rheumatic Diseases 42 (suppl 1)

Kelley W N 1977 Crystal-induced arthropathies. Clinics in Rheumatic Disease 3: 1

II Gout

INTRODUCTION

Uric acid is a metabolic product of the purine residues present in nucleic acid. Most species possess an enzyme, uricase, which catalyses the breakdown of urate into ammonia and carbon dioxide. Man (in common with some birds, reptiles and New World monkeys) has lost this enzyme, and as a result, the sparingly-soluble urate ion is present in significant amounts in all body fluids. It sometimes precipitates to form stable solid phases.

Hyperuricaemia can be defined in one of two ways: 1. as a serum uric acid level above the theoretical solubility of monosodium urate monohydrate in physiological conditions (about 0.42 m.mol/l, or 7 mg/dl); or 2. as a serum uric acid greater than two standard deviations above the mean for the population (about 0.35 mmol/l for women, and 0.42 mmol/l for men).

Only a minority of those with hyperuricaemia suffer from deposition of crystalline material. Two types of crystal can form: (1) monosodium urate monohydrate crystals, which deposit chiefly in connective tissue, commonly those in and around synovial joints, and (2) uric acid crystals, which

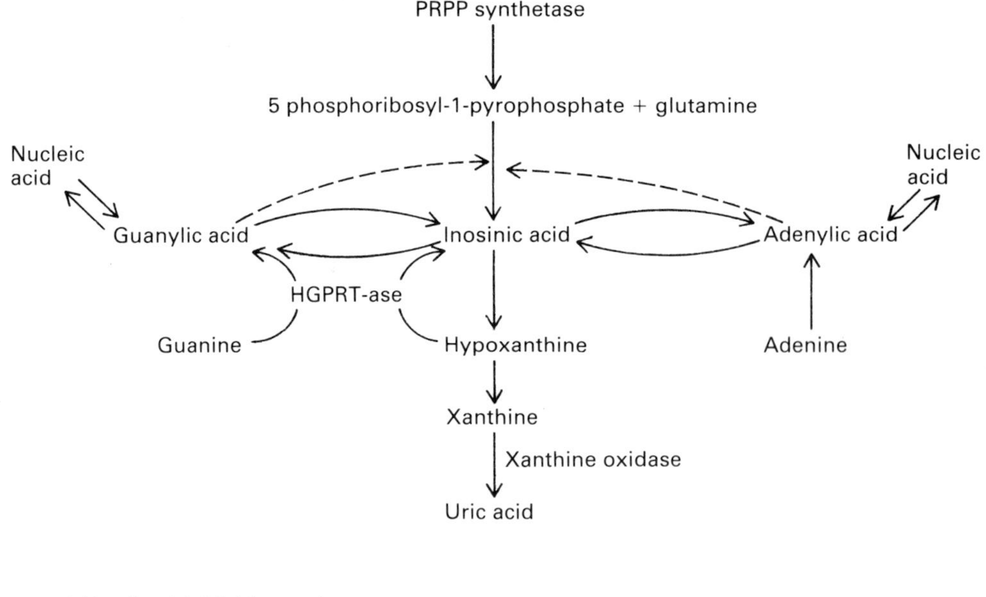

Fig. 9.6 A simplified diagram of some of the metabolic pathways involved in the formation of uric acid

are deposited in the relatively acid pH of the renal collecting ducts, and can contribute to urolithiasis.

Gout can be defined as a pathological reaction of the synovial joints or periarticular tissues, characterised by the presence of crystals of monosodium urate monohydrate.

HYPERURICAEMIA

Metabolism of uric acid

Figure 9.6 is a simplified diagram of some of the metabolic pathways involved in the formation of uric acid. The purine residues adenine and guanine are essential components of nucleic acids and formed principally from inosinic acid; this is manufactured from 5-phosphoribosyl-l-pyrophosphate (PRPP) and glutamine via a pathway controlled by feedback inhibition. Inosinic acid can also be metabolised to uric acid through hypoxanthine and xanthine, although a 'salvage pathway' exists, allowing reconversion of hypoxanthine to inosinic acid. This important salvage pathway is dependent on the enzyme hypoxanthine-guanine-phosphoribosyltransferase (HGPRT), and the breakdown of hypoxanthine to uric acid is catalysed by xanthine oxidase. Several enzyme defects are described and many of the complex pathways have been studied in depth; for further details the reader should consult the quoted references at the end of the chapter.

The total body pool or urate is about 1 g. About one-third of this is derived from the diet and two-thirds from the metabolism of nucleic acid residues outlined above (Fig. 9.7). It is fairly evenly distributed in most body fluids, and mean serum levels in adults are about 0.25 mmol/l for women and 0.30 mmol/l for men. Two-thirds is excreted in the urine via a complex 'four-component' renal mechanism. This involves complete filtration, resorption of most of the urate in the proximal tubule, followed by re-secretion and partial resorption in the distal tubule. One-third is excreted by the gut, where urate is further degraded by bacterially-derived uricase.

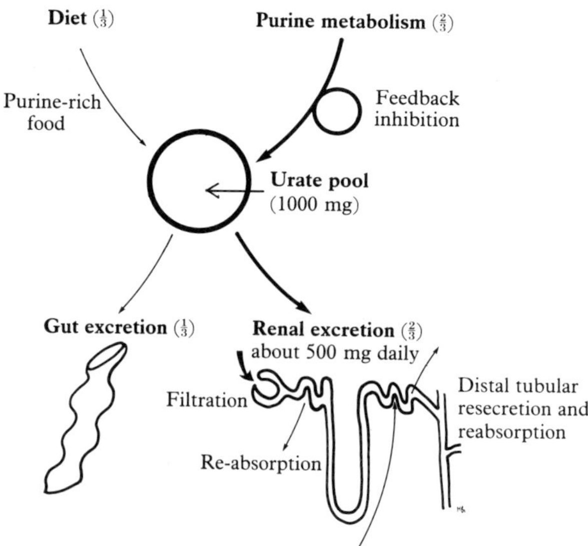

Fig. 9.7 Uric acid metabolism

Causes of hyperuricaemia

Hyperuricaemia can result from dietary excess, from increased synthesis or from reduced excretion of uric acid.

> **Classification of hyperuricaemia**
> 1. Dietary excess
> 2. 'Over-producers' (high renal output of uric acid on low purine diet — rare)
>   a) Increased turnover of nucleic acids, e.g. myeloproliferative disorders
>   b) Abnormal metabolism of uric acid, with or without an identified enzyme defect
> 3. 'Under-secretors' (low renal excretion of uric acid — common)
>   a) Reduced glomerular filtration
>   b) Abnormal tubular handling of uric acid

1. Dietary excess or purines is rarely important, although varying from a high- to a low-purine diet may alter the serum uric acid level by about 25%. Hyperuricaemic individuals are often obese and have a high alcohol intake; both associations may accelerate *de novo* formation of urate rather than acting via increased purine intake.

2. Increased turnover of purines occurs in three contexts:

a) in diseases associated with rapid cellular turnover, especially myeloproliferative diseases such as polycythaemia rubra vera
b) in association with a specific enzyme defect, such as excess PRPP synthetase or a deficiency of HGPRT
c) a mild generalised overactivity of the pathway as probably occurs in some subjects with an inherited tendency to hyperuricaemia in whom no specific enzyme anomaly has yet been found.

3. Decreased excretion of urate via the gut or kidney can also cause hyperuricaemia. The potential contribution of the gut is unknown. Renal excretion is very vulnerable, and makes an important contribution to many cases of hyperuricaemia. The main causes of renal hyperuricaemia are:
a) reduced glomerular filtration (<20 ml/min)
b) competition for tubular excretion by lactic acid or other acids
c) loss of tubular capacity to secrete urate due to damage by drugs toxins, such as lead, or other diseases
d) a genetically-determined tendency to retain more urate than is usual in the kidney

Epidemiology

Serum uric acid levels vary with age, sex and race, and from day to day. Men have higher levels than women, and adults have more urate than children; levels rise in the 20s in men and after the menopause in women. Some races (e.g. New Zealand Maoris) have higher levels than others, and all of us can cause a temporary increase by episodic 'bingeing'.

If hyperuricaemia is defined as a serum uric acid level above 0.42 mmol/l then about 5% of the adult Western male population and 0.5% of females, are hyperuricaemic.

Associations of hyperuricaemia

The associations of hyperuricaemia are the 'associations of plenty'. The significant correlation with

Associations of hyperuricaemia

1. High IQ
2. Driving, 'type A' personality
3. Obesity
4. High alcohol consumption
5. Hypertriglyceridaemia
6. Hypertension
7. Ischaemic heart disease
8. Gout
9. Renal stones

IQ is well established, and may help to explain the high prevalence of gout in our more illustrious ancestors. The relationship with obesity and alcohol intake has already been mentioned, and hyperuricaemia can be reduced by slimming and abstinence alone in many cases. Hyperlipidaemias (mainly type IV) occur in about 50% of gouty patients and in many with hyperuricaemia but no gout. The possible relationships between hyperuricaemia and hyperlipidaemia and their associations with cardiovascular disease remain controversial. Hyperuricaemia is also associated with an increased risk of gout and renal stones, and in both cases the risk is probably proportional to the severity and duration of the raised uric acid levels.

Common causes of hyperuricaemia

1. Diet
   a) Obesity
   b) High alcohol intake
2. Renal
   a) Idiopathic under-secretors
   b) Drugs affecting tubular function
      (i) Diuretics
      (ii) Salicylates (low dose)
      (iii) Anti-tuberculous drugs
      (iv) Others
   c) Renal failure of any cause
3. Increased Turnover of Nucleic Acid
   a) Myeloproliferative Disorders
   b) Haemolytic anaemias
   c) Neoplasia (especially when treated)

Rare causes of hyperuricaemia

1. Enzyme abnormalities
   a) HGPRT deficiency
   b) PRPP synthetase excess
   c) Others
2. Glycogen storage diseases
3. Lactic acidosis
4. Lead intoxication
5. Down's syndrome
6. Severe skin disease

Clinical assessment of hyperuricaemia

In many cases hyperuricaemia is a chance finding of no significance; the product of auto-analysers and over-investigation. 'Non-gout' (a disease characterised by aches and pains and a mildly-elevated uric acid) has become an important condition, causing unnecessary worry for both patient and doctor; it is often misdiagnosed as gout, leading to erroneous and unnecessary use of drugs.

If hyperuricaemia is an issue, three questions need to be asked: 1. Is it really present? 2. What are the causes? and 3. Is it causing any problem?

1. Hyperuricaemia cannot be diagnosed unless two or more fasting serum uric acid levels exceed 0.42 mmol/l. Difference in analytical techniques and in laboratory ranges lead to local variations in this figure.

2. If hyperuricaemia is present the causes must be sought. The history should include a dietary assessment (calories, purine-containing food and alcohol) and a drug and toxins history (diuretics, salicylates, anti-tuberculosis or cancer chemotherapy, lead, others). A full blood count and serum creatinine will help exclude myeloproliferative diseases or significant renal impairment. Further characterisation depends on finding out whether the patient is an 'over-producer' or 'under-secretor'. This is best done by measuring the total urinary excretion of urate while on a low-purine diet, but a quick guide can be obtained from the creatinine/uric acid ratio of spot urine samples (normally less than 0.5).

3. If hyperuricaemia is present the physician is obliged to look for evidence of renal disease (especially stones), cardiovascular disease (especially

hypertension or ischaemic heart disease), hyperlipidaemia and gout. The history, examination, blood pressure and urinalysis are usually sufficient if done thoroughly; further investigation should only be used if there is a high index of suspicion of one or more of the consequences of hyperuricaemia.

Hypouricaemia is an occasional finding, which has a number of known causes.

Causes of hypouricaemia

1. Drugs
   a) Allopurinol
   b) Probenecid
   c) High-dose aspirin
   d) Others
2. Diseases
   a) Xanthinuria
   b) Fanconi Syndrome
   c) Porphyria
   d) Severe hepatic disease
   e) Pernicious anaemia
   f) Isolated tubular defects
   g) Some neoplasia
   h) Others

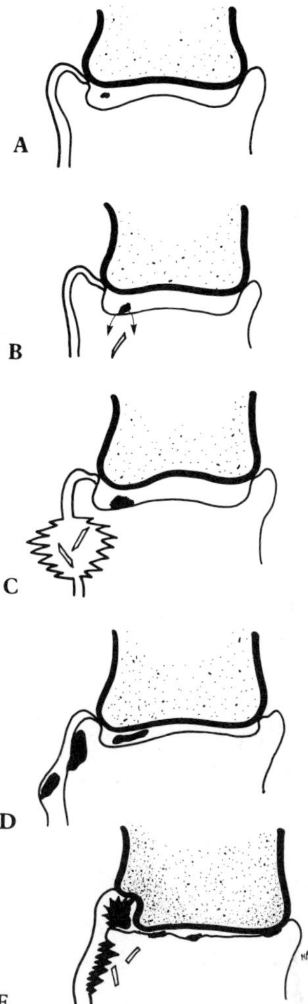

Fig. 9.8 Pathological stages in the development of gout. **A**. Small, asymptomatic crystal deposits in cartilage. **B**. Crystal shedding into joint space. **C**. Free crystals cause acute inflammation of joint lining. **D**. Growth of larger deposits. **E**. Chronic inflammatory changes in soft tissues and bone destruction.

GOUT

Gout is characterised by the presence of crystals of monosodium urate monohydrate in connective tissue and increases in frequency with increasing degrees of hyperuricaemia. However, only a minority of those with hyperuricaemia ever get gout, emphasising the fact that raised uric acid levels are a necessary, but not sufficient, cause.

The pathology and pathogenesis of gout

Crystalline deposits of monosodium urate monohydrate are only found in connective tissue and form preferentially in and around the articular cartilage of synovial joints. The needle-shaped crystals are 2–10 μm long and tend to clump together to form lumps of solid urate (tophi). The natural history of these deposits can be devided into five stages (Fig. 9.8).

1. The growth of small tophi in cartilage
2. Crystal shedding from these deposits
3. Free crystals causing transient inflammatory reactions
4. Growth of larger, more widespread deposits in cartilage and soft tissues
5. Chronic inflammatory and destructive changes associated with large tophi.

1. Growth of small cartilage deposits

Deposition usually starts in the articular cartilage, and the common joint sites are the first metatarso-phalangeal joint and other small joints of the hands, wrists and feet. The diameter of these hard white deposits varies from about 50 μm to 5 mm. The surrounding tissue may appear normal, although osteoarthritic changes are common.

Local factors controlling the site and extent of growth probably include temperature (low temperature favours crystallisation) and depletion of proteoglycan inhibitors. Growth is slow, and it may take years to develop a few small asymptomatic tophi.

2. Crystal shedding

Trauma, local destruction of the surrounding cartilage matrix or a sudden increase in solubility may allow crystals to be shed from the pre-formed deposits. Individual crystals are then found free in the joint space or in periarticular tissues where they may 'seed' further crystal growth or activate inflammatory mediators.

3. Acute inflammation

Acute inflammation in response to urate crystals may occur in joints, bursae or periarticular soft tissues. The tissues are oedematous, hyperaemic and full of polymorphonuclear leucocytes. Individual crystals can be seen in the synovium and the exudate, and phagocytosis by both synovial lining cells and free polymorphs can be observed. There are no other distinctive histological features.

As explained in Chapter 9.I the inflammation is probably mediated by the demonstrable phagocytosis, as well as by direct crystal surface activation of extra-cellular mediators.

4. Tophi and tissue destruction

Over a period of years, larger deposits of urate accumulate in various different sites, including joints and periarticular tissues, the ears, olecranon bursa and Achilles tendon. Less common sites include the eyes, eye-lids, tongue, intestine and penis. These tophi may grow to be several centimetres across. They are surrounded by a low-grade inflammatory cell reaction and encased by fibrous tissue; immunofluorescent staining shows the presence of immunoglobulin around the crystals. Local pressure may cause necrosis of surrounding tissue and the chalky crystalline material may ulcerate through the skin. Joint tophi are associated with destructive changes in the cartilage and periarticular bone, and large cystic, destructive lesions of bone, full of urate crystals, are found.

Tissue damage, especially joint and bone destruction, are striking in chronic tophaceous gout. Local pressure is an insufficient explanation for all the changes seen; the tophi are apparently capable of activating local, presumed enzymatic, mechanisms of joint damage.

Epidemilogy and classification of gout

Gout is principally a disease of men (M:F ratio is 10:1). The mean age of onset is 40 for men and 55 for women. Occasional cases occur in childhood or in relatively young women, and one should then suspect an enzyme defect such as HGPRT deficiency or PRPP synthetase excess.

Gout is usually classified into primary or secondary types.

Classification of gout

Primary: No obvious cause
Secondary: associated with a known cause of hyperuricaemia

Common causes of gout

1. Primary gout
2. Diuretics
3. Myeloproliferative disorders
4. Renal disease

1. Primary gout occurs in the absence of any apparent disease, dietary or drug-related cause. The patients are often obese, hypertensive men with a family history (about 30%) and a high alcohol intake (about 30%, often beer-drinkers).

Most will be found to be mild under-secretors of uric acid (about 70%), and only a small minority have an inherited enzyme abnormality causing significant over-production of urate (less than 5%). An abnormality of connective tissue has been found in these patients, who have high levels of serum uronic acid (a product of proteoglycan metabolism), suggesting that a tissue-factor promoting crystal deposition may be just as important as the hyperuricaemia.

2. Secondary gout can occur in association with any cause of prolonged hyperuricaemia (see p 165). The commonest forms are diuretic-induced and those related to myeloproliferative disorders such as polycythemia rubra vera. Renal failure is an unusual cause, and the oft-quoted association with psoriasis has been shown to be insignificant. Most of the other causes, such as lead poisoning in 'moonshine' drinkers (who distil spirit in lead containers) and glycogen-storage diseases, are rarities in the UK.

Who gets gout?

Gout is well-described in early medical writings, and was known in Ancient Egypt and by Hippocrates. Many famous physicians have suffered from the disease and some, like Thomas Sydenham, have added colourful descriptions to the literature. It was a very common disease in Georgian England, and some of the country's finest politicians, artists and entrepreneurs have suffered its ravages. The caricature of the gout sufferer is of a portly, middle-aged, jolly, port-loving alcoholic. This may have been near to the truth in the past, when purine-rich foods and lead-contaminated wines may have made a significant contribution to hyperuricaemia, but times are changing.

Gout clinics today are visited by many middle-aged, intelligent men, and they often have a high beer intake and mild obesity. But many are abstemious and asthenic, and some are embarrassed by the lingering social stigma of the disease. Increasing numbers of older patients are now getting gout, women as well as men. The cause is often iatrogenic, diuretics playing a major role, and acute attacks are frequently precipitated by intercurrent disease or treatment, including surgery.

Clinical manifestations

Gout is regarded as having four different phases in its clinical history. They reflect the natural history of the pathological changes described and are: 1. asymptomatic hyperuricaemia, generally preceding gout by many years; 2. acute gout; 3. intercritical gout, the phase between acute bouts in which the patient is again asymptomatic; and 4. chronic tophaceous gout.

Clinical phases of gout

1. Asymptomatic hyperuricaemia
2. Acute gout
3. Intercritical gout
4. Chronic tophacous gout

Acute gout

An acute attack of gout is a dramatic, excruciatingly painful condition, requiring immediate attention. Classical attacks are highly characteristic and easy to diagnose from the history and examination; atypical presentations also occur and can cause diagnostic problems.

The classical presentation. The patient, usually a middle-aged man, wakes in the early hours with a feeling of irritation and an ache in one big toe. Over the preceding few days he may have felt irritable or unwell, and the attack might have been precipitated by trauma, an intercurrent illness, surgery, drugs or dietary excess. Within a few hours of onset the base of the toe is swollen, hot and very painful, and the patient cannot bear the weight of the bedclothes on his foot. The inflammation is usually maximal within 24 hours of onset, by which time the joint looks red and angry and a mild pyrexia and malaise may be present. If left untreated the joint slowly returns to normal over the next 5–15 days, often with desquamation and peeling of the overlying skin.

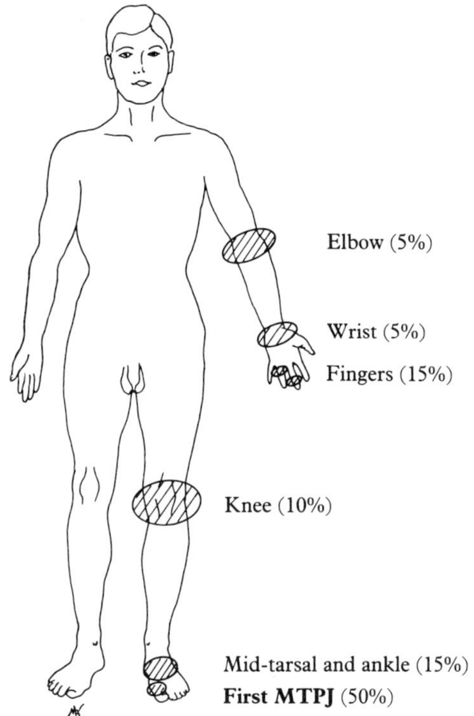

Fig. 9.9 Joint involvement in gout (approximate percentages)

90% of acute attacks of gout are monarticular. About 50% of first attacks and 70% of all attacks affect the first metatarsophalangeal joint. Other commonly affected areas include the ankle, knee, mid-tarsal joints, small joints of the hand, wrist and elbow (in that order). Shoulders and hips are almost never affected (Fig. 9.9).

Atypical acute attacks. Unusual presentations include polyarticular or cluster attacks, gout dominated by a severe systemic reaction and extra-articular inflammation of bursae or subcutaneous tissues.

10% of all attacks involve more than one joint; the distribution is usually patchy and asymmetrical and the synovitis sometimes flits from one joint to another. The olecranon bursa may be the site of acute gout, and involvement of subcutaneous tissues around a joint may mimic streptococcal cellulitis. Any form of acute gout can be associated with high fevers and severe systemic disturbance, causing confusion with septic arthritis. The differential diagnosis is covered in Chapter 22; in practice sepsis and pseudogout cause the most confusion and it is important to be aware that gout can co-exist with either of these conditions.

Atypical presentations of acute gout
1. Polyarticular disease
2. Cluster attacks
3. Periarticuar sites
4. Systemic reactions

Intercritical gout

Some patients get one attack and never have any further trouble. In others, once the disease has started, frequent recurrences of acute synovitis occur. However, the mean interval between attacks is 6–9 months. The phase between these episodes is known as the *intercritical period*.

Most patients are entirely asymptomatic between attacks, although mild aches and pains and early-morning stiffness sometimes occur. If the disease progresses, joint damage from repeated attacks at one site may cause chronic pain to develop; this heralds the onset of the chronic stage of gout.

Chronic tophaceous gout

The natural history of untreated gout depends on the degree and duration of the hyperuricaemia. Persistently elevated levels can result in small chalky deposits appearing on the ears and hands, or around an affected MTP and in the olecranon bursae. If the condition is still not treated, gross knobbly swellings develop and may ulcerate, become secondarily infected and cause severe restriction of movement. With the advent of effective hyperuricaemia therapy, late, severe tophaceous gout has become rare. However, many patients remain unaware of small tophi, and in a few therapy is either ineffective or not used and larger tophi develop.

The chronic gouty patient may present with gross destructive joint disease of the hands, wrists and feet, olecranon bursitis and subcutaneous tophi which can be mistaken for rheumatoid nodules. Acute attacks of synovitis are often less common than in the earlier stages of the disease.

The differential diagnosis of late RA and gout therefore used to present problems, but is now easily solved by identification of crystals from joints or tophi. The chances of the two diseases co-existing is negligible as there is a strong negative correlation between them. Only a handful of patients with both RA and gout have been described, in spite of the fact that they are two common diseases.

Laboratory tests

1. Uric acid

In acute gout the serum uric acid level is nearly always elevated, although occasional cases of normouricaemic gout have been described. In chronic tophaceous gout the total uric acid pool in the body may be 50 or 100 times normal, and high serum levels are the rule. Urinary uric acid excretion is normal or low in under-secretors and elevated in over-producers.

2. Associated metabolic abnormalities

Type 4 hyperlipidaemias are common, and in obese patients glucose intolerance may develop. Heavy beer-drinkers may have a raised γ GT or other disturbances of liver function tests.

3. Synovial fluid

In acute gout the synovial fluid is thin, murky and has a very high total white count, with polymorphonuclear cells predominating. It occasionally looks like infected pus. Polarised-light microscopy reveals large numbers of the typical negatively bifringent urate crystals. In chronic tophaceous gout acute inflammation is less marked, although some crystals can usually be found in any joint or bursal fluid aspirated.

4. Radiology

The radiograph of acute gout is non-specific, showing only soft-tissue swelling and periarticular osteoporosis of affected joints (Fig. 9.10).

In the chronic tophacous phase joint space narrowing and sclerosis and cystic changes develop in the underlying bone (i.e. osteoarthritic changes). A more specific, diagnostic abnormality is the gouty erosion (Fig. 9.11). This is usually para-articular and relatively large, it often has a sclerotic margin and it may have a hook of bone around it. The distinction from rheumatoid erosions is usually easy. The tophi of chronic gout are usually radiolucent, but many calcify due to epitaxial growth of hydroxyapatite on the urate crystals.

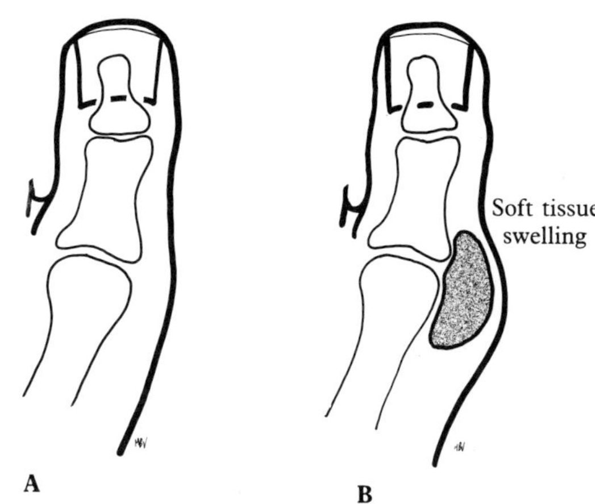

Fig. 9.10 Radiological changes in acute gout. **A**. Normal. **B**. Acute gout of first MTP joint.

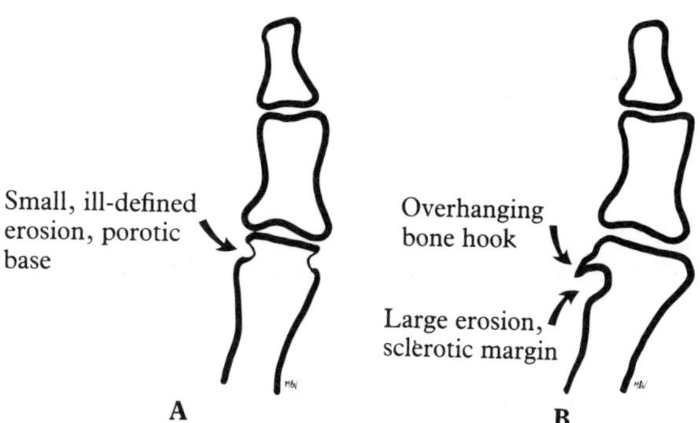

Fig. 9.11 Radiological appearances of erosions in (**A**) rheumatoid arthritis and (**B**) chronic gout

Diagnosing gout

1. Acute gout

The classical clinical features outlined are highly characteristic. However, several other conditions

Differential diagnosis of acute gout of the first metatarso-phalangeal joint ('pseudopodagra')

1. Inflammation of periarticular tissue (bunions, poor man's gout)
2. Pseudogout
3. Psoriatic arthropathy
4. Reiter's disease
5. Septic arthritis
6. Exacerbation of osteoarthritis

occasionally mimic gout of the first MTP ('pseudopodagra') or other joints. The correct diagnosis should be established unless the patient is known to suffer from gout.

Because most hyperuricaemia patients do not get gout, the serum uric acid level is only a guide and is not a confirmatory test. High levels make gout more likely; low levels make it unlikely.

Confirmation of the diagnosis can only be made by identification of crystals in the fluid. Polarised-light microscopy is the usual method used, and well over 90% of cases are unequivocably positive if examined by an experienced person.

Chronic gout

In addition to the clinical features and synovial-fluid urate crystals, the tophi themselves and the radiographs provide further means of diagnosing chronic gout. Tophi often have small surface deposits or tiny ulcerated areas. If a minute amount of the chalky material present can be placed on a glass microscope slide, the crystals can be identified and the diagnosis confirmed. The radiographs, as already explained, are also fairly specific for gout.

Treatment of gout

The management of asymptomatic hyperuricaemia, acute gout and chronic gout are three separate issues that must be kept quite distinct.

1. Asymptomatic hyperuricaemia

Treatment is generally considered to be unnecessary unless there is renal impairment, urolithiasis or levels persistently greater than 0.6 mmol/l (10 mg/dl). There is little evidence to suggest that hyperuricaemia *per se* is damaging, although views about the level at which treatment should be instituted differ. If treatment is given it is as for chronic gout.

2. Acute gout

This is a self-limiting condition, which is however, extremely painful. The treatment is to inhibit inflammation; alteration of uric acid levels is contra-indicated until the attack is over. Resolution and relief of symptoms are aided by rest, and short-term high doses of any non-steroidal anti-inflammatory drug except aspirin (which can raise uric acid levels in small doses but be uricosuric when given in large amounts). Colchicine is also effective, but the dose required often causes diarrhoea; it is a useful alternative when anti-inflammatory drugs are contra-indicated (active peptic ulceration, for example). Joint aspiration also helps relieve symptoms, and in difficult or prolonged attacks intra-articular steroids, or even a short course of ACTH injections are occasionally necessary.

3. Chronic gout

Most authorities agree on the indications for hyperuricaemic therapy.

Indications for hypouricaemic therapy

1. Three or more acute attacks of gout
2. Tophi
3. Bone or cartilage destruction
4. Gout and renal disease
5. Uric acid urolithiasis
6. Very high uric acid levels

In many cases loss of weight and a reduced alcohol intake are all that is necessary. In others removal of an obvious cause such as a diuretic is sufficient. Long-term hypouricaemic drug therapy should not be given lightly and is often unnecessary.

The logical therapeutic approach would be allopurinol (a xanthine oxidase inhibitor) for over-producers and a uricosuric drug for under-secretors. In practice allopurinol is a useful drug for most patients requiring hypouricaemic therapy. It has few side-effects, can be given once daily and the dose can be tailored to achieve effective reduction of uric acid below the solubility limit. Uricosuric drugs must be avoided in over-producers and stone-formers, and patients using them need to maintain a high urine flow. Probenecid or sulphinpyrazone are the drugs usually used. Azapropazone is an alternative, as it combines effective anti-inflammatory activity with mild uricosruricosuric actions; other new non-steroidal anti-inflammatory drugs may have a similar action.

When hypouricaemic therapy is instituted there is a marked increase in the risk of acute attacks in the first few months. This problem requires co-existent therapy with low dose colchicine (0.5 mg b.d. is very effective as a prophylactic drug for a acute attacks) or a non-steroidal anti-inflammatory agent for 2–3 months.

THE KIDNEY

Hyperuricaemia, gout and the kidney are interrelated in several ways.

Interrelationships of gout and the kidney

1. Renal failure can cause gout
2. Gout is associated with vascular disease, including nephrosclerosis
3. Gouty individuals are often under-secretors of uric acid, excrete an acid urine and have mild reduction of glomerular filtration rate
4. Between 10% and 20% of gout patients suffer from uric acid calculi. Hyperuricaemia is also associated with calcium salt urolithiasis
5. A few families with gout and severe premature renal failure are described
6. Hyperuricaemia occasionally leads to acute renal failure associated with crystal deposition
7. Lead poisoning causes renal tubular damage and hyperuricaemia

1. Renal failure can cause gout

If GFR is reduced below about 20ml/min, serum uric acid levels rise. Severe, prolonged renal failure can cause secondary gout, although this is surprisingly rare. When it does occur, the clinical manifestations are no different from those of primary gout.

2. Gouty individuals have abnormal renal function

About 70% of patients with gout tend to secrete urine with a fixed low pH (due to a defect of ammonia excretion) and are under-secretors of uric acid. Thus the majority appear to have a specific abnormality of tubular function contributing to hyperuricaemia. Mild reductions of glomerular filtration are also common, although gout rarely causes severe changes in renal function (see below).

3. Gout is associated with nephrosclerosis

The associations between gout, hyperuricaemia, hypertension and other cardiovascular diseases are reflected in the kidney as elsewhere. Nephrosclerotic changes, attributable to hypertension, are common in the kidney of necropsy specimens from gouty individuals.

4. Gout is associated with urolithiasis

The percentage of patients with gout who also have kidney stones varies in the different series quoted, but is probably in the order of 10%. Stones of uric acid (which crystallises preferentially in the acid medium of the collecting ducts), rather than the sodium salt, are deposited. Hyperuricosuria is also associated with an increased incidence of calcium oxalate stones, although the reasons for this are not yet clear.

5. A few familial cases of renal failure and gout exist

A rare syndrome of premature renal failure and

gout has been described which runs in families. It is probably a distinct subset of secondary gout, although the exact cause is not apparent.

6. *Acute renal failure in gout*

Severe hyperuricaemia (which is usually associated with treatment of myeloproliferative diseases and can be averted by concurrent use of allopurinol) can cause acute renal failure. This is due to crystallisation of masses of urate in the small collecting ducts, literally 'sludging up' the kidney. It can be difficult to diagnose, presenting as an insidious rise in blood urea and reduction in urine flow. Maintaining high flow and alkalinising the urine (to make the uric acid soluble) helps in the treatment.

7 *Lead poisoning*

Lead poisoning causes damage to the renal tubules, resulting in under-secretion of uric acid and sometimes gout (saturnine gout). It can result from industrial exposure (e.g. painters), but is usually seen in 'moonshine' drinkers, and is rare in the UK. High levels of lead in eighteenth-century port may have contributed to the epidemic of gout in upper-class Georgian England.

RARE SYNDROMES ASSOCIATED WITH ABNORMAL PURINE METABOLISM

1. Lesch–Nyhan syndrome

This is a rare syndrome of X-linked recessive inheritance. The enzyme HGPRT is absent, leading to very high uric acid and premature gout. These male children are also mentally-defective and tend to self-mutilation; they may have to be restrained to prevent them biting off their fingers or lips.

Patients with partial defects of HGPRT (heterozygotes) may get early severe gout, but are usually mentally normal. Any young male over-producer should be investigated to aid genetic counselling. The enzyme can be measured fairly easily in erythrocyte preparations.

2. Xanthinuria

A loss of xanthine oxidase leads to excess hypoxanthine and xanthine. Uric acid levels are very low and the main consequence is xanthine renal stones.

3. APD deficiency

Deficiency of the enzyme adenosine phosphoribosyltransferase is a very rare cause of renal stones composed of the adenine product 2-8-dihydroxyadenine.

4. Enzyme deficiencies associated with immunodeficiency

A few rare enzyme abnormalities of purine metabolism are associated with deficient function of T cells, B cells or both. An example is adenosine deaminase deficiency. Although uncommon, these syndromes are of considerable theoretical importance, illustrating ways in which an abnormality of nucleic acid metabolism and a single enzyme defect can cause an abnormal immune response. Exploration of these syndromes may throw new light on a variety of rheumatological diseases and provide new insight into immune response regulation.

FURTHER READING (GOUT)

Emmerson B T 1983 Hyperuricaemia and gout in clinical practice. ADIS Health Science Press, Balgowleh, Australia

Kelley W N 1977 Crystal-induced arthropathies. Clinics in Rheumatic Diseases 3: 1

Scott J T 1978 New knowledge of the pathogenesis of gout. Journal of Clinical Pathology 12: 205–213

Wyngarten J B, Kelley W N 1976 Gout and hyperuricaemia. Grune & Stratton, New York

III Calcification of Articular Tissues

INTRODUCTION

Calcification of connective tissues is an important process contributing to the pathogenesis and clinical outcome of a variety of rheumatic diseases.

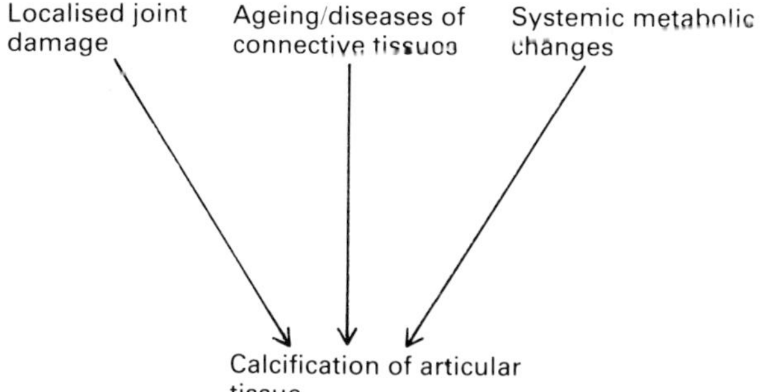

Fig. 9.12 Three different causes of articular calcification

Calcification can be caused by systemic metabolic disease, a generalised defect of connective tissue or localised damage to joints or periarticular tissues (Fig. 9.12).

The presence of calcified tissue may be apparent from radiological shadows of calcific density, which will be seen if enough calcium is present, or from the presence of crystals in synovial fluids or tissue biopsy material. Calcification may also cause a crystal-induced arthropathy — either an acute synovitis or chronic destructive changes (Fig. 9.13). These three effects of articular calcification (X-ray changes, crystals in tissues and arthritis) do not always follow when calcium crystals are deposited, and can occur singly or in any combination (Fig. 9.13).

There are three main types of calcium salt which have been identified in calcified tissue (Table 9.2). The two most important are calcium pyrophosphate dihydrate and hydroxyapatite. Although these two crystals are sometimes found together, and have some similarities in their clinical associations, different causes and effects are apparent, and they are therefore discussed separately.

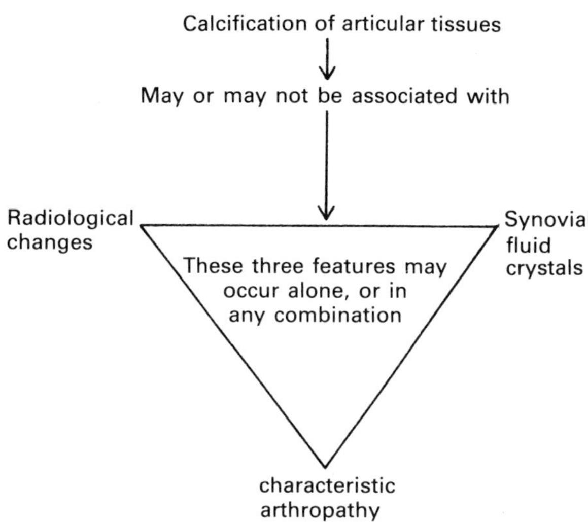

Fig. 9.13 Three different effects of articular calcification

PYROPHOSPHATE DEPOSITION

The deposition of crystals of calcium pyrophosphate dihydrate in human articular cartilage is a common age-related phenomenon. It is a remarkably singular, selective biological event.

1. It only occurs in human joints and periarticular tissue
2. It grows selectively in articular fibrocartilage
3. Only two of many possible salts are deposited.

Pyrophosphate deposition is easy to identify radiologically and has a number of important diseases associations. It is also a marker for a clinically distinctive form of arthritis and has become recognised as an important feature of joint pathology in the elderly.

Table 9.2 The three common salts found in human calcified tissue

	Formula	Bones/teeth	Joints	Periarticular	Other pathological calcification
Hydroxyapatite	$Ca_{10}(PO_4)_6.OH$	+++	+	++	++
Calcium pyrophosphate dihydrate	$Ca_2P_2O_7.2H_2O$	–	++	+	–
Calcium hydrogen phosphate dihydrate (brushite)	$CaHPO_4.2H_2O$	–	+	–	+

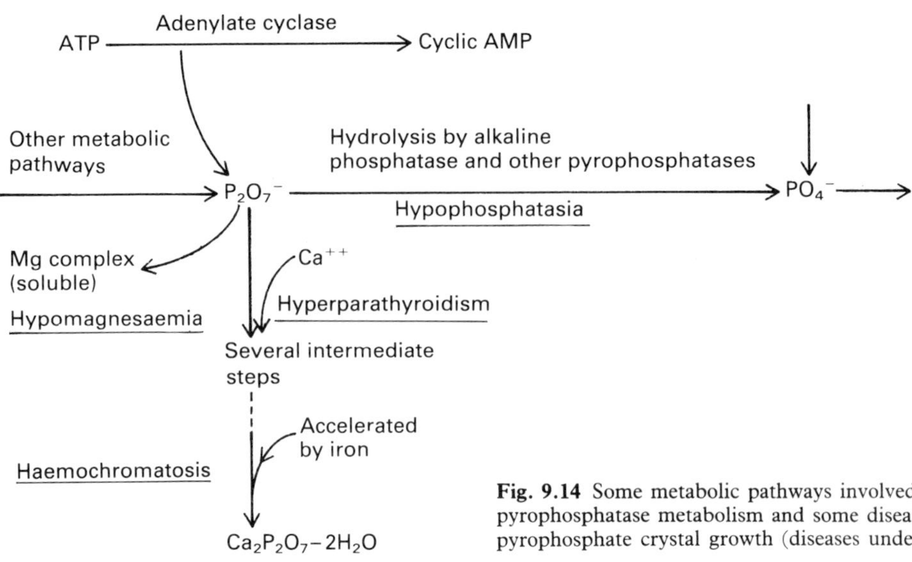

Fig. 9.14 Some metabolic pathways involved in pyrophosphatase metabolism and some diseases promoting pyrophosphate crystal growth (diseases underlined)

Metabolic background

Inorganic pyrophosphate ($P_2O_7^-$) is produced by many energy-generating reactions: one important one is the breakdown of ATP to cAMP (Fig. 9.14). Pyrophosphate is normally hydrolysed to orthophosphate (PO^-), but can combine with magnesium to form a soluble salt. Formation of the much more insoluble calcium salt is favoured by hypercalcaemia, loss of magnesium or of pyrophosphatase enzymes, or the presence of a substance like iron which can promote crystallisation. Some of the metabolic associations of pyrophosphate deposition can be explained in this way (Fig. 9.14).

However, in the majority of patients no obvious metabolic abnormality is present except for a moderate increase in the amount of $P_2O_7^-$ produced locally by the chondrocytes. The association of age and joint damage with a predisposition to form deposits suggests that local changes in the structure of the cartilage may promote crystal formation in many cases. This may be analagous to the abnormality of proteoglycan turnover found in some gout patients (p 169).

Metabolic associations of pyrophosphate deposition

Hyperparathyroidism Hypothyroidism Hyperuricaemia	Uncommon
Haemochromatosis Hypomagnaesaemia Hypophosphatasia	Rare

The crystals and their sites of deposition

The monoclinic and triclinic crystals of calcium pyrophosphate dihydrate vary from about 1–10 μm long. In the polarised-light microscope they look like small bricks and exhibit weak positive bifringence.

The crystals are probably formed initially in close proximity to the chondrocytes. Fibrocartilage is affected more commonly than hyaline cartilage. As the deposits grow they tend to accumulate in the mid-zone of these cartilages, although aggregates are sometimes found in the joint space and synovium due to 'seeding' on crystal derived from the cartilage (Fig. 9.15). The most frequent sites of deposition include knee menisci, the triangular ligament of the wrist, the pubic symphysis and the intervertebral discs.

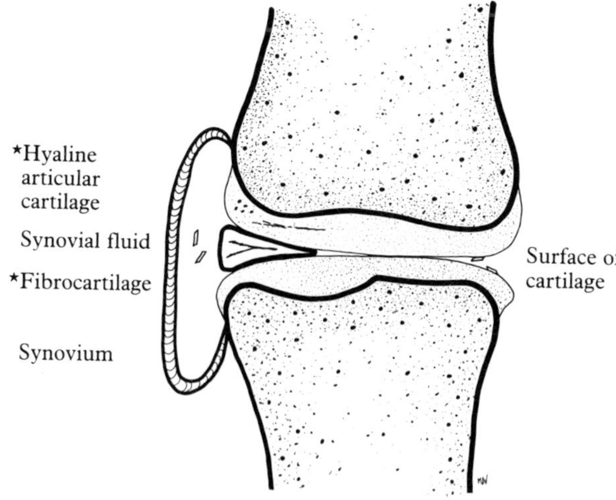

Fig. 9.15 Joint tissue in which calcium pyrophosphate dihydrate crystals may be found.* = probable sites of primary growth of crystals.

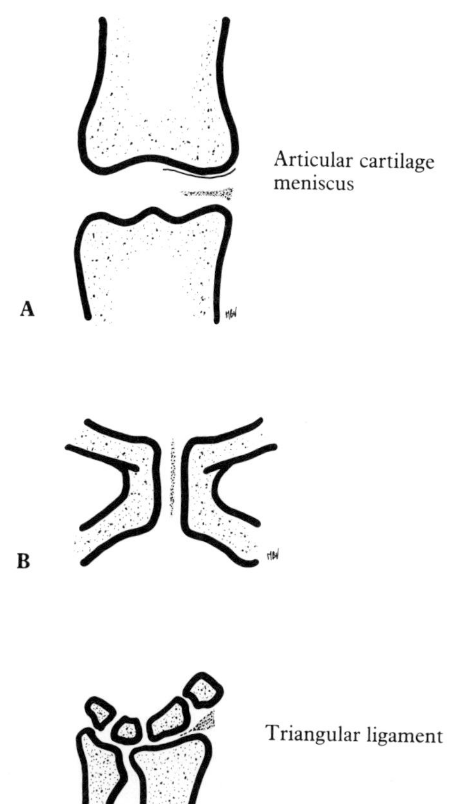

Fig. 9.16 Radiological signs of pyrophosphate deposition in the commonly-involved sites. **A**. Knee. **B**. Pubic symphysis. **C**. Wrist.

Radiographic features

The deposition of linear deposits of the salt in the mid-zone of cartilage gives rise to a characteristic set of radiological changes (Fig. 9.16). An AP view of the knee is the most useful X-ray for the identification. Views of the wrist and pelvis should also be taken. Chondrocalcinosis is often an unimportant incidental radiographic finding, but may be accompanied by X-ray features of the associated arthropathy (see below).

Causes and effects of chondrocalcinosis

If evidence of pyrophosphate deposition is found, either by radiographs or on examination of synovial fluid or joint tissue, two important questions must be asked: 1. What is the cause of the deposition? 2. What effects are the deposits having?

Causes of chondrocalcinosis

A classification of causes of chondrocalcinosis is shown (right).

1. Familial cases are very rare; affected members of the family develop premature chondrocalcinosis and osteoarthritis and a variety of different patterns have been described in different racial groups.

2. A defined metabolic disease can be found as the cause in less than 10% of cases; suspicion is aroused by widespread chondrocalcinosis occuring under the age of 60, or by clinical features of the causative disease.

Classification of cases of pyrophosphate arthropathy
1. Familial (rare)
2. Metabolic (uncommon)
3. Sporadic
   Age-associated (common)
   Secondary to joint damage (common)

3. At least 90% of cases are idiopathic age-associated or 'sporadic'; the knee is commonly the joint in which calcification is seen and may be the only site affected. Age alone appears to be the dominant cause of chondrocalcinosis, the incidence rising in a linear fashion from less than 1% in the under-50s to over 40% in those over 90 (Fig. 9.17).

Metabolic causes (*Fig. 9.14*). Hyperparathyroidism is associated with a marked increase in the incidence of chondrocalcinosis. The frequency and severity of the radiological changes can be correlated with the elevation of parathormone, but the calcification does *not* disappear after parathyroidectomy (which frequently precipitates attacks of pseudogout). Haemochromatosis is another uncommon disease clearly associated with chondrocalcinosis; the hands are often affected (especially the second and third MCPs) and again removing the 'cause' by venesection does not stop the progression of the calcification and associated arthropathy. Both gout and hypothyroidism appear to cause a slight increase in the incidence of pyrophosphate deposition; other suggested disease associations with common conditions like hypertension and diabetes are probably unreal, being caused by the chance concurrence of two common age-related phenomena. A few very rare metabolic aberrations are associated with premature deposition, including hypomagnesaemia, hypophosphatasia (low alkaline phosphatase, skeletal abnormalities) and Baarter's syndrome.

Local causes. Any cause of joint instability or hypermobility may also lead to localised chondrocalcinosis. Unilateral menisectomy, for example, causes a relatively high incidence of calcification of the retained meniscus in the damaged knee when compared with the unoperated side. In patients with pyrophosphate deposition one should therefore look for pre-existing hypermobility, trauma or other joint damage as a possible predisposing cause.

Effects of chondrocalcinosis

Pyrophosphate deposition is associated with some distinctive forms of arthritis which probably result from the presence of the crystals. In common with

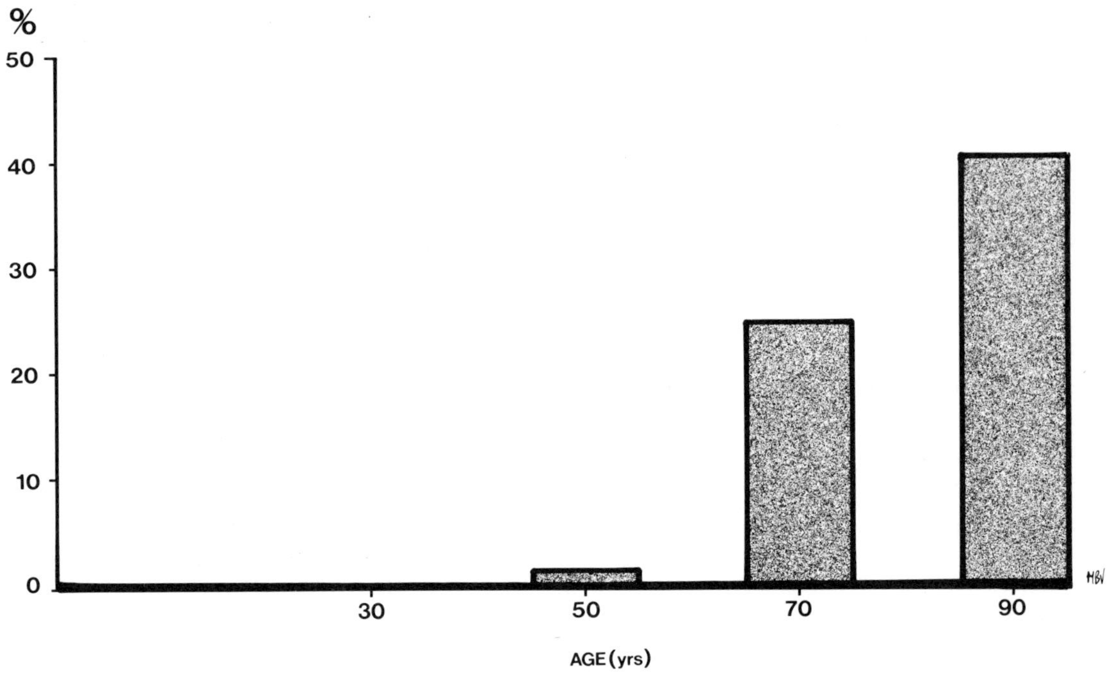

Fig. 9.17 Incidence of radiological chondrocalcinosis in different age-groups

other forms of crystal-related joint disease, these can be conveniently divided into acute self-limiting attacks of synovitis and chronic destructive arthropathies.

Acute synovitis (Pseudogout)

This is a common cause of an acute monoarthritis in elderly people, especially women (F:M ratio is approximately 2:1). It can present in a variety of ways.

Classical pseudogout. The clinical setting is one of an elderly lady who may have minor aches and pains in her joints for a number of years. A minor injury, illness or a hospital admission may precipitate the attack, although there is often no obvious cause. One knee becomes very swollen and painful over a period of about 24 hours. The joints feels tight and is difficult to walk on; it may rupture. If left untreated, the pain and swelling slowly subside over a period of 1–8 weeks. Examination will often reveal widespread changes of osteoarthritis in addition to a large, tense, warm effusion in one knee. Aspiration of synovial fluid will relieve the symptoms and allow crystal identification by polarised-light microscopy. The joint distribution of pseudogout is shown in Figure 9.18.

Atypical presentation. Pseudogout can present in a number of other ways. In about 10% of cases more than one joint is involved. Systemic upset is sometimes great and an incorrect diagnosis of sepsis or traumatic haemarthrosis is often made.

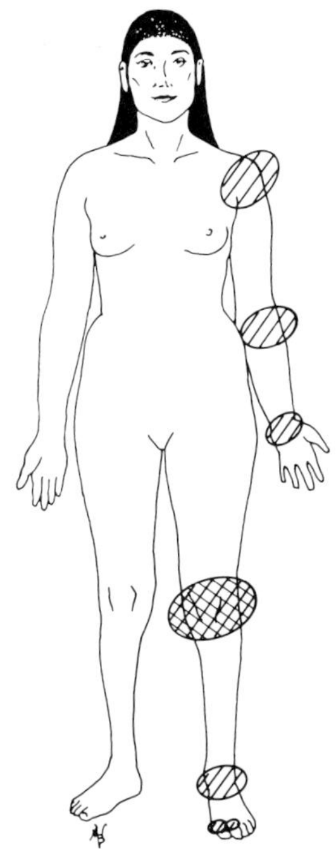

Fig. 9.18 Joint involvement in 'pseudogout'

Atypical presentations of 'pseudogout'
1. Polyarticular acute inflammation
2. Arthritis and pyrexia
3. Haemarthrosis
4. Periarticular inflammation

Chronic destructive arthritis (pyrophosphate arthropathy)

This is a common condition of elderly ladies (F:M ratio is approximately 4:1, mean age 75). The distribution of involved joints is similar to that of pseudogout (Fig. 9.18). A number of variants of this condition have been described.

Typical chronic pyrophosphate arthropathy. A woman in her 70s presents with pain, stiffness and difficulty in moving her knees and wrists. She may also complain of aching in her shoulders, elbows and hips, and other joints, but the knees are her biggest worry. On examination she has bony swelling, warmth and moderate effusions of the knees and perhaps wrists, with marked limitation of movement and severe patello-femoral crepitus. In advanced cases instability and gross varus or valgus deformities develop. Heberden's nodes are often present as well, but the disease is differentiated from generalised osteoarthritis on the basis of its distribution, severity and characteristic radiological and synovial-fluid findings (Table 9.3). Progressive, more destructive, changes may develop over a period of years, although reliable data on outcome is not yet available. The radiographic changes include extensive cystic and destructive changes in bone, associated with chondrocalcinosis and osteoarthritic changes (Fig. 9.19).

Table 9.3 Osteoarthritis and chronic pyrophosphate arthropathy. Generalised OA is very similar, clinically, radiologically and pathologically, to pyrophosphate arthropathy. Some of the features which allow patients with pyrophosphate deposition to be distinguished are listed.

Distinguishing features	Generalised osteoarthritis	Pyrophosphate arthropathy
Joint distribution	Knees, distal interphalangeal joints, carpo-metacarpal joint of the thumb, hips and first metatarso-phalangeal joint	Knees, wrists, ankles, shoulders, elbows, hips and small joints of the hand
Clinical features	Usually modest inflammatory features; joint crepitus, bony swellings and Heberden's nodes common	Often marked inflammatory signs (e.g. large effusions, and hot joints). Other features as in osteoarthritis.
Synovial fluid	Viscous, mononuclear cells predominate; one third contain hydroxyapatite crystals	Variable: usually viscous with mononuclear cells, may be blood-stained or contain many polys. Pyrophosphate crystals usually present.
Radiological signs	Joint-space narrowing, osteophytes, cysts, bone sclerosis and sometimes capsular calcification (loose bodies or ossides)	More variable. As in OA, but cystic and destructive changes in bone often exaggerated. Disproportionate signs in patello-femoral joint. Chondrocalcinosis usually visible.

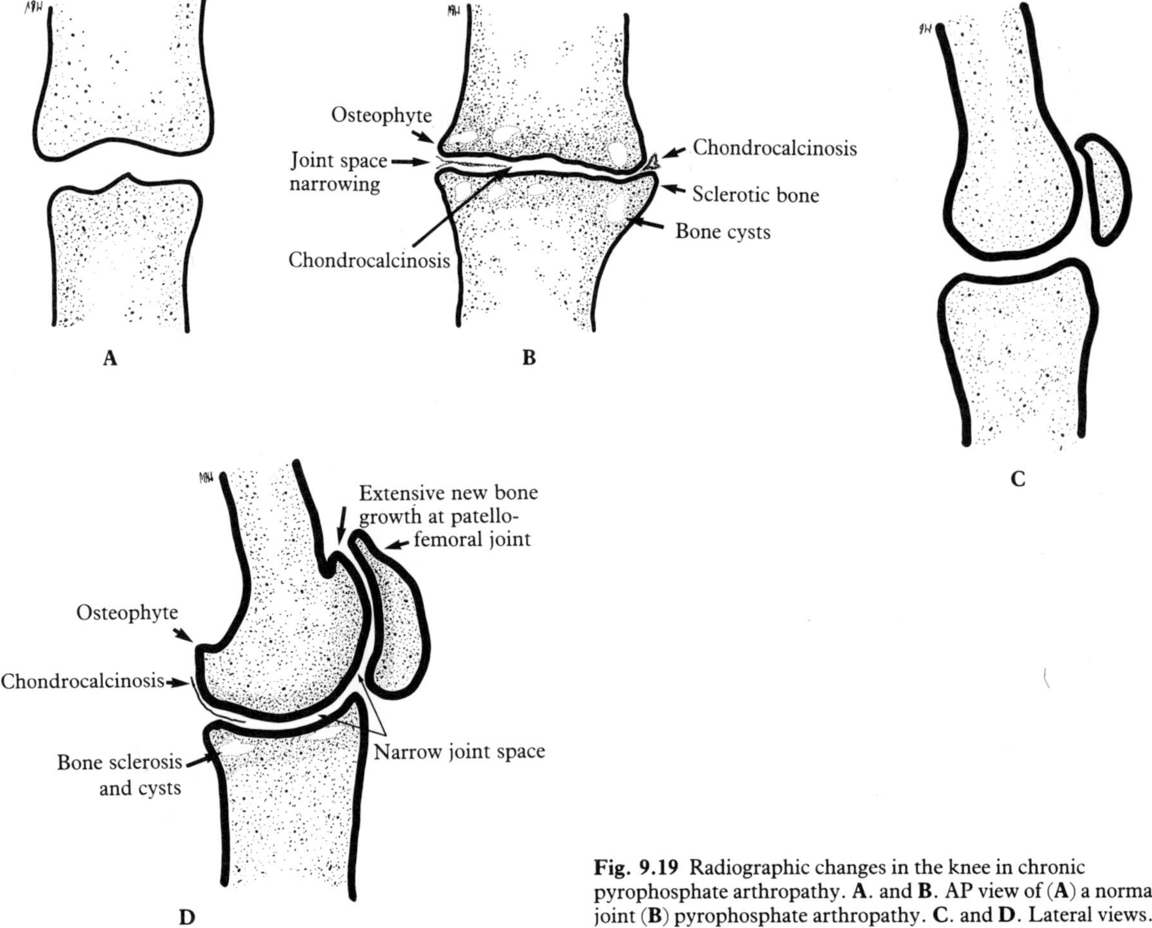

Fig. 9.19 Radiographic changes in the knee in chronic pyrophosphate arthropathy. **A.** and **B.** AP view of (**A**) a normal joint (**B**) pyrophosphate arthropathy. **C.** and **D.** Lateral views.

Atypical presentations. Chronic pyrophosphate arthropathy may mimic a number of other diseases. If the destructive lesions progress in a single joint, the final clinical and radiological picture may resemble a Charcot joint (the so-called *pseudo-neuropathic joint*). If the disease is widespread it may be mistaken for other polyarthropathies. It is most often confused with generalised OA and the two diseases can co-exist. There is some evidence to suggest that OA can promote the development of chondrocalcinosis, which may then accelerate joint damage, so that some authorities regard pyrophosphate arthropathy as a varient of OA rather than a separate disease (see also Chapter 8).

Atypical presentations of chronic pyrophosphate arthropathy

1. Polyarticular inflammatory arthritis mimicking rheumatoid disease
2. With prominent myalgic symtoms and proximal joint involvement, mimicking polymyalgia rheumatica
3. Severe destructive changes mimicking a Charcot joint
4. With destructive changes in the back
5. Indistinguishable from generalised osteoarthritis

Investigations and diagnosis

Patients with radiological *chondrocalcinosis* but no clinical disease usually have no laboratory abnormalities. A minority have a metabolic background for deposition, hypothyroidism and hyperparathyroidism being the commonest causes. The younger the patient and the more extensive the deposits the more need there is for careful investigation. In the elderly patient there is little need to do anything, although a serum calcium and thyroid function tests are warranted if the patient is unwell.

Pseudogout is frequently accompanied by a mild fever, leucocytosis and other haematological and biochemical abnormalities associated with acute inflammation (e.g. high ESR and C-reactive protein). The synovial fluid has a high polymorphonuclear white cell count, and crystals can usually be seen in the polarised-light microscope. Bacteriological examination should be carried out to exclude infection (which can co-exist with pseudogout).

Chronic pyrophosphate arthropathy may cause mild additional signs of chronic inflammation such as a low iron-binding capacity, but laboratory abnormalities are not prominent.

The diagnosis is dependent on 1. a high index of suspicion in the typical clinical setting; 2. a careful search for crystals in the synovial fluid; and 3. the radiological features.

Radiological chondrocalcinosis is so common in the elderly that there is a good chance of it being an incidental finding. Pseudogout or pyrophosphate arthropathy can only be diagnosed if the other clinical and synovial fluid findings are present or if additional radiographic features of joint damage are present.

Treatment

As yet, there is no available means of preventing or treating the crystal deposition *per se*.

Pseudogout. The aim is to reduce symptoms with anti-inflammatory therapy until the self-limiting synovitis receeds. Rest should only be temporary in the elderly because of the extra risks of muscle wasting, thrombo-embolism, pneumonia and other complications. Prompt aspiration of fluid, and injection of steroid if infection has been excluded, is helful. A short course of one of the better tolerated non-steroidal anti-inflammatory drugs may help.

Chronic pyrophosphate arthropathy. There is no definitive treatment for this condition. The approach to therapy is the same as that for osteoarthritis (Chapter 8). Recently, radioactive yttrium injections have also been recommended as a simple way of providing prolonged symptomatic relief, and they may have a place in the treatment of some patients.

HYDROXYAPATITE DEPOSITION

Hydroxyapatite ($Ca_{10}(PO_4)_6OH$) comprises the main mineral of bones and teeth. Most ectopic calcification found in damaged tissue also contains hydroxyapatite (HA) and calcified arteries, lymph nodes and tuberculous lesions are all examples of misplaced hydroxyapatite deposition. Joints and periarticular tissues can also calcify with HA.

Metabolic background

Calcium is a divalent cation which is essential for a variety of metabolic processes. Membrane function is particularly dependant on maintenance of the calcium levels within closely-defined limits. Orthophosphate (PO_4^-) is a product of all cellular reactions, and is essential for the formation of bones and teeth. The product (Ca^{++}) PO_4^-) has to be kept high to maintain the integrity of the skelton, which would otherwise dissolve. Specific cellular mechanisms are available to activate calcification where it is needed (e.g. formation of matrix vessicles in growing cartilage) and tissue factors are available to inhibit its formation in the rest of the body (e.g. $P_2O_7^-$ and aggregated proteoglycans, which probably inhibit calcification of connective tissue).

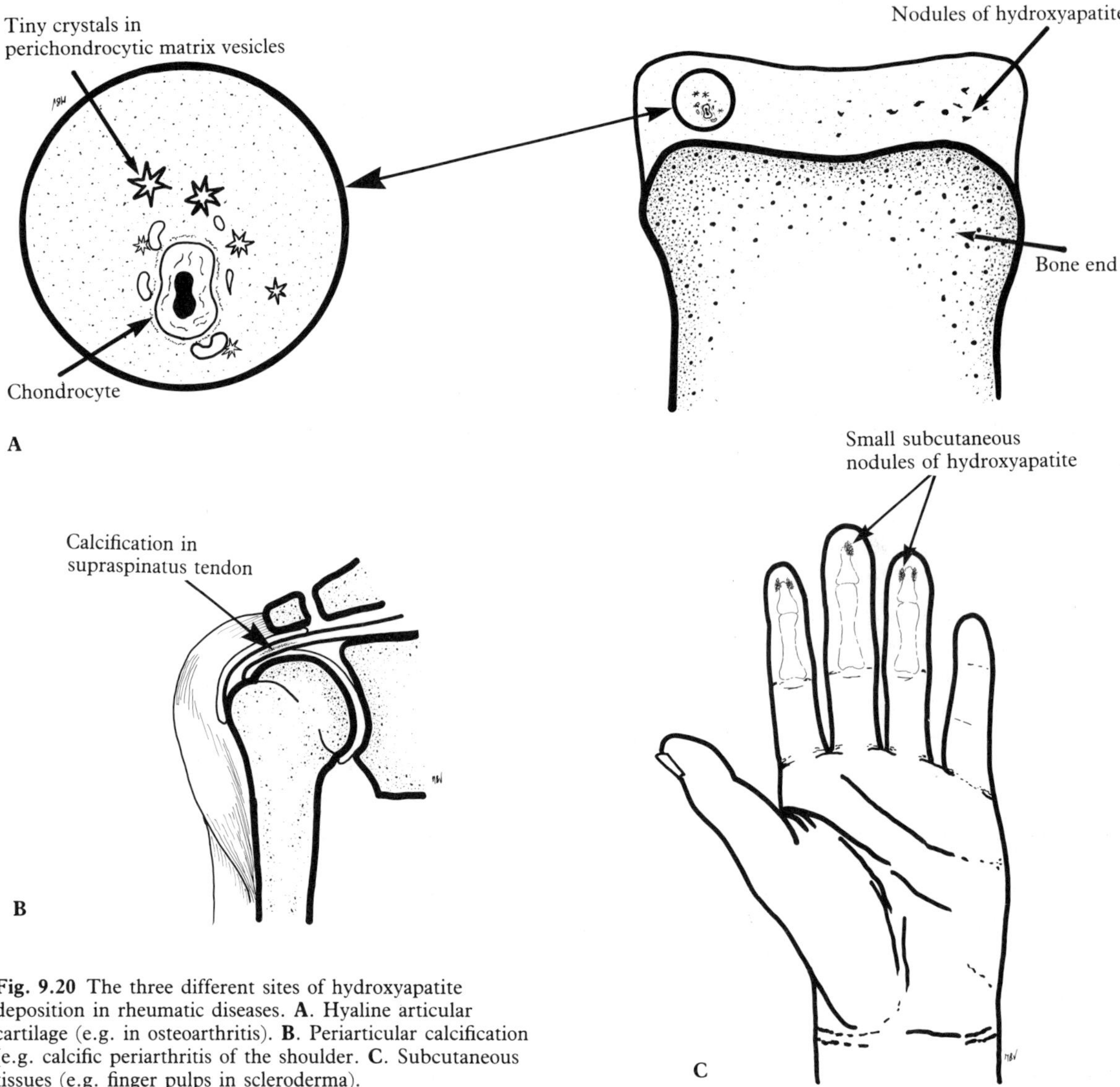

Fig. 9.20 The three different sites of hydroxyapatite deposition in rheumatic diseases. **A**. Hyaline articular cartilage (e.g. in osteoarthritis). **B**. Periarticular calcification (e.g. calcific periarthritis of the shoulder. **C**. Subcutaneous tissues (e.g. finger pulps in scleroderma).

Calcification outside the skeleton can therefore arise from: 1. raising the (Ca) (PO_4) product, resulting in widespread calcification ('metastatic'); 2. local tissue changes which activate deposition, or remove its natural inhibitors ('dystrophic').

The crystals and their sites of deposition

Hydroxyapatite crystals are too small to be seen by light microscopy. Individual particles are about 5–500 nm long, but may aggregate to form round lumps of up to 1μm diameter (spherulites, which are just visible by light microscopy).

There are three different sites of deposition in and around the joints (Fig. 9.20):

1. In hyaline articular cartilage. Crystals form in the perichondrocytic region, and are probably deposited by formation of matrix vesicles as in growth cartilage. They appear in the middle and lower zones of OA cartilage in particular, but may be shed into the synovial fluid.

2. Periarticular capsules, ligaments and tendons. Collagen fibres in these structures probably act as growth sites for dystrophic hydroxyapatite formation. The rotator-cuff tendons of the shoulder are involved more than any other periarticular site.

3. Subcutaneous tissues. Subcutaneous tissues of the extremities and over joints may also calcify in the rheumatic diseases. The hands are the commonest site, although calcific nodules may distribute in an analagous distribution to that of rheumatoid and other nodules.

A further mechanism of calcification of joints is through metaplasia of the synovium, forming cartilage rests which then ossify (see osteochondromatosis, p 228).

Radiological findings

Small areas of calcification in cartilage do not show up on radiographs. Large deposits within the synovium or capsule do, and are usually described as loose bodies or ossicles (Fig. 9.21). They can be distinguished from osteochondromatosis by the absence of trabeculation. Periarticular and subcutaneous deposits are easy to identify on radiographs. The typical appearance of periarthritis of the shoulder is shown in Figure 9.21.

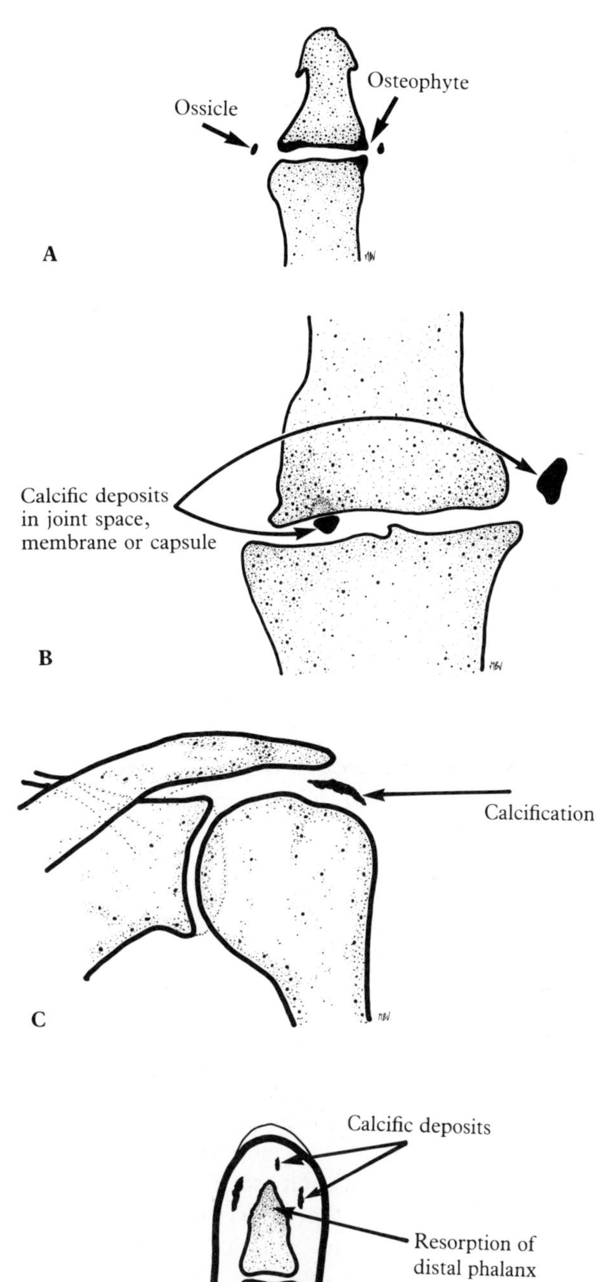

Fig. 9.21 Radiological findings in hydroxyapatite deposition. **A.** Periarticular ossicles in arthritis. **B.** Knee 'loose bodies' in osteoarthritis. **C.** Calcific periarthritis of the shoulder. **D.** Subcutaneous calcification of fingers in scleroderma.

A diagnosis of hydroxypatite deposition can only be confirmed by identifying crystals. More sophisticated apparatus than a light microscope is necessary for this, and it is difficult to tell on either clinical or radiological grounds whether it is present or not.

Cause and effect of hydroxyapatite deposition

Hydroxyapatite deposition may result from both local and systemic disorders and, in common with other major species of crystal deposited in and around the joints, is associated with both an acute inflammatory synovitis and chronic destructive arthritides.

Causes of deposits

Most joint and periarticular deposits are due to a local tissue change resulting in areas of relative avascularity, which seem prone to calcify. However, metabolic diseases occasionally cause deposition at the same sites.

1. Metabolic disorders causing hydroxyapatite deposition. Prolonged hypercalcaemia or hyperphosphatasia may cause ectopic calcification. Hyper- or hypo-parathyroidism, chronic renal failure and Vitamin D excess are rare causes of articular or periarticular hydroxyapatite deposition. Their presence is usually obvious. Diabetes may be associated with an increased incidence of shoulder lesions.

2. Rheumatic diseases causing local hydroxyapatite deposition. Some of the connective tissue diseases lead to dystrophic calcification of periarticular or subcutaneous tissues. The most striking examples are the skin calcification seen in scleroderma hands, especially in the CRST variant (Chapter 7) and calcification of muscle fascia following dermatomyositis (Chapter 7). Similar calcification occasionally occurs in SLE, and relapsing polychondritis may cause calcification of cartilage. Capsular and ligamentous calcification also follows inflammation in some joint diseases, especially ankylosing spondylitis and septic arthritis.

Calcific periarthritis and intra-articular deposition are more commonly related to local areas of damage to a tendon or articular cartilage respectively. Rotator-cuff lesions and osteoarthritic cartilage are probably particularly likely to promote hydroxyapatite crystal formation. Osteoarthritis and skeletal hyperostosis have also been associated with an increased frequency of periarticular deposition.

Causes of hydroxyapatite deposition

1. Systemic metabolic causes which increase the product Ca × PO_4
   a) Hyperparathyroidism
   b) Hypoparathyroidism
   c) Renal failure
   d) Vitamin D excess
   e) (Other causes of hypercalcaemia or hyperphosphatasia)
2. Connective tissue diseases which increase susceptibility of extra-skeletal connective tissue to calcification
   a) Scleroderma
   b) Dermatomyositis
   c) SLE
   d) Polychondritis
   e) (Diffuse, idiopathic, skeletal hyperostosis)
3. Local damage to connective tissues, promoting calcification at a single site
   a) Tendonitis (e.g. avascular supraspinatus tendonitis)
   b) Charcot joints
   c) Septic arthritis
   d) Muscle injury (myositis ossificans)
   e) (Osteoarthritis ?)
4. Idiopathic (sometimes familial) cases

Effects of deposits

Problems encountered in making a positive identification of hydroxyapatite, and the fact that dystrophic calcification can obviously occur as a secondary event in damaged joints make it difficult to unravel the possible role of these crystals as a cause of joint disease.

An uncommon form of self-limiting inflammation of periarticular tissues or joints (calcific

Joint diseases caused by hydroxyapatite crystals

1. *Acute self-limiting inflammatory disorders*
   a) Acute calcific periarthritis (uncommon)
   b) Acute hydroxyapatite synovitis (rare)
2. *Chronic destructive joint disease*
   a) Chronic destructive hydroxyapatite deposition diseases (rare)
   b) (? Osteoarthritis ?)

periarthritis) and rare forms of destructive joint disease are fairly clearly associated with hydroxyapatite crystals. In addition a possible role for these crystals in the pathogenesis of some cases of osteoarthritis has been proposed. Each of these clinical associations is described briefly below.

Acute calcific periarthritis

The deposition of hydroxyapatite in the supraspinatus tendon and elsewhere in the rotator-cuff region, is a common finding in both radiographic and pathological studies (about 7% of adults). It is occasionally associated with a severe acute inflammation of the subacromial bursa, periarticular tissues or the joint itself.

The pain starts suddenly and may be precipitated by trauma; the area is exquisitely tender, hot and red, and a diagnosis of sepsis is often made. The condition may resolve slowly of its own accord over a period of days or weeks and the radiological calcification which helps make the diagnosis often disappears, suggesting that the crystals are shed from the deposit during the attack. If the lesion is aspirated or opened surgically a thick, white fluid containing numerous aggregates of hydroxyapatite crystals, often in spherulites, is obtained. Resolution is accelerated by anti-inflammatory drugs and local depot steroid injections as well as by aspiration. Recovery is usually complete and lasting. Although the shoulder is the commonest site of involvement, the hip (around the greater trochanter) and other sites may be involved (Fig. 9.22) and a few individuals suffer from multiple or recurrent attacks at different sites.

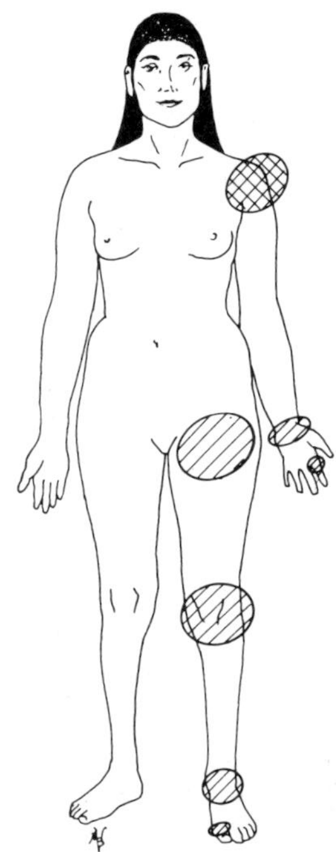

Fig. 9.22 Joint involvement in calcific periarthritis

Chronic destructive hydroxyapatite arthropathy

A few patients have been described with chronic destructive joint disease, accompanied by some cartilage loss and bone erosion in association with hydroxyapatite crystals in the synovial fluid and synovium. This has been observed in the shoulder (a rare sequelae of calcific periarthritis), knee, finger joints and elsewhere. Both clinical and *in vitro* observations suggest that the destruction may be mediated via crystal phagocytosis by synovial lining A cells, with subsequent release of destructive lysomal enzymes in the absence of overt acute inflammation.

Osteoarthritis and hydroxyapatite deposition

Perichondrocytic deposits of hydroxyapatite can frequently be found in osteoarthritic cartilage if it is examined under a high-resolution electron microscope and deposits may also be seen in the synovium and capsule. Several studies have identified these crystals in about a third of osteoarthritis synovial fluids examined. The presence of these crystals correlates poorly with inflammatory features of the disease, but does show some relationship with the severity of the radiological changes.

Crystal deposition in osteoarthritis may be a secondary event, but these findings suggest that hydroxyapatite crystals contribute to the pathogenesis of joint destruction in OA.

Mixed crystal deposition disease

The possible relationship between calcium phosphate crystal deposition and joint destruction is strengthened by the finding of mixtures of pyrophosphate and hydroxyapatite crystals in joints with severe progressive clinical and radiological features of osteoarthritis. Mixtures of these salts are not infrequently found in both advanced OA (where hydroxyapatite may predominate) and chronic pyrophosphate arthropathy.

Occasional cases in which brushite (dicalcium phosphate dihydrate) and other crystals have been identified are also described. However, as mentioned in the introduction, a variety of different salts are likely to be found in small amounts, or in odd deposits, and the exact nature and proportion of each crystal is probably unimportant.

SUMMARY: CALCIUM PHOSPHATE CRYSTAL DEPOSITION AND JOINT DISEASE

The relationship between the deposition of calcium phosphates and joint disease is not a simple one.

From the above outline one can derive the following conclusions:

1. Crystal deposition is not a sufficient cause of arthritis: many elderly people have crystal deposits in otherwise normal joints
2. Crystal deposition is associated with, and is a contribution cause of, several forms of inflammatory and destructive joint disease, such as pyrophosphate arthropathy and acute calcific periarthritis
3. Crystal deposition can result from other joint diseases: menisectomy, for example, predisposes to chondrocalcinosis

In order to accomodate these conclusions, a hypothesis has been proposed which suggests that calcium pyrophosphate and other forms of crystal deposition can act as an amplification loop, accelerating joint damage in many chronic arthropathies (Fig. 9.23).

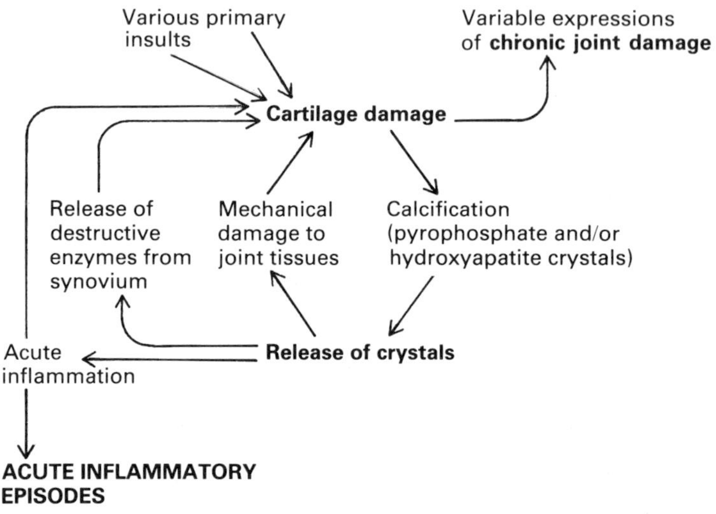

Fig. 9.23 Articular calcification may be an 'amplification loop' accelerating joint damage in many different diseases

FURTHER READING (CALCIFICATION)

Dieppe P A 1978 New knowlege of chondrocalcinosis. Journal of Clinical Pathology 31 (supp 12): 214–222

Dieppe P A, Calvert P 1983 Crystals and joint disease. Chapman & Hall, London

Dieppe P A, Doherty M, Macfarlane D G 1983 Crystal-related arthropathies. Annals of the Rheumatic Diseases 42 (supp 1)

McCarty D J 1976 Calcium pyrophosphate dihydrate deposition disease. Arthritis and Rheumatism 19: 275–285

IV Miscellaneous particles

A variety of miscellaneous crystals and other foreign bodies other than those covered in the preceeding two chapters have also been implicated in the pathogenesis of joint disease. They can be classified as 1. extrinsic particles entering the joint from elsewhere; 2. particles derived from the joint itself; and 3. intrinsic crystals deposited from body fluids (Fig. 9.24).

EXTRINSIC PARTICLES

The differential diagnosis of any acute or chronic monoarthritis must include possible foreign bodies within the joint. Many of the particles implicated cannot be seen radiologically, are easily missed on examination of the synovial fluid and may only be found by careful histological examination of excised synovium. Any history of penetrating trauma is therefore important.

> **Miscellaneous particles found in joints**
> 1. Extrinsic
>   a) Plant thorns
>   b) Other foreign bodies
>   c) Material from joint prosthesis
>   d) Injected corticosteroid crystals
> 2. Derived from the joint
>   a) Cartilate fragments
>   b) Bone fragments
>   c) Fibrin aggregates (rice bodies)
>   d) Strands of fibrin and collagen
> 3. Intrinsic crystal deposition
>   Cholesterol crystals

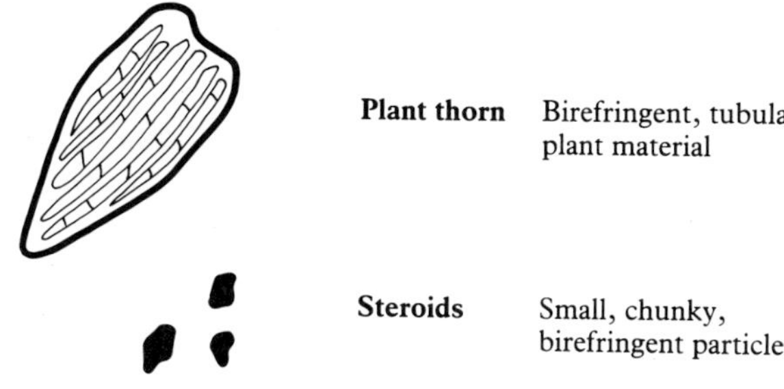

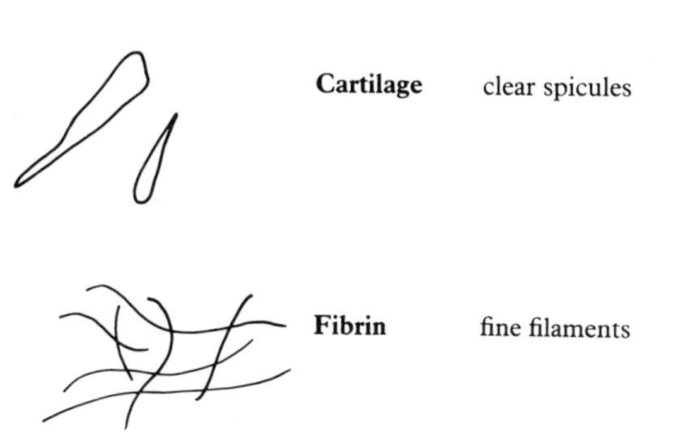

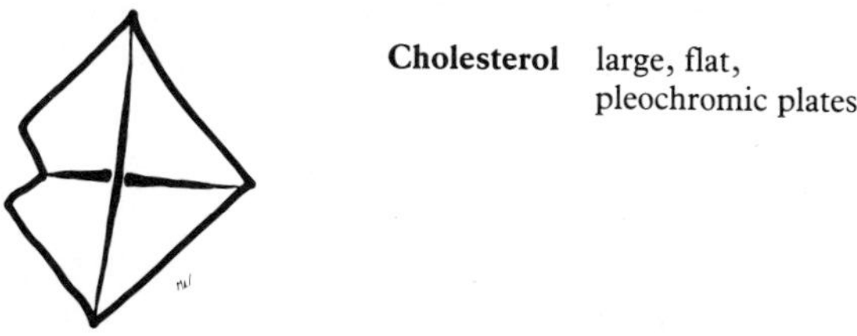

Fig. 9.24 Microscopic appearances of some miscellaneous particles sometimes found in synovial fluids and synovial membrane

1. Plant thorns

Small fragments from the tips of some thorns can cause an inflammatory synovitis. In Europe, the blackthorn and rose thorn are the commonest culprits, whereas in some parts of America palms or cacti (especially the date palm) are important. The fragment penetrates the skin to enter the joint, although the injury may go unnoticed. The knees and small joints of the hand are the commonest sites involved. A short time after the injury an acute self-limiting synovitis occurs; this subsides after a few days but may be followed by a relapsing chronic monoarthritis with synovial hypertrophy. Flexion contractures and small bone erosions may develop. The synovial fluid contains polymorphonuclear cells, and fragments of thorn are sometimes seen on polarised-light microscopy; the synovium shows a chronic granulomatous reaction around the thorn, and the particle may cause a pseudotumour. The condition is cured by synovectomy.

The ability of a single tiny plant fragment to produce first an acute reaction and then a chronic destructive granuloma, with bone erosions, is interesting, and may be analgous to some crystal-related arthritides.

2. Other foreign bodies

Other particles can penetrate the joint via the skin. Some, such as sea-urchin spines, produce a general systemic reaction as well as a local inflammatory reaction; this is probably due to soluble surface toxins. Any foreign body in a joint can cause a low-grade chronic monoarthritis and cause diagnostic confusion.

3. Prosthetic material

Fragments of joint prosthesis and fixing cement have been implicated in late loosening and in chronic inflammatory reactions associated with some joint replacements.

A few prosthetic joints develop severe inflammation, with formation of a large quantity of brown, murky synovial fluid filled with masses of particles. It is important to distinguish this 'foreign-body reaction' from infection.

A reaction to silicone particles is the best established mechanism; they can cause a chronic granulomatous reaction associated with multinucleate giant cell formation and particle phagocytosis. The particles (size ranges from about 5–50 μm) can also cause a reaction in draining lymph nodes. Metal fragments can cause a synovitis, and an immunological reaction due to metal sensitivity has also been suggested as a cause of reactions to prostheses, but is difficult to establish. Skin testing for metal sensitivity does not seem to correlate with reactions in the joints.

4. Corticosteroid cyrstals

Long-acting corticosteroids are frequently used in the treatment of inflammatory synovitis (see Chapter 25). They are crystalline and phagocytosed by synovial lining cells. They can be recognised in the polarised-light microscopy (Fig. 9.24), and may persist for 2–3 months after an injection. These crystals sometimes cause a transient painful increase in inflammation before having a beneficial effect. This may depend on the batch, type and particle size of the preparation, and is infrequent. Patients should be warned that the pain occasionally gets worse for the first 24 or 48 hours before getting better.

PARTICLES DERIVED FROM THE JOINT

Fragments of cartilage are frequently seen in synovial fluid. They are particularly obvious in osteoarthritis and other destructive forms of arthropathy. They have a characteristic appearance (Fig. 9.24). Bone particles may occur but are difficult to identify. Aggregates of fibrin can form large, round bodies (*rice bodies*) and strands of collagen fibrin and other fibres may also be identified. Fibrin is particularly common in rheumatoid arthritis.

The relevance of this 'joint detritus' is unclear. Fragments are phagocytosed by synovial lining cells and may cause a low-grade inflammatory reaction; they could also cause direct damage to the joint surface. Fibrin and other insoluble material might activate other mediators of joint damage (the complement cascade, for example). Thus particles derived from damaged joints could be helping to perpetuate or accelerate joint damage in a number of diseases.

CRYSTALS

Sparingly soluble products of purine metabolism (Chapter 9.II) and a variety of calcium salts

(Chapter 9.III) are often found in articular tissues The only other important crystal implicated in joint disease contains cholesterol.

Cholesterol crystals

These crystals have a characteristic appearance (Fig. 9.24), and are easily identified by polarising-light microscopy (p 160). Occasional particles are seen in the synovial fluid in various different diseases. Rarely, the fluid is so full of cholesterol crystals that it appears milky; RA is usually the underlying disease. Most patients with cholesterol joint effusions are normolipidaemic. Hyperlipidaemias can be associated with joint disease (Chapter 16.IV) but cholesterol crystals have not been identified in that context and there is no evidence that they have any role in the pathogenesis of these conditions.

Experimental work suggests that cholesterol crystals can cause chronic granulomatous reactions and florid fibrosis, and they have also been suggested as a possible contributory cause of synovial and capsular reactions in both RA and OA.

FURTHER READING (MISCELLANEOUS PARTICLES)

Dieppe P A, Doherty M 1982 The role of particles in the pathogenesis of joint disease. Current Topics in Pathology, Bone and Joint Disease 71: 199–234

10 Infections and arthritis

INTRODUCTION

There are several mechanisms whereby microbial agents can give rise to arthritis. Direct invasion of joints may result in acute or chronic joint disease, and such 'infective' or 'infectious-agent' arthritis will form the major subject of this chapter. Infection elsewhere in the body, however, can also lead to arthritis in the absence of joint invasion. If this occurs during the course of infection, as with infective endocarditis, microbial antigen or 'debris' can often be demonstrated within the joint, suggesting a type III reaction, and eradication of the microbial agent will result in cessation of joint inflammation. If, on the other hand, the arthritis occurs after elimination of the responsible organism, as in Reiter's disease, then microbial antigen is not recoverable from the joint and the 'reactive' synovitis may become recurrent or chronic in the absence of further microbial stimulation. Some infections can give rise to more than one type of arthritis, (e.g. *Salmonella*, p 84).

The present chapter is concerned primarily with direct infection of joint tissues. The concept of 'reactive' arthritis is fully described in Chapter 5 (p 66). Although 'infective' arthritis is one of the few rheumatological conditions amenable to cure, improper management can result in disaster for the patient. General considerations will first be presented and then specific infections described.

Association between microbial infection and arthritis

1. 'Infective' arthritis (microbes directly invading joints)
   a) Bacterial (including mycobacteria)
   b) Viral
   c) Fungal, protozoal and worm infections
2. Sterile arthritis associated with infection outside joint
   a) Arthritis occurring during course of systemic infection (antigen often isolated from joint)
      (i) Hepatitis B virus (possibly other viruses also)
      (ii) Infective endocarditis
      (iii) Whipple's disease (p 324)
      (iv) Arthritis associated with jejuno-ileal bypass (p 68)
      (v) Lepromatous 'Lepra reaction'
   b) 'Reactive' arthritis occurring after subsidence of initiating infection (antigen not demonstrated within joint)
      (i) Rheumatic fever (p 412)
      (ii) Reiter's syndrome and reactive arthritis associated with *Shigella*, *Salmonella* and *Yersinia* infection (p 80).

ACUTE SUPPURATIVE ('SEPTIC') ARTHRITIS

This condition is a medical emergency, requiring early recognition and prompt treatment if joint destruction and deformity are to be prevented. Despite the recent availability of potent anti-bacterial drugs, the incidence of septic arthritis remains unchanged, although there has been a shift in the spectrum of hosts and organisms involved. Previously considered a condition primarily of children, a significant incidence of septic arthritis is now seen in the elderly, the chronically debilitated and the immunologically-compromised, and although staphylococci still remain the commonest causative agent, Gram-negative infections have become increasingly prevalent, particularly in the compromised adult. Gonococcal arthritis presents distinctive clinical features and will be considered separately.

Predisposing factors

Apart from penetrating injury or contiguous spread from osteomyelitis infection usually reaches the synovium via the blood, so that any condition commonly associated with bacteraemia is liable to predispose to joint sepsis. Bacteraemia, however, is only rarely followed by joint infection, suggesting that breakdown in local joint defence mechanisms is an important factor. Although apparently normal joints may become infected, especially by *Staphylococcus* or *Gonococcus*, joints already affected by rheumatic disease, particularly RA, appear particularly predisposed.

In the absence of obvious underlying disease, involvement of normal joints in the adult, recurrent joint sepsis, or infection with less common agents should trigger investigation of host defences. Although sophisticated techniques are required for detailed study of immune competence, routine testing and clinical examination can provide a ready assessment.

Examples of conditions that predispose to septic arthritis

1. Joint disease — particularly rheumatoid arthritis
2. Diabetes mellitus
3. Any chronic, debilitating illness: e.g. uraemia, malabsorption, liver disease
4. Chronic alcoholism
5. Intravenous drug abuse
6. Neoplastic disease — especially acute leukaemia, lymphoma, myeloma
7. Iatrogenic factors
   a) Corticosteroids and immunosuppressive drugs
   b) Intra-articular injection
   c) Joint prosthesis

Assessment of host defence

1. Polymorphonuclear leukocytes
   a) White cell count + differential
   b) Stain secretions/exudates for PMN
   c) Nitroblue tetrazolium reduction (indicates normal hexose monophosphate shunt activity)
2. Humoral immunity
   a) Serum protein electrophoresis
   b) Quantitation of immunoglobulins
   c) Isoagglutinins
3. Cellular immunity
   a) Lymphocyte count
   b) Delayed skin tests
4. Serum complement

Causative organisms and pathogenesis

Although septic arthritis can be caused by a wide variety of bacteria, in practice only a few agents are commonly encountered and these show differential predilection for certain age groups (Table 10.1). Particular host circumstances are also associated with certain organisms — a Gram-negative bacillus, for example, is a rare cause of septic arthritis, but is the most likely agent in a patient with acute leukaemia, while Staph. aureus is the most likely agent in a patient with RA.

Once joint invasion has occurred, it is the enzymes released from PMN and synoviocytes,

Table 10.1 Relative frequency of major bacteria causing septic arthritis, according to age

Organism	Age (years) <2	2–15	16–50	>50
Staph. aureus	++	+++	+	+++
H. influenzae	++	+	–	–
N. gonorrhoeae	–	+	+++	–
Strep. pneumoniae	+	+	–	+
Strep. pyogenes	+	++	+	+
Gram-negative bacilli	+	+	+	++

rather than toxic bacterial products, that are mainly responsible for subsequent joint damage. Three stages of articular cartilage destruction are distinguished:

1. Early release of proteolytic enzymes resulting in rapid removal of proteoglycan (reversible)
2. Chondrocyte damage caused by alteration in proteoglycan support, progressing to chondrocyte death and subsequent inability to reconstitute proteoglycan (irreversible)
3. Synovial proliferation and enzyme release, causing destruction of collagen and residual proteoglycan, with resultant deformity

Once chondrocyte death has occurred, joint damage may still progress even after the infection has been curtailed: cessation of the process in the first stage is therefore necessary if full recovery is to be allowed. Marked fibrosis and ankylosis may occur during the recovery phase and be a major case of impaired joint function.

Clinical features

The classic presentation is with acute onset of pain and swelling in a single large joint, particularly the knee. Examination reveals joint-line tenderness, effusion, overlying erythema and restriction of both active and passive movement, and aspiration of pus containing bacteria on Gram staining rapidly confirms the diagnosis. In practice, however, symptoms and signs are often less dramatic and the key to diagnosis usually resides in a high index of clinical suspicion. Features that should suggest the possibility of acute joint sepsis are outlined below.

Features that should suggest the possibility of acute joint infection

1. Rapidly progressive mono or oligo arthritis
2. Involvement of 'odd' joints
   a) Sternoclavicular joint
   b) Unilateral SIJ
3. Sequential, additive, joint involvement
4. Disproportionate symptoms in one or more joints in patient with RA
5. Joint symptoms in 'at risk' patient, e.g.
   a) Drug addict
   b) Patient with leukaemia
   c) Any ill, debilitated patient
6. Erythema overlying a joint
7. Marked lymphadenopathy in region draining an inflamed joint
8. Fever in patient with joint symptoms

The adult knee and childhood hip are most frequently involved, but other common sites include ankles, elbows, wrists and shoulders (Fig. 10.1). Large joints are predominantly

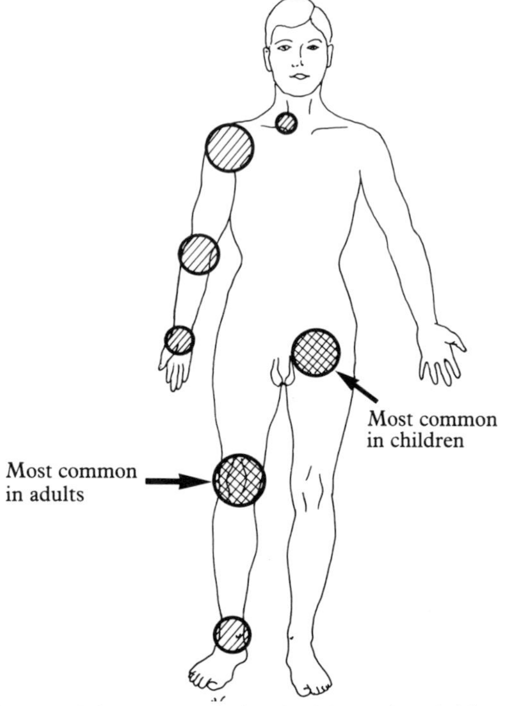

Fig. 10.1 Joints commonly involved in septic arthritis

affected and sepsis in small joints of hands and feet is rare except by local extension (e.g. infected ulcers in a diabetic foot). Involvement of 'odd' joints infrequently affected by other diseases may occur, and a symptomatic sternoclavicular or sacroiliac joint should always raise suspicion. Polyarticular involvement is well-recognised and all joints must be carefully examined. Sequential, additive joint involvement is particularly suggestive of infection e.g. pain and swelling in a knee which persists and is followed by pain and limitation of movement in the ipsilateral hip (Fig. 10.2).

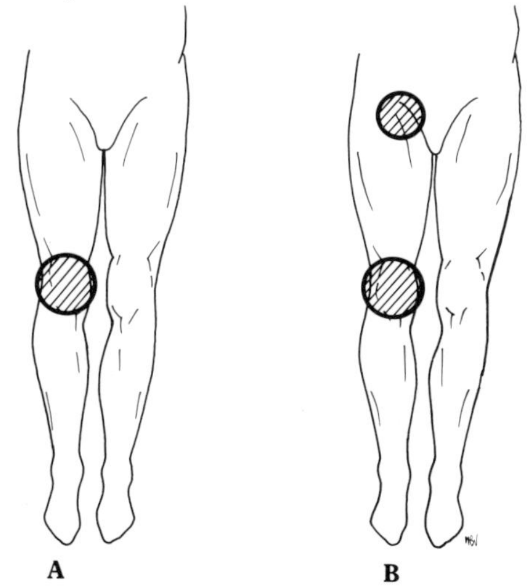

Fig. 10.2 Example of additive joint involvement, within a region, that suggests sepsis. **A**. Day 1. **B**. Day 3.

Systemic features may include anorexia, nausea and low-grade fever, but rigors are rare. A diligent search for the portal of entry (including skin, respiratory tract, urinary tract, gut) may reveal the source of infection and aid in appropriate antibiotic selection.

Investigations

Although several non-specific laboratory findings are characteristic of septic arthritis, the diagnosis can only be confirmed by synovial fluid staining and culture. Every suspicious joint should be aspirated and the SF promptly examined.

In the absence of prior antibiotic therapy, the initial Gram stain will reveal organisms in the majority of cases and provide a sound basis for appropriate antibiotic treatment. The subsequent yield of positive cultures will depend on the care with which samples are obtained: transportation, preferably in a pre-warmed transport medium, must be rapid, and both aerobic and anaerobic culture techniques should be used. Special techniques are employed for fastidious organisms, e.g. gonococcus, if the clinical situation is appropriate (p 197).

Characteristic, but undiagnostic, laboratory findings in septic arthritis

1. *Synovial fluid*
   - a) Macroscopic appearance
     - (i) Turbid
     - (ii) Decreased viscosity
     - (iii) Poor mucin clot
   - b) Cells
     - (i) Raised, $>50\,000/mm^3$
     - (ii) Marked predominence of PMN ($>90\%$)
   - c) Chemistry
     - (i) Low glucose, $<50\%$ of serum values
     - (ii) Raised lactate, >100 mg/dl
2. *Peripheral blood*
   - a) Cells
Leukocytosis, predominantly PMN
   - b) Viscosity
Raised

Blood cultures are positive in up to 75% of patients. Urine, sputum, urethral, cervical, stool, wound or nasopharyngeal cultures should also be obtained, as appropriate, prior to antibiotic treatment.

Speed in confirmation of diagnosis and initiating treatment is all important, but if the gram stain is negative, cultures will take 24–48 hours to provide a result. In recent years several techniques have been tried in an attempt to: 1. speed diagnosis; or 2. confirm an infective aetiology in situations where antibiotics have already been given. Such techniques may come to play an increasingly important role in diagnosis and include the detec-

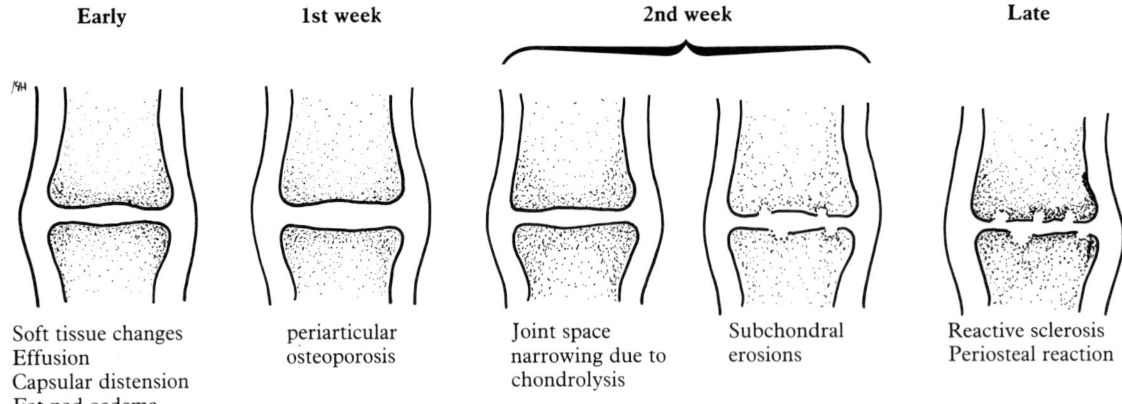

Fig. 10.3 Sequence of radiographic changes in septic arthritis

tion of bacterial antigens by radioimmunoassay and counterimmunoelectrophoresis, and the determination of volatile products of microbial metabolism by gas chromatography.

X-rays are generally unhelpful in confirming the diagnosis, but should be taken of both the involved and the contralateral normal joint as a base-line for future studies. The earliest findings (within the first 7–10 days) include effusion, soft-tissue swelling and juxta-articular osteopenia (Fig. 10.3). Subluxation of the shoulder or hip may occur as an early sign due to tense effusion, especially in young children, and anaerobic infection may rarely produce gas in the joint and periarticular tissues. Later findings may include joint space narrowing, subchondral bone destruction, periosteal reaction and, rarely, periarticular calcification (especially following capsular rupture with pneumococcal infection). Gallium or technetium scintigraphy may be useful in demonstrating unsuspected sites of involvement and have been reported to be of particular use in suspected sepsis of the axial and pelvic skeleton.

Management

Any delay in initiating treatment will adversely affect the long-term outlook. There are three major aspects to management:

1. Appropriate antibacterial agents in effective doses
2. Adequate joint drainage
3. Correct local physical treatment and subsequent physiotherapy

Antibiotics should be started as soon as samples for culture have been taken. The choice of antibiotic is determined by the clinical situation and initial Gram stain (Table 10.2): antibiotics may later be changed according to culture sensitivities. Most parenterally administered antibiotics freely enter the inflamed synovial joints: intra-articular instillation may provoke a chemical synovitis, is unnecessary and should therefore be avoided. There are no set guidelines to govern the duration of antibiotic therapy but in practice parenteral administration for 2 weeks, followed by oral administration for 2–4 weeks, is usual, though longer treatments may be given to particularly compromised patients. The antibacterial activity in synovial fluid and serum can easily be monitored and drug dosages can be altered accordingly.

Adequate drainage is essential to relieve intra-articular pressure and to remove damaging enzymes and debris. The choice between closed needle aspirations (using a wide-bore needle, once or twice a day) and open surgical drainage remains controversial. Open drainage allows thorough saline lavage to be performed, but needle aspiration alone is frequently sufficient and usually allows more rapid mobilisation. Definite indications for surgical drainage include:

Table 10.2 A suggested choice of initial antibiotic based upon Gram stain and age

	Presumed organism	Drug of choice	Alternative
Gram-positive cocci			
Any age	*Staph. aureus*	*P-r penicillin	Cephalosporins
Gram-negative cocci			
Adolescent/Adult	*N. gonorrhoeae*	Penicillin G	Tetracycline, erythromycin
Young child	*H. influenzae*	Ampicillin	Chloramphenicol
Gram-negative bacilli			
Adult	*Ps. aeruginosa*, *E. coli* *S. marcescens*	Gentamycin + carbenicillin	cephalosporins
Child	*Ps. aeruginosa*	Gentamycin + carbenicillin	cephalosporins
No organisms seen			
Healthy adult	*N. gonorrhoeae*	Penicillin G	cephalosporins
Compromised adult, Neonate	*Staph. aureus* or Gram-negative bacilli	*P-r penicillin + gentamycin	cephalosporins and carbenicillin
Child > 1 month old	*Staph. aureus* or *H. influenzae*	*P-r penicillin + ampicillin	cephalosporins and chloramphenicol

*P-r = penicillinase resistant

1. Inability to completely aspirate pus (due to loculation or high viscosity)
2. Inaccessibility of joint (hip, SIJ)
3. Persistent reaccumulation of pus and lack of improvement despite adequate antibiotic treatment.

If the joint is readily accessible it therefore seems sensible to use repeated needle aspiration first: regular review of the situation, however, should lead to prompt surgical intervention if complete aspiration is not possible or if no improvement is seen within 48 hours.

Splinting of the affected joint and avoidance of weight-bearing are recommended initially, but passive range-of-motion exercises, to maintain mobility and prevent flexion contractures, should be started as soon as pain is subsiding (usually within 36–48 hours). Active joint motion is then instituted and increased as symptoms improve: early active motion undoubtedly improves the final outcome for the joint.

'Post-infectious synovitis' is an occasional feature of treated septic arthritis which may cause confusion. The joint again becomes warm and tender and develops a sterile effusion with a PMN-predominant leukocytosis. Recrudescence of infection is always suspected, but cultures are repeatedly sterile and synovial biopsy reveals synovial cell hyperplasia and a mixed mononuclear/PMN infiltration. The condition is usually self-limiting and its mechanism is not understood — development of this synovitis appears unrelated to the severity of infection or previous status of the joint.

The final outcome for the patient will depend on many factors, the most important being the speed with which appropriate therapy is instituted. Frequently, however, the acute infection is cured but the joint is left with impaired function due to deformity, fibrosis or ankylosis, and is predisposed to later, progressive, changes of osteoarthritis.

Special problems

Septic arthritis in childhood

Although this may occur at any age, it is particularly seen in children under 2, and is two to three times more common in boys. The hip is most commonly involved, then the knee and elbow: multiple joint involvement is rare. Although direct spread from osteomyelitis may occur in this age group, haematogenous spread from a focus in the middle ear, respiratory tract or skin is most usual. An underlying generalised abnormality is uncommon.

Onset of symptoms is often abrupt and usually relates to the affected joint, which is tender, warm, swollen and held in a position that maximises the capsular volume (the hip in abduction, flexion and external rotation: the knee in 40° flexion). The infantile hip, the commonest joint involved, is particularly vulnerable to long-term complications because of its precarious blood supply. Persistent dislocation, subluxation, osteonecrosis, femoral head and neck deformity, leg-shortening and joint fusion may all occur if treatment is inadequate. Surgical decompression and drainage should therefore always be performed in this situation.

Acute hip sepsis frequently presents diagnostic problems, mainly because of joint inaccessibility. Transient hip synovitis, which may well be viral in origin, is not uncommon, but before this is diagnosed bacterial infection must be excluded.

Sepsis in a rheumatoid joint

Many factors predispose patients with RA to joint sepsis: for example, lowered anti-bacterial activity in SF, reduced neutrophil chemotaxis, Felty's syndrome, steroid or immunosuppressive treatment. Septic arthritis particularly affects elderly, seropositive, nodular rheumatoid patients with a long history of joint disease. Onset is frequently insidious with malaise, anorexia or confusion, so that a high index of suspicion must be maintained. Disproportionate symptoms in one or a few joints in a patient with RA should always lead to aspiration of the affected joints. Although the knee is most commonly involved, multiple joint involvement is well recognised, and infection in nodules and bursae frequently co-exists. The majority of infections are due to *Staph. aureus*, but Gram-negative organisms are becoming increasingly common.

Delay in diagnosis is presumably responsible for the high mortality with which this complication is usually associated. If treated early and correctly, however, the prognosis is favourable.

Disc space infection

This most commonly is due to *Staph. aureus* and arises by haematogenous spread from a distant focus, particularly in children, or as a consequence of disc surgery in adults. The lumbar spine is particularly affected. Presentation is often insidious with progressive back pain, frequently persistent at night. Localised tenderness and paravertebral spasm are usual. Differentiation is from other causes of back pain (p 399). The plasma viscosity is usually raised but early X-rays may be normal. Later, progressive loss of disc height and irregularity of both vertebral end plates may be demonstrated (Fig. 10.4). Gallium scintigraphy may aid in early detection.

Aspiration biopsy will confirm the diagnosis and treatment aims at 6–12 weeks of immobilisation. Antibiotics are usually given, though evidence that they alter the outcome is incomplete, resolution frequently occurring following immobilisation alone. The intervertebral space often fuses following infection.

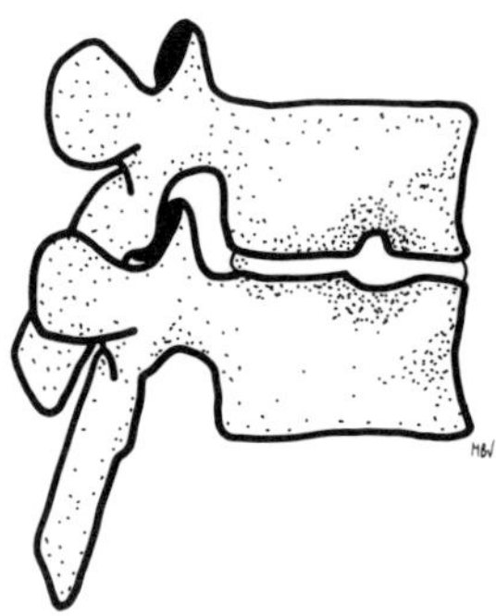

Fig. 10.4 Discitis — late appearance

Septic arthritis in intravenous drug abusers

Intravenous drug abusers, especially heroin addicts, appear particularly predisposed to septic arthritis, perhaps related to contamination from skin, tap water or injection paraphernalia. The arthritis differs from that seen in non-drug users in that: 1. *Pseudomonas aeruginosa* and *Serratia marcescens* are particularly common culprits; 2. Infection occurs in atypical joints — e.g. sternoclavicular and SIJ. Monoarticular involvement is usual and the outcome is generally favourable compared to Gram-negative joint sepsis in patients with chronic underlying disease.

Viral hepatitis, infective endocarditis and osteomyelitis are other well-recognised infective complications in such individuals.

Infection after prosthetic joint surgery

Immediate postoperative infection has been greatly minimised by scrupulous aseptic technique and peroperative antibiotic cover, but joints that have undergone previous surgery remain particularly prone to this complication. Delayed infection may present months or years later with joint loosening or abscess formation in the vicinity of the joint, infection being confirmed at re-operation. Although irrigation, drainage and prolonged antibiotic therapy are employed for both immediate and delayed infections, the vast majority ultimately require removal of the prosthesis.

Secondary bacterial 'seeding' of a previously sterile prosthesis may occur at any time, and a history of preceding infection, particularly in the urinary tract, is frequently implicated. Rheumatoid patients are particularly prone. Prompt antibiotic treatment and continuation for 6–12 months may allow retention of the prosthesis in some cases. All patients with artificial joints should be warned to take prophylactic antibiotics before extensive dental work, urinary tract instrumentation or other invasive procedures, and any infections, however minor, deserve vigorous antibiotic and, when necessary, surgical treatment to prevent such haematogenous spread.

GONOCOCCAL ARTHRITIS

Although antibiotics have reduced the proportion of gonococcal infections that progress to systemic dissemination and arthritis (c. 0.3%), the dramatic increase in prevalence of gonorrhoea has made gonococcal arthritis the commonest form of infectious agent arthritis in many countries, notably the U.S.A. The arthritis of disseminated gonococcal infection presents a distinctive clinical picture which usually can be readily differentiated from other forms of acute infective arthritis (Table 10.3): characteristic features include marked female predominance, multiple joint involvement (upper and lower limbs), tenosynovitis, dermatitis (the 'dermatitis-arthritis' syndrome) and rapid response to therapy.

Arthritis most commonly occurs within the first two weeks following infection. Young women under 40 are predominantly affected (F:M = 4:1), presumably because they form the largest reservoir of asymptomatic, untreated infection. Presentation within the first week of menstruation or during pregnancy is often noted, suggesting that physiological factors, such as vaginal pH, may enhance the tendency to dissemination. Gonococcal arthritis is being increasingly recognised in homosexual males and may also rarely occur in children and older adults (over 50). Usual sites of primary infection are the urethra in males, the cervix in females, and throat and rectum in both sexes (eye and skin infection can occur in infants).

Pathogenesis

This continues to be a subject of some controversy, principally because gonococci are only infrequently cultured from SF or skin. Although a hypersensitivity mechanism or immune-complex interaction have both been suggested, a direct toxic effect of viable, or even non-viable, organisms on the tissues seems most likely.

Table 10.3 Clinical distinctions between gonococcal and other acute bacterial arthritides

	Gonococcal arthritis	Other organisms
Predominant age	15–40	Child or elderly
Sex	F ≫ M	Slight male predominance
Joint distribution	Usually polyarticular Large and small joints Upper and lower limbs	Usually monoarticular Large joints Lower limbs
Tenosynovitis	Common	Rare
Skin lesions	Common	Rare
SF organisms on Gram stain	Uncommon	Usual
Response to appropriate antibiotic	Rapid (2–4 days)	Slower (pain often persists 7–10 days)

Two apparently distinct forms of gonococcal arthritis have been suggested, primarily on clinical grounds:

1. A 'bacteraemic' form: occurring early in the illness with fever, chills, dermatitis, polyarthritis with minimal effusion and positive blood cultures
2. A 'septic' form: with mono-/oligoarthritis and positive SF culture but minimal toxic symptoms, no skin lesions and negative blood cultures

However, correlation between clinical and bacteriological features is, in general, poor and evidence to support such a clinical distinction is far from complete.

Clinical features

The typical presentation of an acute onset, migratory polyarthritis affecting upper and lower limbs in a young female with fever, tenosynovitis and/or typical peripheral skin lesions, is distinctive and should always lead to consideration of disseminated gonococcal infection as the cause of the illness.

Arthritis

This is the commonest major manifestation of disseminated gonococcal infection and classically presents as an asymmetrical and migratory polyarthritis which may subsequently localise to one or more joints. Presentation as a pure monoarthritis, however, is uncommon. Onset is often sudden and severe and effusions may be marked. An important diagnostic feature is frequent involvement of both upper and lower limbs, with knees, wrists and ankles most commonly affected, followed by small joints of hands and feet, elbows and shoulders (Fig. 10.5). Any joint, however, including hips and TMJ, may be involved.

Tenosynovitis, particularly affecting the dorsum of hands and feet, wrists and Achilles tendon, is common (c. 70%), and has been proposed as a major diagnostic feature.

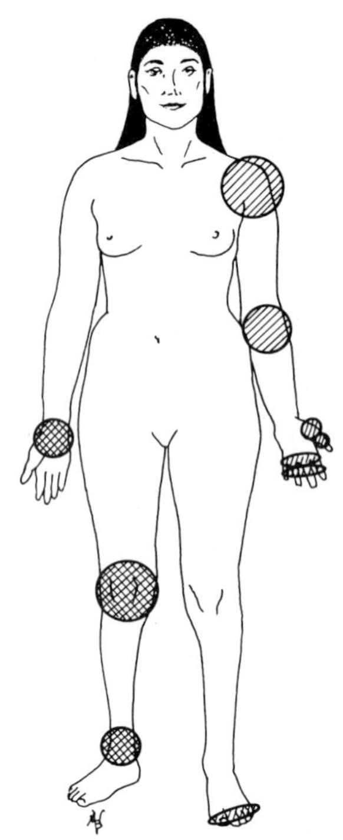

Fig. 10.5 Joints commonly involved in gonococcal arthritis

Skin manifestations

Although rarely numerous, typical skin lesions are frequently present (c. 70%). They usually start as small red papules or petechiae which either disappear or evolve through vesicular and pustular stages to develop a characteristic grey, necrotic, umbilicated centre on a haemorrhagic base. Frequently tender, they tend to distribute on distal aspects of the limbs.

Other systemic manifestations

Fever may be absent, low-grade or significantly elevated: rigors are reported in around 50%. Pericarditis, myocarditis, endocarditis, meningitis and osteomyelitis are all fortunately rare, but may complicate the occasional patient in whom disseminated infection is not recognised and treated promptly. Perihepatitis, due to peritoneal spread from a pelvic focus, may occur, but subclinical hepatitis from bacteraemic spread is more common (elevated transaminases and mild jaundice may cause confusion with viral hepatitis).

Diagnosis

The clinical picture of dermatitits, arthritis, tenosynovitis and fever should strongly suggest the correct diagnosis, but confirmation requires culture of the organism.

Because of the fastidious nature of *N. gonorrhoea*, correct culture techniques are of paramount importance. Cervical, urethral, rectal and pharyngeal cultures should all be taken into Theyer–Martin plates, (containing agents which inhibit contaminants), but chocolate agar is more appropriate for blood, skin and SF samples. The SF is usually inflammatory, showing a predominence of PMN, but even under optimal conditions SF cultures are positive in only 50%, so that in the appropriate clinical setting a positive culture from any of the cultured sites may be considered as confirmatory for diagnosis. Fluorescent antibody techniques may further help demonstrate the presence of the organism. Skin lesions histologically show non-specific small-vessel vasculitis with leukocytoclasis and haemorrhage; Gram stains and immunofluorescent techniques may demonstrate the organism but direct culture is only occasionally positive. Gonococcal serological studies at present do not distinguish recent and distant infection and are therefore of little diagnostic value.

The differential diagnosis may include other infectious agent arthritides, rheumatic fever, viral hepatitis, rheumatoid arthritis and SLE. Contrasting features with Reiter's syndrome, which may occur in a similar clinical situation, are outlined in Table 10.4.

Treatment

This follows the same general lines as for any other septic arthritis, but specific points include:

1. Antibiotic choice. Disseminated gonococcal infection is extremely sensitive to antibiotics. Unlike isolated genitourinary infection, there are as yet no reports of penicillin resistant strains causing disseminated disease. The most widely used regimen is penicillin G 10 million units IV daily until symptoms subside, followed by oral ampicillin (2 g daily) for 10 days, but even only 3 days of parenteral penicillin may be effective in this situation. The rapid response to treatment (2–3 days) has been suggested as a further diagnostic feature of this syndrome.

2. Social aspects. These include patient education and contact tracing.

In general recovery is excellent. As with any septic arthritis, however, failure to institute rapid, effective therapy will lead to joint destruction and later possible bony fusion. Recurrent disseminated gonorrhoea and arthritis should lead to investigation for deficiency of the complement components C6, C7 or C8, since these may predispose to gonococcal infection. (Formation of the C5–C9 membrane attack complex appears crucial in handling Neisserial infection.)

Table 10.4 Differences between gonococcal arthritis and Reiter's syndrome

	Gonococcal arthritis	Reiter's syndrome
Sex distribution	F > M	M > F
Migratory arthritis	+	–
Joint distribution	Lower and upper limb	Lower limb
Back pain	–	+
Course	Acute	Recurrent/chronic
Achilles tendinitis	±	+
Plantar fasciitis	–	+
Conjunctivitis	Rare	Common
Uveitis	–	+
Balanitis	–	+
Mouth ulcers	–	+
Keratoderma	–	+
HLA B-27 positive	5–10%	70–90%
Personal or family history of arthritis	–	+
Response to penicillin	++	–

MENINGOCOCCAL ARTHRITIS

Arthritis complicates about 5% of all meningococcal infections but appears particularly common in adults, affecting 30% of patients over 30. The commonest form is an oligoarthritis, predominantly affecting knees, ankles and elbows, which occurs as the systemic or meningeal infection is improving. Persistent, purulent effusions may develop which seem uninfluenced by antibiotic treatment but which rarely result in permanent joint damage. SF cultures are inevitably sterile and the pathogenesis appears to be a hypersensitivity reaction involving deposition of meningococcal antigen, IgG, IgM and complement.

Rarer presentations include an oligoarthritis without meningitis, osteomyelitis in infants and a 'dermatitis-arthritis' syndrome similar to that seen in disseminated gonococcal infection (tenosynovitis, however, is invariably absent). Treatment is with high-dose penicillin.

TUBERCULOUS ARTHRITIS

Previously a not uncommon condition of children and young adults, tuberculous arthritis may now be seen at any age but is rare, occurring in less than 1% of patients with TB. Only 20% of patients with osteoarticular disease have active pulmonary lesions, but another 30% show abnormal chest films. Multiple articular involvement occurs in up to one third of cases but other extrapulmonary disease (usually involving urinary tract or lymph nodes) is only occasionally present.

The commonest predisposing factors appear to be trauma and a compromised host status, e.g. drug abuse, diabetes, steroids. Tuberculous arthritis is relatively more common in Asian immigrants, in whom it may show special features including a tendency to multiple joint involvement, frequent tendon-sheath infection and childhood dactylitis.

Pathogenesis and distribution of joint involvement

Osteoarticular involvement usually follows reactivation of a haematogenously seeded focus in para-articular bone or synovium, first colonised during primary lung infection. Reactivation results in a chronic, granulomatous reaction, with or without caseation. Although any bone, joint, bursa or tendon may be infected, tuberculous arthritis shows definite preference for vertebrae and weight-bearing joints.

Vertebral involvement

Infection particularly occurs in the thoracolumbar spine, starting anteriorly as a single focus close to the intervertebral disc, which is soon destroyed, and then spreading as a 'cold abscess' under the anterior longitudinal ligament to involve adjacent vertebrae (Fig. 10.6). Chronic destruction typically results in anterior collapse and kyphosis.

Peripheral joint involvement

Weight-bearing joints such as hips, knees and ankles are most commonly involved, followed by wrists and elbows. Infected synovium forms into a chronic granulomatous pannus that slowly erodes cartilage, peripherally at first, and then bone. Further spread eventually leads to involvement of surrounding structures such as capsule, tendons and bursae.

Clinical features

Presentation is typically with long-standing back pain or chronic pain and swelling in a single joint in an otherwise apparently healthy individual.

Back pain is the commonest symptom of vertebral involvement and may be present for months or years before prominent angulation ('gibbus') develops. Rarely, sinus formation or pressure on surrounding structures (e.g. paraplegia) may lead to the diagnosis.

Pain is also the commonest symptom of synovial joint involvement. A marked discrepancy is usually present in that the joint is only mildly tender and warm yet shows massive synovial proliferation and effusion, marked restriction of movement and gross muscle wasting. Involvement of surrounding tendons, particularly extensors at

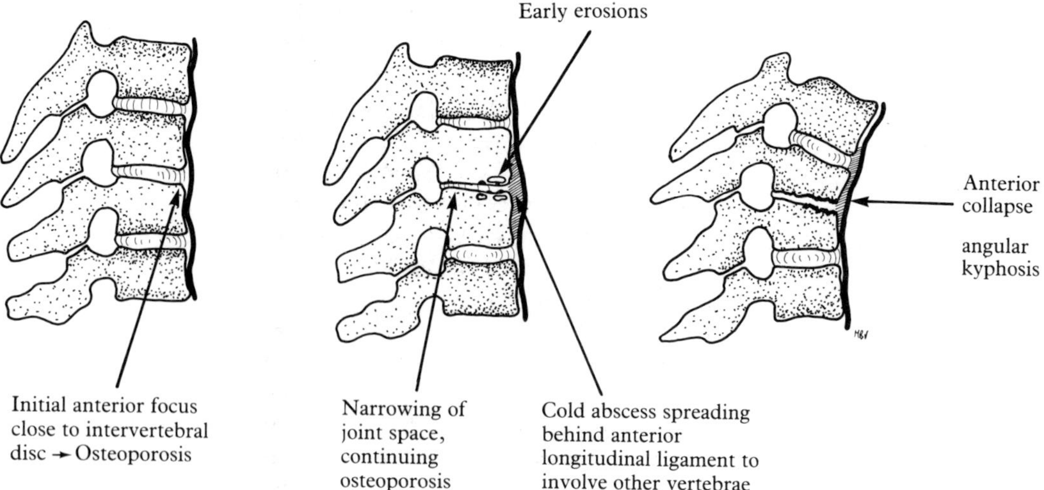

Fig. 10.6 Progression of spinal TB

the wrist, may also occur, and flexor tendon inflammation may produce carpal tunnel syndrome.

Mild fever and weight loss may be present, but night sweats, rigors, severe malaise and anorexia are unusual except in the rare situation where pulmonary or miliary TB co-exists.

Tuberculous dactylitis (infection of the short tubular bones of hands and feet, usually without joint involvement) is rare and virtually confined to children, presenting as a painless, swollen metacarpal, metatarsal or phalanx.

Investigations and diagnosis

Because of its chronic nature, X-rays are usually abnormal at presentation (Figs 10.6 and 10.7). Non-weight-bearing surfaces of articular cartilage are affected first, resulting in soft-tissue swelling with initial preservation of joint space. Bone haziness progresses to irregular, peripheral erosions and osteoporosis is often marked. Cystic lesions with sclerotic margins; and calcification of caseous material, may rarely occur. Eventually widespread joint destruction will result, followed by bony ankylosis.

The most reliable diagnostic investigation is open biopsy; histology may reveal caseating granulomata and positive results from staining and culture are higher than those obtained from SF alone. A strongly-positive Mantoux test is usual (if negative the diagnosis is unlikely).

Because of its relative infrequency, chronic

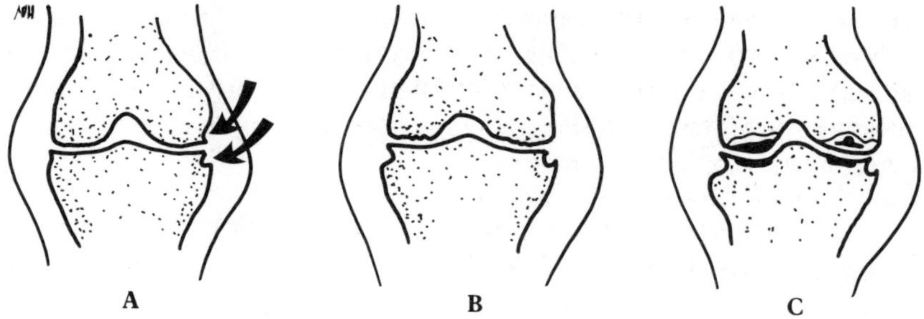

Fig. 10.7 Progressive changes in tuberculous arthritis affecting a synovial joint. **A**. Soft tissue swelling; effusion; marginal destructive lesions (arrowed); osteoporosis. **B**. Progressive joint space narrowing; subchondral irregularity. **C**. Isolated foci of bone showing increased density ('kissing' sequestra).

course and lack of pathognomonic features, long delay in diagnosis is usual (12–18 months) — the commonest misdiagnosis being monoarticular onset of RA or a spondyloarthritic variant. Certain features, however, should lead to consideration of tuberculous arthritis and to early, invasive investigation to confirm or exclude the diagnosis:

1. Insidious onset of monoarthritis
2. Marked synovial proliferation
3. Involvement of adjacent tendons (tenosynovitis ± rupture)
4. Osseous erosion on X-ray

Management

Treatment is with combination chemotherapy, continuing with two agents for at least 18 months. Surgery is reserved for drainage of large abscesses and fixation of unstable spines, and should only be performed after commencing chemotherapy. Since destruction of weight-bearing cartilage is a late occurrence, early diagnosis and treatment may in fact lead to good restoration of function. However, because of the usual long delay in diagnosis, the ultimate outcome is often poor.

Atypical mycobacteria

These are ubiquitous, generally saprophytic organisms of low pathogenicity which can produce disease that is indistinguishable from TB. Periarticular and articular involvement is rare, occurring particularly in compromised hosts, especially those with pre-existing joint disease.

Chronic involvement of tendon sheaths of fingers and wrists is most common, but articular infection, particularly of fingers and knees, may also occur. Unlike TB, atypical mycobacteria commonly show multifocal involvement. Although trauma or penetrating injury is frequently implicated, haematogenous infection is probably most usual.

Diagnosis is by culture of infected tissue or SF, and treatment must be based on sensitivity testing. Drug resistance is common and a combination of four or five drugs and/or synovectomy may be necessary.

FUNGAL ARTHRITIS

Because of the rarity and indolent nature of fungal arthritis, long delay in diagnosis is usual, resulting in frequent irrreversible joint destruction. Mycotic infections are endemic in some parts of the world and may affect apparently healthy individuals, but in non-endemic areas infection, particularly with *Candida*, is predominantly seen in compromised hosts. Certain features should raise suspicion of fungal arthritis and lead to use of selective media for culture.

Features that suggest the possibility of fungal arthritis

1. Chronic, indolent synovitis of joint or tendon sheath
2. Marked synovial proliferation with few inflammatory features
3. Arthritis in a compromised host (especially *Candida* infection)
4. History of recent travel in endemic area

NB Features 1 and 2 also suggest tuberculous infection, which is often closely mimicked by fungal infections

Most cases result from direct extension from an osteomyelitis focus, but haematogenous spread from a pulmonary focus may also occur. Amphotericin B is frequently required to effect a cure and, in addition, surgical drainage, débridement or even amputation may be necessary. Erythema nodosum is an additional, rare cause of joint problems in patients with disseminated mycotic infection (particularly coccidiodomycosis).

Although all are rare, the following infections are most commonly encountered.

Superficial 'maduramycoses'

Actually a mixed infection of fungi and bacteria these cause skin, subcutaneous tissue and bone infection with sinus formation, swelling and disfigurement of the feet. The condition is often surprisingly painless.

Coccidiodomycosis (SW USA)

Up to 80% of people in endemic areas may be infected at some time, but chronic pulmonary disease and dissemination is rare. Transient arthralgias are common during acute infection and may be accompanied by erythema nodosum, both probably representing a hypersensitivity reaction. Persistent bone and joint infections are often multiple and show predilection for bony prominences such as elbows, knees and malleoli. Previously healthy individuals may be affected.

Blastomycosis (N America, S Africa)

Joint involvement is almost always accompanied by skin lesions and lung involvement. Special features include an occasional acute onset and usual ease of demonstration of organisms in SF.

Sporotrichosis

Disseminated disease with skin lesions and polyarthritis usually occurs only in compromised hosts, but insidious monoarthritis or tenosynovitis may occasionally occur in healthy adults following direct implantation into skin from soil and decaying vegetable matter.

Candidiasis

Joint involvement usually follows haematogenous infection in compromised hosts. Unlike other fungal infections, surgical drainage can often be avoided since contiguous bone involvement is unusual.

Brucellosis

Joint involvement is uncommon during infection by *B. abortus* from cattle or *B. suis* from pigs, but occurs quite frequently (85%) in undulant fever due to *B. melitensis* from sheep and goats. Joint complications are rarely seen in the UK since *B. abortus* is the commonest of the three organisms to cause infection. Brucellosis, however, should be considered as a possible cause of atypical back or joint pain, particularly in those at special risk of infection e.g. farmers, butchers, veterinary surgeons, country dwellers, travellers from endemic areas.

Two types of joint involvement are recognised:

1. Widespread arthralgia, occasionally migratory, causing back and limb pains during febrile episodes (usually transient)
2. A mono- or oligoarthritis, particularly affecting knees, hips, shoulders, SIJ or spine, which usually resolves after several weeks without residua.

Arthritis is occasionally more persistent and may result in X-ray changes of localised porosis and cartilage and bone destruction, followed later by sclerosis and osteophyte formation. Spondylodiscitis (disc space narrowing with destructive changes in adjacent vertebrae) is particularly common in the lumbar spine and may later give rise to characteristic large anterior spurs.

Brucella are very slow-growing organisms and are cultured from SF of affected joints in only a few cases. Blood cultures are more commonly positive, but the diagnosis is often based on high or rising agglutinin titres. Treatment is with Co-trimoxazole but relapse is not uncommon.

Viral arthritis

Although arthralgia and myalgia are a feature of many virus infections, arthritis is unusual. In contrast to infectious arthritis caused by bacteria or fungi, viral arthritis shows two characteristic features: 1. a greater tendency to polyarticular than to mono- or oligoarticular disease; 2. a negligible risk of chronicity and tissue necrosis.

Immune complexes appear to cause the synovitis in most polyarticular forms of viral arthritis. In hepatitis B and adenovirus arthritis for example both serum and SF contain cryoprecipitates (composed of immunoglobulin, complement and viral antigen), and hypocomplementaemia accompanies the arthritis. In the less common oligo- or monoarticular forms, however, tissue inflammation may be caused directly by viral replication. In rubella, the ease with which virus is recovered from joint fluid suggests that it may replicate within synovium.

Although great variability is seen among, and even within, the viral arthritides, certain features should suggest that joint symptoms may be due to viral infection:

1. A non-specific prodrome is common e.g. malaise, fatigue, headache, stiff neck, sore throat, nausea
2. There is often a rash — usually macular or papular
3. Low-grade fever and lympadenopathy are frequently present
4. The clinical situation may be suggestive, e.g.
   Recent immunisation against rubella
   Drug abuse with hepatitis B
   Seasonal onset and exposure to endemic area for arbovirus and Lyme arthritis
5. Arthralgia or arthritis is inevitably short-lived and reversible

The arthritis syndromes associated with rubella, serum hepatitis and mumps deserve special consideration since they are relatively common and may cause diagnostic confusion with early rheumatoid disease. An infective aetiology for RA continues to receive considerable attention and Lyme arthritis will therefore be described as an example of a persistent arthritis resulting from a chronic spirochaete infection.

Rubella

Arthritis may occur in up to 30 per cent of women with naturally acquired rubella infection but is an uncommon complication in children or men. Sudden onset of pain and stiffness usually follows the rash by 1–7 days and typically affects large and small joints symmetrically. Fingers, wrists and knees are particularly involved, often without objective signs of inflammation. The arthritis lasts only 2–3 weeks and diagnosis is confirmed by rising titres in convalescent serum.

Arthritis occurring 2–6 weeks following vaccination with attenuated strains is also common (1–10 percent), but differs from that seen with naturally occurring infection in that monoarticular involvement, particularly of the knee, is frequent, and children may also be affected. Although the arthritis lasts only 1–3 weeks, recurrences, particularly in the knee, are common, occurring with decreasing frequency over months or years.

Viral hepatitis

Arthralgia and polyarthritis are well recognised prodromal features of hepatitis-B infection and appear to result from circulating immune complexes formed during the pre-icteric phase of antigen excess.

Onset of pain and stiffness is characteristically sudden. Usually polyarticular and symmetrical, PIPs and MCPs are most commonly affected, but almost any joint, including TMJs and spine, may be involved. Half the patients have a concomitant, often pruritic, rash that is occasionally urticarial.

LFTs are inevitably abnormal at presentation and HBsAg is usually recoverable from the blood. The arthritis seldom lasts more than a few weeks, does not recur and leaves no residua.

Mumps

Arthritis occurs in $< 1\%$ of cases but is particularly common in men. Joint symptoms usually follow parotitis by 1–2 weeks and predominantly involve large peripheral joints, often in migratory fashion. The arthritis resolves completely after 2–3 weeks.

Lyme arthritis

This condition, first recognised in Lyme, Connecticut, appears to be due to a spirochaete, the ixodes dammini spirochaete, transmitted by tick-bite.

Erythema chronicum migrans — a red macule that expands with central clearing into a large, indurated lesion — characteristically precedes the arthritis by several weeks. Joint symptoms are abrupt in onset and may be migratory, affecting one or a few large joints, commonly knees. Attacks last 1–2 weeks but are recurrent and may result in chronic, persistent synovitis, particularly in the knee. Cardiac conduction defects and neurological abnormalities may occasionally occur.

Cryoprecipitates are found in high titre in SF and serum, and immune complexes have been implicated in the pathogenesis of the synovitis, which may be histologically indistinguishable from RA. Antibiotic therapy is beneficial in early disease, and often prevents major late complications such as chronic arthritis. Tetracycline appears to be the most effective drug, although penicillin and erythromycin also help. Synovectomy has been tried, with some success, in those with persistent and troublesome effusions.

Infective endocarditis

This condition may give rise to several musculoskeletal complications.

1. Arthralgia and arthritis

Joint pains occur in up to 25% of patients with subacute endocarditis and are a frequent presenting feature, particularly in the elderly. Myalgia is a common accompaniment but may occur alone as a major symptom.

Arthralgia is typically asymmetrical and affects several large joints, most commonly knees, elbows, ankles or wrists. Pain is often severe and affected joints may show signs of inflammatory synovitis. Symptoms and signs are characteristically episodic, occurring in attacks which last several days to a few weeks.

Features that suggest the diagnosis of infective endocarditis in a patient with joint pains

1. Recurrent, self-limiting attacks of asymmetrical oligoarthritis lasting 4–14 days
2. Arthralgia/arthritis in a patient with fever and a heart murmur
3. Recent history of dental extraction/operation/instrumentation
4. The presence of associated features, e.g.
   a) Mild splenomegaly
   b) Splinter haemorrhages
   c) Petechiae, purpura, Osler's nodes
   d) Retinal or conjunctival haemorrhage
   e) TIA or cerebral 'embolism'
   f) Microscopic haematuria
   g) Clubbing

A heart murmur, which may alter during the illness, is present in over 95% of patients. Fever, similarly, is present in almost all cases but is typically irregular and remittent and may therefore be missed. Infective endocarditis should always be considered in a patient with joint symptoms, fever and a murmur. Less common, but characteristic, associations may also be present to aid in diagnosis. Osler's nodes appear as transient crops of small, firm, pink nodules in the skin of the finger tips and toes, and similar lesions may be palpable on palms and soles (Janeway lesions).

Echocardiography usually demonstrates vegetations on an abnormal valve and the diagnosis is confirmed by positive blood cultures. Non-specific findings may include anaemia, peripheral leukocytosis (± monocytosis), raised viscosity and hyperglobulinaemia, and rheumatoid factors are present in 50%. Joint X-rays are normal and synovial tissue shows only minimal non-specific inflammatory changes.

Joint, skin and renal lesions appear to result primarily from a vasculitis induced by circulating immune complexes, and SF cultures are inevitably sterile. Joints recover completely following appropriate treatment with antibacterial agents.

2. Septic arthritis

This is uncommon but may occur in acute endocarditis due to virulent organisms, e.g. *Staph. aureus*.

3. Clubbing and secondary hypertrophic osteoarthropathy

This may occur as a very rare, late manifestation of untreated endocarditis (p 292).

A rare condition that may mimic infective endocarditis and present as a rheumatic illness is atrial myxoma. This benign tumour usually causes dyspnoea, weakness or syncope, but occasionally presents with:

1. Joint pains — usually bilateral and symmetrical, affecting small joints of hands, knees and ankles

2. Malaise and weight loss
3. Pulmonary or systemic emboli (small emboli may produce splinters or digital infarcts)
4. Raynaud's phenomenon

Variable signs of mitral or tricuspid stenosis may be found on examination and a raised viscosity is usual. Blood cultures, however, are sterile and echocardiography will reveal the correct diagnosis. Complete recovery follows removal of the tumour.

Leprosy

Two major forms of joint involvement are recognised:

1. The commonest occurs secondary to peripheral neuropathy and affects distal joints of hands and feet. A Charcot-type joint may rarely be produced (p 231) but more commonly there is marked osteolysis associated with trophic ulceration. Sepsis is a major complication and eventual complete loss of fingers, toes, hands and feet may occur.

2. A large-joint arthritis is an occasional feature of the *lepra* reaction. This consists of showers of painful, red, indurated nodules over the extremities and occasionally the trunk, accompanied by fever, general malaise, painful neuritis and rarely lymphadenitis, iritis and orchitis. It appears to be an Arthus-like reaction secondary to release of mycobacterial antigen and occurs primarily during early treatment of lepromatous leprosy patients. Such episodes may be isolated or occur continuously over months and years. Severe reactions may require treatment with thalidomide, clofazimine or steroids.

Syphilitic arthritis

Several forms of joint involvement are recognised but all are rare.

1. Congenital syphilis

'Clutton's joints' affect older children (8–15 years) or young adults, presenting as stiffness and swelling, usually of both knees. Effusions may be marked, fever is common and stigmata of congenital infection are usually present (interstitial keratitis, Hutchinson's incisors and Moon's molars, nerve deafness, periostitis of the tibia). The pathogenesis is unclear: treponemes are not recoverable from the joints and the synovitis is unaffected by penicillin. Complete recovery is usual in 3–12 months.

Rarer manifestations include spindling of fingers and toes due to phalangeal involvement (syphilitic dactylitis) and 'pseudoparalysis' with distal periarticular swelling due to epiphysitis.

2. Secondary acquired syphilis

Arthralgia is common in early contagious syphilis, occurring with fever, mucocutaneous lesions and lymphadenopathy. Response to penicillin is usually rapid and complete.

Painless knee synovitis, unresponsive to penicillin, may occur with late secondary or early tertiary syphilis. As with Clutton's joints, spirochaetes are not recoverable from the joints and complete recovery is usual within 12 months.

Spondylitis, confined to one to five vertebrae and particularly affecting the cervical spine, is a rare, late manifestation that causes pain, stiffness and localised tenderness. Although progression to vertebral body destruction is usual, cord compression is rare. Penicillin is usually effective.

3. Tertiary acquired syphilis

Gummatous lesions may cause a relatively painfree, progressive, chronic monoarthritis of large joints such as the knee. X-rays show characteristic localised bone destruction and periosteal reaction. Penicillin is usually effective.

Periostitis is the commonest skeletal lesion of late syphilis and particularly affects the tibia (*sabre tibia*) and shoulder girdle. Penicillin produces rapid resolution.

Charcot joints may complicate tabes dorsalis and are characterised by joint disorganisation and sclerotic remodelling, with exuberant osteophytosis and periarticular calcification. The cause of such 'neuropathic' joints is unclear (p 231).

FURTHER READING

Brogadir S P, Schimmer B M, Myers A R 1979 Spectrum of the gonococcal arthritis-dermatitis syndrome. Seminars in Arthritis and Rheumatism 8(3): 177–183.

Hyer F H, Gottlieb N L 1978 Rheumatic disorders associated with viral infection. Seminars in Arthritis and Rheumatism 8(1): 17–31.

Infectious Arthritis 1978 In: Schmid F R (ed) Clinics in rheumatic diseases. W B Saunders, London

Ward J R, Atcheson S G 1977 Infectious arthritis. Medical Clinics of North America 61(2): 313–329

11 Immunodeficiency diseases

Immunodeficiency as a cause of disease may occur as a direct result of some primary defect in the body's immunological mechanisms or secondary to a change in immunological function caused by other disease processes or their treatment. While immunodeficiency due to the latter is quite common, cases of primary immunodeficiency are rare. The description of these uncommon conditions is relevant in the context of the rheumatic diseases, however, since not only are some of these primary deficiency states associated with an increased frequency of connective tissue diseases but also some are closely linked to the deficiency of purine salvage pathway enzymes.

PRIMARY IMMUNODEFICIENCY

CLASSIFICATION

Table 11.1 shows a list of primary deficiency states based on the WHO classification. They include disorders primarily of B-lymphocyte function, such as Bruton's agammaglobulinaemia; disorders primarily of T-lymphocyte function, such as the DiGeorge syndrome; combined immunodeficiency syndromes, and a large heterogeneous rag-bag, 'common variable immunodeficiency', representing the largest group of all.

Figure 11.1 shows the interactions between the naturally-occurring and the adaptive arms of the immune systems and it can be seen that a defect in one area will have far-reaching effects on other functional components. As the precise site of the various defects becomes known the classification shown here will be considerably modified.

Table 11.1 Classification of primary immunodeficiency disorders

Type	Predominant cellular defect	
	B cell	T cell
1. Bruton's agammaglobulinaemia	+	
2. Selective IgA deficiency	+	
3. Immunodeficiency with elevated IgM	+	
4. Transient hypogammaglobulinaemia of infancy	+	
5. Antibody deficiency with near-normal immunoglobulins	+	
6. Thymic hypoplasia (DiGeorge)		+
7. Nezelof's syndrome		+
8. Severe combined immunodeficiency without ADA deficiency	+	+
9. Severe combined immunodeficiency with ADA deficiency	+	+
10. Reticular dysgenesis	+	+
11. Wiskott–Aldrich syndrome	+	+
12. Ataxia telangiectasia	+	+
13. Common variable immunodeficiency	+	±

INCIDENCE

The exact incidence of these disorders is not known, but they are rare. Selective deficiency of

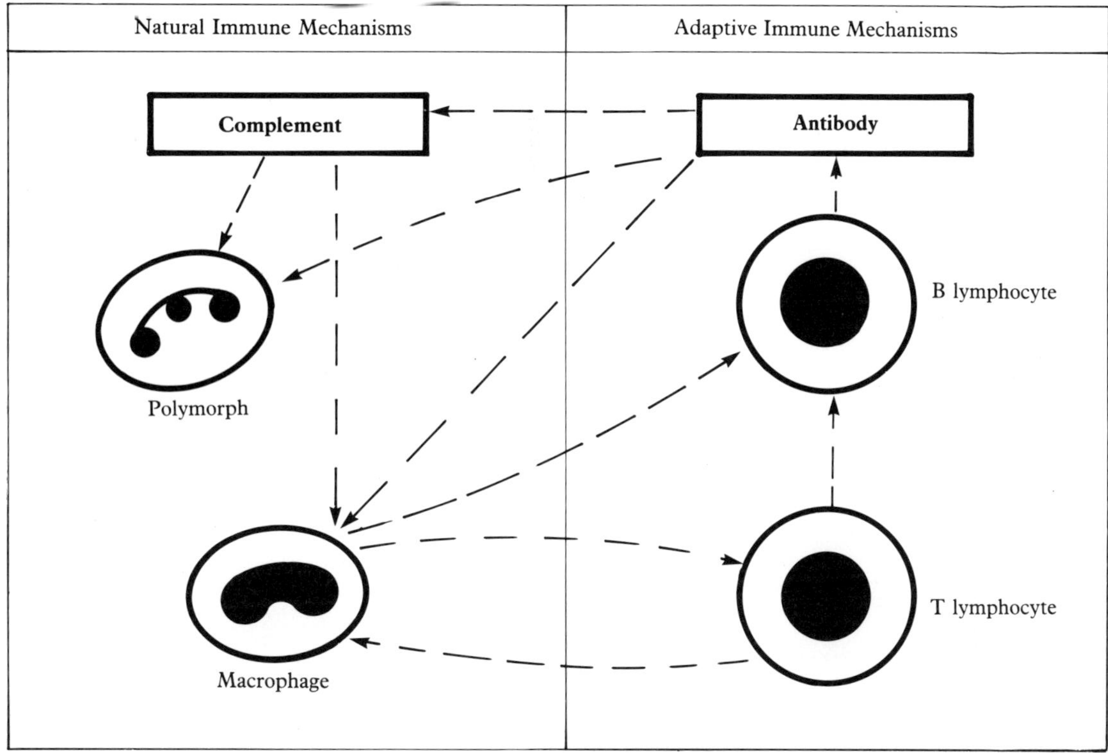

Fig. 11.1 Interactions between the naturally-occurring and the adaptive arms of the immune system

IgA is the most common form of a primary immunodeficiency with a prevalence reported between 0.05 and 0.9%. In childhood, males are affected five times more than females, while in adults the sex incidence is equal.

AETIOLOGY

Most of the primary immunodeficiency diseases appear to result from the absence of particular immunological functions associated with the failure to develop specific functionally competent cell populations, but often the precise biological defect is not known. In the minority of cases, however, the cause has been established. In DiGeorge's syndrome there is thymic dysplasia due to a defect in the embryological development of the third branchial arch. Recently, other syndromes have been associated with the deficiency of key enzymes in the purine salvage pathway.

Enzyme defects in the purine salvage pathway associated with immunodeficiency (Fig. 11.2)

A gross deficiency of each of three sequential enzymes involved in the catabolic degradation of purine nucleotides has been reported in patients with immunodeficiency.

1. Adenosine deaminase (ADA) deficiency is associated with severe combined immunodeficiency due to the impaired function of T and B cells
2. Purine nucleoside phosphorylase (PNP) deficiency has been associated with an isolated defect in T cells
3. Purine ecto-5′-nucleotidase activity is low in a proportion of patients with X-linked agammaglobulinaemia and common variable immunodeficiency.

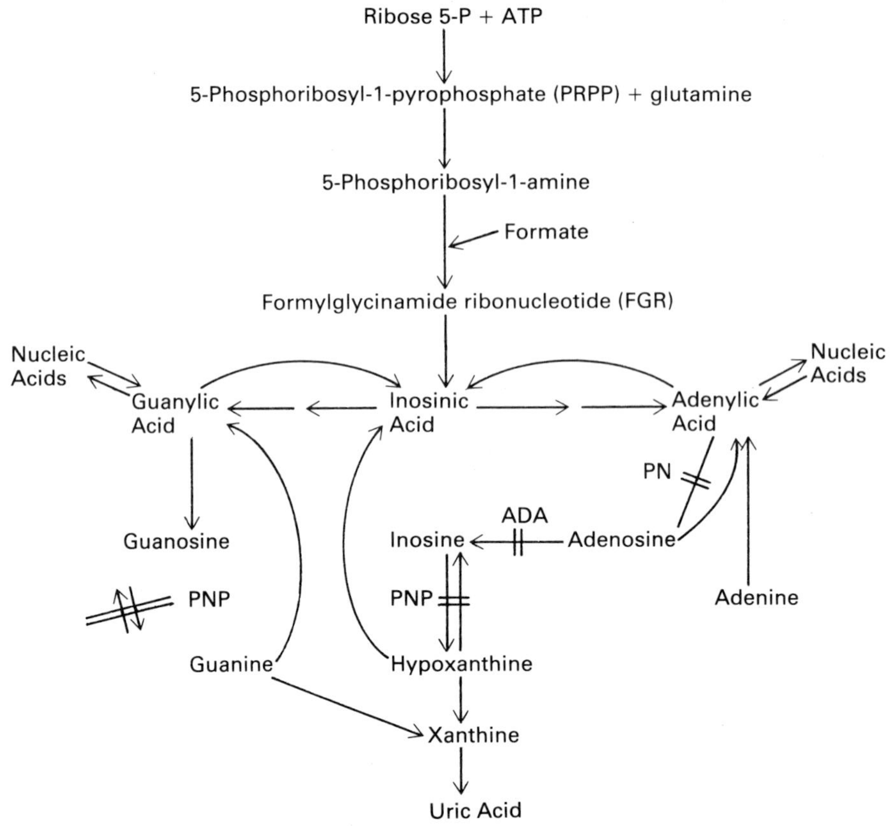

Fig. 11.2 Enzyme defects in purine metabolism associated with immunodeficiency (ADA = adenosine deaminase; PNP = purine nucleoside phosphorylase; PN = purine ecto-5'-nucleotidase)

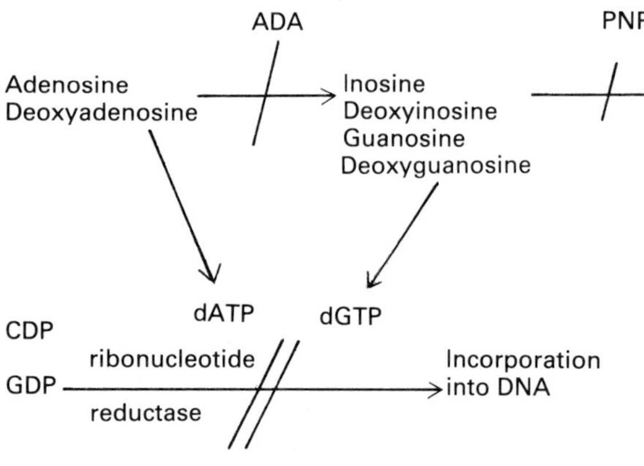

Fig. 11.3 Effect of ADA- and PNP-deficiency on purine metabolism

The absence of ADA and PNP leads to an accumulation of the substrates for these enzymes with enhanced accumulation of dATP and dGTP respectively in cells such as erythrocytes and lymphoid cells. Both dATP and dGTP are potent inhibitors of ribonucleotide reductase resulting in inhibition of DNA synthesis (Fig. 11.3). *In vitro* studies have shown that the build-up of deoxyadenosine and deoxyguanosine is more toxic for T cells than B cells. Deoxyadenosine also inactivates other enzymes, such as S-adenylhomocystein hydrolase (SAM), which are not affected by deoxyguanosine. This may account for the additional effect of ADA deficiency on B cells and chondrocytes.

It is not known whether or not the deficiency of purine ecto-5′-nucleotidase seen in some patients with agammaglobulinaemia is the cause or the result of deficient B cells.

CLINICAL MANIFESTATIONS

Recurrent infection is the hallmark of primary immunodeficiency states, reflecting the importance of the immune system in dealing with micro-organisms. The nature of the immune deficit determines in part the spectrum of infections that may be encountered. Thus, abnormalities of B-cell function and deficiency of specific complement components is accompanied by infection by organisms that are largely disposed of by opsinisation such as encapsulated bacteria (pneumococci, staphylococci etc). T-cell dysfunction, on the other hand, is associated with intracellular infections with viruses, fungi and certain bacteria such as *Mycobacterium tuberculosis*.

Certain of these immunodeficiency disorders are associated with an increased frequency of polyarthritis, connective-tissue diseases and other autoimmune manifestations (Table 11.2). This association may be due to the abnormal immune regulation inherent in the defect, or the result of persistent infection as the result of the immunodeficiency.

Clinical characteristics of antibody and cellular deficiency

Antibody deficiency

1. Recurrent infections with extracellular encapsulated bacteria, e.g. *Pneumococcus, Staph., Strep., Haemophilus*.
2. Chronic sinopulmonary disease
3. Susceptible to enterovirus infections but not to other viruses or fungi
4. Growth retardation not marked
5. Antibody deficiency in serum and secretions
6. May or may not lack circulating B cells
7. Hypoplasia of lymphoid and nasopharyngeal tissue in X-linked agammaglobulinaemia, with lymphocyte depletion of B cell dependent areas of lymph node and spleen
8. Increased risk of autoimmune disorders or malignancy

Cellular deficiency

1. Recurrent infections with opportunistic agents such as viruses, fungi or *Pneumocystis carinii*
2. Growth retardation, short life span, wasting and diarrhoea
3. Fatal reactions from live virus or BCG vaccination
4. Anergy

Table 11.2 Immunodeficiency disorders and associated autoimmune disease

Disorder	Frequency of associated auto-immunity
X-linked agammaglobulinaemia	++
Selective IgA deficiency	+++
Thymic hypoplasia	0
Severe combined immunodeficiency	0
Wiskott–Aldrich syndrome	+
Ataxia telangiectasia	+
Common variable immunodeficiency	+++
Complement-component deficiency	+++

+++ = frequent
++ = occasional
+ = rare

1. Disorders characterised by abnormal B-cell function

a) X-linked agammaglobulinaemia (Bruton's agammaglobulinaemia)

This rare condition predominantly affects males, and study of various kindreds suggests an X-linked mode of inheritance. The majority of affected children remain well for the first 6–9 months of life, by virtue of maternal immunoglobulin acquired via the placenta, but thereafter they suffer repeated infections with extracellular pyogenic organisims such as pneumococci, streptococci and *Haemophilus* resulting in manifestations such as sinusitis, pneumonia, otitis, meningitis or septicaemia. There is also an increased risk of viral hepatitis and infection with adenoviruses, suggesting a major role for secretory IgA in the host defense against these viruses. Other viral infections and chronic fungal infections are generally not seen. Those who survive infection have an increased frequency of polyarthritis resembling rheumatoid arthritis, dermatomyositis and an increased incidence of lymphoreticular malignancy.

Fully developed B lymphocytes and plasma cells are absent or greatly reduced in the blood and blood-forming organs resulting in absent or reduced production of all classes of immunoglobulin and absence of antibodies both to naturally-occurring blood-group antigens (isohaemagglutinins) and in response to antigenic stimulus. Lymphopenia is not a feature and while B lymphocytes are absent the number of circulatory T cells is normal or increased. *In vitro* studies show an absence of B-cell function but normal T-cell activity. Similarly, the T-cell-dependent areas of lymph nodes and spleen are normal, while B-cell-dependent areas are depleted, with hypoplasia of adenoids, tonsils and peripheral lymph nodes and absence of Peyer's patches.

b) Selective IgA deficiency

This is the most common of the defined immunodeficiency disorders, the prevalence varying in different populations form 1/300 to 1/3000. There is a strong familial tendency, and the deficiency appears to be inherited, although the mode of inheritance is unknown.

Many people with selective IgA deficiency are asymptomatic but it is commonly associated with ill-health:

(i) Chronic or recurrent infections of mucosal surfaces. Patients show an increased susceptibility to infections especially of the respiratory, gastro-intestinal and urinary tracts. Common manifestations are recurrent sino-pulmonary infections and chronic diarrhoea, often caused by infection with *Giardia lamblia*. This reflects the importance of secretory IgA in combating pathogens at the portal of entry. These manifestations also occur in the rare patient who lacks secretory piece, and therefore secretory IgA, but has normal serum IgA levels.

(ii) Atopy is present in 50% and may be due to the fact that antigens normally excluded by IgA react with IgE bound to mast cells to produce an immediate hypersensitivity reaction.

(iii) There is an increased incidence of connective tissue diseases and other auto-immune phenomena

(iv) There is an increased incidence of malignancy, including tumours of the lung, gastrointestinal tract and lymphoreticular system.

Auto-immune diseases associated with selective IgA deficiency

1. SLE
2. RA
3. JCA
4. Gluten-sensitive enteropathy
5. Pernicious anaemia
6. Thyroiditis
7. Chronic active hepatitis
8. Dermatomyositis
9. Idiopathic Addison's disease
10. Sjögren's syndrome
11. Autoimmune haemolytic anaemia
12. ITP
13. Myaesthenia gravis
14. Vitiligo
15. Diabetes mellitus

There are absent or very diminished amounts of IgA in the serum and external secretions but usual levels of other immunoglobulin types and normal cell-mediated immunity. The biological defect is unknown, although in some cases specific T-cell suppression of IgA production has been demonstrated. Antibody to IgA is found in over half of the cases and, while its aetiological significance is unknown, it has clinical relevance since it can be the cause of severe or even fatal anaphylactic reactions to intravenous administration of blood products.

c) Common variable immunodeficiency

This is a rag-bag which encompasses a spectrum of disorders with varying degrees of hypogammaglobulinaemia and abnormal T-cell function producing immunodeficiency which is characteristically variable over time. There is a variable age of onset but this is most commonly between the

Auto-immune diseases associated with common variable immunodeficiency

1. Rheumatoid arthritis
2. SLE
3. Sjögren's syndrome
4. Auto-immune haemolytic anaemia
5. ITP
6. Alopecia areata
7. Vitiligo
8. Pernicious anaemia
9. Thyroiditis
10. Myaesthenia gravis

Contrasting features of the arthritis of hypogammaglobulinaemia with typical RA

1. Equal sex distribution
2. Sparing of finger and toe joints
3. Non-deforming
4. Non-erosive
5. Rare rheumatoid nodules
6. Absent rheumatoid factor
7. Atypical synovial histology
8. Favourable response to gammaglobulin administration in adults

ages of 15 years and 35 years, and an equal sex distribution is seen.

Clinically, patients resemble children with Bruton's agammaglobulinaemia, and the predominant manifestation is recurrent infection. They frequently have gastrointestinal symptoms, especially chronic diarrhoea and recurrent infection with *Giardia*. These patients also have a high incidence of circulatory auto-antibodies and an increased frequency of auto-immune disease and malignancy.

Unlike children with X-linked agammaglobulinaemia, those with common variable immunodeficiency have circulating B cells even though the reduction in serum immunoglobulin levels can be profound. Similarly most patients have well developed lymphoid tissue with normally populated B- and T-cell areas. *In vitro* tests vary; B cells of some patients synthesise immunoglobulin on exposure to mitogenic factors but are unable to secrete it, while B cells of others neither synthesise nor secrete immunoglobulin. The primary defect is unknown and probably varies from patient to patient. In some there appears to be excessive activity of T-suppressor cells.

d) Arthritis associated with hypogammaglobulinaemia

The association of a polyarthritis resembling rheumatoid arthritis and primary hypogammaglobulinaemia was first described in children, 50% of whom are affected, but has since been recognised in adults with common variable immunodeficiency.

The features of most common forms of polyarthritis seen in these conditions are listed. It shows important differences from typical rheumatoid arthritis. While there is symmetrical involvement, the polyarthritis of hypogammaglobulinaemia initially affects larger joints such as the knees, ankles and wrists but spares the fingers and toes, although tenosynovitis of the hands and feet can be prominent. The arthritis is usually non-deforming and radiological erosions are rare. Subcutaneous nodules are also rare and rheumatoid factor is absent. The synovial membrane shows a mononuclear cell infitrate but not the degree of lymphoid hyperplasia seen in rheumatoid arthritis.

The arthritis of common variable immunodeficiency responds to immunoglobulin administration while that associated with Bruton's agammaglobulinaemia does not.

Other forms of arthritis are also seen occasionally. There are rare cases of typical erosive rheumatoid arthritis and equally rare cases of Whipple's disease. Septic arthritis may be a serious complication of the immunodeficiency state.

2. Disorders characterised by abnormal T-cell function

Well-defined syndromes which appear to affect primarily the T cells include DiGeorge's syndrome and Nezelof's syndrome. Although immunoglobulin levels are usually normal or even elevated in these conditions, B-cell function is also depressed presumably as the result of defective T-helper cell function. These are rare and severe conditions and it is unusual for affected individuals to survive beyond infancy or childhood.

a) DiGeorge syndrome

This rare condition is due to the abnormal embryonic development of the third and fourth pharyngeal pouches. Failure of development of the thymus and parathyroid glands is responsible for the major clinical manifestations but associated features include a characteristic facies, cardiovascular anomalies and oesophageal atresia.

Features of DiGeorge's syndrome

1. Failure of thymus to develop
   Diminished CMI and recurrent infection
2. Failure of parathyroids to develop
   Hypocalcaemia
3. Characteristic facies
   a) Notched pinnae
   b) Hypotelorism
   c) Bowed mouth
4. Cardiovascular anomalies
   a) Right side aortic arch
   b) Atrial and ventricular septal defects
5. Oesophageal atresia

The diagnosis is first suggested by hypocalcaemic seizures during the neonatal period but the subsequent course is dominated by often overwhelming infections leading to death in infancy. Most infections are with fungi, particularly candidiasis, or viruses although Gram-negative bacterial infections also occur. Infection with the opportunistic pathogen *Pneumocystis carinii* also occurs.

As the result of thymic deficiency, thymus-dependent areas of lymph nodes and spleen are depleted of lymphocytes, and although peripheral lymphopenia is usually not marked, there is a reduced proportion of lymphocytes with T-cell markers. There is reduced T-cell function demonstrated by both *in vivo* and *in vitro* tests. Although serum immunoglobulin levels are normal, the capactiy for most antibody responses to specific antigens is often depressed.

b) Nezelof's syndrome

This rare condition affects young children from 6 months of age and is characterised by thymic dysplasia and neutropenia but normal or even elevated immunoglobulin levels. In contrast to DiGeorge's syndrome there are no endocrine or cardiovascular abnormalities, and children present with failure to thrive and recurrent infections with opportunistic pathogens, often resulting in death before the age of 4. There is often a familial history, and an autosomal recessive mode of inheritance has been identified in some and X-linked inheritance in others.

c) Purine nucleoside phosphorylase (PNP) deficiency

Certain patients with severe T-cell defects but normal B-cell function have been described with a total lack of PNP activity in their red blood cells.

3. Disorders characterised by severe combined defects of B-cell and T-cell function

a) Severe combined immunodeficiency (SCID)

Though rare, this represents the most severe of all immunodeficiencies and death usually occurs within the first year of life. Babies present within 6 months of birth with failure to thrive and recurrent severe infections caused by viruses, fungi and other opportunistic pathogens such as *Pneumocystis carinii*. Lymphopenia is often marked and B- and T-cell areas of peripheral lymphoid tissue and spleen are depleted of lymphocytes. Parameters of both B- and T-cell function are markedly depressed.

The mode of inheritance in the majority is autosomal recessive (Swiss-type agammaglobulinaemia) or X-linked recessive. In 15% a complete lack of ADA can be identified in the erythrocyte. In addition to immunodeficiency, these children have a high frequency of skeletal abnormalities such as cupping and flaring of the anterior rib ends due to chondro-osseous dysplasia involving the costo-chondral junctions.

b) Reticular dysgenesis

Children born with this rare condition are both lymphopenic and neutropenic and suffer from severe immunodeficiency involving both T-cell and B-cell function. They succumb to overwhelming infection within the first few weeks of life.

4. Disorders characterised by partial immunodeficiency associated with other conditions

a) Wiskott–Aldrich syndrome

Children with this rare syndrome, which is transmitted as an X-linked recessive trait, present early in life with the clinical triad:

1. Undue susceptibility to infection, initially with high-grade extracellular encapsulated pathogens such as *Pneumococcus*, and later with opportunistic infections
2. Eczema
3. Thrombocytopenia, usually causing petechiae or bloody diarrhoea but occasionally fatal complications such as intracranial bleeding

Those children who survive to their teens often die from lymphoreticular malignancies.

Serum IgM levels are often low while other immunoglobulin types are normal or even elevated. Defective T-cell function becomes more marked with time. Characteristically there is a reduced ability to form antibodies to specific antigens, especially polysaccharide and small protein antigens, and it is hypothesised that the site of the defect is at the level of antigen recognition.

b) Ataxia telangiectasia

This rare condition is inherited as an autosomal recessive trait and characterised by:

1. Progressive cerebellar ataxia during the first few years of life
2. Oculo-cutaneous telangiectasia
3. Immunodeficiency leading to well established sino-pulmonary disease by 5 years of age

Other features include insulin resistance, hepatic abnormalities, testicular and ovarian dysgenesis and premature ageing with greying hair and atrophy of the skin. There is an increased incidence of lymphoreticular malignancies with age.

Immunological abnormalities include selective IgA deficiency in the majority, impaired ability to form antibody to antigenic challenge and impaired cell-mediated immunity which becomes increasingly more marked.

Chromosonal abnormalities have been described, and the primary defect is thought to be an impaired ability to repair DNA.

5. Disorders characterised by specific complement-component deficiencies

In recent years selective deficiences of components of the complement system have been described. They appear to be rare but are associated with immunodeficiency, leading to an increased susceptibility to infection and with an increased frequency of connective-tissue diseases depending on which complement component is lacking (Table 11.3). Inheritance of these conditions appears to be Mendelian, with two co-dominant

Table 11.3 Complement deficiencies associated with rheumatic diseases

Complement component	Associated disease
C1q	Severe combined immunodeficiency
C1r	SLE, glomerulonephritis
C1s	SLE
C4	SLE
C2	SLE, DLE, RA, JCA Dermatomyositis, glomerulonephritis Henoch–Schonlein purpura, Hodgkin's disease
C3	Infections, SLE
C5	Infections, SLE
C6	Gonococcaemia
C7	Gonococcaemia, systemic sclerosis
C8	Gonococcaemia, SLE
C1 1NH	Hereditary angio-oedema, SLE
C3b INA	Infections

genes controlling synthesis of the complement component. Heterozygotes therefore synthesise approximately half-normal levels.

Deficiency of early components of the classical complement pathway such as C1, C4 and C2 are associated mainly with connective tissue diseases, especially SLE-like disorders

C2-deficiency is the most common component deficiency with a prevalence of approximately 1% in the heterozygous state and a predicted prevalence of 0.0025% for the homozygous state. Associations have been drawn between homozygous deficiency and SLE, DLE, RA, JCA, vasculitis and glomerulonephritis. Significant associations have also been made between the heterozygous state and SLE and JCA. The SLE accompanying C2-deficiency resembles other forms of SLE but tends to be milder, with less renal disease but more cutaneous disease, and often with low or absent ANA.

Deficiency of C3 is associated with an increased susceptibility to life-threatening bacterial infection. Deficiency of the terminal components (C5 to C8) appears to be associated with an increased susceptibility to infections such as recurrent or disseminated gonococcal infections where bacterial lysis is important for elimination of the pathogen.

Deficiencies of inhibitors of the complement pathway are also recognised. In fact, the commonest genetic defect of the complement system is impaired synthesis of C1 esterase inhibitor. Patients present with hereditary angioneurotic oedema characterised by episodic attacks of non-painful, non-pruritic oedema lasting 2–4 days and affecting mainly the limbs, trunk and neck. The greatest danger is from airways obstruction due to involvement of tissues of the upper airway. During the attack C4 and C2 are depleted, and while levels usually rise between attacks C4 almost always remains depressed. Absent or, more commonly, depressed levels of C1 esterase inhibitor confirm the diagnosis. The minority however, have normal levels but the protein is non-functional. It is of interest that this condition is also associated with SLE.

The link between complement-deficiency states and connective-tissue disease is not clear. One hypothesis relates this increased susceptibility to the role of complement in neutralising viral agents and in enhancing the clearance by the reticulo-endothelial system of circulating immune complexes. Since genes regulating the synthesis of C2 and C4 are located in the HLA complex on chromosome 6, another hypothesis is that the link with connective-tissue disease is through a common association with certain Ir genes in the HLA complex.

SECONDARY IMMUNODEFICIENCY

Alteration of immunological function as a result of a disease process or as the result of treatment is a much more common cause of immunodeficiency. It can occur during the course of certain viral infections, in malnutrition and in malignancy,

Table 11.4 Some causes of secondary immunodeficiency

	B cell	T cell
Lymphoproliferative diseases		
Chronic lymphatic leukaemia	++	+
Myeloma	++	
Hodgkin's disease	±	++
Infections e.g.		
Bacteria		
TB		+
Syphilis		+
Leprosy (lepromatous)		++
Parasites		
Malaria	+	
Viruses		
Epstein-Barr		+
Measles		+
Cytomegalovirus		+
Acquired immunodeficiency syndromes (AIDS)		++
Chronic inflammatory disorders e.g.		
SLE		+
Sjögren's	+	+
Sarcoid	+	+
Decreased systhesis or increased loss of immunoglobulin		
Protein-calorie malnutrition	+	
Nephrotic syndrome	+	
Dystrophia myotonica	+	
Drugs e.g.		
Corticosteroids		
Cytotoxics		
Azathioprine	+	++
Cyclophosphamide	++	++
Methotrexate	++	++

particularly leukaemias, lymphoreticular malignancy and Hodgkin's disease (Table 11.4). In most cases immunological disturbance is minor, but occasionally the severity of the immune defect can dominate the underlying disease. Patients with SLE and severe forms of Sjögren's syndrome have an increased frequency of infections, both with common pyogenic micro-organisms and opportunistic infection, which cannot be entirely accounted for by immunosuppressive therapy. Patients with active SLE have diminished cell-mediated immunity and serum factors are present, probably circulating immune complexes, which interfere with opsonisation. However, the commonest cause of severe secondary immunodeficiency, particularly in the context of the rheumatic diseases, is iatrogenic with the use of high-dose steroids and cytotoxic drugs. These agents affect the function of various cellular components of the immune system, including polymorphs and macrophages as well as lymphocytes, and patients are at risk of developing unusual opportunistic infections such as *Pneumocystis carinii* pneumonia.

Acquired immunodeficiency syndrome (AIDS)

The acquired immunodeficiency syndrome (AIDS) has only recently been recognised and is characterised by a profound disturbance of cell-mediated immunity. Patients present with *Pneumocystis carinii* pneumonia or with Kaposi's sarcoma or both, frequently accompanied by various other infections involving intracellular micro-organisms. There is often a preceding illness with fever, weight loss, diarrhoea and lymphadenopathy. Patients are lymphopenic with a loss of T-helper cells so that the normal helper:suppressor ratio is reversed. They are anergic, and *in vitro* tests of T-lymphocyte function are abnormal. Humoral immunity is largely normal. The patients are most commonly male homosexuals or drug abusers or both, but cases have also been described amongst haemophiliacs. Though initially described in urban USA, cases are now seen in other parts of the world. A striking feature of AIDS is that it appears to be communicable, probably principally by sexual contact. There are preliminary reports that a retrovirus may be involved which is capable of infecting T cells and inducing immunosuppression.

EVALUATION OF IMMUNODEFICIENCY

The hallmark of immunodeficiency is recurrent infection, and the diagnosis may be suggested by features in the history and examination such as age and sex of the patient, the family history, the type of infection and the presence of associated clinical abnormalities. Tests of B and T lymphocytes, macrophages and complement function confirm the diagnosis.

B-lymphocyte function can be assessed *in vivo* by quantitation of serum immunoglobulin, the detection of naturally-occurring antibodies such as blood group isoagglutinins and the detection of antibody after immunisation, e.g. with the Schick test. *In vitro* tests include the quantitation of circulating lymphocytes with B-cell markers and assessing the ability of lymphocytes to synthesise immunoglobulin after stimulation with mitogens such as pokeweed mitogen.

In vivo tests of T-cell function include the response to a battery of skin tests using PPD, *Candida* and SK-SD. In addition, delayed skin hypersensitivity may be actively evaluated by sensitisation with DNCB, a strong inducer of cell-mediated immunity.

In vitro tests include the peripheral lymphocyte count, quantitating the lymphocytes with T-cell markers and measuring the proliferative response of lymphocytes to mitogens such as PHA and ConA, or specific antigens such as PPD.

Assessment of the complement system is carried out *in vitro* either by functional assays or by immunochemical quantitations of individual components. The CH50 (p 466) is a functional assay of the classical pathway which requires the presence of each factor. Absence of one factor results in zero or very low values. Quantitation of individual complement components can be carried out using immunoassays and in specialised laboratories results can be confirmed by functional tests for individual proteins.

Other tests include the evaluation of migration

Evaluation of immunodeficient patients

HISTORY OF RECURRENT

CLINICAL EVALUATION

1. Age and sex
2. Family history
3. Type of infection
4. Associated abnormality
5. Underlying disease
6. Presence or absence of lymphoid tissue
7. Routine blood studies
   a) Lymphopenia
   b) Granulocytopenia

Evaluate B cell function

In vivo tests

1. Serum Ig levels
2. Blood group isoagglutinins
3. Anti viral antibody titre, e.g. Schick test after previous diphtheria immunisation
4. Antibody response to new antigens, e.g. Ø 174

In vitro tests

1. Surface markers — number of Ig^+ cells
2. Pokeweed mitogen stimulation
   Specific antigen stimulation

Evaluate T cell function

In vivo tests

1. Skin tests: PPD, *Candida*, SK-SD
   Skin tests with DNCB

In vitro tests

1. Surface markers
   — number of SRBC rosette-forming cells
   — number OKT3, T4 and T8 + cells
2. PHA and ConA stimulation
   Specific antigen stimulation

Evaluate complement function

1. CH50
2. Immunoassay of specific components

Other tests

Evaluation of macrophage and neutrophil function

a) Migration and chemotaxis
b) Phagocytosis

and phagocytic capacity of macrophages and polymorphs.

TREATMENT

Commercial gammaglobulin is effective in preventing recurrent pyogenic infections in patients with hypo- or agammaglobulinaemia. In adults with common variable immunodeficiency this therapy is also effective for the polyarthritis. The exception is selective IgA deficiency in which gammaglobulin should not be used because of the risk of severe hypersensitivity reactions due to the presence of antibody to IgA.

Other forms of immunodeficiency present a greater challenge to treatment. Some cases of DiGeorge's syndrome have been successfully treated with transplantation of thymus from allogeneic embryos which has corrected the T cell deficiency and the defective immunological function. Histocompatible bone marrow transplants have been successful in some individuals with SCID and Wiskott-Aldrich syndrome. Transfusion of irradiated normal red cells produces temporary improvement in patients with ADA and PNP deficiency.

REFERENCES

Asherson G L, Webster A D B 1980 The diagnosis and treatment of immunodeficiency diseases. Blackwell, Oxford

12 Polymyalgia rheumatica

Polymyalgia rheumatica (PMR) is a clinical syndrome, comprising aching and stiffness in the proximal part of the limbs and trunk, especially in the shoulder girdles, constitutional features such as depression and weight loss and a rapid sedimentation rate, which occurs predominantly in patients over the age of sixty. It may develop as a presentation of an underlying disease , particularly giant cell arteritis, but most commonly it occurs in isolation. Its importance lies in its frequency in the elderly population and in its responsiveness to small doses of corticosteroids.

INCIDENCE

PMR occurs predominantly in the elderly population. The mean age of onset is 70 and the vast majority of cases develop between the ages of 60 and 90. Rare cases, however, have been reported in the fifth decade. Women are affected twice as commonly as men and there is a striking predilection for Caucasians. This is particularly noticeable in studies reported from the USA, where it is only rarely seen in American Blacks. Its incidence is not well defined, although it has been estimated to be approximately 40 cases per 100 000 per year.

AETIOLOGY

The aetiology of PMR is unknown. Constitutional factors appear to be important. There is a strong relationship to the ageing process and a genetic predisposition is suggested by the racial incidence and the reports of familial aggregation. Attempts to look for an infective aetiology have failed. Although there is one report of a high incidence of hepatitis-B virus antibody in patients with PMR, this finding has not been substantiated in other studies. Non-specific immunological abnormalities, such as hyperglobulinaemia and the presence of circulating immune complexes, have been reported during active phases of disease. However the part played, if any, by immunological mechanisms is not known.

PATHOLOGY

20% of patients with PMR have typical changes of giant cell arteritis in temporal artery biopsies. Otherwise there are very few abnormal pathological findings. Muscle biopsies looking for the cause of the marked myalgia are either normal or show non-specific type II muscle fibre atrophy. There are reports, however, of lymphocytic infiltration in synovial biopsies from the sterno-clavicular joints, shoulder and knee.

CLINICAL FEATURES

Presentation

The typical presentation is an elderly women who develops pain and stiffness in the limb girdle and spinal muscles accompanied by marked constitutional symptoms over two to three weeks. Often, however, the onset is abrupt.

Clinical features of polymyalgia rheumatica

1. Disease of the elderly. F: M 2: 1
2. Onset: subacute or abrupt
3. Pain and stiffness in girdle and spinal muscles
4. Marked morning stiffness
5. Constitutional features: fatigue, anorexia, weight loss, depression
6. Raised ESR
7. Mild to moderate anaemia
8. Raised alkaline phosphatase
9. Responsive to small doses of prednisolone (10 mg/d)

Musculoskeletal manifestations

The clinical syndrome is dominated by pain and stiffness in the neck, shoulders and back, upper arms and thighs. The symptoms are bilateral and usually symmetrical. Prominent features are pain at night and marked morning stiffness with difficulty in getting out of bed. In marked contrast to the severity of the symptoms there is a paucity of physical findings. There may be bilateral tenderness in the upper arms but muscle weakness is not a feature. A proportion of patients have a peripheral synovitis. Late features are generalised muscle atrophy and signs of adhesive capsulitis of the shoulders.

Systemic manifestations

These are often marked and include fatigue, anorexia, weight loss and depression.

LABORATORY FINDINGS

The ESR is almost invariably raised, often markedly so. A mild to moderate normochromic anaemia is common and other non-specific findings include elevated $\alpha 2$- and gammaglobulins. Liver function tests are abnormal in 50%, usually an elevated alkaline phosphatase. Liver biopsy, however, is generally normal. Synovial fluid from inflamed knees shows an elevated WBC (1000–5000/mm^3; 50% polymorphs) and joint scans using pertechnitate (^{99m}Tc) have demonstrated isotope uptake by the shoulder and acromio-clavicular joints in a large proportion of cases.

DIAGNOSIS

The diagnosis of PMR depends on recognising the features that make up the clinical syndrome. The most valuable features are shown below.

Helpful features in diagnosis of PMR (after Bird et al 1979)

1. Bilateral shoulder pain and/or stiffness
2. Onset of illness of less than 2 weeks' duration
3. ESR greater than 40 (Westergren)
4. Duration of morning stiffness greater than 1 hour
5. Age 65 or more
6. Depression and/or weight loss
7. Bilateral tenderness in upper arms

DIFFERENTIAL DIAGNOSIS

PMR needs to be distinguished from conditions shown opposite. Local disorders of the shoulder (Chapter 21.III) are usually unilateral and not accompanied by systemic illness. Viral myalgia is generalised and short lived and rarely lasts more than two weeks. Prominence of peripheral joint involvement and muscle weakness distinguishes rheumatoid arthritis and polymyositis from PMR respectively.

Differential diagnosis of PMR
1. Local disorders of the shoulder
2. Viral myalgia
3. Rheumatoid arthritis
4. Occult malignancy
5. Metabolic disorders, e.g. thyrotoxicosis
6. Parkinson's disease

CONDITIONS THAT MAY PRESENT WITH PMR

Polymyalgia may be the presenting feature of a number of underlying diseases shown below.

Diseases associated with polymyalgia rheumatica
1. Giant cell arteritis
2. Rheumatoid arthritis
3. SLE
4. Carcinoma
5. Lymphoma

PMR occurs in half of those with clinical features of giant cell arteritis. Conversely, histological evidence of giant cell arteritis in temporal artery biopsies in the absence of symptoms is seen in up to 20% of PMR patients. Although there is no evidence that PMR is due to vasculitis some suggest that PMR is a manifestation of giant cell arteritis, while others view them as separate entities which tend to occur together.

Polymyalgia may be the presenting feature of rheumatoid arthritis. The prominence of synovitis affecting peripheral joints and positive tests for rheumatoid factor are clues to this association.

Rarely, polymyalgia may be the presenting feature of SLE in the elderly or of more serious underlying diseases such as carcinoma or lymphoma.

TREATMENT

PMR responds to small doses of corticosteroids of the order of 10 mg/day. Often the clinical improvement is dramatic and occurs within 48 hours, but sometimes on this dose it may take up to 1 week. This response to steroids has some diagnostic importance, and an underlying disorder such as giant cell arteritis should be suspected in those who do not respond. When there is a question about the diagnosis a single-blind therapeutic trial can be performed during two two-week periods when the patient either takes prednisolone 10 mg/day or ascorbic acid. The response to treatment is assessed from symptomatic improvement and by change in the ESR.

After resolution of the symptoms and a fall in the ESR, the dose of prednisolone is gradually reduced by no more than 10% of the total every 2 weeks as gauged by the symptoms and ESR. This allows identification of the minimum supressive dose.

PROGNOSIS

PMR generally follows a self-limited course over several months to several years. Corticosteroids can be withdrawn within 5 years in the majority. However, a few patients develop clinical features of giant cell arteritis during the course of PMR and the clinician should remain alert to this possibility.

REFERENCES

Coomes E N, Ellis R M, Kay A G 1976 A prospective study of 102 patients with polymyalgia rheumatica syndrome. Rheumatology and Rehabilitation 15: 270–276

Ettlinger R E, Hunder G G, Ward E L 1978 Polymyalgia rheumatica and giant cell arteritis. Annual Review of Medicine 29: 15–22

Hunder G G, Hazelman B L 1981 Giant cell arteritis and polymyalgia rheumatica. In: Kelley W M, Harris E D, Ruddy S, Sledge C B (eds) Textbook of Rheumatology W B Saunders, Philadelphia, pp 1189–1196

13 Miscellaneous rheumatic disorders

I Behçet's Syndrome

Behçet's syndrome is a multi-system disorder of unknown aetiology which was originally described as a triple symptom complex: recurrent oral and genital ulceration and relapsing iritis (Behçet 1937). Besides this triad additional features including cutaneous vasculitis and meningoencephalitis are recognised as part of the syndrome. It is most commonly seen in Greece, Turkey, Cyprus, the Middle East and Japan and is uncommon in Europe and North America. The pattern of disease expression appears to vary somewhat in different parts of the world.

INCIDENCE

Behcet's syndrome shows a striking geographical distribution. In Japan the prevalence is 1/1000 and is a common cause of blindness, while it is uncommon in Britain. In most parts of the world men are affected twice as commonly as women, though in North America females are more commonly affected. The peak age of onset is in the third decade.

AETIOLOGY

The basic lesion is Behcet's syndrome is vasculitis and there is evidence that immune-complex disease plays an important part in the pathogenesis of this syndrome. Some investigators have reported the isolation of a virus from Behcet's, but evidence for a specific viral aetiology is unconvincing. Genetic factors related to the HLA complex have been associated with Behcet's and various clinical patterns of disease have been related to different histocompatability antigens: HLA-B5 with ocular disease; HLA-B27 with arthritis; HLA-B12 with mucocutaneous involvement. It is of interest that HLA-B12 is also associated with idiopathic recurrent oral ulceration. Not all investigators find these HLA associations, however.

PATHOLOGY

The histology of the mucosal ulcers is that of chronic inflammation and is identical to that of idiopathic aphthous ulcers. Necrotizing vasculitis can be found in vessels of the skin, vulva, retina and brain.

CLINICAL FEATURES

1. Presentation

The earliest presenting feature is oral and genital ulceration, usually accompanied by fever, malaise and arthralgia. These manifestations are followed within days or sometimes years by involvement of the eyes, skin, blood vessels and CNS. The two most important complications are uveitis and meningoencephalitis.

2. Involvement of individual organ systems

The common manifestations are summarised below.

Clinical features of Behçet's syndrome

1. Buccal ulceration (aphthous)
2. Genital ulcers
3. Skin lesions: pyoderma; erythema nodosum
4. Eye lesions: iritis (with hypopyon); episcleritis; conjunctivitis; keratitis; papilloedema and optic atrophy
5. Arthritis
6. Vascular disease: migrating superficial phlebitis; major vessel thrombosis; aneurysms; peripheral gangrene
7. CNS lesions: brain-stem syndrome; confusional states; meningomyelitis
8. Gastrointestinal lesions: colonic ulcers

a) Mucous membranes

Aphthous ulceration of the mouth is an early and almost constant feature. It occurs on the buccal mucosa, lips, tongue and pharynx. In full-blown cases ulcers extend from the lips to the fauces and are deep and painful. These deep ulcers sometimes heal with scarring.

Genital ulcers resemble oral aphthae and occur on the vulva and vagina of females, and on the scrotum and penis in males.

b) Eyes

A variety of ocular lesions occur, but iritis with pus in the anterior chamber (hypopyon) is highly characteristic. However, the major cause of blindness is posterior uveitis with involvement of the vitreous body and retina. Eye complications rarely occur as initial manifestations but usually several years after the onset of the disease.

c) Joints

Polyarthritis develops in about half the cases, predominantly affecting the knees, ankles, wrists and elbows. Permanent joint changes are rare, although radiological changes of sacro-iliitis have been reported.

d) Skin

A variety of skin lesions are seen including pustules, nodules and papules. Tender subcutaneous nodules may occur on the lower extremities clinically identical to erythema nodosum. A characteristic skin lesion is the development of a pustule at the site of skin puncture, such as a venesection site.

e) Blood vessels

Vascular complications include migratory superficial thrombophlebitis, deep venous and arterial thromboses, aneurysms and occlusion of major vessels producing features such as an aortic arch syndrome.

f) CNS

Involvement of the nervous system in some patients determines the prognosis and includes brain stem syndromes, organic confusional states, corticospinal tract signs, meningitis and myelitis.

g) Other features

These include colonic ulcers and occasionally pericarditis.

Laboratory findings

Laboratory findings are non-specific and include a raised ESR, mild to moderate anaemia and hyperglobulinaemia.

Circulating immune complexes are detected in over half the cases of active disease and sometimes cryoglobulins are found.

Synovial fluid shows an elevated white count (5–10 000) of which most are neutrophils. In CNS disease the CSF shows a moderate lymphocytosis.

Diagnosis

There are no pathognomonic pathological or

laboratory features of Behçet's syndrome and the diagnosis is entirely a clinical one. At present there are no standardised diagnostic criteria. One proposed set of criteria suggests the presence of at least three of the following six features: recurrent aphthous stomatitis; genital ulcers; uveitis; synovitis; cutaneous vascultis; meningo-encephalitis. Under this scheme the presence of recurrent aphthous stomatitis is mandatory.

Conditions commonly considered in the differential diagnosis are shown below. Since idiopathic aphthous stomatitis has been associated with HLA-B12, at least some cases may represent a forme fruste of Behçet's syndrome.

Differential diagnosis of Behçet's syndrome

1. Idiopathic aphthous ulceration
2. Reiter's syndrome
3. Disseminated sclerosis
4. Crohn's disease

The pattern of synovitis resembles that of spondyloarthropathies such as Reiter's syndrome.

REFERENCES (BEHCET's SYNDROME)

Chajek T, Fainaru M 1975 Behçet's disease. Report of 41 cases and a review of the literature. Medicine 54: 179–196

O'Duffy J D, Lehner T, Barnes C G 1983 Summary of the Third International Conference on Behçet's Disease. Journal of Rheumatology 10: 154–158

Wright V A, Chamberlain M A 1978–1979 Behçet's syndrome. Bulletin on the Rheumatic Diseases 972–977

II Relapsing Polychondritis

This uncommon systemic disorder, which may occur alone or complicate other connective tissue diseases, is characterised by recurrent inflammatory lesions involving cartilaginous structures, organs of special sense (eyes, ears, nose) and the cardiovascular system. The clinical and pathological features suggest a primary acquired disease affecting tissues rich in glycosaminoglycans (GAG) and proteoglycans. Polychondritis thus stands apart from other inflammatory joint diseases in appearing to result from a primary inflammatory response directed against cartilage.

PATHOLOGY AND AETIOLOGY

The earliest change in cartilage is patchy loss of GAG, resulting in diminished matrix basophilia, with perichondral small-cell infiltrates, progressing to chondrocyte degeneration and cartilage replacement by invading granulation tissue. Fibrosis, with or without calcification, and cystic spaces filled with gelatinous material represent end stage disease. A mild, non-specific inflammatory synovitis may accompany joint involvement.

Although the aetiology of polychondritis remains obscure, an immunological mechanism is suggested by its co-existence with other 'immunological' diseases and by the production of polychondritis-like disease in animal models following intra-articular or i.v. hyaline cartilage preparations and anti-proteoglycan sera. The trigger agent, however, remains unknown, and although antibodies to cartilage, proteoglycan aggregates, subunit and link protein fractions have been described they are not specific to patients with polychondritis and may merely represent secondary phenomena to cartilage damage.

CLINICAL FEATURES

The disease has been reported in all races but occurs predominantly in whites with equal sex incidence. Onset is at any age, most commonly 20–60. Chondritis, arthritis and ocular inflammation are the usual presenting features (Fig. 13.1).

Chondritis

Auricular inflammation is the most consistent feature (85%) presenting typically with sudden onset of pain and tenderness in one or both external pinnae. A diffuse violaceous or red swelling may be seen to overlie the cartilaginous (upper two-thirds) of the ear (Fig. 13.2), and inflammatory encroachment upon the external meatus may impair hearing and occasionally result in a clear,

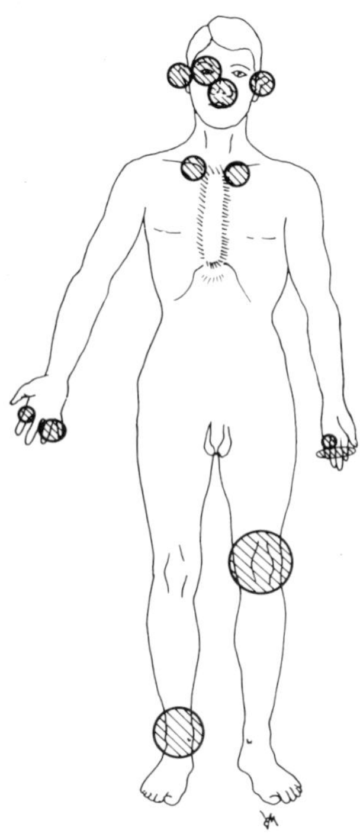

Fig. 13.1 Sites of involvement in polychondritis

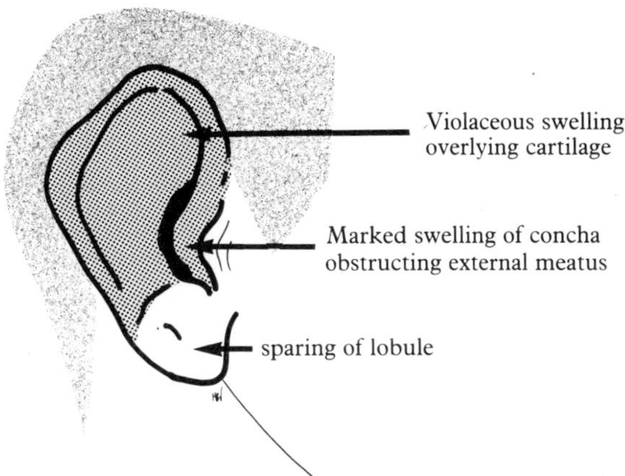

Fig. 13.2 Acute auricular chondritis

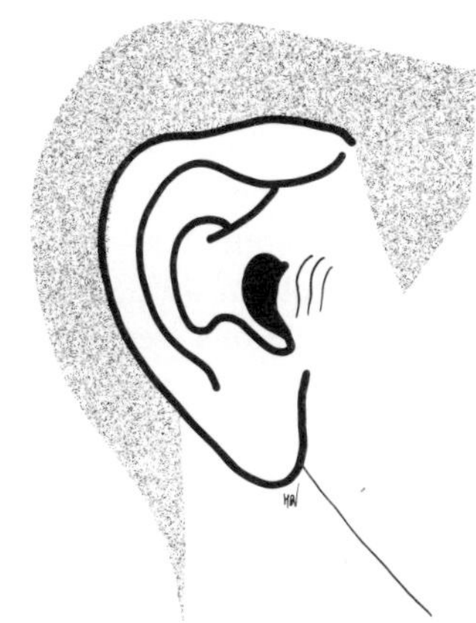

Fig. 13.3 Late result of auricular chondritis — 'floppy ear'

serous discharge. Attacks last several days or weeks before subsiding spontaneously. Severe or recurrent episodes may lead to weakening and loss of cartilage and a floppy, drooping ear (Fig. 13.3).

Nasal chondritis (70%) may also present acutely with pain and tenderness, nasal stuffiness, rhinorrhoea or epistaxis. Saddle-nose deformity may follow repeated attacks but occasionally develops in the absence of overt inflammation.

Hoarseness and tenderness over the thyroid cartilage and anterior trachea, accompanied by cough, dyspnoea or inspiratory stridor, signify laryngotracheal involvement and a poor prognosis. In severe cases oedema from glottic and laryngeal inflammation may necessitate tracheostomy, though concommitant collapse of tracheal and bronchial rings may cause difficulty in establishing adequate ventilation. Secondary infection and recurrent attacks may eventually lead to loss of structural support and death from asphyxiation.

Arthritis

Next to ear involvement this is the commonest presenting feature, eventually appearing in 80% of patients. Presentation is classically with episodic pain and swelling affecting a few joints in an otherwise fit adult. Small joints of hands, knees and ankles are most commonly involved in a symmetrical fashion (Fig. 13.1). Response to NSAIDs is good, and signs usually resolve spontaneously over several weeks, to reappear after variable intervals in other joints. Deformity and symmetrical polyarticular disease are uncommon but may particularly occur when polychondritis complicates other diseases.

Parasternal inflammation may accompany the peripheral arthritis and result in chest pain, xiphisternal tenderness and painful swelling and instability of costochondral, sternomanubrial and sternoclavicular joints. Destruction is rare but may cause a flail chest. There appears to be no temporal correlation between joint involvement and other features of the disease.

Eye inflammation

This eventually occurs in two-thirds of cases. Although all layers of the eye may be affected, presentation is most commonly with episcleritis, scleritis, conjunctivitis or iritis.

Other features

Fever, myalgia and non-specific cutaneous lesions are occasionally present. Inner and middle ear disease, characterised by auditory and/or vestibular dysfunction, is infrequent at the onset but subsequently appears in about 40%.

Cardiovascular complications develop in up to a quarter of established cases, particularly men, presenting most commonly with aortic incompetence secondary to dilatation of the valve ring and ascending aorta. Aneurysms involving any region of the aorta may also be present and occasionally rupture. Mitral and tricuspid incompetence, pericarditis and conduction defects are less common.

Other connective-tissue diseases, particularly RA, JCA, Sjögren's and SLE, may co-exist and usually antedate the onset of polychondritis by months or years. Although numbers of reported cases are small, there is also a suggested association with thyroid disease and malignancy.

INVESTIGATIONS

There are no specific laboratory tests. Raised viscosity, normocytic normochronic anaemia and modest leukocytosis reflect disease activity and eosinophilia is not uncommon.

X-rays of affected joints may show juxta-articular osteopenia and occasionally joint space narrowing in the absence of erosions. When another disease (e.g. RA) co-exists, severe destructive changes may occur, with characteristics of the accompanying disorder.

Tracheal tomograms and cine bronchography may be of use in demonstrating tracheo-bronchial narrowing. Cartilage calcification of the pinnae, nose, trachea or larynx is occasionally seen but is not specific.

Synovial fluid is generally 'non-inflammatory' with no specific features, and cartilage biopsy will reveal the changes already described.

DIAGNOSIS

Conspicuous inflammatory lesions involving cartilage of ears, nose and laryngobronchial system are distinctive, and the diagnosis of polychondritis is usually made clinically: biopsy of involved cartilage may be supportive. Diagnostic criteria proposed by McAdam (1976) are outlined opposite.

Joint, eye, nose and ear disease may also occur in PAN and Wegener's granulomatosis, though the presence of pulmonary and renal disease (and neurological disease in PAN) should allow differentiation. Co-existence of eye, joint and valve disease requires differentiation from RA, Behçet's sarcoid and seronegative spondarthritides: CNS and mucosal lesions of Behçet's and lung and skin changes of sarcoid, however, are not components of polychondritis, and sacro-iliitis and axial disease are rare. Patients with RA and scleritis are commonly strongly seropositive and demonstrate erosive, symmetrical disease which usually precedes ocular involvement by some years.

PROGNOSIS AND TREATMENT

The clinical course is variable but is usually characterised by episodic flares that result in progressive tissue damage. Prognosis is made difficult by reporting of only florid cases which not uncommonly proceed to death from respiratory tract or cardiovascular disease. It is likely, however, that in the majority of cases the outlook is less ominous.

Proposed diagnostic criteria for polychondritis
Definite Polychondritis = 3 or more of the listed clinical features

CLINICAL MANIFESTATIONS
1. Bilateral auricular chondritis
2. Nasal chondritis
3. Non-erosive, seronegative inflammatory polyarthritis
4. Ocular inflammation
5. Laryngeal and/or tracheal chondritis
6. Auditory and/or vestibular dysfunction

PLUS*
Cartilage biopsy confirmation of compatible histology from ear, nose or respiratory tract.

* If the diagnosis is clinically obvious biopsy confirmation is unnecessary

NSAIDs commonly control less serious manifestations but steroids may be required in acute inflammatory phases and are usually successful. In severe, uncontrolled disease, however, azathioprine, cyclophosphamide or other cytotoxic agents should be tried. There is no evidence that any of these agents modify the natural history of the condition.

Successful surgical treatment of aortic aneurysms and valve disease has been reported, as has airway reconstruction for severe tracheal disease. Treatment must be tailored to the individual, however, and careful and prolonged follow up is advised.

FURTHER READING (RELAPSING POLYCHONDRITIS)

McAdam L P, O'Hanlon M D, Bluestone R, Pearson C M 1976 Medicine 55: 193

III Tumours of Joints

Neoplastic disorders of joints are rare. This is surprising since the synovium is such an active vascular tissue. Benign tumours occur more frequently than malignant ones and secondary deposits are even rarer. The main neoplastic condition of joints are listed below.

Principle neoplastic condition of joints
Primary
1. Benign
   a) Pigmented villonodular synovitis
   b) Osteochondromatosis
   c) Giant-cell synovial tumour
   d) Xanthomata, haemangiomata, lipomata
2. Malignant
   Synovial sarcoma

Secondary
1. Carcinoma: colon, breast lung
2. Sarcoma: osteogenic
3. Myeloproliferative: leukaemia, lymphoma

PIGMENTED VILLONODULAR SYNOVITIS (PVNS)

PVNS is a rare tumour found mainly in the weight-bearing joints, usually the knee. Young adults are most often affected and some series show a male preponderance. It is usually thought of as a benign tumour but it is not entirely certain that the underlying process is truly neoplastic. The macroscopic appearance is striking: the synovial tissue is grossly hypertrophied and discoloured reddish brown; some of the villi develop long projections which tangle and knit together to form a shaggy carpet; other areas form nodules which are sessile or become pedunculated and hang down like grapes. Very rarely an areas of PVNS-like synovium has been reported in a bursa or tendon sheath not connected to a joint cavity. The pathological tissue may be confined to one area or spread diffusely throughout the joint. Occasionally there is infiltration into adjacent bone and soft tissue. Microscopically, there is a surface covering of synovial lining cells. The connective tissue stroma contains numerous thin-walled blood-vessels and a varible population of polyhydral cells, cholesterol-containing foam cells and multinucleated giant cells. Brown haemosiderin granules are prominent in cells and impart the characteristic colour. Occasionally areas of exuberant growth will contain many mitoses, suggestive of a malignant lesion, but metastases have not been described.

PVNS causes pain, swelling and effusion in the affected joint, usually the knee, but symptoms may be mild and intermittent so that diagnosis is typically delayed for several years. Background ache, stiffness and swelling is often punctuated by sudden episodes of locking and acute severe pain due to crushing of a frond of hypertrophied synovium between the articulating surfaces. Such episodes are followed by a period of increased pain and swelling. The effusion is nearly always blood-stained and persistent aspiration of a sero-sanguinous synovial fluid is often the main clue to the correct diagnosis.

Plain X-ray will usually reveal an effusion and area of soft-tissue swelling and occasionally there is also pressure osteoporosis and erosion of adjacent bone. Arthrography will outline the extent of the growth but the diagnosis should be confirmed by biopsy, if possible done under arthroscopic control, particularly to exclude synovial sarcoma.

The course of PVNS is slow and variable but usually progressive. A radical synovectomy is advisable, since there is a high risk of recurrence if any abnormal tissue is left behind. Occasionally, persistent recurrent cases are treated with radiotherapy or intra-articular radioisotopes.

GIANT-CELL SYNOVIAL TUMOUR

This is thought to represent a local form of PVNS and may arise in the joint or in tendon sheaths. The knee is the most commonly affected joint. There is one large sessile or pedunculated mass, often arising from the junction of the capsule and meniscus. Locking of the knee is the single most common complaint but occasionally the mass may become trapped, producing acute pain and swelling. Treatment is by excision after the nature of the mass is confirmed histologically. Tendon-sheath giant-cell tumours occur commonly on the flexor surface of the hands of middle-aged women. They are non-tender swellings which gradually increase in size, stretching the skin and interfering with function. Pressure on the neighbouring bone may give the radiographic appearance of scalloping and waisting of the bone. Excision is usually curative.

OSTEOCHONDROMATOSIS

In this condition, foci of cartilage develop in the synovial membrane of a joint, usually the knee, but occasionally another large joint such as the hip or elbow. Pieces of cartilage may become detached and enter the joint cavity forming loose bodies. Since there is metaplasia of the connective tissue under the synovial cells this disorder is classified as neoplastic. The cause is unknown.

Osteochondromatosis is usually diagnosed in the middle-aged and elderly and men are more commonly affected than women. There is often a long history of intermittent monoarticular joint pain accompanied to varying degrees by swelling, locking and grating. Joint movement may be restricted and the cartilage bodies can sometimes be palpated, particularly in the suprapatella pouch.

Since the cartilage is usually either calcified or ossified, X-ray examination is most helpful and typically shows fuzzy radio-opacities in the soft tissues. If ossified, they may have the radiographic appearance of trabecular bone. Very rarely, the bodies contain no calcium and so are not visible on X-ray but they can be seen on arthroscopy.

Treatment consists of clearing the joint of the loose bodies and removing the synovium, if this abnormal, to prevent them forming again.

SYNOVIAL SARCOMA (SYNOVIOMA)

This is a rare tumour of young adults which is believed to arise from synovial tissue near to but not actually in the joint space. It is virtually confined to the extremities and 70% are found in large lower-limb joints. It presents as a mass which is often painless and slow-growing. Those near the surface present earlier than those situated more deeply within a joint.

A synovial sarcoma appears a well-demarcated pink/yellow fleshy mass of tissue often adhering to the joint capsule. It may feel gritty in parts because of the presence of calcium. The histological appearance is variable, with a mixture of spindle and polygonal cells. It does not usually invade locally but metastasises readily and the prognosis is grim. The overall mortality rate is 90% and mean survival, from presentation to death, about 7 years. Because the tumour is slow-growing and symptoms mild there is often a long delay from onset to diagnosis, by which time spread to lung, lymph node, chest wall, bone and brain has often occurred. For this reason patients presenting with a joint soft-tissue mass need prompt attention. Speckled calcification is frequently seen on X-ray and is a useful clue, but the diagnosis must be confirmed by a biopsy before proceeding to surgery. The main differential diagnosis is PVNS. Local excision of the tumour is a disaster since it encourages metastasis and recurrence is inevitable. The only hope of effecting a cure is radical amputation at a level far away from the tumour.

SECONDARY MALIGNANCY

Synovium is a highly vascular tissue and yet secondary carcinoma appears to be rare. This is either because joints are not often examined at necropsy or because they are protected from metastases. There have been reports of secondaries occurring with lung, colon and breast primaries. Leukaemia, particularly in children, is important as a cause of joint pain, often from bleeding due to low platelets but also due to true synovitis from leukaemic infiltration. Bone tumours arising near joints may be locally invasive and spread to the synovium.

FURTHER READING

Schajowicz D 1981 Tumours and tumour-like lesions of bone and joints. Springer, Berlin

IV Epiphyseal Dysplasias

Epiphyseal dysplasias are a subgroup of genetically-determined bone dysplasias which affect the development of the osseous skeleton. In this subgroup the abnormal bone growth involves the epiphyses of the vertebrae, wrist, tarsus and long bones, and sometimes the neighbouring metaphyseal region. Like other forms of bone dysplasia, these conditions are very rare and exist in many clinical forms with variable genetic transmission, and are classified on the basis of clinical and radiological findings. They resemble mucopolysaccharidoses in their skeletal manifestation but can be distinguished from mucopolysaccharidoses by the lack of both visceral involvement and well-defined biochemical abnormalities. Depending on the severity of the dysplasia, affected individuals present in infancy or childhood with dwarfism or abnormal gait, or in the third decade with precocious osteoarthritis affecting the hips.

CLINICAL TYPES

Epiphyseal dysplasia can broadly be divided into two groups: multiple epiphyseal dysplasia and spondylo-epiphyseal dysplasia, the latter being characterised by predominant involvement of the vertebrae.

1. Multiple epiphyseal dysplasia

Multiple epiphyseal dysplasia is a rare disorder inherited as an autosomal dominant.

The patient presents as a child, usually between the ages of 5 and 10 years, with joint pain and limited joint movement especially affecting the hips knees and shoulders, resulting in a waddling gait and difficulty climbing stairs or running. Alternatively, the patient presents as a young adult in his 20s or 30s with premature osteoarthritis of the hips and, to a lesser extent, of the other joints. Several clinical variants are seen:

a) Involving mainly the elbow and knee
b) Involving metaphyseal development as well as epiphyses resulting in dwarfing, though this is not usually severe

c) Involving the shoulders and hips together with vertebral abnormalities resembling pronounced Schmorl's nodes.

Radiological findings

Radiological findings in the child are characteristic and consist of bilateral, symmetrical irregularity and under-development of the epiphyseal ossification centres, predominantly in the hips (Fig. 13.4), knees, hands (Fig. 13.5) and ankles. In the adult the appearance is of osteoarthritis.

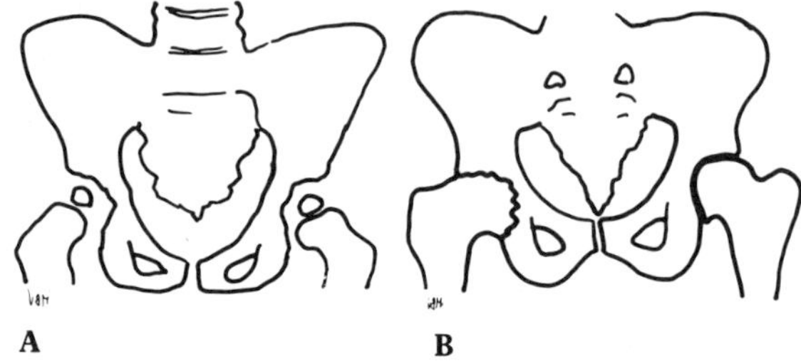

Fig. 13.4 Multiple epiphyseal dysplasia. **A.** Child, showing small femoral capital epiphyses and irregularities of the acetabulum. **B.** Adult, showing advanced degenerative changes.

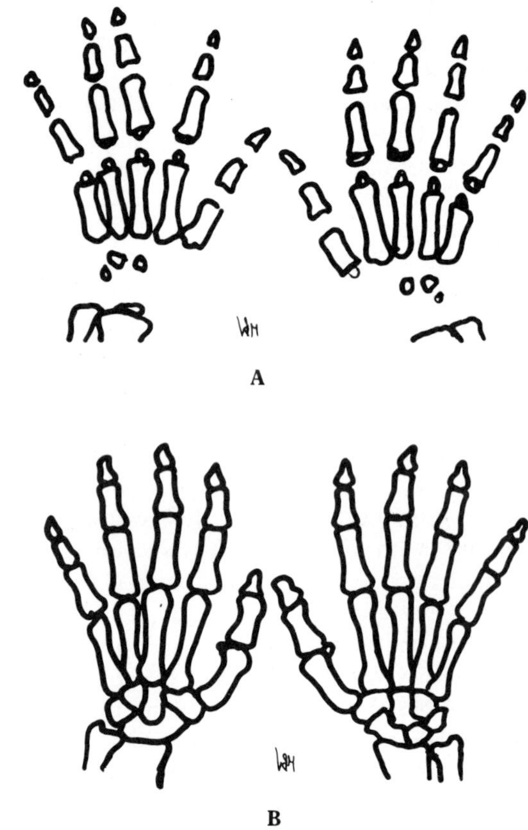

Fig. 13.5 Multiple epiphyseal dysplasia. **A.** Child, showing dysplastic epiphyses and delayed development of carpal bones. **B.** Adult, showing degenerative changes with joint-space narrowing.

2. Spondylo-epiphyseal dysplasia

Spondylo-epiphyseal dysplasias comprise two forms:

a) Congenital

This is transmitted as an autosomal dominant or recessive trait. The vertebrae are predominantly affected, but there may be peripheral joint involvement. This is located particularly in the hips and shoulders, but can be more extensive, and in some families there are metaphyseal abnormalities. Affected individuals present in childhood with growth defects, musculoskeletal pain and difficulty in standing and walking.

b) Spondylo-epiphyseal dysplasia tarda

This form is transmitted as an X-linked recessive and is seen in males who present in their teens or early adulthood with pain, stiffness and limited movement in their spine and hips. Involvement of other peripheral joints is uncommon.

Radiological findings

The vertebrae in pre-pubertal children show a distinctive anterior tongue due to delayed development of the annular cartilage (the ring epiphyses) (Fig. 13.6a). Subsequently there is flattening of the vertebrae with irregularity of the superior and inferior vertebral plates and a characteristic humping up of the middle and posterior portion of the vertebral body, leaving a fish-mouth-shaped area anteriorly on lateral views (Fig. 13.6b).

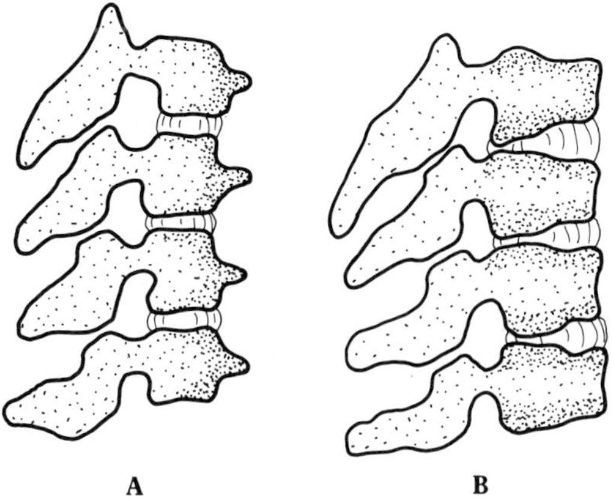

Fig. 13.6 Spondylo-epiphyseal dysplasia. **A**. Child, showing anterior tongue due to belated development of ring epiphyses. **B**. Adult, showing platyspondyly, irregularity of end plates and heaping-up of middle and posterior portions of vertebral bodies.

DIAGNOSIS

Classically these conditions present with precocious osteoarthritis of the hips. Features that point to the diagnosis of epiphyseal dysplasia include short stature, characteristic radiological abnormalities and a positive family history. Depending on the age of presentation it must be distinguished from conditions such as those listed below.

Differential diagnosis of epiphyseal dysplasia
1. Mucopolysaccharidoses
2. Achondroplastic dwarfism
3. Osteochondritis
4. Ankylosing spondylitis
5. Polyarthritis
6. Ochronosis

TREATMENT

There is no definitive treatment for these conditions and therapy consists of physiotherapy to improve posture and mobility, symptomatic treatment of pain, and arthroplasty for those with severe osteoarthritis of the hips.

FURTHER READING (EPIPHYSEAL DYSPLASIAS)

Kahn M F, de Seze S 1975 Rheumatic manifestations of heritable disorders of connective tissue. Clinics in Rheumatic Diseases 1(1): 3–36
McKusick V A 1972 Heritable disorders of connective tissue, 4th edn. C V Mosby, St Louis

V Neuropathic (Charcot) Joints

INTRODUCTION

The term 'Charcot joint' was originally used to describe an arthropathy occuring in the lower limbs of patients with tabes dorsalis. It is applied more widely now to describe any joint in which an exaggerated form of osteoarthritis is associated with loss of pain and/or position sense, although similar clinical and radiological features can be found in a joint even when denervation is not clinically apparent. The mechanism of destruction in neuropathic joints is not clearly understood. One theory is that impaired innervation causes mild functional instability which results in repeated minor trauma to the joint. Alternatively, as Charcot himself believed, the nerves may supply a trophic factor which is required to maintain the integrity of a joint. Pyrophosphate deposition occurs frequently in neuropathic joints and may lead to further alteration in the physical properties of the cartilage and accelerate destruction.

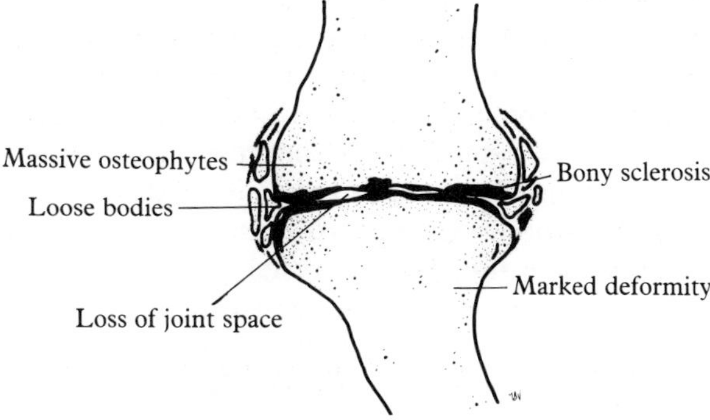

Fig. 13.7 Radiological features of a Charcot joint

Tabes dorsalis is very rare nowadays but other conditions are associated with the development of Charcot joints.

Conditions predisposing to neuropathic joints

1. Tabes dorsalis (knees, ankles, feet, spine)
2. Diabetic polyneuropathy (feet, ankle, spine)
3. Alcoholic neuropathy
4. Syringomyelia (wrist, elbow)
5. Marie–Charcot–Tooth (ankle, knee)
6. Leprosy
7. Congenital insensitivity to pain
8. Other spinal cord and peripheral nerve lesions

CLINICAL FEATURES

Patients usually present with a chronic monoarthritis or dislocation, the joint being determined by the site of greatest sensory loss, characteristically the elbow and wrist in syringomyelia, the knee in tabes dorsalis and the foot in diabetes. The highest frequency occurs in syringomyelia and leprosy where 20–30% of patients will develop neuropathic joints, and the figures for tabes dorsalis is 4–10%, and for diabetes 0.2%. The most striking clinical feature is that the signs are disproportionately greater than the symptoms would suggest. The joint is swollen and often dislocated with an effusion, crepitus, instability and often marked deformity. It may eventually become flail and the affected limb may consequently become shortened. Spinal involvement may result in spinal cord compression. Although there is usually surprisingly little discomfort, occasional bouts of pain do occur as a result of bleeding into the joint, a crystal-related synovitis or trapping of a loose body between the articular surfaces. The course is usually one of chronic and progressive joint destruction which is punctuated by episodes of acute inflammation.

The joint fluid is usually grossly abnormal and is best described as 'filthy'. It may be cloudy, bloodstained and contain a large amount of debris and crystals of both pyrophosphate and hydroxyapatite may be detected by the appropriate techniques.

The radiological features can be summarised as gross destruction associated with profuse new-bone formation and remodelling.

Radiological features of Charcot joints

1. Joint space narrowing
2. Bony sclerosis
3. Profuse new bone formation
4. Loose bodies
5. Periarticular calcification
6. Subluxation and dislocation
7. Fractures
8. Gross deformity

Useful investigations for diagnosing the underlying cause of neuropathic joints include WR, glucose tolerance test, myelogram for syringomyelia and nerve-conduction studies and nerve biopsy for the other neuropathies.

MANAGEMENT

The underlying pathology of neuropathic joints is usually irreversible and treatment is largely symptomatic. During acute flares the joint should be rested and aspiration of a large effusion may shorten the duration and reduce the severity. Diabetic should have their blood sugar level tightly controlled and the foot symptoms may be helped by moulded footwear. Unstable joints should be splinted to aid control of a limb and reduce trauma. Surgical removal of large foreign bodies is occasionally indicated and arthrodesis will relieve severe pain and gross instability.

FURTHER READING (CHARCOT JOINTS)

Bruckner F E, Howell A 1972. Neuropathic joints. Seminars on Arthritis and Rheumatism 2: 47

VI Reflex Sympathetic Dystrophy Syndrome

This uncommon disorder of regional periarticular soft tissue is known by a variety of names. It is characterised by pain, swelling, vasomotor disturbances and trophic skin changes, usually involving a whole hand or foot. About 50% of cases are idiopathic, and in 50% there is a clear preceding cause. These causes include trauma, neurological damage (especially root or peripheral-nerve lesions) and ischaemic heart disease. There is an equal sex incidence, and the syndrome can occur in all ages.

Reflex sympathetic dystrophy syndrome – alternative terminology

1. Sudeck's atrophy
2. Causalgia
3. Shoulder–hand syndrome
4. Algodystrophy
5. Regional migratory osteoporosis
6. (and many others)

The main clinical features of reflex sympathetic dystrophy syndrome

At onset

1. Severe pain
2. Generalised bone, joint and periarticular tenderness
3. Oedema
4. Vasomotor disturbance
5. Involvement of a region (usually a hand or foot)

Late stage

1. Atrophic skin and subcutaneous tissue
2. Flexion contractures

CLINICAL FEATURES

The clinical course of the disorder can be divided into three overlapping stages; the acute, dystrophic and atrophic phases. The *acute phase* is characterised by pain, tenderness, swelling and vasomotor changes in the affected area, developing slowly within weeks of any preceeding injury. Severe burning pain is the main symptom, and this, combined with extreme tenderness throughout the whole area, prevents normal use. If the foot is involved, weight-bearing is usually impossible and affected hands are functionally useless. Hand disease is often combined with stiffness of the ipsilateral shoulder (shoulder–hand syndrome). Generalised oedema and vasomotor changes causing coldness (less commonly a hot, flushed limb) are also present. After some weeks or months the pain and swelling subside and trophic changes appear in the skin, with flaking and atrophy (the *dystrophic stage*). After a further period of 3–6 months subcutaneous atrophy and flexion contractures may develop (the *atrophic stage*). The course is very variable, and early treatment may prevent subsequent atrophy.

INVESTIGATIONS

There are no biochemical or haematological abnormalities, and no evidence of systemic inflammation. However, plain radiographs and bone scans usually show characteristic changes aiding diagnosis. Within the first few weeks patchy osteoporosis develops throughout the affected region; this is associated with increased uptake of bone-seeking isotopes such as technetium-labelled diphosphonates. The radiographic changes slowly resolve over a period of months as the condition improves.

TREATMENT

The syndrome is rare and very variable, making the assessment of treatment difficult. It is generally agreed that early mobilisation during the acute phase is essential. A course of steroids (often given as ACTH) often helps, and sympathetic blockade relieves pain and swelling in some cases. Many other therapeutic manoeuvres have been attempted, with relatively little success.

Occasional cases recur, with different sites of involvement, after intervals of months or years (regional migratory osteoporosis). In these and other forms of the syndrome, the pathogenesis remains obscure. Most authors favour a primary aetiological role of autonomic nerve disturbance, hence the name, but the intense, active changes in bone remain unexplained.

FURTHER READING

P Doury, Y Dirheimer S Paltin 1981 Algodystrophy. Springer, Berlin

SECTION THREE

Rheumatology and general medicine

14 Rheumatology and general medicine: introduction

Rheumatology has been defined as that branch of medicine which deals primarily with disorders of the musculoskeletal system, including all diseases of the joints and periarticular tissues. The division of medicine into specialities according to different systems is obviously useful but it is also artificial, as all of the different systems interact and many diseases have no respect for a single specialist interest.

Any attempt to subdivide the rheumatic disorders further according to their effects on different organs of the body has obvious problems, especially when so many of the diseases are of unknown aetiology and pathogenesis. There are, however, obvious differences between conditions like osteoarthritis, which mainly affect the synovial joints and periarticular tissue, and a disease such as haemophilia where a known defect in another system can cause major damage to the synovial joints. Between these extremes lie many of the idiopathic rheumatic diseases like rheumatoid arthritis — a multi-system disease in which the musculoskeletal system is most severely affected. Therefore three broad divisions of rheumatic disorder can be recognised.

Categories of rheumatic disease

1. Disorders which mainly affect the joints and periarticular tissues, e.g.
   a) Osteoarthritis
   b) Pigmented villonodular synovitis
2. Multisystem diseases of unknown aetiology which affect the musculoskeletal system, e.g.
   a) Rheumatoid arthritis
   b) Systemic lupus erythematosus
      (Most of the major rheumatic diseases)
3. Disorders of other systems which can affect the joints, e.g.
   a) Haemophilia
   b) Acromegaly

RHEUMATIC DISEASE AFFECTING OTHER SYSTEMS

In Chapter 15 the effects of rheumatic diseases on other systems in the body is considered. Disorders which mainly affect the joints occasionally present with symptoms or signs referrable to another system — ulnar nerve compression secondary to osteoarthritis of the elbow, for example — and most of the major rheumatic diseases are multisystem disorders which frequently affect organs other than the musculoskeletal system. Clinical problems often develop from these extra-articular features and knowledge of what may or may not be related to the presence of a known rheumatic disease is therefore vital.

SYSTEMIC DISEASES AFFECTING THE MUSCULOSKELETAL SYSTEM

Chapter 16 covers a number of diseases which primarily affect other organs or systems in the body, but which may also result in musculoskeletal disorders. Many systemic diseases can present with joint pains or other rheumatic signs and symptoms, and patients with neoplasia, endocrine disease, blood dyscrasias and other conditions may be seen first by a rheumatologist. Knowledge of the pattern and type of joint disease which may arise from these diseases is therefore necessary.

INTERACTION BETWEEN RHEUMATIC AND OTHER DISEASES

Synovial joints are complex organs composed of many different cellular, chemical and functional elements (Chapter 1). Any condition which generally affects bone, muscles or any of the fibres and cells of connective tissue is therefore likely to affect the joints. The special vascular pattern in synovial tissue may also make joints peculiarly susceptible to systemic disease. The functional aspects of joints include their role in the reticulo-endothelial system, and large fluxes of cells, proteins and other particles and chemicals pass through synovial tissue. This may explain in part the effects which joint disease can have on other systems and vice versa. Many investigators of systemic disease are looking to the joints for answers to pathogenesis, and in many rheumatic diseases the changes seen in organs such as the kidney, eye or skin is providing clues to further understanding.

RHEUMATOLOGY IN MEDICINE

It has been estimated that about 20% of general-practice consultations in the UK concern rheumatic complaints. One recent survey suggested that rheumatic disorders were also a major feature in patients admitted to hospital with acute medical emergencies. Patients under the care of rheumatologists often have problems in other systems. In our own practice, for example, about 30% of out-patients and about 75% of in-patients have significant medical problems outside the musculoskeletal system, and in many cases these problems are directly related to a primary rheumatic disease. General medicine is therefore an integral part of rheumatology and vice versa.

15 Other systems involved in joint disease

I The Skin and Mucous Membranes

Certain lesions of the skin and appendages are so typical that their identification helps to establish the diagnosis of certain rheumatic diseases (Fig. 15.1). Examination of the skin, hair, nails and mucous membranes should therefore be as careful as that of the joints. Aids to examination include adequate illumination, a magnifying glass and a microscope slide to press the skin in order to distinguish the blanching of erythema from a purpuric lesion. Microscopy of nail scrapings treated with potassium hydroxide will differentiate fungal infection from other nail disorders and biopsy of lesions elsewhere, such as nodules, may also be required to establish the diagnosis.

Skin rashes characteristic of certain rheumatic diseases (Table 15.1)

1. Psoriasis

Psoriatic arthritis develops in 7% of those with psoriasis (p 86). Classical psoriasis appears as demarcated raised erythematous plaques covered with layers of scales. Plaques occur anywhere, but especially over the elbows, knees, lumbosacral area and scalp. Extent of involvement is variable, and sometimes it is limited to a small patch in the umbilicus or gluteal cleft.

2. Keratoderma blennorrhagica

Keratoderma blennorrhagica is the characteristic skin lesion of Reiter's syndrome. It begins as a vesicle with an erythematous base and develops into a sterile pustule. Subsequently it evolves into a keratotic lesion mainly on plantar surfaces, especially the soles, toes and fingers. Less commonly it occurs on other sites such as the scalp and umbilicus. These lesions are very similar to pustular psoriasis both clinically and histologically.

Table 15.1 Skin rashes characteristic of certain rheumatic diseases

Skin lesion	Rheumatic diseases
Psoriasis	Psoriatic arthritis
Keratoderma blenorrhagica	Reiter's disease
Discoid lupus erythematosus	DLE/SLE
Butterfly rash	SLE/dermatomyositis
Heliotrope	Dermatomyositis
Palpable purpura	Vasculitis
Livedo reticularis	Vasculitis
Evanescent erythematous macular rash	Still's disease
Erythema marginatum	Rheumatic fever
Pustules at sites of trauma (venesection sites)	Behçet's disease

3. Discoid lupus erythematosus

The discoid lupus lesion starts as a circumscribed indurated erythematous plaque which develops a central area of hyperkeratosis, follicular plugging and atrophy. Plaques generally occur on the face, behind the ears and on the scalp, but may be widespread. The histology is very characteristic and shows epidermal atrophy, liquefaction-degeneration of the epidermal basal layer and a patchy

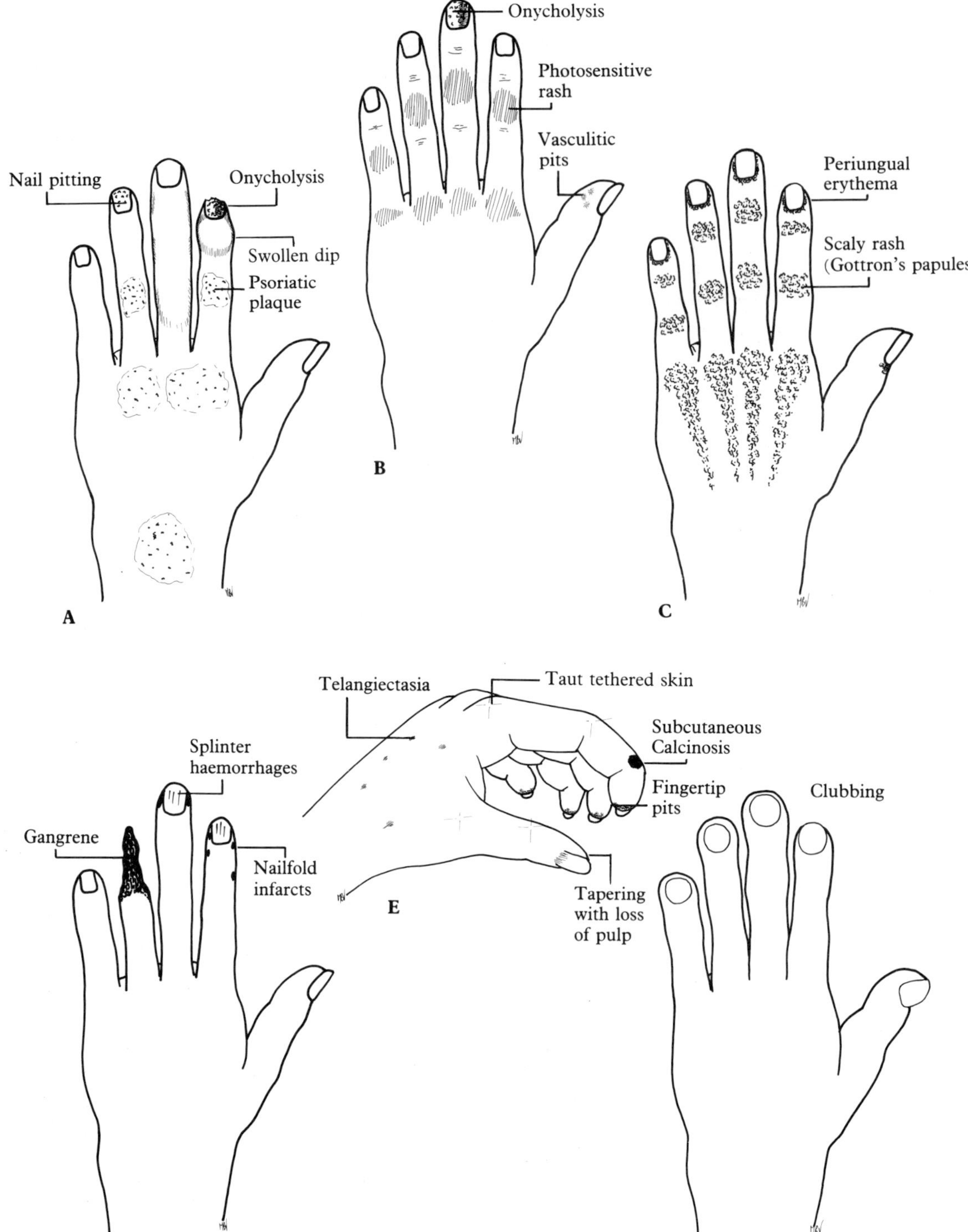

Fig. 15.1 Hands showing skin and nail changes in certain rheumatic diseases. **A**. Psoriasis. **B**. SLE. **C**. Dermatomyositis. **D**. Vasculitis. **E**. Scleroderma. **F**. HPOA.

lymphocytic infiltrate. Granular deposits of immunoglobin and complement are seen along the dermo–epidermal junction when the biopsy is examined by immunofluorescence. These lesions occur in 10% of patients with SLE, but may also represent the only manifestation of the disease which is then termed discoid lupus erythematosus (DLE).

4. *Butterfly rash*

An erythematous butterfly rash affecting the malar region and the bridge of the nose is a well known feature of SLE occurring in 30% of patients, usually during an exacerbation. It may be photosensitive, when it is often accompanied by a maculo-papular eruption in light-exposed areas, including the dorsal surface of the fingers between the joints.

A similar butterfly rash, which may also exhibit photosensitivity is seen in dermatomyositis. In this disease, however, skin lesions tend to involve extensor surfaces, with the formation of atrophic scaly plaques (Gottron's sign) over the extensor surface of the knuckles.

A different butterfly rash is produced by acne rosacea and is characterised by a marked pustular inflammatory component and seborrhoeic dermatitis, which produces a dry or greasy lesion, often with glabellar and nasolabial accentuation.

5. *The heliotrope*

The heliotrope rash is the most characteristic cutaneous feature of dermatomyositis. It consists of purple-red colouration of the upper eyelid which is often associated with periorbital oedema.

6. *Cutaneous manifestations of vasculitis*

The clinical picture of vasculitis is described in Chapter 7.V. When the skin is involved the manifestations depend on the depth and calibre of the affected vessel. They include small nailfold or digital infarcts, nodules, pustules, vesicles and ulcers. Two characteristic manifestations are:

a) Palpable purpura is the result of vasculitis affecting small cutaneous vessels, especially the post capillary venule, leading to endothelial swelling, infiltration by leukocytes and extravasation of erythrocytes. This occurs predominantly on the lower extremities and over dependent parts and can be distinguished from thrombocytopaenic purpura, and purpura due to increased capillary fragility due to corticosteroid therapy.
b) Livedo reticularis is a reticular blotchy pattern of dusky erythema which occurs especially on the trunk and lower extremities and is due to alteration in the cutaneous blood supply.

7. *The rash of Still's disease*

A characteristic erythematous rash accompanies Still's disease consisting of salmon or erythematous macules on the limbs, trunk and face. Large lesions have a central pallor. The rash is evanescent and appears at the height of fever usually in the afternoon or evening and disappears by morning.

8. *Erythema marginatum*

Erythema marginatum is an uncommon but specific lesion of active rheumatic fever. It occurs as erythematous rings on the trunk and extremities and the hallmark is rapid progression and resolution.

9. *The rash of Behçet's syndrome*

Pustules occurring at the site of trauma, characteristically at a venepuncture site, is reported to be a characteristic feature of Behcet's syndrome. In practice, it is an uncommon manifestation of a rare disease.

In addition to these typical lesions, a host of non-specific rashes can be seen often as a result of a drug reaction. These include exanthema, urticaria, lichenoid and pityriasis rosea-like eruptions, and occasionally exfoliative dermatitis.

Sclerosis of the skin

Causes of tightness, induration and tethering of the skin are shown overleaf. Scleroderma is the

Mucocutaneous reactions to drugs used in arthritis

Erythematous rash
- Non-steroidal anti-inflammatory agents (NSAID)
- Gold
- Penicillamine
- Anti-malarials
- Allopurinol

Exfoliative dermatitis
- Gold
- Anti-malarials (especially in psoriasis)

Lichenoid eruptions
- Gold
- Anti-malarials

Pityriasis rosea-like eruption
- Gold

Purpura
- Corticosteroids
- Gold
- Penicillamine
- Immunosuppressive drugs

Urticaria
- NSAID
- Allopurinol

Skin pigmentation
- Gold
- Anti-malarials

Stomatitis
- Gold
- Penicillamine
- Immunosuppressive drugs
- NSAID

commonest cause. It may be a manifestation of systemic sclerosis or a form of scleroderma localised to the skin such as morphea or linear localised scleroderma. These conditions are discussed in Chapter 7.III.

In systemic sclerosis skin involvement may be generalised, when it is often associated with severe internal organ involvement and a poor prognosis, or restricted to the acral regions (hands, feet and face). An early sign of skin involvement is indolent non-pitting oedema.

Plaques of morphea are usually single or few in

Sclerosis of the skin

Scleroderma
1. Localized
   (a) Morphea
   (b) Linear localized scleroderma
2. Systemic sclerosis

Scleroderma variants
1. Eosinophilic fasciitis
2. Polyvinyl chloride disease

Sclerodactyly associated with SLE, RA and polymyositis
Cheiroarthropathy
Scleroedema
Phenylketonuria
Carcinoid syndrome
Porphyra cutania tarda
Cutaneous amyloidosis
Werner's syndrome
Progeria

number. Occasionally they are multiple. The lesion consists of a circumscribed area which is often elevated and indurated with an atrophic, ivory-coloured centre and a mauve-coloured periphery. Linear localised scleroderma has a band-like distribution with involvement of underlying tissues, including muscle and bone, and often affects the lower extremity. Extreme cases occurring in childhood can lead to hemiatrophy.

Rarer causes of sclerotic changes include cheiroarthropathy. This term describes limited joint mobility in the hands associated with thick, waxy skin which has been reported in up to one-quarter of adolescent diabetics. Its presence has been associated with the presence of microvascular complication of diabetes. (p 302)

Pigmentary changes

Causes of hyperpigmentation are shown opposite. Hyperpigmentation or hypopigmentation frequently develops at sites of inflammatory skin lesions in SLE.

Striking hyperpigmentation may occur in scleroderma. This usually accompanies sclerosis but may precede it, and occurs especially over the

Causes of hyperpigmentation
Systemic lupus erythematosus
Scleroderma
Dermatomyositis
Felty's syndrome
Haemochromatosis
Ochronosis
Drugs — e.g. Gold
Chloroquine

extremities and anterior chest. It may be as intense as in Addison's disease but there is no mucous membrane pigmentation. Often the appearance is stippled with hypo- and hyperpigmentation.

Poikiloderma refers to a cutaneous response to inflammation leading to patches of reticular hyperpigmentation associated with skin atrophy and telangiectasia which is particularly characteristic of dermatomyositis.

Brown pigmentation over the exposed surfaces especially the tibia, develops in some patients with Felty's syndrome.

The majority of patients with haemochromatosis develop bronzing of the skin, especially over exposed parts due to excessive quantities of melanin. In a proportion of these, haemosiderin is also present giving the skin a slate-grey appearance.

Patients with alkaptonuria develop skin pigmentation which results from deposition of the brown-black homogentisic acid polymer in the cartilage and dermis. It is most marked in the ear, end of the nose and costochondral junction, where the colour is transmitted from underlying cartilage. The skin is pigmented to a lesser extent over the malar areas, nose, axilla and groin.

On rare occasions hyperpigmentation occurs with the use of drugs such as gold and chloroquine.

Non-tender nodules

Subcutaneous nodules arising from changes in the connective tissues such as in RA, from deposition of uric acid, from metastatic calcification in systemic sclerosis and polymyositis, or from xanthomas in hyperlipidaemic states, tend to occur over areas subject to pressure and trauma, especially the elbow, back of the forearm, lumbosacral region and around joints.

Some of the causes of non-tender nodules
1. Nodules over pressure points
   Common
      Rheumatoid arthritis
      Chronic gout
   Uncommon
      Xanthomas
      Calcinosis
      SLE
      Rheumatic fever
      Juvenile chronic arthritis
2. Others
      Amyloidosis
      Multicentric reticulohistiocytosis

Tender nodules

Causes of tender nodules are shown below.

Erythema nodosum consists of painful red nodules usually over the shin but may be more

Causes of tender nodules
Erythema nodosum
Streptococcal infections
Drug reactions — e.g. Sulphonamides
Oral contraceptives
Sarcoidosis
Chronic inflammatory bowel disease
Tuberculosis
SLE
Acute rheumatic fever
Behçet's syndrome
Leprosy
Lymphoreticular malignancy

Panniculitis
Weber–Christian disease
Lupus profundus

Sweet's syndrome

widespread occurring most often in young women. They are often accompanied by mild constitutional symptoms, arthralgias and occasionally painful arthritis of the ankles and knees. It represents a hypersensitivity reaction to a number of systemic antigens, though often no underlying cause is found. A chest X-ray should be performed to exclude sarcoidosis or TB

A biopsy of a nodule shows acute inflammation with a lymphocytic infiltrate around the septal veins of the subdermal fat, and sometimes when sarcoidosis is the cause, a sarcoid granuloma.

Weber–Christian disease is a clinical syndrome which occurs predominantly is young or middle-aged women characterised by crops of tender nodules. These occur mainly on the thigh, trunk and on the breasts and are due to inflammation of the subcutaneous fat. Their appearance is accompanied by mild constitutional symptoms including arthralgias.

Panniculitis is also a rare complication of SLE causing tender nodules on the face, buttocks and upper arms. This manifestation is termed 'lupus profundus' and resolves leaving a depressed scar.

Sweet's syndrome is a rare condition often following a 'flu-like illness which is characterized by raised painful skin lesions accompanied by fever, leukocytosis and often an acute arthritis of peripheral joints. Biopsy of the skin lesion shows a dense infiltration of neutrophils.

Nail changes

Nail changes seen in rheumatic disease are listed below. In psoriasis the arthritis is more closely related to nail changes than to the skin lesions. Often the severity of nail involvement parallels the severity of the arthritis, and there may be a topographical relationship between nail changes and distal interphalangeal joint involvement.

Nail lesions have recently been recognised in SLE and include pitting and onycholysis (separation of the nail from the underlying nail-bed).

Periungual erythema is a striking feature in cases of poly- and dermatomyositis and in some patients with SLE.

Characteristic alterations in the morphology of nailfold capillaries are seen in systemic sclerosis and polymyositis. In these diseases, large dilated capillary loops can be seen with microscopy often adjacent to the areas of absent nailfold capillaries (p 261).

Nail changes in rheumatic diseases

Pitting	Psoriasis
Onycholysis	Psoriasis Reiter's disease SLE
Subungual hyperkeratosis	Psoriasis Reiter's disease
Clubbing	HPOA
Periungual erythema	SLE Polymyositis
Nailfold telangiectasia	Systemic sclerosis Polymyositis SLE

Abnormalities of the hair and scalp

Alopecia is a common feature of SLE and is usually diffuse. It often accompanies a clinical exacerbation and may be the first manifestation of a flare-up of the disease. Hair will regrow when the disease improves.

Abnormalities of the hair and scalp

Alopecia	Diffuse: SLE Focal with scarring: SLE; DLE
Lupus hair	SLE
Psoriasis	
Scalp tenderness (and ocassionally necrosis)	Giant cell arteritis

Focal alopecia in association with discoid lupus lesions is seen in both DLE and SLE and is associated with irreversible scarring of the scalp.

Another characteristic feature of SLE is fragmentation of the frontal hairs leading to a receding hairline with shortened, broken-off hair, known as *lupus hair*.

Scalp involvement is common in psoriasis, and scalp tenderness is a common feature of giant cell arteritis, which in rare cases may be complicated by areas of scalp necrosis.

Lesions of the mucous membranes

1. Oral ulceration

Oral ulceration is a common clinical feature of a number of rheumatic disorders.

Oral ulcers in the rheumatic diseases

Superficial, painless	Reiter's syndrome
Superficial, painful	Gonorrhoea SLE Drugs
Aphthous	Inflammatory bowel disease Behçet's syndrome

It occurs in at least 40% of patients with Reiter's syndrome. Lesions are often asymptomatic and occur anywhere on the palate, tongue, buccal membrane and gingival surface. They differ from aphthous ulcers in being superficial, diffuse rather than circumscribed, and having an erythematous margin.

Typical aphthous ulcers occur in 30% of patients with ulcerative colitis and Crohn's disease. These patients tend to develop extra-bowel features such as polyarthritis.

In gonococcal infection, inflammation of the tongue, palate and pharynx may occur as the result of direct sexual contact. These lesions are more painful than those of Reiter's syndrome which often represent the main differential diagnosis.

Ulceration of the oral mucosa is common in SLE. Often it is painful, but asymptomatic ulceration of the hard palate is a very frequent finding.

Aphthous ulcers with or without genital lesions are the hallmark of Behçet's syndrome. They occur on the buccal mucosa, lips, tongue and pharynx, and in full-blown cases ulcers extend from the lips to the fauces and are deep and painful. Sometimes these deep ulcers heal with scarring.

Oral ulceration may also represent a side effect of drug therapy.

2. Other oral lesions

The oral mucous membranes are almost always involved in systemic sclerosis and become indurated and less flexible. Macular telangiectasia may develop on the lips and tongue and are prominent in the CREST variant of systemic sclerosis.

Loss of saliva leading to xerostomia is one of the hallmarks of Sjögren's syndrome. There is often rampant caries, and in severe cases the buccal membrane is parched.

3. Genital lesions

Balanitis develops in 25% of patients with Reiter's syndrome. Superficial ulcers develop on the glans penis which evolve into hyperkeratotic lesions (balanitis circinata) on the circumcised penis.

In Behçet's syndrome genital uclers resemble oral aphthae and occur on the vulva and vagina of females and on the scrotum and penis in males. Similar lesions may occur in Crohn's disease.

FURTHER READING (SKIN)

Callen J P 1982 Cutaneous lesions in the connective tissue disorders. Clinics in Rheumatic Diseases 8: 327–520

II The eye

INTRODUCTION

Eye disease is a common occurrence in many of the rheumatic diseases and may occasionally be the

Table 15.2. Preferential sites of ocular involvement in the rheumatic diseases

Disease	Conjunctiva	Episclera	Sclera	Cornea	Iris	Retina
RA	0	+++	+++	+	+	+
AS	0	0	0	0	+++	0
SLE	+	0	0	0	0	+++
Reiter's	+++	0	0	0	+	0
PAN	+	+++	+++	+	+	
Wegener's	0	0	+++	++	0	++
JCA	0	0	0	++	+++	+
Polychondritis	++	+++	+	+	+++	++
Sjögren's	+++	0	0	+++	0	0
Temporal arteritis	+	+	+	0	0	+++
Behçet's	0	+	+	0	+++	+++

presenting complaint (Table 15.2). With the exception of the retina and optic nerve, the tissues of the eyes and joints share a common mesodermal origin, which may be part of the explanation for this high frequency. These tissues, excluding the avascular cornea, are capable of mounting the entire range of inflammatory responses at a site where they can be directly observed. Ophthalmology has developed into a highly specialised branch of medicine but it is important for anyone looking after patients with rheumatic disorders to have a working knowledge of the field to avoid missing useful diagnostic clues or failing to recognise and treat correctly a potentially sight-threatening lesion.

The eye is composed of several closely applied layers (Fig. 15.2). The conjunctiva covers the exposed anterior surface and the inner part of the eyelids. Under this is a loose vascular network of connective tissue called the *episclera* whose main function is to supply nutrition to the underlying, relatively avascular, sclera. The *sclera* is the tough, white covering of the eye which becomes the transparent cornea anteriorly. Under the sclera is the uveal tract, a highly-vascular pigmented layer which forms the iris and ciliary body anteriorly and the choroid layer posteriorly. Inflammation of the entire tract is called *uveitis*. *Iritis* implies inflammation of the iris alone, while *anterior uveitis* or *iridocyclitis* is reserved for inflammation of the iris and ciliary body, but excludes the rest of the choroid. Although these anatomical distinctions can be made, in practice several different layers may be involved in an inflammatory process; for example, scleritis is usually accompanied by episcleritis and, if severe, may progress to involve the underlying uveal tract producing sclero-uveitis.

Some types of eye inflammation can look very dramatic but are relatively harmless. The presence of a serious eye condition is suggested if there is pain, impairment of vision or abnormality in the shape or response of the pupil and if the condition is unilateral.

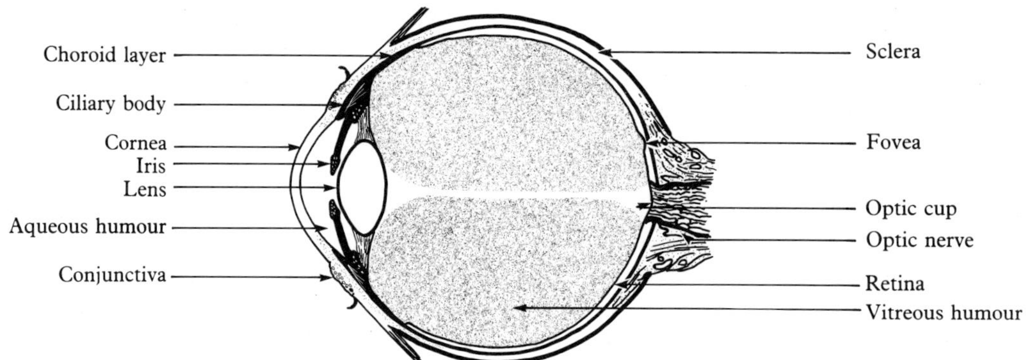

Fig. 15.2 Basic anatomy of the eye

THE RED EYE

There are four main conditions to be considered in a patient with a rheumatic disease who presents with a red eye: conjunctivitis, episcleritis, scleritis and acute iritis. Iritis and scleritis are usually painful, whereas conjunctivitis causes mild irritation and episcleritis is asymptomatic. Iritis is usually unilateral, although each eye may be affected in turn during separate episodes but the other conditions are frequently bilateral.

Conjunctivitis

The eyes feel itchy and irritated rather than painful and are diffusely red due to engorgement of a fine network of vessels and there is often a mucopurulent discharge (Fig. 15.3). The redness of conjunctivitis can be distinguished from episcleritis and scleritis because it extends over the bulbar surface of the eyelids and the vessels can be moved over the surface of the eye using a suitable applicator.

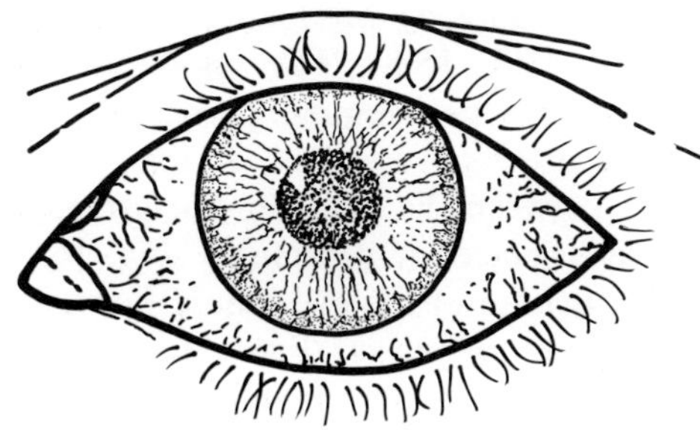

Fig. 15.3 Conjunctivitis

Conjunctivitis forms part of the diagnostic triad of Reiter's syndrome. Patients with RA who have dry eyes are also susceptible to bacterial conjunctivitis, often with *Staphylococcus aureus*, which can cause corneal abscesses if not treated promptly with antibiotic eye drops. Where indicated the eyes should be swabbed for bacteria to exclude infection. When the conjunctivitis is part of a reactive arthritis, it will usually settle without treatment or with a topically applied NSAI ointment such as oxphenbutazone.

Episcleritis

Episcleritis tends to occur in self-limiting episodes which last 7–10 days and are often asymptomatic. The eyes are flushed bright red and individual blood vessels can be clearly seen. The inflammation may be diffuse or isolated to certain areas — *nodular episcleritis* (Fig. 15.4). In contrast to conjunctivitis, the vessels cannot be moved over the surface of the eyeball but will constrict with adrenaline eye drops. Recurrent attacks of episcleritis are common in RA and do not indicate severe systemic disease; treatment is usually not required. If an episode is prolonged or uncomfortable it may be relieved by oxyphenbutazone eye ointment. Steroids should be avoided.

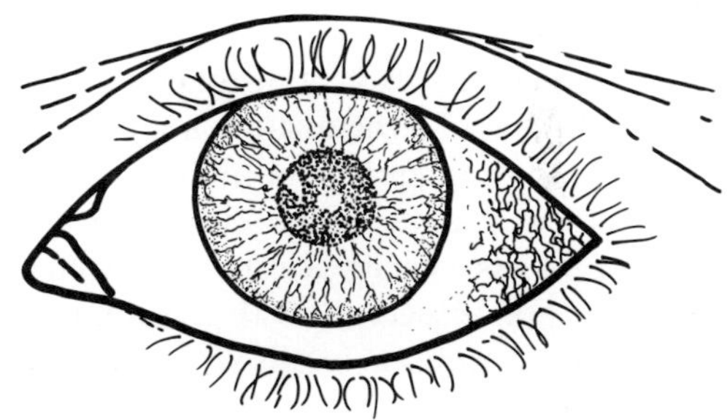

Fig. 15.4 Nodular episcleritis

Scleritis

This is a serious condition which requires urgent treatment. It is usually accompanied by episcleritis and it is important to distinguish between the two. Pain is common in scleritis and may be very severe. The scleral vessels lie deep and impart a dark purple hue to the eye in contrast to to bright red flush of episcleritis. This difference can be best appreciated by examining the eye in natural daylight. Doubtful cases can be further distinguished by instilling adrenaline eyedrops (1:1000) which will constrict the episcleral vessels only. Several forms of scleritis are recognised. In nodular scleritis a localised area of intensely painful vascular congestion is associated with a raised lesion caused by scleral oedema. The inflammation produces a change in the biochemical structure of the proteoglycans of the sclera so

Types of scleritis
1. Anterior
   Diffuse
   Nodular
   Necrotising (including scleromalacia perforans)
2. Posterior

that it becomes transparent. When the attack resolves, this leaves a characteristic slate-grey area in the white sclera where the underlying pigmented choroid shows through. In diffuse scleritis pain is less severe but the inflammation may involve the cornea, causing keratitis and keratolysis ('corneal melt').

Necrotising scleritis is the most serious form of scleritis. Granulomas with a histological appearance similar to that of a rheumatoid nodule form in the sclera, causing intense local inflammation and pain and result in thinning of the sclera. One characteristic form of necrotising scleritis, scleromalacia perforans, is not associated with severe pain or inflammation. Instead, a localised nodule in the sclera insidiously breaks down, producing a hole in the sclera through which the choroid is visible. The contents of the orbit rarely bulge through the defect unless there is a rise in the intra-occular pressure. Posterior scleritis can be difficult to diagnose clinically because nothing is apparently amiss at the front of the eye. Instead there may be pain and visual disturbance from retinal detachment caused by the intense inflammatory exudation.

Scleritis is estimated to occur in about 0.6% of patients with RA and usually indicates severe disease with systemic features such as vasculitis, pleural effusion and pericarditis. It predicts an unfavourable outcome with nearly a quarter of affected patients dead at 5 years. The outlook for sight is also not good, with 40% having reduced visual acuity due to sclerosing keratitis or secondary glaucoma. Scleritis is also common in the systemic vasculitides and may be the presenting feature, particularly of Wegener's granulomatosis, where it may cause ring corneal ulceration and retinal detachment.

Mild cases of scleritis may respond to local or systemic nonsteroidal anti-inflammatory treatment but usually systemic steroid therapy is required since local drops do not penetrate the sclera adequately. Doses as high as 60 mg per day may be required initially, reducing rapidly as the inflammation subsides. If there is a poor response and the pain and inflammation does not settle within a few days it may be necessary to add a cytotoxic drug such as azathioprine or cyclophosphamide. Corneal or scleral grafting can be performed to make good any defects in the surface of the eye. Secondary glaucoma may follow an attack of scleritis and further impair visual acuity.

Acute iritis

Patients with acute iritis present very quickly for medical attention because of severe, throbbing pain. This is associated with lacrimation, photophobia and blurring of vision. Usually only one eye is affected at any one time and shining a light into the good eye will cause increase in pain as the inflamed iris constricts. The small vessels of the limbus are engorged, producing a characteristic ciliary flush (Fig. 15.5). The pupil is small and spastic and may be irregular particularly if there have been previous episodes of iritis producing adhesions between the posterior surface of the iris and the lens (posterior synechiae) (Fig. 15.6). Slit lamp examination of the eye should be carried out to confirm the diagnosis. The aqueous is cloudy due to the large numbers of white cells which may adhere to the back of the cornea in clumps and be visiable as keratitic precipitates. The white cells may also fall to the bottom of the anterior chamber

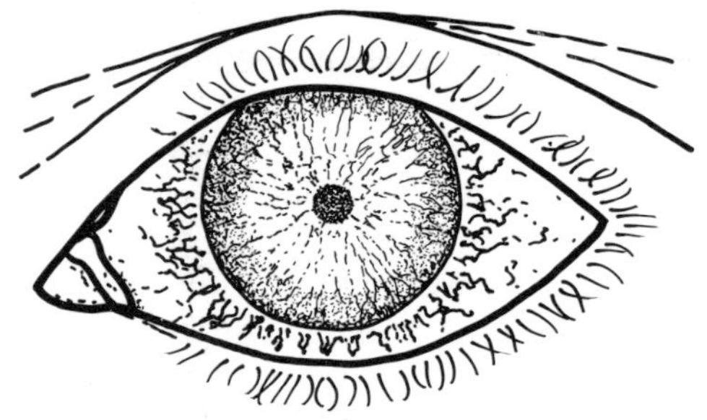

Fig. 15.5 Acute anterior uveitis

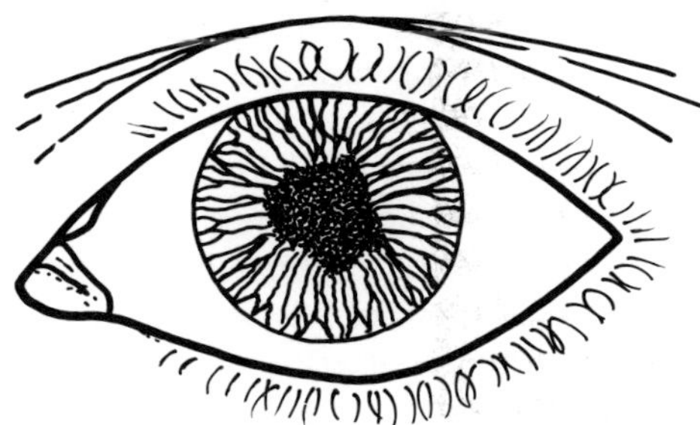

Fig. 15.6 Posterior synechiae

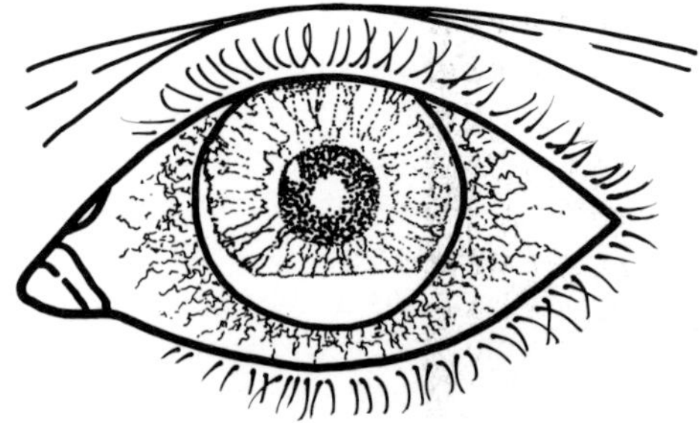

Fig. 15.7 Acute iritis: hypopyon

piling up to form a collection of pus called a *hypopyon* (Fig. 15.7).

Acute iritis must be treated promptly in order to avoid formation of adhesions which can later obstruct the flow of aqueous humour causing secondary glucoma and visual loss, by using mydriatics and steroid drops.

DRY EYE

Keratoconjunctivitis sicca (KCS)

Sjögren's syndrome is the association of dry eyes and mouth with a connective tissue disease. It is found in nearly a quarter of patients with RA and is also common in SLE, scleroderma and polymyositis and results from lymphocytic infiltration and destruction of secretory glands. In the early stages of lacrimal gland involvement there may be a parodoxical increase in tear secretion, causing watering of the eyes but once the condition is established tear secretion is reduced so that the surface of the eye dries out, particularly in the exposed interpalpabral region. The secretions produced by the mucus glands of the cornea also become abnormal and tenacious due to lack of a watery component from the lacrimal glands. This mucus tends to stick to the surface of the cornea, pulling off strips of epithelium when the eyes are blinked, a condition called *filamentous keratitis.* Dry eyes are prone to bacterial infection due to lack of lysozyme which is present in the normal tears. Corneal shrinkage, ulceration and scarring may also occur.

Patients rarely notice that the eyes are dry but instead complain that they feel gritty and are difficult to open first thing in the morning. The condition may be asymptomatic and ideally all susceptible patients should be screened for KCS annually. The Schirmer paper test is only a crude guide, but less than 15 mm of wetting of the paper strips after 5 minutes is suggestive and these patients should be referred for fuller assessment to an ophthalmologist. Slit-lamp examination will show an abnormal tear film and punctate areas of epithelial loss can be demonstrated by staining the eye with 1% Rose Bengal drops. The presence of this punctate keratitis plus diminished tear secretion will confirm the diagnosis of KCS. The Rose Bengal stain often causes severe discomfort in patients with KCS and should usually be used in conjunction with local anaesthetic drops.

Treatment of KCS is unsatisfactory. The tears can be replaced by regular use of lubricating artificial tears such as hypromellose drops. More severely affected patients may need to have the lacrimal ducts obstructed surgically to prolong the time the tears, both natural and artificial, remain in the conjunctival sac. A simple lubricating eye ointment may prevent sticking of the eyelid to the cornea at night.

LOSS OF VISION

There are six occular conditions associated with loss of vision which are relevant to the rheumatic diseases.

Chronic iritis

There is a chronic form of iritis which may be so insidious that it passes unnoticed by the patient or

Causes of visual loss
1. Chronic iritis
2. Glaucoma
3. Ischaemic optic neuropathy
4. Cataract
5. Hyperviscosity
6. Retinopathy

doctor until it causes severe visual impairment from glaucoma, corneal opacification and cataract. Girls of 7 years and above with JCA are prone to this complication, particularly if they are ANF positive and may become blind as a consequence. These children must have regular 6-monthly slit-lamp examinations until adulthood even though they are asymptomatic. Local steroid drops may halt the progression of the disease. A late complication of this form of iritis is band keratopathy in which corneal scars become calcified and visible as white bands which obscure vision. It is now possible to remove some of these by special surgical techniques.

Chronic glaucoma

This results from obstruction to the circulation of the aqueous humour and is usually secondary to a disturbance elsewhere in the eye. A common cause is pupillary adhesions from iritis or as a consequence of topical and systemic steroid therapy. Chronic glaucoma is usually asymptomatic until the damage inside the eye is advanced and the patient notices marked reduction in central vision. Signs at this late stage are large defects in the visual fields, enlargement and excavation of the optic cup and raised intra-occular pressure. Treatment is aimed at reducing the pressure using constricting drops, topical beta-blocking agents and acetazolamide and where possible eliminating the underlying cause.

Ischaemic optic neuropathy

Occlusion of the vessels supplying the optic nerve can cause sudden complete blindness in one eye. The optic disc is swollen but pale and the ischaemic retina is pale with a prominent cherry-red spot. This is a dreaded complication of temporal arteritis, but may also occur in patients with polymyalgia rheumatica even if their musculoskeletal symptoms have been well-controlled on a small dose of steroid. Treatment with a much higher dose (e.g. 60 mg) is indicated once the diagnosis of temporal arteritis is suspected.

Cataracts

Cataracts are opacities in the lens which are unnoticed when small but which may eventually increase in size sufficiently to diminish vision. Cataracts can be seen silhouetted against the red reflex through the dilated pupil when looking through an opthalmoscope held about 20 cm away from the eye. Corticosteroid therapy is associated with the development of cataracts in the back of the lens just under the capsule and their presence is an indication to try to withdraw the drug. Cataracts are also a common occurrence in children with chronic iritis in JCA.

Hyperviscosity

This is a characteristic syndrome associated with a markedly elevated plasma and whole-blood viscosity. One feature is blurring of vision due to sludging of blood in the retinal vessels. This process can actually be observed in the vessels as a segmentation of the column of blood the so called 'trucking' or 'string of sausages' sign.

Retinopathy

Hydroxychloroquine is a useful second line drug in the treatment of RA and SLE but in high doses over a prolonged period of time it can rarely cause visual impairment due to a direct toxic effect on the retina. The frequently mentioned 'bull's eye' macula is extremely rare and only seen in the severest cases which now almost never occur due to closer monitoring of the eyes of patients who are put on this drug and to the use of lower doses for a shorter time. Vasculitis in RA and other systemic vasculitides can occasionally produce haemorrhages and exudates which may threaten vision if they occur in the region of the macula.

ASYMPTOMATIC ABNORMALITIES IN THE EYES

Occasionally when examining the eye of a patient with a rheumatic disease, abnormalities are seen which may be diagnostically helpful. This is particularly true for the patients with SLE who may have a systemic flare of the disease and be found to have soft fluffy white spots (histologically called *cytoid bodies*) on the posterior part of the retina due to focal infarction from vasculitis. Occasionally frank flame-shaped haemorrhages may be apparent. The features of hypertensive retinopathy haemorrhages, exudates and even optic nerve head swelling — may appear quite suddenly in a patient with scleroderma or polyarthritis nodosa, who develops a hypertensive crisis secondary to renal failure. A list of some useful diagnostic clues which may be detected in the eye is given below.

Useful diagnostic clues found in the eye

Ochronosis	Black sclera
Osteogenesis imperfecta	Blue sclera
Hypoparathyroidism	Corneal calcification
Pseudoxanthoma elasticum	Angiod streaks
Marfan's syndrome	Dislocated lenses
Mucopolysacharridoses	Corneal clouding
Wilson's disease	Keyser–Fleischer rings

FURTHER READING (EYE)

Miller D 1979 Ophthalmology: the essentials. Houghton Mifflin, Boston

Henkind P, Gold D H 1973 Occular manifestations of rheumatic disorders: natural and iatrogenic. In: Ehrlich G E (ed) Rheumatology annual review. S Karger, Basel

Epstein W V 1979 The eye and connective tissue diseases In: Cohen A S (ed) Rheumatology and immunology. The science and practice of clinical medicine 4. Grune & Stratton, New York

III The blood and reticulo-endothelial system

BLOOD

All of the blood components can be affected by rheumatic disease or by drugs used in their treatment. Haematological abnormalities frequently reflect disease activity but they are occasionally the presenting feature or initial clue that leads to correct diagnosis e.g. thrombocytopenia or lymphopenia in a febrile patient with malaise and arthralgia should suggest lupus.

Many of the abnormalities listed in the following sections are drug-induced and it should be remembered that marrow toxicity is the commonest life-threatening side effect of anti-rheumatic agents.

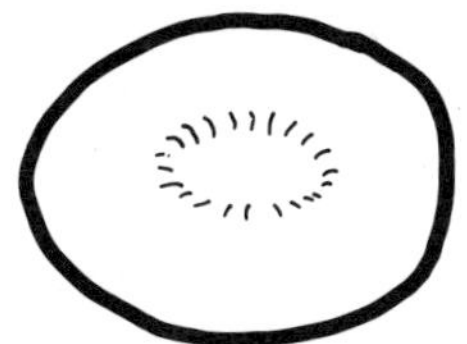

Fig. 15.8 Erythrocytes

Red cells (Fig. 15.8)

Anaemia is a frequent feature of RA and other inflammatory diseases and occasionally is severe. Several factors in the inflammatory process, especially increased RES activity, interfere with normal iron metabolism to result in:

1. Impaired re-utilisation of iron. Most iron in serum originates from haemoglobin breakdown in the RES — impaired re-utilisation is therefore commonly reflected by reduction in serum iron levels.
2. Abnormal distribution of iron in tissues. Increased iron, mainly stored within the protein apoferitin as ferritin, is found not only in usual storage sites (liver, spleen, bone-marrow) but also in lymph nodes and synovium.
3. Decreased production and increased degradation of transferrin. This is reflected indirectly by a low serum TIBC.

The drop in serum iron correlates closely with the activity of the inflammatory process, but hypoferraemia in association with anaemia may cause confusion and result in unnecessary, possibly harmful administration of iron products in the mistaken belief that iron deficiency is present. Contrasting features of pure iron-deficiency anaemia and anaemia associated with inflammatory disease are shown in Table 15.3.

Table 15.3 Contrasting features of iron deficiency anaemia and anaemia due to inflammatory disease (e.g. active RA)

	Iron deficiency	Inflammatory disease
Red cell variables and film	Hypochromic	Normochromic
	Microcytic	Normocytic
Serum iron	↓	↓
Serum TIBC	High	Low
% saturation	↓ ↓	Variable
Serum ferritin	<15 μg/1	15–250 μg/1
Marrow stores	↓/Absent	Normal/ ↑
Absorption of iron	↑ ↑	Normal
Effect of iron replacement on anaemia	Beneficial	No effect

Neutrophils (Fig. 15.9)

Although a raised peripheral neutrophil count is a common feature of several rheumatic diseases, a marked and persistent neutrophil leukocytosis, in the appropriate clinical setting, may support or suggest the diagnosis of two rare conditions — PAN (p 129) and Still's disease (p 93). The possibility of sepsis, however, should always be considered.

Drug-induced neutropenia may be marked and result in predisposition to life-threatening infection, the risk and severity of complications being related to the degree of neutropenia (unlikely with counts of 1000/μl or more, but almost certain with counts of 500/μl or less). The mechanism of injury is often unclear but may involve direct toxicity or leukocyte agglutinins.

Felty's syndrome is a variant of seropositive RA with splenomegaly and granulocytopenia of less than 2000/ul. Various factors may be involved in the pathogenesis, including decreased neutrophil production, increased margination and sequestration, and impairment of neutrophil function (p 56). Unlike the situation with drug toxicity, susceptibility to infection is less predictable, some patients appearing prone to repeated, severe infection with near-normal white counts, while others with profound neutropenia are apparently unaffected. Such disparity stresses the importance of the function, as well as the numbers, of circulating neutrophils, and also the role played by other host-defence mechanisms (p 208).

Abnormalities affecting neutrophil function are difficult to quantify but may involve:

1. Extracellular factors, e.g. circulating anti-neutrophil antibodies in SLE.
2. Drug effects, e.g. binding of colchicine to tubulin with subsequent suppression of chemotactic factor synthesis and release.
3. Constitutional factors, e.g. impaired phagocytosis in neutrophils of HLA-B27-positive individuals.

Eosinophils (Fig. 15.10)

Eosinophils are particularly involved in tissue responses evoked by Type I hypersensitivity reactions, and appear to perform several major functions including:

INCREASED NUMBERS

PAN
Still's disease
Septic arthritis
Crystal synovitis
Rheumatic fever
Behçet's
Steroids

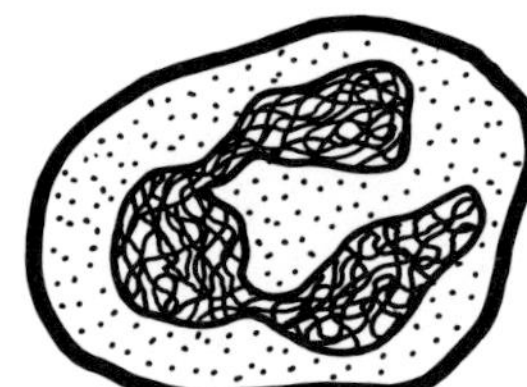

DECREASED NUMBERS

Felty's syndrome
Drugs
- Cytotoxic drugs
- Levamisole
- Gold
- Penicillamine
- Phenylbutazone
- Allopurinol

Fig. 15.9 Neutrophils

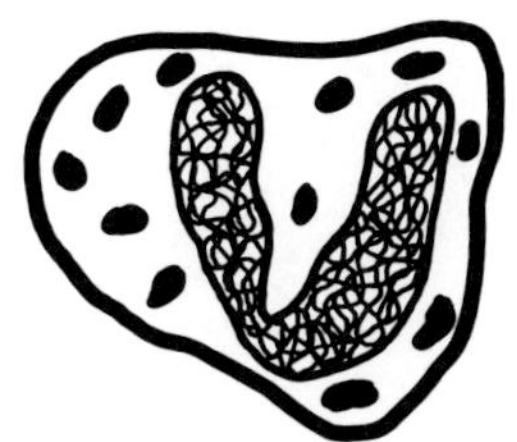

Fig. 15.10 Eosinophils

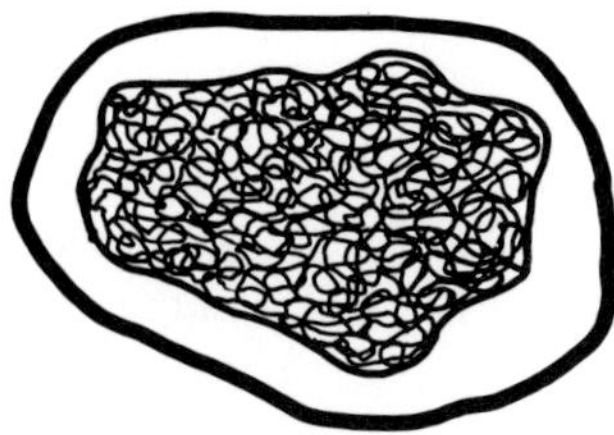

Fig. 15.11 Monocytes

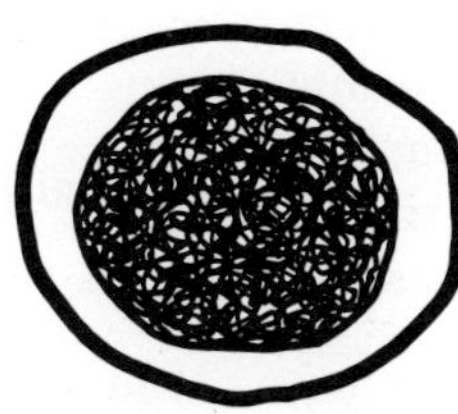

Fig. 15.12 Lymphocytes

1. Release of enzymes (e.g. histaminase) that degrade mediatiors released from basophils and mast cells
2. Preferential phagocytosis of extruded mast cell granules
3. Ability to damage non-phagocytosable parasites
4. Phagocytosis of soluble immune complexes

In patients with RA moderate eosinophilia may be induced by immune complexes and appears to show some correlation with systemic disease. Marked eosinophilia, however, is a characteristic finding in Churg–Strauss vasculitis, PAN with pulmonary involvement and eosinophilic fasciitis, and has been used in support of theories invoking hypersensitivity in the pathogenesis of these disorders.

Monocytes (Fig. 15.11)

Compared to granulocytes, monocytes have a much smaller marrow reserve, a more limited capacity to augment production under stress, a longer intravascular half-life, and a proportionately large extra-vascular compartment. Measurement of circulating blood monocytes is therefore usually of little diagnostic value.

Lymphocytes (Fig. 15.12)

Lymphocytes are believed to play a major role in many rheumatic diseases (p 16) but alteration in circulating numbers is uncommon except as a consequence of treatment or in SLE, when it may help to suggest the diagnosis. Reports that esti-

INCREASED NUMBERS
RA
Still's disease
Wegener's granulomatosis

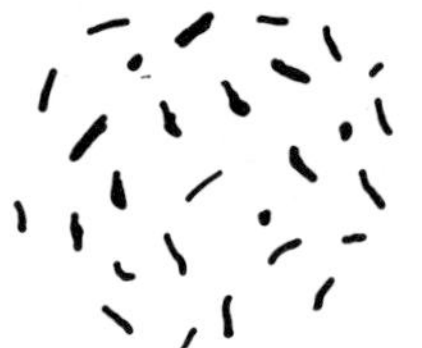

DECREASED NUMBERS
SLE
Felty's syndrome
Drugs
- Gold
- Penicillamine
- Azathioprine
- Methotrexate
- Chlorambucil
- Allopurinol
- Phenylbutazone
- Indomethacin

Sjögren's syndrome
Meningococcaemia
Infective endocarditis

Fig. 15.13 Platelets

mation of circulating lymphocyte subsets, according to function, may be of value in diagnosis of disease awaits further confirmation.

Platelets (Fig. 15.13)

Although active lupus is probably the commonest rheumatic disease to cause thrombocytopenia, drugs are by far and away the most frequent cause of low platelet counts in patients with rheumatic disease, and administration of gold, penicillamine, cytotoxic and immunosuppressive agents should always be accompanied by regular counts to allow early detection of falling platelet numbers. Easy bruising, spontaneous petechiae or purpura of skin and mucous membranes, and haemorrhage, are rarely seen unless the platelet count falls below 20 000/mm^3. Easy bruising is also seen in conditions that weaken connective tissue support, e.g. corticosteroids, RA, osteomalacia.

Abnormalities of clotting

Predisposition to thrombosis is a clinical feature of Behçet's syndrome and SLE. A definite hypercoagulable state that predisposes to large-vessel thrombosis and ulceration may occur in Behcet's due to a decrease in fibrinolysis (demonstrated by prolonged euglobulin lysis time and undetectable FDPs) perhaps related to low factor XII levels. The situation in SLE is more complex but may involve a lupus anticoagulant and subsequent overcompensation by normal thrombotic mechanisms resulting in predisposition to large vessel (usually venous) thrombosis.

Bleeding due to factors directed against the clotting cascade — usually factors VIII, IX, XII — is uncommon in SLE but may be a cause of major bleeds following operative procedures, particularly in lupus patients with co-existent platelet abnormalities. Drugs such as aspirin may also predispose to bleeding by effects on clotting and other factors, and many NSAIDs will displace oral anticoagulants from binding sites on albumin.

Clinical problems

Anaemia in a patient with polyarthritis

Mild to moderate anaemia, with a normochromic normocytic film, commonly reflects active inflammatory disease. Abnormal red cell indices, marked anaemia or anaemia that appears disproportionate to clinical serological or radiological indices of inflammation, however, should always be investigated along the usual lines.

A common clinical problem is to decide whether a patient with inflammatory arthritis, usually RA, has anaemia due to active disease, blood-loss from the gut, or both. This situation is especially confusing since:

1. Faecal occult bloods are often positive in patients taking NSAIDs
2. Presence or absence of upper GI symptoms bears little relationship to blood loss
3. Both conditions may produce a low serum iron and occasional thrombocytosis

The indices listed in Table 15.3 may aid in differentiating active disease from blood-loss if they

Main causes of anaemia, with appropriate screening investigations

Blood loss
- Red cell indices, serum iron/TIBC
- Serum ferritin, faecal occult bloods

Haemolysis
- Reticulocyte count
- Serum haptoglobins
- Coomb's test

Malabsorption
- Red cell folate, B12
- Serum calcium
- Serum β carotenoids

Decreased production
- White cell and platelet count
- Urea and electrolytes
- Consider marrow aspiration

occur separately, but in practice such distinctions show considerable overlap, especially when both occur together or blood-loss is acute. Frequently the issue can only be resolved by upper GI endoscopy or barium studies. Several factors, however, should suggest the possibility of blood loss from the gut in a patient with rheumatic disease and anaemia:

1. Anaemia that appears disproportionate to clinical, biochemical or radiological indices of inflammation
2. A rapid fall in haemoglobin
3. A TIBC in the upper half of the normal range and a serum ferritin of <55 μg/l, (the latter is an appropriate lower limit of normality, since inflammation may directly stimulate apoferritin production and it is apoferritin that is normally measured in serum 'ferritin' estimations)
4. A previous history of peptic ulceration

Hyperviscosity

Hyperviscosity syndrome is a rare complication of RA (p 41) and Sjögren's syndrome (p 140). It may present with diverse features that include dyspnoea, confusion, ataxia, visual blurring, paraesthesiae, epistaxis, skin haemorrhages, menorrhagia or rectal bleeding. Fundal examination may reveal engorgement of large, tortuous veins and occasionally haemorrhages, exudates or papilloedema. Hyperviscosity syndrome is most commonly caused by diseases characterised by large amounts of monoclonal cryoglobulins e.g. Waldenström's macroglobulinaemia, myeloma and lymphoma. Cryoglobulins occurring in RA and Sjögren's, however, are polyclonal and represent true immune complexes, containing rheumatoid factors, IgG and frequently complement. Marked cryoglobulinaemia in these diseases more usually present as immune complex vasculitis than with complications due to viscous flow.

RETICULO-ENDOTHELIAL SYSTEM (RES)

The pathology of many of the rheumatic diseases is intimately involved with activity of the RES components (p 16), and it is therefore not surprising that systemic lymphadenopathy and minor hepatosplenomegaly are commonly found in the following diseases:

- RA
- SLE
- Sjögren's syndrome
- Still's disease

Increased RES activity is evidenced by enhanced clearance of particulate matter from the circulation in patients with RA and SLE. Such increased activity may certainly play a part in the neutropenia and thrombocytopenia of Felty's syndrome (p 56) and may also help explain the increased iron retention in spleen and marrow so characteristic of these disorders.

Reticulo-endothelial clearance may occasionally be reduced in patients with active SLE or systemic rheumatoid disease, and it has been suggested that excessive loading may result in RE 'blockade', allowing subsequent overspill of complexes back into the circulation with resultant systemic effects. There is some evidence to suggest that plasmaphoresis may temporarily reduce this load and allow the RES to recover.

Clinical problems

Lymphadenopathy in a patient with a rheumatic disease

When lymphadenopathy occurs in the diseases listed above, its distribution does not closely reflect the pattern of joint involvement, and, clinically, enlarged axillary nodes are most frequently detected (necropsy studies in RA show frequent additional enlargement of para-aortic nodes). When lymphadenopathy is present it is usually symmetrical and nodes are mild to moderate in size, soft or firm, and freely mobile. Occasionally, however, especially in RA, lymphadenopathy is sufficiently pronounced as to suggest malignancy. Lymphangiography is unhelpful in such cases since appearances are usually indistinguishable from lymphoma. Biopsy in a patient with RA will reveal cortical follicular hyperplasia (occasionally so massive as to obliterate interfollicular tissue and resemble follicular lymphoma), macrophage accumulation in the sinuses (sinus 'histiocytosis') and lymphocytic and fibroblastic infiltration of the capsule. During active disease oedema and focal PMN aggregates are characteristic.

Given that lymphadenopathy may be part of the disease process in RA, SLE, Sjögen's syndrome and Still's, the problem arises as to when to biopsy an abnormal looking node in a patient with such a disease. Decisions are made difficult when one considers that:

1. Sjögren's syndrome (particularly primary) predisposes to malignancy
2. There is evidence suggesting that drugs such as alkylating agents that are used in these patients may predispose to malignancy
3. Unrelated malignancy, e.g. Hodgkin's, carcinoma, may occur by chance and escape early detection
4. Non-invasive procedures are inevitably inconclusive and, although needle biopsy may occasionally be sufficient, removal of the whole node is often required to exclude malignancy.

Faced with this problem, which usually arises in a patient with RA or Sjögren's, it seems sensible to proceed to node biopsy in the following circumstances:

1. If a node is hard and fixed
2. Marked enlargement and asymmetry
3. Rapid increase in size of a node or regional group
4. In a patient with Sjögren's syndrome and marked lymphadenopathy who demonstrates a fall in serum immunoglobulins from previously elevated levels (p 140)

Splenomegaly in a patient with a rheumatic disease

Clinically detectable splenomegaly is not uncommon in RA, SLE, Still's disease and Sjögren's syndrome. Splenomegaly in a patient with RA raises the possibility of:

1. Active disease
2. Felty's syndrome
3. Amyloid

A differential WBC and the other characteristic clinical features may allow a diagnosis of Felty's (p 56) and urinalysis and rectal biopsy should be performed if amyloid is a clinical possibility (p 63).

Splenomegaly in a patient with arthralgia and fever should suggest the possibility of:

1. Infective endocarditis
2. SLE
3. Infectious mononucleosis, brucellosis and other infections

IV Arteries, Veins and Lymphatics

Local changes in the flow of blood and lymphatic fluid are usual at the primary target site of any rheumatic disease, being integral parts of the inflammatory process. Many rheumatic diseases also affect vessels more generally, producing alterations in their function or integrity. Some of the anatomical sites and the pathological processes involved are outlined in Figure 15.14.

Increased flow within a vessel is due to dilatation or a hyperdynamic circulation and is usually unimportant. Decreased flow can result from several

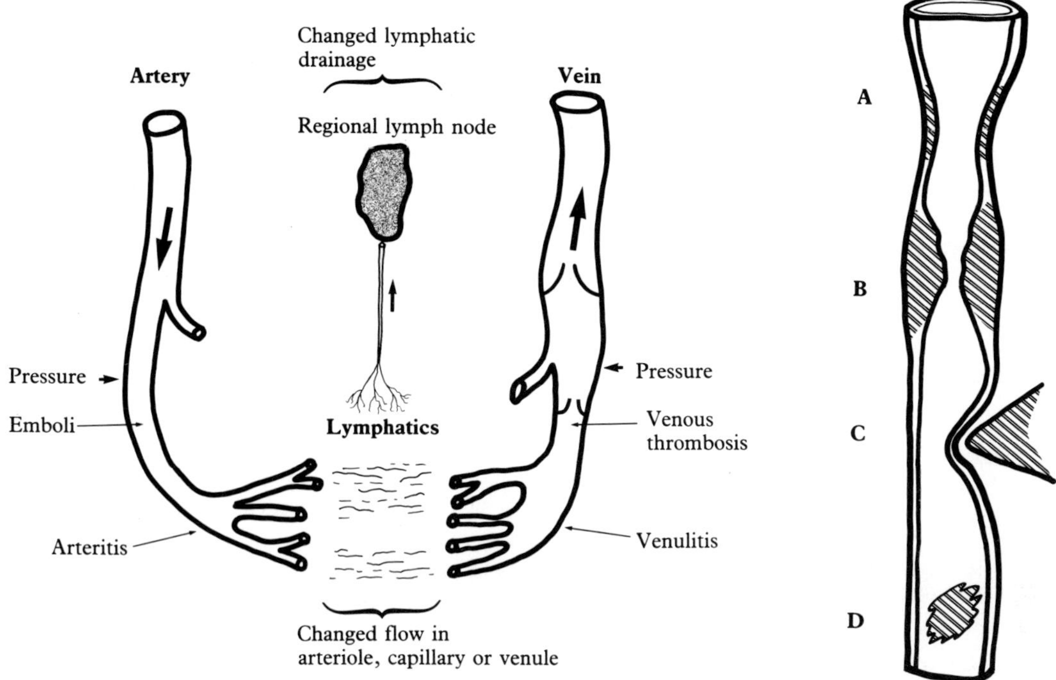

Fig. 15.14 Arteries, veins and lymphatics: sites of damage in rheumatic diseases

Fig. 15.15 Causes of reduced flow in blood vessels. **A**. Active constriction of vessel wall (e.g. Raynaud's phenomenon). **B**. Disease of vessel wall (e.g. vascultitis). **C**. Pressure from outside (e.g. osteophytic pressure on vertebral arteries). **D**. Obstruction within the lumen (e.g. hyperviscosity syndrome).

different causes (Fig. 15.15), and often results in major clinical problems.

ARTERIAL DISEASE

Most arterial disease is due to atherosclerosis. However, arteritis, described in Chapter 7 is an important pathological feature of rheumatic diseases. Severe joint deformity occasionally causes pressure on arteries, the only significant examples being osteophytic obstruction of the vertebral arteries producing a vertebro-basilar syndrome, and the contribution of spinal artery obstruction to spinal cord compression. Emboli are not a feature of rheumatic diseases, although the combination of arthritis and peripheral emboli might suggest the possibility of rheumatic fever, subacute bacterial endocarditis or an atrial myxoma.

Clinical problems

1. Raynaud's phenomenon

Raynaud's phenomenon can be defined as paroxysmal digital ischaemia, it is usually exacerbated by cold and less often by emotion. The affected area goes through a characteristic sequence of changes: it first goes white and numb, then becomes painful and blue, and finally becomes red as reactive hyperaemia terminates the attack. The pathological basis of the phenomenon remains unknown; the arterioles are apparently unduly sensitive to cold, pressure and other stimuli, and contract at the initiation of attacks. The hands are usually affected and women between puberty and the menopause are the chief victims.

Raynaud's phenomenon may be idiopathic (Raynaud's disease), or due to a large number of causes including several rheumatic diseases. An underlying cause is more likely to be obvious in

Causes of Raynaud's phenomenon

Rheumatic diseases

1. *Common*
   - Systemic sclerosis
   - Mixed connective-tissue disease
   - SLE
2. *Rare*
   - Rheumatoid arthritis
   - PAN
   - Sjögren's
   - Aortic arch syndrome
   - Algodystrophy

Others (mostly rare)
- Arteriosclerosis
- Buerger's disease
- Embolus, thrombosis, stenosis in arteries
- Cervical rib
- Hyperabduction syndrome, other mechanical obstructions
- Vibrating machinery
- Ergot poisoning
- Smoking
- Cold agglutinins
- Dysproteinaemias
- Polycythaemia
- Paralysis or disuse of limb

Idiopathic (common)
- Raynaud's disease

a man (especially use of vibrating machinery) or if the patient is over 40. However, the common clinical problem concerns the young woman presenting with Raynaud's of the hands: is there any apparent cause, and will she develop a connective-tissue disease in the future?

A thorough history and examination will exclude most of the common non-rheumatic causes such as drugs, arteriosclerosis, vibrating machinery and cold injury. An X-ray of the thoracic inlet to exclude cervical rib, and blood tests for cold agglutinins, dysproteinaemias and polycythaemia, exclude other possible causes. In the majority none of these things is abnormal, and the problem of diagnosis remains. Raynaud's is rare in rheumatoid arthritis, common but usually mild in SLE and sicca syndrome, and severe and often the presenting feature of systemic sclerosis or MCTD, preceding other manifestations by months or even many years. About 10% young women with severe Raynaud's will eventually develop one of the latter two diseases. An abnormal pattern of nail-fold capillaries (see below) and anti-nuclear antibodies are the only known predictors of a connective-tissue disease. Speckled ANA and a high titre of anti-RNP suggests that MCTD might develop; whereas anti-centromere antibody is more indicative of forthcoming scleroderma.

2. *Peripheral ulcers and ischaemic lesions*

Peripheral ischaemia may cause gangrene, a variety of different skin ulcers, paronychiae, skin thinning and hair-loss, or pain influenced by posture and exercise. In patients with a rheumatic disease one has to differentiate between a coincidental cause (such as arteriosclerosis, thromboangiitis obliterans or arterial emboli) and a complication of the primary disease (e.g. vasculitis or an intravascular occlusion).

Peripheral ischaemic lesions of the hands are common in scleroderma and MCTD. Gangrene of an isolated area in the hands and feet occurs in rheumatoid vasculitis; it is also seen, but is surprisingly unusual, in PAN and SLE. Peripheral ulcers, especially of the legs, are common in RA and may be due to a combination of thin skin, venous stasis and dependency of the limb, as well as arteritis. Deep 'punched-out' ulcers in unusual sites are more likely to have a vasculitic basis than the usual shallow ulcers over the ankle, but it is often difficult to differentiate them on clinical grounds alone.

Factors which will help to differentiate between vasculitis and arteriosclerosis are shown. Clinical and laboratory evidence of widespread small-vessel vasculitis is often apparent in patients with a connective-tissue disease who present with ischaemic lesions, whereas the arteriopath usually has signs of long-standing large-vessel disease, and venous ulcers have their own clinical features. In difficult cases non-invasive studies of flow such as Doppler wave-form analysis may help; arteriography is rarely necessary.

Factors which help to differentiate vasculitic skin ulcers in RA

Systemic features of vasculitis
- Weight-loss
- Malaise
- Nail-fold lesions
- Other vasculitic skin rashes

The ulcer:
- Deep, punched-out ulcer
- Unusual sites (e.g. dorsum of foot, back of calf)
- Sudden onset

Large vessels normal
- Peripheral pulses normal
- No signs of general limb ischaemia
- No evidence of venous disease

Investigations suggestive of active vasculitis
- High ESR
- High titre rheumatoid factor (especially IgG subclass)
- High titre anti-complementary activity or other tests of circulating immune complexes
- Vasculitis on rectal biopsy

VENOUS DISEASE

Venules, as well as arterioles, are often affected by the vasculitis of connective tissue diseases (Chapter 7). Venous obstruction can also result from pressure on the vessel wall or from thrombosis. Venous thrombosis is a feature of some systemic rheumatic diseases. Patients with Bechçet's syndrome sometimes have a prolonged euglobulin lysis time, suggesting that reduced fibronolysis may be the cause. Some SLE patients have an abnormal anticoagulant ('lupus anticoagulant') but thrombosis rather than bleeding may result. Hyperviscosity, due to dysproteinaemias, thrombocytosis or polycythaemia, may also complicate a rheumatic disease and predispose to venous thrombosis.

Patients with long-standing RA often have thin, friable veins that are difficult to find but bleed easily; the cause is unknown.

Rheumatic diseases which can predispose to venous thrombosis

1. Systemic lupus erythematosus
2. Behçet's syndrome
3. Hyperviscosity
4. Immobility caused by severe disability
5. Pressure on veins from joint cysts or deformity

Clinical problems

DVT or ruptured Baker's cyst? (Table 15.4)

The sudden onset of pain, tenderness and swelling in one calf, with some oedema of the foot and calf pain on dorsiflexion of the ankle (Homan's sign), is very common. The main differential diagnosis of the presentation is between vein thrombosis (d.v.t.) or a ruptured Baker's cyst at the back of the knee. The signs and symptoms below the knee may be identical, and mistakes are frequently made. Patients are often misdiagnosed as having a d.v.t. and anti-coagulated; this can cause bleeding into the diseased knee joint and calf, with secondary muscle necrosis and shortening, or Sudek's atrophy.

A good history and examination of the knee joint will allow the correct diagnosis to be made

Table 15.4 Differential diagnosis of deep vein thrombosis and ruptured Baker's cyst

d.v.t.	Ruptured joint
Factors predisposing to thrombosis may be apparent (e.g. 'the Pill')	Previous joint swelling often noticed. May be an obvious generalised arthropathy.
Onset often gradual	Onset often sudden (patient may feel something give way at back of knee)
Knee joint usually normal	Effusion in knee joint and palpable Baker's cyst usually present
Tenderness maximal over deep veins in back of calf	More generalised tenderness, often includes joint line and back of knee.
Other symptoms and signs in calf and leg are similar in the two conditions	

in the majority of cases (Table 15.4). A ruptured Baker's cyst usually occurs in a patient who has been aware of knee swelling and a fulness at the back of the knee for weeks or months. A history of a sudden pain while climbing stairs, followed by a feeling of fluid running down the leg, is not unusual (such patients still get anti-coagulated!). An arthrogram, if done early, will confirm the presence of a cyst, and its rupture (Fig. 15.16). However, the defect may seal off within days, and inability to show the dye running down the calf does not exclude the diagnosis. A synovial cyst, with or without rupture, occasionally results in a d.v.t. by causing pressure on veins, and the two diagnoses occasionally co-exist; venography may then be useful. However, patients with a rheumatic disease known to cause synovitis of the knee joint should be regarded as having a ruptured Baker's cyst until proved otherwise.

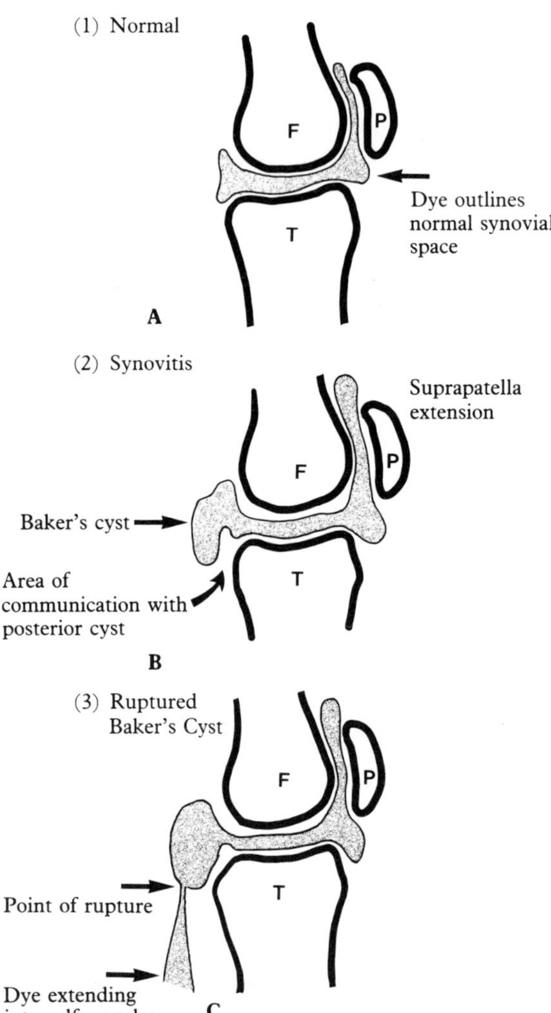

Fig. 15.16 Diagrammatic representation of lateral knee radiographs after intrasynovial injection of radio-opaque dye (arthrography). **A**. Normal. **B**. Synovitis. **C**. Ruptured Baker's cyst. (F = femur; T = tibia; P = patella.)

LYMPHATIC DISEASE

Normal lymphatic drainage increases if extra demands are made, as in the case of local inflammation in a limb, increasing the volume of extravascular fluid. Joint inflammation, especially in RA, may result in excess fibrin formation, which can block lymphatic drainage and predispose to oedema. Any co-existent lymphatic problem, for example congenital lymphatic hypoplasia, may also result in oedema of a limb developing when joints or extra-articular tissues become inflamed.

Clinical problems

Oedema in rheumatoid arthritis

Peripheral oedema can complicate any rheumatic disease, and if generalised the usual causes must be considered (cardiac failure, nephrotic syndrome, liver disease, malabsorption etc.). Nephrotic syndrome and malabsorption are rare complications of many connective-tissue diseases.

Oedema of the limbs is a particularly common problem in RA. The likely causes depend on whether it is unilateral or bilateral. Swelling of one limb suggests venous or lymphatic blockade or joint rupture. Generalised oedema raises the possibility of nephrotic syndrome (drugs or amyloid?) or congestive cardiac failure, and the usual clinical and urinary protein tests quickly sort the problem out. However, oedema of the hands, and to a lesser extent the feet, is often due to disease activity alone with no other apparent predisposing cause. This is especially common in early inflammatory synovitis, in older patients and in acute-onset RA. Oedema may be the presentation of RA, and other clinical signs of synovitis may be masked.

Causes of oedema in rheumatoid arthritis

1. Localised oedema in one limb
   a) Joint rupture
   b) Venous obstruction
   c) Lymphatic obstruction
2. Generalised oedema
   a) Active synovitis alone
   b) Hypoalbuminaemia
      (i) Nephrotic syndrome (think of drugs or amyloid)
      (ii) Malabsorption
      (iii) Severe systemic disease
   c) Congestive cardiac failure

HYPERAEMIA IN RHEUMATIC DISEASES

Bone and joint disease are associated with a localised increase in blood flow in the affected tissues. This is most striking in joint synovitis and in Pagetic bone, and a variety of imaging techniques used in rheumatology are based on this increased blood flow (Chapter 24.II).

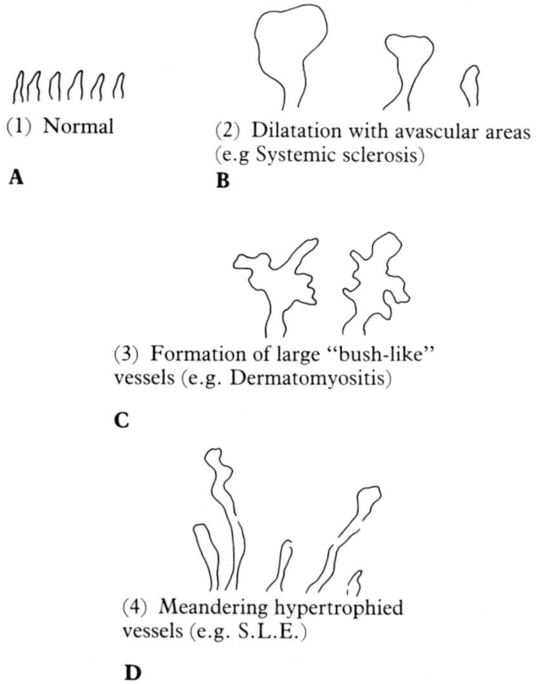

RA and the connective-tissue diseases can also cause a more generalised hyperaemia, involving capillary beds not directly involved by the inflammatory process. Palmar erythema and redness around the nail-folds and finger pulps is especially common in active RA. Nail-fold capillary hyperaemia is also a marked feature of scleroderma, dermatomyositis and to a lesser extent SLE. In these diseases capillary abnormalities with growth of new loops, as well as increased blood-flow, contribute to the abnormality. The nail-bed should be examined by dropping oil onto the area and then, under bright light, observing the vessels with a magnifying glass. As an alternative, the oil and an opthalmoscope can be used. Some of the typical changes seen are shown in Figure 15.17. The mechanism of these hyperaemic changes remains unknown, although the speculation that vascular changes and a variety of angiogenic factors have an important role in rheumatic diseases is of great interest.

(1) Normal

A

(2) Dilatation with avascular areas (e.g Systemic sclerosis)

B

(3) Formation of large "bush-like" vessels (e.g. Dermatomyositis)

C

(4) Meandering hypertrophied vessels (e.g. S.L.E.)

D

Fig. 15.17 Patterns of vascular abnormality in nailfold capillary beds in patients with connective-tissue disorders. **A**. Normal. **B**. Dilatation with avascular areas (e.g. systemic sclerosis). **C**. Formation of large 'bush-like' vessels (e.g. dermatomyositis). **D**. Meandering hypertrophied vessels (e.g. SLE).

FURTHER READING (ARTERIES, VEINS AND LYMPHATICS)

Mariq H R, Spencer-Green G, Le Roy E C 1980 Skin capillary abnormalities as an indication of organ involvement in scleroderma (systemic sclerosis) and related disorders. Arthritis and Rheumatism 23: 183–189

Birnstingle M 1971 The Raynaud syndrome. Postgraduate Medical Journal 47: 297–310

Hughes G V R, Pridie R B 1970 Acute synovial rupture of the knee — a differential diagnosis from deep vein thrombosis Proceedings of the Royal Society of Medicine 63: 857–860

V The Heart

All three layers of the heart may be involved by several of the rheumatic diseases and heritable disorders of connective tissue (Fig. 15.18). In addition, several conditions predispose to premature atherosclerosis or hypertension, and cardiac function may further be compromised by drugs used in treatment.

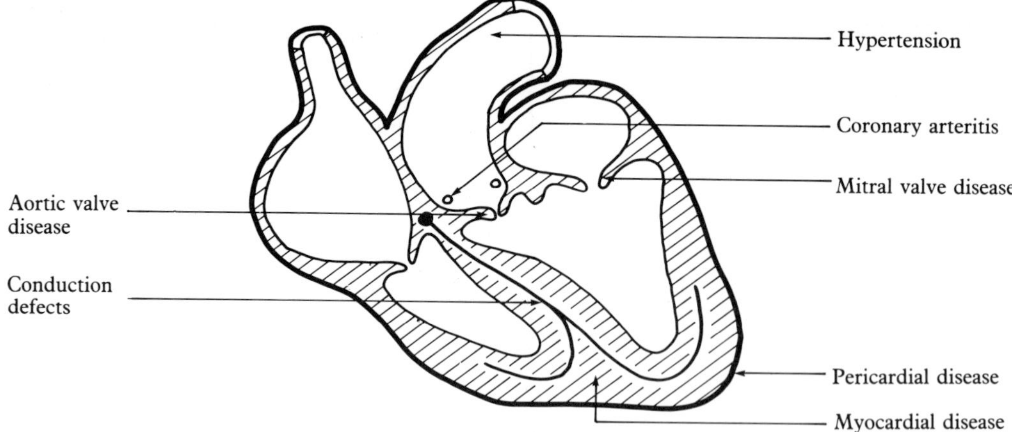

Fig. 15.18 Diagrammatic representation of the heart showing important sites of involvement by rheumatic diseases

Rheumatic diseases and drugs used in treatment that predispose to hypertension, atherosclerosis and fluid retention

1. *Hypertension*
   a) Polyarteritis nodosa
   b) Scleroderma
   c) Pseudoxanthoma elasticum
   d) Steroids
2. *Premature Atherosclerosis*
   a) Pseudoxanthoma elasticum
   b) Hyperuricaemia
   c) (? Steroids in SLE)
3. *Fluid retention/cardiac decompensation*
   a) Phenylbutazone/indomethacin and other NSAIDs
   b) Salicylates
   c) Steroids

Cardiac involvement by rheumatic disease is often insignificant and asymptomatic, requiring thorough examination if it is to be detected. Recognition of cardiovascular involvement, however, is important since:

1. It may be an important feature that aids in diagnosis (e.g. pericarditis in Still's disease)
2. Cardiac disease may occasionally be a serious, life-threatening complication of rheumatic disorders (e.g. constrictive pericarditis in RA, myocardial disease in scleroderma)
3. Early correction of certain complications (e.g. fluid retention with phenylbutazone) may prevent serious consequences developing

Pericardial disease

Pericardial involvement in rheumatic disease is probably common, though clinical and post-mortem studies suggest that it is usually asymptomatic and of little consequence. Acute peri-

Rheumatic diseases that may cause pericarditis

1. *Commonly associated*
   a) Rheumatoid arthritis
   b) Still's disease
   c) SLE
   d) Mixed connective tissue disease
   e) Rheumatic fever
2. *Rarely associated*
   a) Ankylosing spondylitis
   b) Reiter's disease
   c) Scleroderma
   d) Dermato-myositis
   e) (Polyarteritis nodosa)
   f) (Polychondritis)

Rheumatic diseases that may cause myocarditis

1. *Commonly associated*
   a) Rheumatic fever
   b) Still's disease
   c) Rheumatoid arthritis
2. *Uncommonly associated*
   a) Scleroderma
   b) Amyloid (restrictive cardiomyopathy)
   c) SLE
   d) Mixed connective tissue disease
   e) (Haemochromatosis)
   f) (Sarcoid)

carditis may predate diagnosis of the underlying disease, particularly in RA and SLE, and may be an important feature in diagnosis (e.g. Still's disease, rheumatic fever). Treatment is aimed at rest, pain relief and control of the underlying disease.

Myocardial disease

Post-mortem studies reveal varying degrees of mononuclear cell infiltration of the myocardium in several rheumatic diseases, particularly RA, but the frequency and importance of subclinical myocarditis remains unknown.

Acute myocarditis is particularly a feature of rheumatic fever and Still's disease and usually presents with symptoms and signs of right and left heart failure. The ECG commonly shows minor ST and T-wave changes but rhythm and conduction disturbances, frequently just prolongation of the P–R interval, may also occur. Treatment is rest and diuretics with attention to the underlying disease, (possibly involving aspirin or steroids).

The chronic myocardial disease of rheumatic fever (p 412), scleroderma (p 117) and amyloid (p 318) are discussed elsewhere. Granulomatous or interstitial myocarditis with subsequent scar tissue involving the specialised conduction tissues may result in varying degrees of heart block — a complication especially noted with ankylosing spondylitis.

Rheumatic diseases that may produce conduction defects

1. *Commonly associated*
   Rheumatic fever
2. *Rarely associated*
   a) Ankylosing spondylitis
   b) Reiter's disease
   c) Rheumatoid arthritis
   d) Amyloidosis
   e) Dermato-myositis
   f) (Sarcoidosis)
   g) (Polychondritis)

Endocardial disease

The frequency of valvular disease in almost all rheumatic syndromes is disputed. Studies are made difficult by the common finding of 'benign' systolic murmurs (e.g. prolapsing mitral leaflet) in apparently normal individuals, and echocardiography has further increased the incidence of minor abnormalities detected.

Despite such difficulties, however, there does appear to be an association between valve disease and the conditions listed below. It should

Rheumatic diseases associated with aortic valve disease

1. *Stenosis*
   Rheumatic fever
2. *Incompetence*
   a) *Definitely associated*
      (i) Rheumatic fever
      (ii) Ankylosing spondylitis
      (iii) Reiter's disease
      (iv) Marfan's syndrome
      (v) Juvenile chronic arthritis
   b) *Probable/rare association*
      (i) SLE
      (ii) Mixed connective tissue disease
      (iii) Rheumatoid arthritis
      (iv) (Polychondritis)
      (v) (Morquio's and Sheie's syndromes)

be noted that, unlike uveitis 'lone', aortic incompetence shows no association with HLA-B27 and is therefore not considered a forme fruste of the seronegative spondarthritides.

Acute valve damage in association with rheumatic diseases is decidedly unusual, and rapidly changing murmurs with cardiac decompensation should always raise suspicion of infective endocarditis (p 205). Valve lesions should be treated surgically as required, bearing in mind any special operative or post-operative risks attendant on the underlying disease (e.g. cervical or temporomandibular disease, steroid treatment, Felty's syndrome).

Coronary arteritis

This is a rare but commonly fatal complication of:

Polyarteritis nodosa
Rheumatoid vasculitis
Giant cell arteritis
Muocutaneous lymph node syndrome

Clinical problems

Heart failure in a patient with rheumatic disease

Assessment of cardiac status in a patient with rheumatic disease frequently presents difficulties. Exertional symptoms, for example, may go unnoticed due to immobility, and fatigue and ankle swelling may be blamed on active disease. Interpretation of the JVP is difficult in the presence of severe cervical involvement, and hepatomegaly and oedema are frequent findings in patients with active RA. Further problems in assessment may be caused by concommitant lung disease.

Faced with such difficulties the following may in general be recommended:

1. Maintain a high index of suspicion of cardiac involvement
2. Perform as always, a full and careful examination
3. Do not place too much reliance on negative clinical findings in patients in whom signs are difficult to elicit — be prepared to investigate appropriately with chest X-ray, ECG or echocardiography
4. Always consider the possibility of drug induced fluid retention (a common cause of cardiac decompensation in elderly rheumatic patients)

Chest pain in a patient with rheumatic disease

As in non-rheumatic patients, correct diagnosis of chest pain requires a careful history and examination supplemented by a chest X-ray, ECG and other investigations as appropriate. In patients with rheumatic disease, however, concomitant joint and lung disease may cause particular difficulties in diagnosis of cardiac pain.

Chest pain due to pericardial disease is usually central but may radiate to the shoulder and upper arm and cause confusion with shoulder pain in a patient with active RA or SLE. The sharp quality of the pain, its accentuation on inspiration and lying flat, and inability to reproduce the pain on shoulder examination should, however, allow distinction. The definitive sign is a pericardial rub which is frequently localised and varies with time and position, but pleurisy commonly co-exists, especially in RA and SLE, and may cause difficulty in auscultatory diagnosis. The chest X-ray and echocardiogram are unhelpful except in the presence of an effusion, and the abnormality may only be shown on an ECG.

Patients with PAN, rheumatoid vasculitis or giant cell arteritis may present with chest pain and all the features of myocardial infarction, and in this situation differentiation from coronary insufficiency due to non-vasculitic causes is a difficult problem. Although angiography may demonstrate aneurysm formation in PAN, arteritis itself shows no distinctive angiographic features and the diagnosis is usually only made with confidence after death. In practice, the assumption that myocardial damage is due to vasculitis is usually made clinically because of the presence of marked disease activity elsewhere, and steroids are either instituted, or the existing dose increased. Evidence for benefit from steroids in this situation, however, is lacking and a careful watch must be kept for fluid retention.

Constrictive pericarditis

Constriction is uncommon but particularly occurs with RA. Chronic pericardial thickening is also a possible component of 'scleroderma heart' (p 117). Symptoms of constriction are predominantly those of right-sided failure (fatigue, exertional dyspnoea, ankle swelling, abdominal fullness), but these commonly go unnoticed in a severely affected patient with RA. Similarly, although sinus tachycardia, atrial fibrillation and small volume pulse (± paradox) should easily be detected, interpretation of the JVP (for rapid y descent and Kussmaul's sign) in a patient with severe neck involvement is difficult, and hepatomegaly and ankle oedema are often blamed on active rheumatoid disease. Difficulty with clinical signs in this situation, the insidious nature of the complication and the fact that the chest X-ray is unhelpful (showing a small or normal-sized heart, rarely pericardial calcification) usually results in a long delay in diagnosis. Catheterisation is required to confirm the diagnosis but differentiation from constrictive cardiomyopathy may be difficult (the latter usually gives rise to some cardiomegaly). Medical treatment of failure due to constriction is usually unsuccessful and pericardiectomy should be considered in the light of a full cardiac study and overall assessment of the patient's condition.

VI The Lung

The pleura, lung parenchyma and pulmonary vasculature may be involved in many of the rheumatic diseases as shown in Figure 15.19. In some conditions the pulmonary involvement is an integral part of the disease and is discussed fully in the relevant disease section. However, there are more general clinical problems related to the chest which recur time and again in rheumatological practice and often cause diagnostic and management difficulties.

PLEURAL EFFUSION

Pleural inflammation is common in RA, SLE and JCA. It may present as a sharp knife-like pain which is aggravated by breathing and coughing

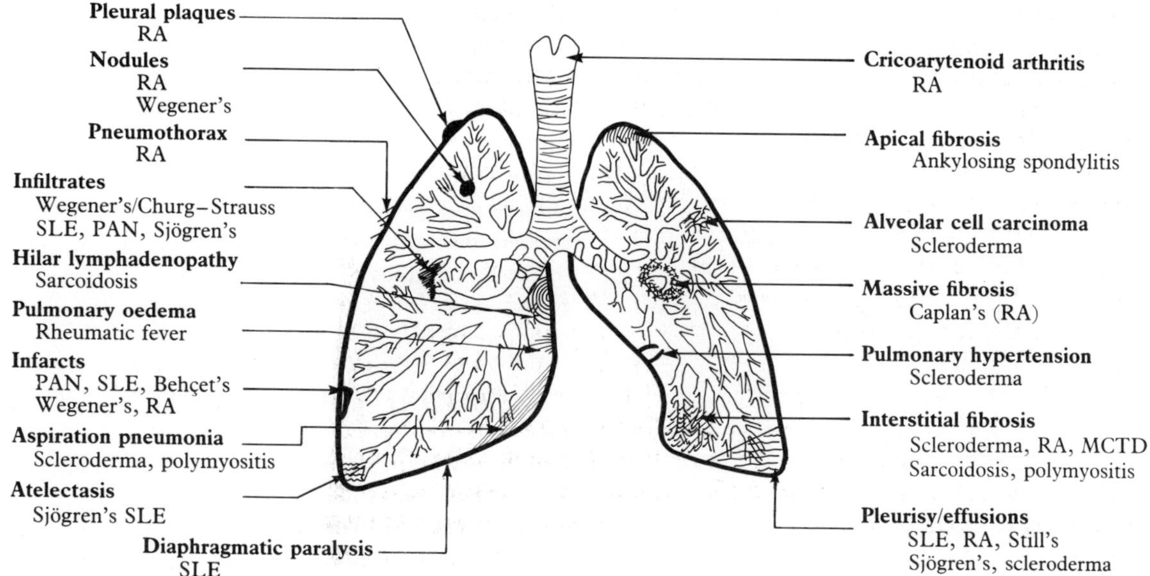

Fig. 15.19 Pulmonary involvement in rheumatic diseases.

and be accompanied by a pleural rub. Sometimes a rub is heard in the absence of pain and occasionally a large pleural effusion is found incidentally on clinical examination. This is particularly true in middle-aged men with acute systemic RA whose dominant features are weight-loss and anaemia, with relatively little joint disease in the early stages. This clinical picture may suggest a diagnosis of bronchial carcinoma or infection, particularly TB and a diagnostic aspiration is the single most useful test for sorting these out. The fluid should be sent for culture, cytology, biochemical analysis for sugar, LDH, protein and immunological analysis for rheumatoid factor, complement and immune complexes. The characteristics of a rheumatoid effusion are listed below. Occasionally there is still diagnostic uncertainty and this can usually be resolved by a pleural biopsy which often shows infiltration of plasma cells and lymphocytes in RA and sometimes a histological appearance indistinguishable from a rheumatoid nodule. Rheumatoid effusions are best left alone unless they are causing symptoms because they tend to recur rapidly and because, in a debilitated patient who may be receiving immunosuppressive drugs, there is a real risk of introducing infection. The fluid often becomes encysted if repeatedly aspirated and there also appears to be an increased risk of pneumothorax and bronchopleural fistula. The effusion is usually resorbed as the disease activity abates.

Characteristics of rheumatoid pleural fluid

1. Thick, yellow, cloudy appearance
2. High numbers of mononuclear cells
3. Comet cells on cytology
4. High LDH and protein
5. Low sugar and C3
6. Rheumatoid factor and immune complexes may be detected

PULMONARY FIBROSIS

In some rheumatic diseases e.g. scleroderma and polymyositis, pulmonary fibrosis occurs so frequently that it is considered to be a feature of the disease. Pulmonary fibrosis also occurs in patients with RA but there is still much discussion as to whether it is a disease feature, occurs by chance or is related to drug therapy. One study compared the chest X-ray appearance of patients with RA and matched controls but could find no difference in the incidence of pulmonary fibrosis in the two groups. Another study of patients with cryptogenic fibrosing alveolitis found that 16% of these patients had a seropositive polyarthritis indistinguishable from RA compared to an expected prevalence of 4%. Patients with RA often have reduced gas transfer on formal lung function testing in the presence of a normal chest X-ray, which implies that mild subclinical pulmonary fibrosis may be quite common. In practice there seem to be two distinct groups: those in whom pulmonary fibrosis is detected as a chance finding with fine late-inspiratory crepititions associated with reticulonodular shadowing on X-ray and those who present with breathlessness, clubbing and cynosis. Patients with symptoms usually follow a rapid downhill course and are dead on average within 5 years of onset, whereas the subclinical group seem to remain fairly static over many years. There is no accepted conventional treatment which will reverse the process in the badly-affected. Steroids are widely used but results are conflicting. It may be that those patients with a desquamative interstitial pneumonitis do better than those with established fibrosis but the two types can only be differentiated by bronchial lavage or lung biopsy. Penicillamine and cytotoxic drugs have also be used to treated pulmonary fibrosis but there are no good controlled studies on their usefulness.

SHADOW ON A CHEST X-RAY

Many types of shadow can occur on the chest X-ray of patients with rheumatic diseases. The recognition of these is often a matter of considerable practical importance since the patients are sometimes subjected to an unnecessary exploratory thoractomy to make a diagnosis.

Nodular shadows in lung parenchyma

Intrapulmonary nodules are a well-documented occurrence in patients with seropositive RA. They may be single or multiple and usually have a round or lobulated appearance. They do not invade the surrounding pulmonary tissue or cause distal collapse and are not necessarily associated with the presence of pleural disease. Although they can occur throughout the lungs there is a predilection for the upper lobes. They may come and go spontaneously and can occasionally break down, as do rheumatoid nodules elsewhere in the body, resulting in cavitation and haemoptysis. In the right clinical setting these nodules need usually just be observed on serial X-rays. Rarely, the pulmonary nodules appear before synovitis or nodules elsewhere and in these patients rheumatoid factor is usually negative. In such difficult cases, differential diagnosis must include carcinoma, lung abscess or hamartoma and sputum culture, cytology, bronchocopy and tomography may be needed alone or together to arrive at the correct answer. Only rarely will a biopsy be necessary. As a general rule it is better not to tamper with these nodules unless absolutely necessary because this may encourage them to break down and cause persistent bronchopleural fistulae.

There is a well-described limited form of Wegener's granulomatosis which presents with asymptomatic nodular shadows that are often found by chance on a chest X-ray. Biopsy is necessary to make the diagnosis since they have the same histological appearance as Wegener's granulomatosis elsewhere, namely necrotising granulomatous vasculitis. These patients rarely develop widespread systemic disease and the outlook is excellent.

Massive fibrotic nodules may develop in patients with RA who are exposed to inorganic dusts such as coal, silica or asbestos. The dust particles are thought to act as a nidus around which the fibrotic lesions develop.

Nodular fibrotic lesions are also a rare complication of ankylosing spondylitis. The apices of the lungs are affected, usually bilaterally. When these lesions were first described they were thought to be due to tuberculosis, but they are now recognised to be a feature of AS and may be related to the fixed rigid chest that is found in the more severely affected patients. These fibrotic lesions may cause parenchymal destruction and cyst formation. The cavities are prone to infection with *Aspergillus fumigatus*.

Pulmonary infiltrates

Areas of pneumonitis can occur in all forms of systemic vasculitis, particuarly SLE, PAN and Wegener's granulomatosis and Churg–Strauss syndrome and are also rarely a feature of Sjögren's syndrome. These areas are seen on a chest X-ray as patchy infiltrates which may come and go from day to day. Clinically, such pneumonitis may be asymptomatic or give rise to cough, mild dyspnoea or pain, accompanied by a local area of crepitation or reduced breath sounds.

Pulmonary infiltration also characterises the chronic form of sarcoidosis. The mid-zones are usually involved, giving a striking mottled appearance on the X-ray, but there is little disturbance of respiratory function. About a quarter of patients go on to develop true fibrosis, again usually in the midzones but this is associated with a better prognosis than diffuse idiopathic pulmonary fibrosis.

Pleural plaques

Thickened areas of pleura are common in patients with RA and scleroderma. In RA they are usually asymptomatic and are sometimes associated with intrapulmonary nodules or pleural effusions. In scleroderma they may give rise to coarse, creaking pleural rubs.

Pulmonary infarcts

Peripherally-placed wedge-shaped shadows are characteristic of pulmonary infarction and may occur in patients with systemic vasculitis, particularly SLE, PAN, Wegener's granulomatosis and rheumatoid disease. In Behcet's syndrome thère is, in addition, a hypercoagulability state. Patients with a pulmonary infarct present with pleuritic

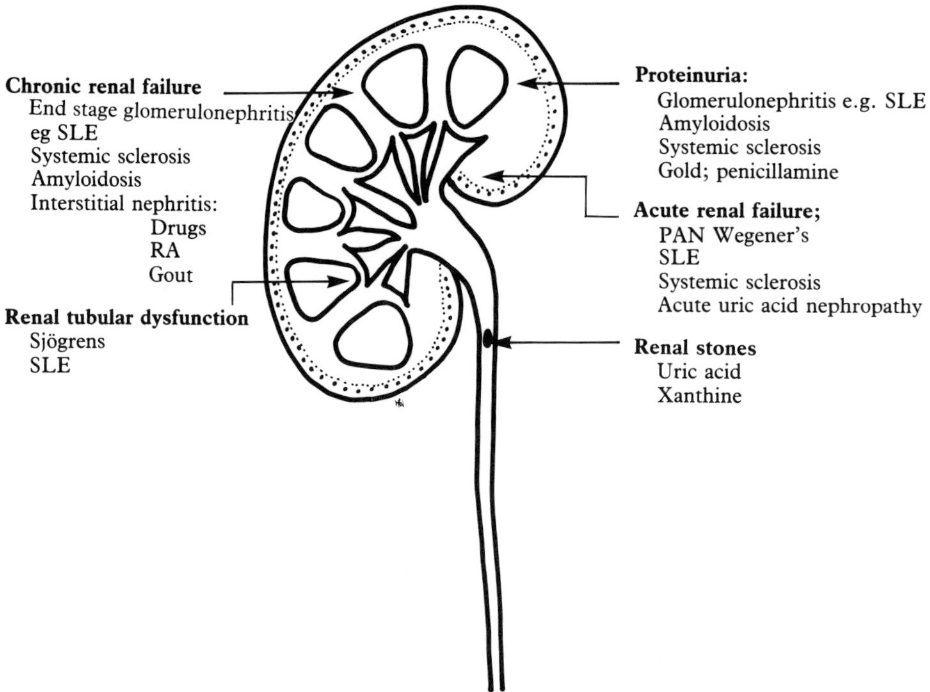

Fig. 15.20 Renal involvement in the rheumatic diseases

chest pain occasionally accompanied by cough and haemoptysis. It may be very difficult clinically to distinguish between pulmonary infarction and pleural disease and the chest X-ray appearance and lung scan will help. Even when infarction is established as the cause of the symptoms, it may be due to local vasculitis in the pulmonary vessels or result from embolisation from a venous thrombosis. By assessing the activity of the underlying disease and looking for evidence of a deep venous thrombosis it may be possible to decide between these two possibilities but sometimes patients have to be treated as if they had both to be on the safe side. Recurrent small pulmonary infarcts are thought to be one cause of the 'shrinking lung' syndrome in SLE.

FURTHER READING (LUNG)

Epler GR 1979 Pulmonary manifestations of connective tissue diseases. In: Cohen AS (ed) Rheumatology and immunology. The science and practice of clinical medicine Grune & Stratton, New York.

VII The Kidney

Certain rheumatic diseases commonly affect the kidney (Fig. 15.20). This is particularly true for the rarer systemic rheumatic diseases such as systemic lupus erythematosus (SLE), progressive systemic sclerosis (PSS) and the systemic vasculitides. On the other hand, rheumatoid arthritis rarely affects the kidneys although drugs used to treat this disease may do so.

PROTEINURIA

Proteinuria poses an important diagnostic problem in rheumatology. Major causes are listed below and may be due to the disease itself, to the development of a complication such as amyloidosis or as a result of treatment such as gold or penicillamine.

Causes of proteinuria in rheumatic diseases

1. Glomerulonephritis
   a) Common
      (i) SLE
      (ii) PAN
      (iii) Wegener's granulomatosis
      (iv) Henoch-Schönlein purpura
   b) Rare
      (i) Polymyositis
      (ii) Sjogren's syndrome
      (iii) Rheumatoid arthritis
2. Drugs
   a) Gold
   b) Penicillamine
3. Amyloidosis
   a) RA
   b) Ankylosing spondylitis
   c) JCA
   d) FMF
4. Systemic sclerosis

1. Glomerulonephritis

Proteinuria is the commonest manifestation of glomerulonephritis which frequently complicates SLE and the systemic vasculitides such as PAN and Wegener's granulomatosis. Mild to moderate proteinuria (up to 3 g per day), frequently accompanied by microscopic haematuria, is often the only clinical feature of lupus nephritis but sometimes marked proteinuria leading to the nephrotic syndrome may occur. Severe lupus nephritis is accompanied by renal failure, and progressive renal impairment is the rule in PAN and Wegener's. Glomerulonephritis is an uncommon manifestation of other systemic rheumatic diseases such as polymyositis and Sjögren's syndrome and is a rare feature of rheumatoid disease. In RA the much more likely cause of proteinuria is toxicity due to gold or penicillamine, or the development of amyloidosis.

2. Gold and penicillamine

Treatment with both gold and penicillamine can be complicated by an immune-complex glomerulonephritis manifested predominantly by proteinuria. 5–10% of patients on gold and 10–15% on penicillamine develop proteinuria which may reach nephrotic proportions. It is usually not accompanied by renal impairment and is generally reversible on discontinuing the drug, although resolution may take many months.

3. Amyloidosis

Amyloidosis is a complication seen in up to 5% of RA patients but may also develop during the course of other chronic rheumatic diseases such as ankylosing spondylitis and chronic juvenile arthritis. It is also a major complication of FMF. It results in progressive proteinuria often leading to the nephrotic syndrome and subsequently progressive renal impairment and death from renal failure.

Diagnosis of proteinuria

Once common causes of proteinuria such as urinary tract infection, and non-renal causes such as congestive cardiac failure, have been excluded, persistent proteinuria, which always has pathological significance, needs further investigation. Finding red-cell casts on examination of the sediment from a mid-stream specimen of urine is an important clue to glomerular injury but other investigations such as differential protein clearance have very limited diagnostic value in this situation and renal biopsy is essential to the diagnosis of proteinuria in these diseases. When proteinura develops in rheumatoid patients treated with gold or penicillamine renal biopsy should be performed if there is renal impairment or if proteinuria persists unchanged for 3 months after the drugs are stopped. When PAN is suspected some advocate the use of angiography prior to blind renal biopsy because of the risk of rupturing a micro-aneurysm.

The renal biopsy should, if possible, be examined by immunofluorescence and electron microscopy as well as by light microscopy. The histology of these conditions is described in other chapters. A wide variety of histological lesions are seen on light microscopy in lupus nephritis, including minimal mesangial proliferation, severe glomerular inflammation with prominant intracapillary cellular proliferation, areas of fibrinoid necrosis, epithelial crescent formation and diffuse thickening of the glomerular basement membrane with no proliferative changes. However, the major feature of lupus nephritis, common to all these histological types, is the prominent granular deposition of immunoglobulin and complement in the mesangium and in the capillary loops, which can be demonstrated by immunofluorescence. In contrast, the glomerulonephritis of PAN and Wegener's is not characterised by these marked findings on immunofluorescence microscopy.

In drug-induced nephropathy gold deposits have been demonstrated in the renal tubules and interstitial tissues but the major lesion in gold nephropathy is a membranous glomerulonephritis with deposition of immunoglobulin and complement in the glomeruli. In penicillamine nephropathy light-microscopic changes are often minimal, though subepithelial deposits are demonstrated by EM and consist of immunoglobulin and complement. Occasionally a Goodpasture-like syndrome is seen with penicillamine.

RENAL IMPAIRMENT

1. Acute renal failure

Acute renal failure is a major complication in PAN and Wegener's granulomatosis and occurs in some patients with severe lupus glomerulonephritis. Clinical renal disease in systemic sclerosis usually takes the form of highly-malignant arterial hypertension leading to rapidly progressive and irreversible renal failure. This often occurs early in the course of the disease. Although hypertension and high plasma renin levels are the rule, renal failure sometimes occurs with normal blood-pressure.

Causes of acute renal failure in rheumatic diseases

1. Acute glomerulonephritis:
   PAN
   Wegener's granulomatosis
   SLE
2. Systemic sclerosis
3. Acute uric acid nephropathy
4. Severe interstitial nephritis: SLE

Anuria is rarely seen but may occur in acute uric acid nephropathy in which precipitation of uric acid crystals in the collecting tubules and ureters leads to obstruction. This uncommon complication most often occurs in patients with a profound overproduction of uric acid secondary to leukaemia or lymphoma, particularly when receiving treatment. Rarely, it occurs in other situations, such as gouty patients with marked uricosuria and in individuals following severe and unaccustomed exercise or convulsions.

Occasionally NSAIDs cause a marked but reversible reduction in glomerular filtration rate and renal blood flow, probably via inhibition of prostaglandin synthetase.

2. Chronic renal failure

Progressive renal failure is the rule when the kidneys are involved in Wegener's granulomatosis and PAN. In these conditions renal failure is the commonest cause of death. It is also a major cause of death in SLE, although a smaller proportion with renal involvement progress to chronic renal failure. A small proportion of patients with Henoch–Schonlein purpura are now known to develop severe and permanent renal damage.

Causes of chronic renal failure in rheumatic diseases

1. End-stage glomerulonephritis
2. Systemic sclerosis
3. Amyloidosis
4. Interstitial nephritis: Drugs
   Gout
   RA

The development of amyloidosis during the course of a chronic rheumatic disease is associated with a poor prognosis, since virtually all develop progressive renal impairment.

Causes of chronic renal failure in RA other than amyloidosis are rare, although death from chronic renal failure is more common in RA than in the general population, and in one large series accounted for 17% of deaths. To what extent these changes are due to the disease *per se* or due to the drugs used to treat it is not known. Most, if not all, non-steroidal anti-inflammatory agents are potentially nephrotoxic and produce renal papillary necrosis in animals. However, with the exception of mixtures of aspirin and phenacetin, they have only rarely been associated with renal papillary necrosis, and there is little convincing evidence that they cause significant renal damage in the majority of patients.

The finding of an increased urinary excretion of the lysosomal enzyme p-N-acetyl glucosaminidase (NAG), an indicator of renal parenchymal damage, in patients with untreated RA suggests that interstitial nephritis may be a feature of the disease *per se*. Similarly, there is an increased incidence of impaired renal function in patients with gout. Longstanding advanced tophaceous gout with hyperuricaemia and marked uricosuria may be acompanied by a urate nephropathy which contributes to the deteriorating renal function. In such cases deposits of uric acid can be found in the renal interstitial tissue sometimes with associated inflammation. In lesser degrees of hyperuricaemia the contribution of raised serum uric acid levels *per se* to renal impairment as opposed to accompanying age-related changes and nephrosclerosis due to hypertension is contraversial.

RENAL STONES

5–10% of all urinary calculi in the UK and USA are composed of uric acid, although the proportion is higher in other parts of the world, such as Israel (40%). Very few of those with stones have gout, oversecretion of uric acid being a feature of stone-formers and undersecretion being common in patients with gout (see Chapter 9). Hyperuricosuria predisposes to calcium-containing stones as well as to urate calculi.

The prevalence of renal calculi in gouty subjects is falling. Previous estimates suggested that about 20% of patients developed stones, but recent surveys put the figure well below this. The rare 'over-producer' is at risk, but the under-secretors rarely develop problems. Occasionally xanthine or oxipurinol calculi have been described in patients treated with the xanthine oxidase inhibitor allopurinol.

RENAL TUBULAR DYSFUNCTION

Renal tubular abnormalities are one of the systemic manifestations of Sjogren's syndrome and result from a chronic interstitial nephritis with infiltration of the interstitium with vast numbers of lymphocytes and plasma cells. The commonest defect is inability to concentrate or acidify the urine, but a more global tubular defect may occur with amino aciduria, glycosuria and phosphaturia. Similar abnormalities are rarely seen in SLE.

FURTHER READING (KIDNEY)

Bacon P A, Hadler N M 1982 The kidney and rheumatic diseases. Butterworth, London

VIII The Gastrointestinal Tract and Liver

GASTROINTESTINAL TRACT

The gastrointestinal tract may be directly involved by the pathological process of a rheumatic disease or as a consequence of therapy. A list of common gastrointestinal symptoms and some causes are given in Figure 15.21.

Dysphagia

This may occur as a result of arthritis affecting the TMJ, which makes chewing painful. Patients with a dry mouth from sicca syndrome, which is particularly common in patients with RA, scleroderma, lupus and MCTD, find chewing and swallowing very difficult unless water is drunk along with each mouthful of food. In the most severe cases, even talking is difficult and the teeth decay rapidly. Oral ulceration is a feature of SLE,

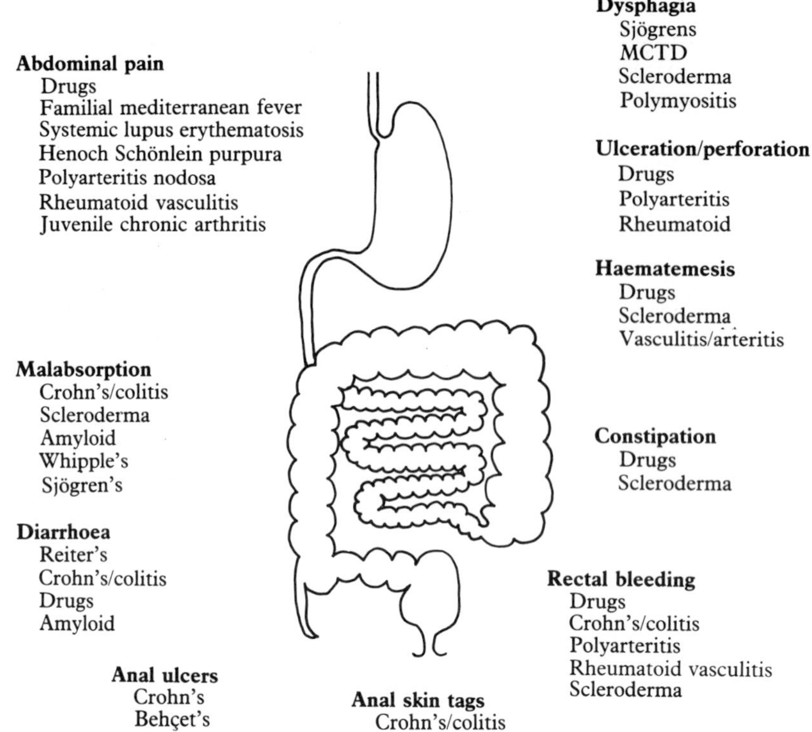

Fig. 15.21 Gut involvement in the rheumatic diseases

Reiter's, Behçet's and may be a sign of vascultis in RA. Gold therapy may cause stomatitis and severe oral ulceration and many patients find that in the early stages of taking penicillamine they lose their sense of taste and hence their interest in food. Patients with scleroderma may have several problems combining to cause dysphagia. Tightening of the skin round the mouth may be so severe that the mouth can barely be opened wide enough to eat. Lack of saliva may make swallowing difficult and further down the oesophagus, fibrosis and stricture may cause solid food to stick. The oesophagus is often atonic and dilated so that the food residue may reflux into the lungs, particularly at night, causing atelectasis and infection which may cause further respiratory problems in patients already predisposed by their disease to pulmonary fibrosis. In order to detect mild degrees of oesophageal involvement in scleroderma a barium swallow should be done with the patient lying slightly head down and prone in order to demonstrate pooling and reflux. Polymyositis may also cause dysphagia and aspiration of food due to weakness of the muscles of the pharynx and larynx.

Abdominal pain

Abdominal pain is very common in patients with rheumatic diseases. By far the commonest cause is gastritis or peptic ulceration as a result of treatment with NSAIDs or steroids, although there is some evidence that patients with RA may be predisposed to develop peptic ulceration even in the absence of treatment. The symptoms may range from vague generalised discomfort in the abdomen to more typical frank peptic ulceration with localised epigastric pain accompanied by nocturnal waking and relieved with food. Many patients obtain relief of symptoms by changing or reducing the tablets or adding an antacid. It is often difficult to decide which patients warrant further investigation. Duration and severity of symptoms, together with other features such as anaemia and epigastric tenderness, are the best guidelines. The results of barium meal or endoscopy are not predictable on the basis of the clinical symptoms in many cases. Some patients with the worst symptoms have normal endoscopic examination or show just a few shallow erosions. Ulcers in patients on NSAIDs are often large and located in the prepyloric region, although this is by no means a specific feature.

Patients with scleroderma may have episodes of generalised abdominal discomfort due to pseudo-obstruction of the bowel.

Abdominal crisis

Sudden severe abdominal pain accompanied by collapse is very likely to be due to perforation of the stomach or duodenum secondary to peptic ulceration. In diseases such as PAN, severe rheumatoid vasculitis or other arteritides, infarction of the bowel would also be high on the list of differential diagnoses. The cytotoxic drug azathioprine is increasingly used to treat a number of rheumatic diseases and this has been reported to cause severe upper abdominal pain and vomiting in a few patients shortly after starting treatment. The serum amylase is raised, suggesting that the underlying cause may be drug-induced acute pancreatitis. Severe abdominal pain is a feature of Henoch–Schönlein purpura and is probably due to involvement of the bowel by vasculitis. Intermittent self-limiting attacks of severe cramping abdominal pain and fever mimicking peritonitis are characteristic of FMF. Osteoporotic collapse of vertabrae in patients treated with steroids may cause referred pain in the abdomen.

Weight-loss

When an inflammatory polyarthritis such as RA is very active there may be considerable systemic disturbance with marked weight-loss. The degree of emaciation may be so severe that it resembles the cachexia of malignant disease. Such patients usually have anaemia, raised plasma viscosity and ESR, elevated acute phase proteins, alkaline phosphatase and platelet count and high titres of rheumatoid factor. Weight will not normally be regained until the disease activity is brought under control with drugs or subsides spontaneously. If a patient with long-standing RA suddenly starts to lose weight out of proportion to the activity of the disease the possibility of amyloidosis, lymphoma (particularly in those with sicca syndrome), occult joint sepsis, depression or Felty's syndrome should be considered as well as other general causes of weight-loss such as carcinoma and hyperthyroidism.

In scleroderma, the bowel wall may become thickened, dilated and poorly peristaltic resulting in a blind-loop syndrome from bacterial overgrowth and this causes considerable weight-loss from malabsorption. The dilated loops of bowel may also undergo episodes of pseudo-obstruction in which the abdomen becomes distended and uncomfortable. Marked weight-loss is also a feature of Whipple's disease and is caused by malabsorption due to infiltration of the intestinal mucosa by rod-shaped organisms.

Crohn's disease and ulcerative colitis may initially present to the rheumatologist with an arthritis or arthralgia without diarrhoea or abdominal pain. There may, however, be weight-loss and subtle evidence of malabsorption such as anaemia and a low serum folic acid.

Gastrointestinal bleeding

Studies have shown that nearly all patients on NSAIDs lose blood from the stomach, in the order of 5 ml a day, in the absence of frank peptic ulceration or erosions. Tests for blood in the motions of such patients are therefore likely to be positive. Bleeding may become much heavier when there is ulceration or erosion and can present as haematemesis, melaena or anaemia. Occasionally, the lower end of the oesophagus may bleed catastrophically in scleroderma.

Rectal bleeding may be a feature of Crohn's disease or ulcerative colitis and can also follow bowel infarction in the vasculitic disorders, particularly PAN, rheumatoid vascultis and Henoch–Schönlein purpura.

Diarrhoea

If a patient with an acute arthritis, particularly of the Reiter's type, develops diarrhoea, the possibility of a specific gut infection, particularly with *Shigella* or *Campylobacter* should be considered. A large joint lower-limb arthropathy associated with sacro-iliitis may occur in Crohn's disease and ulcerative colitis and occasionally the arthritis presents before the intestinal disease is apparent. The presence of erythema nodusum or pyoderma gangrenosum, uveitis, oral lesions or anal skin tags, weight-loss and anaemia may be useful additional clues. Amyloid disease may cause diarrhoea, either by direct infiltration of the mucosa of the bowel wall or indirectly as part of an automonic neuropathy. Sclerodermatous involvement of the small bowel may result in poorly-peristaltic loops of bowel which may become contaminated by bacteria causing bouts of malabsorption and diarrhoea and may improve following a course of antibiotics to clear the bowel.

Whipple's disease causes fatty diarrhoea and may present with an arthritis mimicking RA. Rod-shaped organisms can be detected in the jejunal mucosa and the affected synovium. Although Whipple's is a rare disease, it is an important diagnosis since antibiotic therapy is curative.

Drugs, particularly colchicine and the fenamates, cause diarrhoea as a side-effect, and occasionally a proctitis results from the use of anti-inflammatory suppositories.

Constipation

Patients with painful joints often have difficulty getting to the toilet to respond to the call to defecate and consequently are prone to constipation. Drugs, particularly DF118 and other codeine derivatives, are also constipating. Sclerodermatous involvement of the large bowel may also cause sluggish colonic peristalsis and severe constipation.

LIVER

Below are listed some recognised associations between liver disorders and the rheumatic diseases.

Hepatic involvement in rheumatic diseases

1. *Generalised disorders affecting both liver and joints*
   a) Haemochromatosis
   b) Sarcoidosis
   c) Mucopolysaccharidoses
   d) Amyloidosis
   e) PAN
   f) Temporal arteritis/polymyalgia rheumatica
   g) Infections — infectious mononucleosis, hepatitis B, TB, syphilis, gonorrhoea (perihepatitis)
2. *Rheumatological disease with recognised hepatic involvement*
   a) Rheumatoid arthritis
   b) Adult-onset Still's disease (hepatomegaly, hepatitis)
3. *Hepatic disease with recognised rheumatological manifestations*
   a) Primary biliary cirrhosis PBC) (arthralgia, ± hypercholesterolaemic arthropathy)
   b) Chronic active hepatitis (CAH) (arthralgia, necrotising vasculitis, mixed essential cryoglobulinaemia)
   c) Wilson's disease (osteoporosis, chondrocalcinosis, osteoarthritis)
   d) Alcoholic cirrhosis (polyarthritis, Dupuytren's contracture)
4. *Disease associations*
   a) PBC + CRST syndrome
   b) PBC/CAH + Sicca/Sjögren's syndrome
5. *Hepatotoxic agents used in treatment of rheumatic diseases*
   a) Aspirin (marked sensitivity in SLE)
   b) Phenylbutazone (hepatitis)
   c) Gold (hypersensitivity cholestasis)
   d) Penicillamine (hepatitis + cholestasis)
   e) Azathioprine/chlorombucil/6MP (allergic hepatitis)
   f) Methotrexate (hepatitis progressing to diffuse fibrosis)
   g) Allopurinol (granulomatous hepatitis + jaundice)
   h) Benoxaprofen (now withdrawn)
6. *Acute-phase protein response by liver*
   Abnormal response in SLE, scleroderma

Hepatomegaly

A soft hepatomegaly may be detected clinically in patients with an active arthritis, particularly RA, and may reflect increased activity of the RES. A firm liver is often palable in patients with Felty's syndrome and amyloidosis.

Abnormal liver function tests

A mild disturbance of liver function is common in patients with an active rheumatic disease. The alkaline phosphatase behaves very much like an acute-phase reactant and rises and falls with disease activity and this is frequently accompanied by a reciprocal fall in the serum albumin. A marked persistent elevation of liver enzymes should raise the possibility of primary biliary cirrhosis or serum hepatitis, which may present with an arthritis. Patients with SLE who are treated with salicylates often develop abnormal liver function and this type of drug should probably be avoided. The NSAIDs as a group can also cause mild disturbance of liver function in some patients and in this situation the drug should be changed to one from another pharmacological group. Experience with the drug benoxaprofen has taught that the elderly in particular may be susceptible to liver damage on long-acting NSAIDs and should be monitored for this. If an elderly housebound patient with rheumatoid or some other form of disabling arthritis has persistently marked and inappropriate elevation of the alkaline phosphatase the iso-enzymes should be requested since osteomalacia is common in this sort of patient as a result of dietary vitamin D deficiency.

REFERENCES (GASTROINTESTINAL)

Gastrointestinal disease and arthritis. In: Cohen A S (ed) Rheumatology and immunology. The science and practice of clinical medicine 4. Grune & Stratton, New York 1979

Hawkins C F 1978 Rheumatic disease and the alimentary tract. In: Arthritis and Rheumatism Council for Research Reports on the rheumatic diseases. London

IX The central nervous system

Rheumatic diseases can affect various different anatomical sites within the central nervous system (Fig. 15.22). Intracranial lesions can result from vascular events complicating some of the connective tissue disorders. Lesions of the foramen magnum, spina cord and cauda equina may be secondary to diseases of the vertebral column causing instability, or space-occupying lesions. Psychiatric disturbances also result from chronic rheumatic conditons, either directly via organic brain damage or indirectly from pain and disability.

CLINICAL PROBLEM: EXAMINATION OF THE CNS IN PATIENTS WITH RHEUMATIC DISEASES

The neurological examination presents special problems in patients with disorders of muscles and joints. *Sensory* testing is usually straightforward, although atlanto-axial subluxation in rheumatoid arthritis can present with symptoms and signs similar to those of a peripheral neuropathy, and it may be difficult to differentiate those from other causes of sensory disturbance. Tingling and numbness in the hands or feet present the biggest problems: a numb hand may be due to entrapment of the median or ulna nerve (or sometimes both at the wrist), cervical root pressure, cord compression, mononeuritis multiplex of peripheral nerves, or a sensory polyneuropathy. Careful analysis may be difficult in a deformed, immobile rheumatic hand which is sometimes ulcerated, or painful due to active joint disease.

Motor testing is even more difficult. Joint disorders cause painful restriction of movement and reflex wasting and inhibition of muscles, making a complete assessment of power impossible. Coordination is also impaired when there is severe muscle-wasting and joint restriction of movement. Reflexes may be absent if joints are ankylosed or the tendons impeded. The commonest examples are absence of the knee jerk due to severe patello-femoral disease or an abnormal quadriceps tendon,

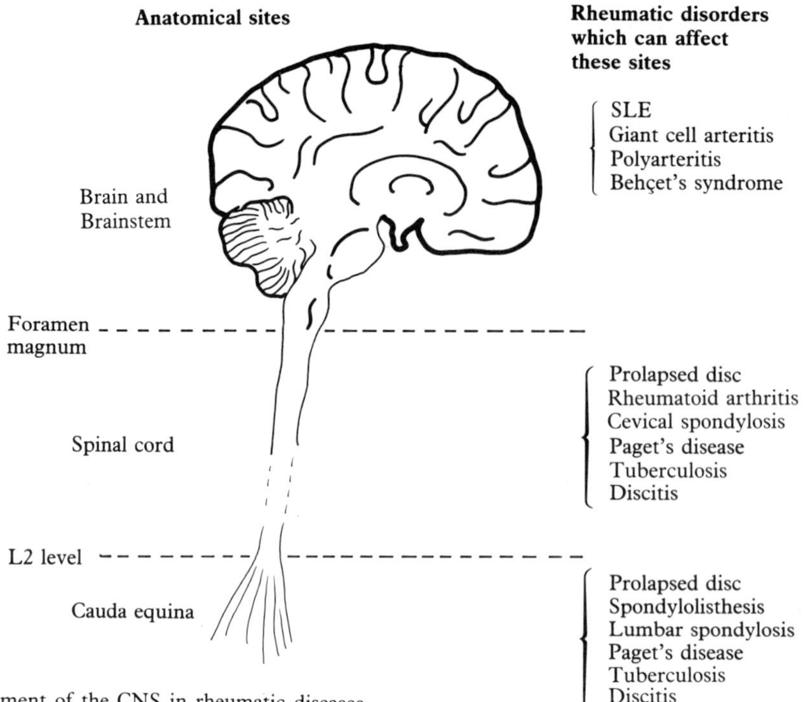

Fig. 15.22 Involvement of the CNS in rheumatic diseases

a lost ankle jerk in severe hindfoot disease and absence of finger jerks and Hoffman's sign due to deformity and immobility of the fingers. The plantar response may be impossible to elicit or even misleading in advanced forefoot disease, especially if there has been surgical intervention (e.g. a Keller's or Fowler's operation). Some rheumatic diseases cause a combination of joint and muscle disease, making neurological assessment even more difficult, and combinations of central (cord or root) and peripheral (nerve entrapment or neuropathy) lesions affecting the limb may occur. The patient with advanced destructive joint disease, in whom increasing weakness raises suspicion of possible compression of the cord (often at the atlanto-axial region) can present a particularly difficult and worrying diagnostic problem.

INTRACRANIAL LESIONS

Diseases which cause a vasculitis can affect intracranial blood vessels and result in a variety of focal neurological lesions. SLE can also cause diffuse brain damage and a wider spectrum of neuropsychiatric disturbances.

Giant cell arteritis often involves the superficial temporal and retinal arteries, and the commonest neurological lesion is visual disturbance or sudden blindness due to occlusion of ciliary or retinal vessels. Cerebral arteries may be involved, resulting in a 'stroke'. Cerebrovascular accidents are also rare complications of PAN, SLE, Wegener's granulomatosis and Behçet's syndrome. Hyperviscosity syndromes complicating connective-tissue disease can block small intracranial blood

Rheumatic disorders which can result in focal intracranial ischaemic lesion

1. Giant cell arteritis
2. Polyarteritis nodosa
3. SLE
4. Behçet's syndrome
5. Wegner's granulomatosis
6. Hypervisocisty syndrome

vessels, giving rise to a variety of different neurological signs.

CNS involvement occurs in over half of all SLE patients. A wide variety of syndromes have been described. Psychiatric disturbances are frequent and range from mild depression or depersonalisation to a frank psychosis. Migraines and personality changes during active phases of the disease are prominent and may be a helpful guide to the disease state. Epilepsy and damage to cranial nerves of the eye are not infrequent. Hemiplegia, paraplegia, chorea, cerebellar ataxia and other cranial nerve lesions are rare but well-recognised features of the disease.

Clinical manifestations of CNS involvement in SLE

1. Common
   a) Psychiatric disturbance
   b) Depression
   c) Epilepsy
   d) Migraine
   e) Occular cranial nerve lesions
2. Uncommon
   a) Psychosis
   b) Hemiplegia
   c) Paraplegia
   d) Cerebellar ataxia
   e) Chorea
   f) Other cranial nerve lesions
   g) Meningitis
   h) Coma

Behçet's syndrome can also cause a wide variety of CNS manifestations. A meningitic picture, with chronic headaches and possible cranial nerve or long tract signs, may develop, and involvement of the brain stem, ophthalmoplegias and Parkinsonian changes can also occur.

LESIONS AROUND THE FORAMEN MAGNUM AND UPPER CERVICAL SPINE

The complex anatomy of this region contributes to its susceptibility to damage from a special group of disorders of the musculoskeletal system.

1. Basilar impression

This is the extension of the arch of the atlas into the foramen magnum. It is associated with the odontoid peg of the axis compressing the lower part of the brain stem and can also result in lesions of the long sensory tract of the fifth cranial nerve (especially the ophthalmic divison, causing loss of sensation over the forehead and depression of the corneal reflex), the lower cranial nerves, upper cervical roots and cord. A wide variety of neurological signs occur. The causes include congenital malformations of the occipital condyles, osteogenous imperfecta, Klippel–Feil syndrome, Paget's disease and rheumatoid arthritis with vertical atlanto-axial subluxation. The radiological features of basilar impression (platybasia) can occur in the absence of any neurological lesion.

Causes of platybasia

1. Osteogenesis imperfecta
2. Congential malformations of occipital condlyes
3. Klippel–Feil syndrome
4. Paget's disease
5. Rheumatoid arthritis

2. Atlanto-axial subluxation

This is caused by rheumatoid arthritis, severe neck trauma or, very rarely, as a complication of ankylosing spondylitis. It can damage C2 nerve roots, the vertebral arteries and the upper cervical cord.

Causes of atlanto-axial subluxation

1. Trauma
2. Rheumatoid arthritis
3. Ankylosing spondylitis (rare)

Cord compression due to atlanto-axial subluxation classically presents with quadraplegia and a high sensory level. However, the onset is often insidious, symptoms may be confined to the hands or feet and the signs may be subtle or suggestive of a higher or lower level of cord damage. The sensory divison of the fifth cranial nerve and C2 roots are often affected, and neck pain and stiffness are usual. Some involvement of the spinal blood vessels may contribute to the patchy, variable and confusing neurological signs that sometimes occur. Examination is particularly difficult in the chronic severe rheumatoid patient on steroids who is susceptible to this complication. A high level of clinical suspicion, and myelography in the presence of definite neurological signs, are necessary to establish the level and nature of the lesion. Neurological involvement correlates poorly with the degree of instability seen on plain flexion and extension radiographs.

3. Vertebro-basilar insufficiency

Transient interruption of blood flow in the vertebral arteries can also result from lesions around the foramen magnum and upper cervical spine. Causes include cervical spondylosis and rheumatoid arthritis as well as many other disease of the blood vessels, bones and joints of the spine.

A variety of brain stem structures may be involved, and the features include vertigo, diplopia, transient hemianopia or blindness and parasthesiae or weakness of a limb. Attacks are sometimes induced by neck movements (especially extension), and a reduced, painful range of motion of the cervical spine is usually present.

THE SPINAL CORD AND CAUDA EQUINA

Spinal cord compression can result from a variety of diseases within the spinal canal and cord itself, as well as from disorders of the vertebral column. The commoner vertebral causes are listed. The likely pathology depends partly on the level of involvement. Cervical cord compression (usually around C5 and C6) may be due to a central disc protrusion, cervical spondylosis or rheumatoid arthritis. Damage to the thoracic or lumbar cord can be caused by infections including tuberculosis (Pott's disease of the spine) and discitis as well as disc disease and spondylitis. Cauda equina lesions are usually associated with a congenitally narrow canal which becomes further compromised by a spondylolisthesis, disc protrusion or spondylosis.

Rheumatic disorders which can cause spinal cord compression

1. Spondylosis
2. Spondylolisthesis
3. Central disc prolapse
4. Paget's disease
5. Spinal tuberculosis
6. Staphylococcal discitis
7. Rheumatoid arthritis

Paget's disease and primary or secondary neoplasms of the vertebral bodies can affect any level of the spinal cord. Severe trauma to the vertebral column is one of the commonest causes of spinal compression. Osteopaenic vertebral collapse rarely causes cord damage, although nerve roots are frequently involved.

Clinical features depend on the level of the lesion, the rate of onset and the degree of interference with the blood-supply to the spinal cord. Involvement of the spinal roots at the level of the compression causes radicular symptoms and signs, and interruption of the long ascending and descending tracts produces variable sensory and upper motor neurone changes below. A slowly progressive lesion tends to cause pyramidal tract involvement first and posterior column loss next; spinothalamic and sphincter disturbances are late features.

The neurological signs may be accompanied by signs in the back itself. Flexion may produce pain shooting down the spine below the lesion (Lhermitte's sign); local tenderness is indicative of an inflammatory or neoplastic lesion of vertebral bodies; painful restriction of movement is usually present and may be accompanied by deformities such as a kyphoscoliosis; rheumatoid subluxation or a lumbar spondylolisthesis may be palpable; overt swelling or heat over the spine are occasionally present.

The likely diagnosis depends on the age and sex of the patient, on the presence of any known disease such as RA, and on the level of damage. Plain radiographs are essential, but myelography is usually necessary to outline the exact level involved. Spinal cord compression is an emergency situation that requires prompt investigation and surgical intervention when possible.

Intermittent claudication of the cauda equina

Damage to the cauda equina can cause particular diagnostic difficulty. The common presentation is with aching in the calves, paraesthesia in the legs on exercise and/or foot-drop in an elderly person. A mixture of variable upper and lower motor neurone signs in the legs and sphincter disturbance are often present. In many cases signs and symptoms only develop on exercise and are relieved by rest. This is probably due to a combination of postural changes (the lumbar lordosis is exaggerated on on standing and exercising) and oedema of the canal causing direct pressure, as well as vascular insufficiency of the spinal arteries. Riding a bicycle (the lumbar spine is flexed) is usually asymptomatic, and symptoms may be relieved by bending forwards. The patients are usually elderly, and the syndrome may be confused with vascular claudication of the legs. However, neurological signs such as reduced reflexes and sensory loss may appear transiently after exercise, and peripheral pulses are generally normal. Plain radiographs usually show a narrow canal with lumbar spondylosis or spondylolisthesis; rarely a variety of other vertebral or canal lesions induce the syndrome.

PSYCHIATRIC CHANGES

Psychiatric abnormalities in patients with rheumatic disorders may be due to the disease affecting the brain, to drugs or to inability to cope with the pain, disability or deformity present.

SLE frequently causes psychiatric changes due to direct involvement of the cerebral cortex; Behçet's syndrome and PAN occasionally have similar effects. Drugs which can cause problems include steroids (mania, depression or psychosis), indomethacin (confusion, dizziness and depression, especially in the elderly) and others.

Some degree of depression, anger, frustration and resentment is normal in patients with a chronic painful disabling disease like RA. Quite severe depression can occur and is more common when inflammatory disease is active. The patient's outcome, in terms of his ability to function and cope with life in spite of his disability, is very dependent on the personality and degree of psychiatric disturbance produced by the disease. Management includes treatment of the inflammatory disease process, helping with the functional difficulties and discussing the problems with the patient and his family. Formal anti-depressant therapy is sometimes useful to lift mood, and may also reduce musculoskeletal pain.

TWO CLINICAL PROBLEMS

1. Headache

Headaches are a common complaint in all clinics. In patients with rheumatic disorders the physician needs to be aware of a number of special causes. Unilateral frontal headaches, often with scalp tenderness, may be due to temporal arteritis — a medical emergency. Occipital headaches can result from compression of the C2 nerve root, indicating significant changes in the neck. Late-onset migraine may be a feature of SLE or other vasculitic disorders, and anti-rheumatic drugs (e.g. indomethacin) can cause severe generalised headache. Thus, although tension and anxiety are probably the commonest causes, headaches must be treated seriously in patients with rheumatic diseases, and a full history and examination must be carried out.

2. Depression

Depression presents in a variety of ways, including lethargy, lack of interest, sleep disturbance, weight-loss, increased musculoskeletal pain or with symptoms of anxiety. In a rheumatology clinic awareness of depression, both as a cause of somatic symptoms and a result of disease, is needed.

Depression may increase pain, and alter physical signs, with exaggeration of tender periarticular spots (see the 'Pain-amplification syndrome', p 360). It may be the only cause of rheumatic symptoms such as arthralgia. Mood changes can also tip the balance between independence and dependency; the lethargy and lack of drive of depression resulting in a disabled patient 'giving up'. It is often difficult to establish the extent to which psychiatric and personality factors contribute to disability in an individual patient.

Depression can also arise as a result of the disease or its treatment. Persistent active inflammation of any cause is debilitating and 'depressing'. In some disorders, especially SLE, neuropsychiatric disturbances are a more prominent and direct result of the disease (see above). Drugs (e.g. steroids, some non-steroidal anti-inflammatory agents) can cause depression, but so can the frustration of constant pain and disability. Factors such as sexual frustration or inability to continue a favourite sport or pastime may be a major factor. A sympathetic history and careful counselling may help untangle the problems of depression in rheumatic diseases.

FURTHER READING (CNS)

Walton J N 1975 Essentials of neurology, 4th edn. Pitman Medical, London

Bland J H 1974 Review: rheumatoid arthritis of the cervical spine. Journal of Rheumatology 1: 319

Klippel J H, Zvaifler N J 1975 Neuropsychiatric abnormalities in SLE. Clinics in Rheumatic Diseases 1: 621

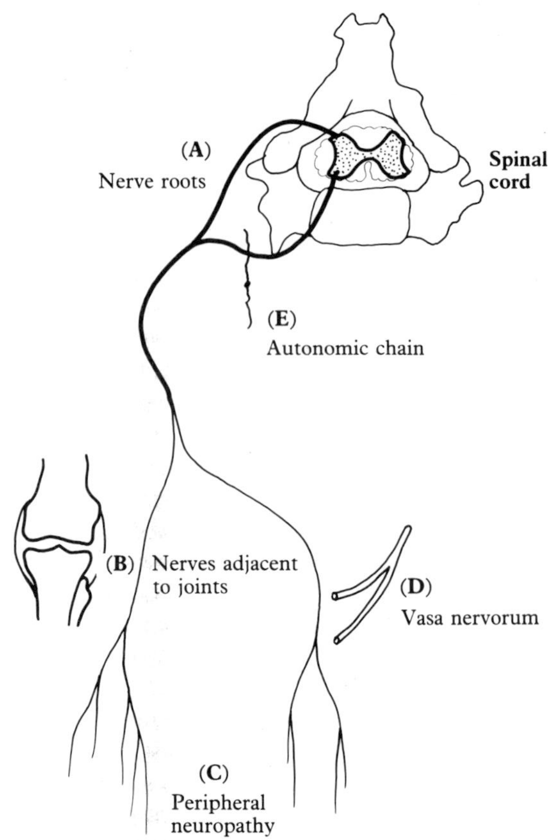

Fig. 15.23 Sites and causes of damage by rheumatic disease. Machanical lesions — (**A**) root pressure; (**B**) entrapment and compression neuropathies. (**C**) peripheral neuropathies; (**D**) mononeuritis multiplex; (**E**) autonomic neuropathy.

X The Peripheral Nervous System

Rheumatic diseases can cause damage to peripheral nerves at four principal sites between the spinal cord and nerve endings (Fig. 15.23). The autonomic nervous system is occasionally involved.

Pressure on spinal nerve roots is common, and is usually due to disc prolapse or osteophytosis. More distal entrapment and compression neuropathies are also frequent both as presenting features and complications of rheumatic diseases. These mechanical lesions usually cause a reversible neuropraxia rather than permanent interruption of nerves.

Connective tissue diseases are among the more important causes of peripheral neuropathies, and occasionally cause mononeuritis multiplex or an autonomic neuropathy. These types of nerve injury are probably due to damage to the vasa nervorum and ischaemia of peripheral nerves.

ROOT PRESSURE

Pressure on spinal nerve roots tends to occur where spinal movement is greatest, i.e. in the mid-cervical, mid-thoracic and low lumbar regions. It can result from narrowing of the exit foramina between the vertebrae or from space-occupying lesions.

The commonest cause in young people is a posterio-lateral protrusion of the intervertebral disc. The usual site is L4–L5, and manual workers are often affected. In older people severe osteophytic lipping around damaged intervertebral discs or osteoarthritis of the apophyseal joints are the most important causes, and commonly affect C5–C6 roots. Rheumatoid arthritis often affects the cervical spine and may cause pressure on the C2 nerve root, with atlanto-axial subluxation, or on lower cervical nerve roots. Other bone and joint lesions such as spondylolisthesis, Paget's disease of vertebrae, ankylosing spondylitis and many more occasionally present with a spinal root syndrome.

Symptoms at the site of spinal involvement are often mild or absent. Patients present with pain referred to a myotome and paraesthesia in the corresponding dermatome. Symptoms are usually exacerbated by appropriate spinal movement and sometimes by coughing and sneezing, which raise the intrathecal pressure (impulse pain, see also Chapter 22.II). Sensory loss in the dermatome, and weakness and decreased reflexes of corresponding muscles may develop.

Referred root pain often causes diagnostic confusion. Reproducing the pain by spinal movement and eliciting an appropriate area of sensory disturbance, may allow the correct diagnosis to be made on clinical grounds. However, these signs may be minimal, and the plain X-ray is often normal. Radiculography to outline the nerve-root sheaths may be necessary to demonstrate the lesion. Some common misdiagnoses are listed (Table 15.5); many patients with root pressure have had unnecessary tablets for migraine or arthritis, and some have had inappropriate coronary angiography.

Table 15.5 Some common sites for root pressure

Site (Common cause)	Common misdiagnosis
L5 (L4–L5 disc)	Local disease of knee, leg or foot
L3 (L2–L3 disc)	Hip disease, meralgia parasthetica
T6 – T10 area	Pleurisy, angina, disease of chest wall
C5 (Cervical spondylosis)	Shoulder lesions, 'fibrositis'
C2 (Atlanto-axial subluxation in RA)	Occipital headaches, migraine

ENTRAPMENT AND COMPRESSION NEUROPATHY

Compression neuropathies occur where a nerve passes over a bony area close to the skin. Entrapment neuropathies develop where the nerve is enclosed by a tight soft-tissue band (Fig. 15.24).

The usual presentation is with insidious onset of pain and parasthesiae in the distribution of a peripheral nerve; weakness is sometimes the main problem. The site and extent of nerve damage can usually be assessed clinically, but electromyography is helpful in difficult cases.

Carpal tunnel syndrome

The patient, usually a middle-aged woman, develops pain and parasthesiae in the hand, particularly at night. The dominant hand is usually affected first, and she may have to shake it and hang it out of bed to relieve symptoms. Use of the wrist may exacerbate symptoms in the day. Early signs include slight loss of sensation over the medial 3½ digits, and parasthesiae on pressure on percussion over the dorsum of the wrist (Tinel's sign). Protracted nerve compression causes weakness of abductor pollicis brevis, resulting in wasting of the thenar emminence and difficulty with pinch grip. Symptoms may spread into the whole hand, or up the forearm to the elbow, but signs are usually confined to the anatomical distribution of the nerve (Fig. 15.24E).

Rheumatoid arthritis frequently presents with carpal tunnel syndrome, and any wrist arthropathy may lead to compression. Carpal tunnel syndrome

Causes of carpal tunnel syndrome

1. Idiopathic
2. Rheumatoid arthritis
3. Other arthropathies
4. Colles fractures
5. Myxoedema
6. Acromegaly
7. Pregnancy
8. Obesity
9. Amyloidosis

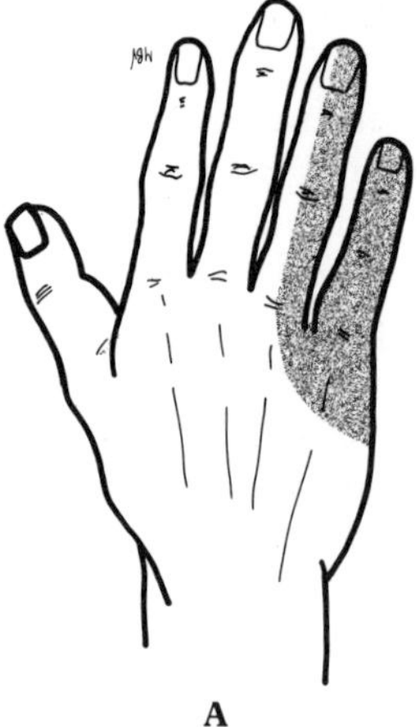

A
Sensory loss resulting from compression at the elbow

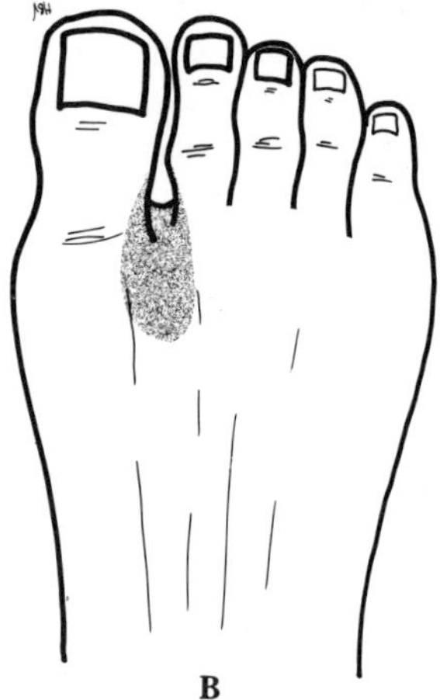

B
Sensory loss resulting from compression at the knee

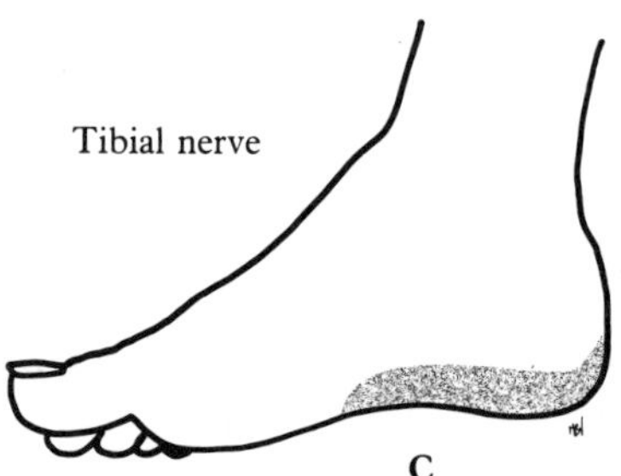

C
Sensory loss resulting from nerve entrapment at the ankle

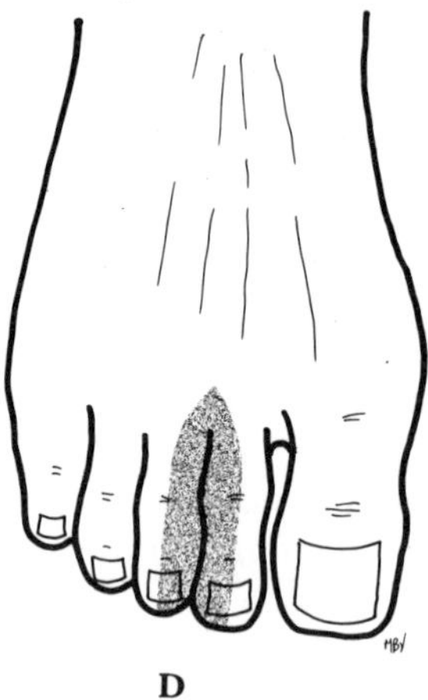

D
Sensory loss resulting from a neuroma in the web space in the forefoot (Morton's metatarsalgia)

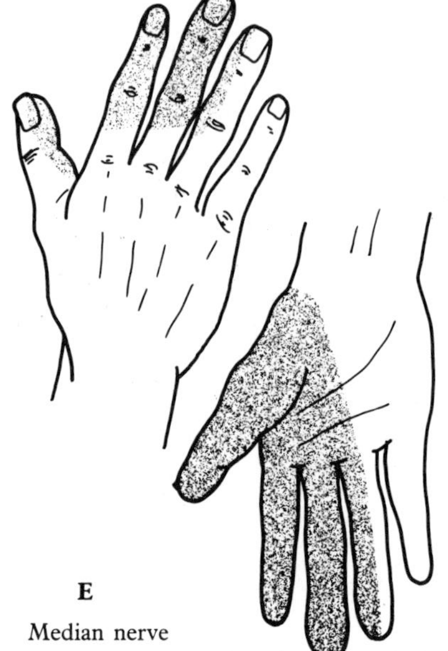

E
Median nerve

F
Lateral cutaneous nerve

Fig. 15.24 Peripheral neuropathies. **A**. Ulnar nerve. **B**. Common peroneal (lateral popliteal) nerve. **C**. Tibial nerve. **D**. Interdigital nerve. **E**. Median nerve. **F**. Lateral cutaneous nerve of the thigh

is also a rare presenting feature of primary amyloidosis. However, many cases are idiopathic and there are several other non-rheumatological causes. In view of the association with myxoedema and acromegaly, the facies and tongue, as well as the joints, must be part of a general examination to look for causes.

Ulnar nerve lesions

The ulnar nerve can be trapped at the elbow, forearm or in various sites in the wrist and hand. The commonest areas of compression are around the medial epicondylar groove at the elbow (usually with advanced RA or OA), or in Guyon's canal at the wrist. Symptoms are referred to the lateral one and a half fingers, and the long flexors and intrinsic muscles of the hand related to these two digits may get weak and wasted. Prolonged pressure leads to clawing of the little and ring fingers (Fig. 15.24A).

Meralgia parasthetica

Pain parasthesia and sensory disturbances over the anterior aspect of the thigh may be due to pressure on the lateral cutaneous nerve. Alternative diagnoses include hip pain, L3 root pain, adductor tendinitits or trochanteric bursitis. Obesity or tight clothes are the usual causes of this lesion (Fig. 15.24F).

Common peroneal nerve

This nerve is vulnerable where it winds round the head of the fibula. Pressure may arise from a mechanical abnormality of the knee or a gross destructive joint lesion. Calipers, knee splints, pressure on radiography or operating tables and direct trauma may also cause damage.

Patients often present with foot-drop and have weakness of the dorsiflexors and evertors of the ankle. There is usually a small patch of sensory loss on the dorsum of the foot between the first and second toes (Fig. 15.24B).

Tarsal tunnel syndrome

The tibial nerve is enclosed by the flexor retinaculum at the ankle. Pressure causes tingling, pain and numbness in the foot which may be worse on standing or at night. The diagnosis may be missed because foot pain is thought to arise from the joint and periarticular structures. Tarsal tunnel syndrome is not uncommon in RA.

Morton's metatarsalgia

Patients present with pain in the MTP joint and toe, exacerbated by weight-bearing. There may be parasthesiae in the toes and sensory loss. Careful palpation of the web space between the toes may uncover the neuroma on the interdigital nerve and pressure there may reproduce the symptoms. Morton's metatarsalgia is often confused with articular causes of metatarsalgia.

Management of entrapment neuropathies

Establishing the correct cause of pain and/or sensory disturbance is critical and may be difficult where nerve pressure is caused by painful arthritis. Clinical suspicion must always be high, especially in RA, and conduction studies of the nerves may help establish the diagnosis.

Removal of any obvious cause of compression (a caliper for example) and resting splints at night (especially for carpal tunnel) may relieve symptoms. Local injections of a small quantity of long-acting steroid in the area adjacent to an entrapment neuropathy often helps by reducing inflammatory oedema around the nerve. Surgical decompression or transposition of nerves is sometimes necessary, particularly if motor signs are developing.

PERIPHERAL NEUROPATHY

Sensory, or mixed motor and sensory peripheral neuropathies, occur in the connective tissue diseases, usually with a glove and stocking distribution.

Patients present with tingling, burning pain, sensations of walking on cotton wool or wearing gloves, difficulty or unsteadiness in walking, or band-like pains at the wrist or ankle. If this occurs in the context of an active arthropathy, there is obviously scope for overlooking it as another manifestation of joint disease. However, careful examination should reveal peripheral sensory impairement. In difficult cases conduction studies may be warranted to establish the diagnosis.

The connective tissue diseases which can produce a peripheral neuropathy are listed below. The cause is probably a vasculitis of the vasa nervorum. RA is the commonest cause: a sensory neuropathy is a frequent cause of distressing symptoms but is usually benign; a mixed sensory-motor lesion indicates active systemic vasculitis and the patient should be treated accordingly (Chapter 7).

Connective tissue diseases causing peripheral neuropathy

1. COMMON
   RA (sensory)
2. UNCOMMON
   a) RA (mixed sensor-motor)
   b) SLE
3. RARE
   a) PAN
   b) Sjögren's
   c) Wegner's granulomatosis
   d) Scleroderma
   e) Drugs
      (i) Chloroquine
      (ii) Dapsone

In a patients with an active long-standing rheumatic condition like RA it is unnecessary to look hard for another cause of a peripheral neuropathy, although awareness of a possible coincidental diabetic or malignant neuropathy is essential.

MONONEURITIS MULTIPLEX

Mononeuritis multiplex is caused by vascular lesions of discrete areas on several different peripheral nerve trunks. The presentation is variable. In some cases insidious onset of damage to one nerve trunk heralds the condition and is followed by other lesions months or years later. In other patients the onset is dramatic, with several different nerves being affected over a short time period.

The sites of involvement are commonly those of the compression or entrapment neuropathies, and the signs and symptoms similar. The same connective tissue diseases that cause a peripheral neuropathy can result in this syndrome, although it is particularly a feature of PAN.

Mononeuritis multiplex

Causes include

1. Diabetes
2. Rheumatoid vasculitis
3. Polyarteritis nodosa
4. SLE
5. Amyloidosis
6. Alcohol
7. Leprosy
8. Sarcoidosis

There are a small number of important alternative causes. Any patient with mononeuritis multiplex must be fully investigated. Nerve biopsy may be necessary and the condition must be remembered as a frequent presentation of PAN and a rare complication of other connective tissue diseases.

AUTONOMIC NEUROPATHY

Autonomic neuropathy is a rare complication of any connective tissue disease. It may present with dryness or sweating of extremities, postural hypotension, impotence, sphincter disturbances or alteration in bowel habit. Sinus arrhythmia is lost; this can be detected by loss of beat to beat variation on an ECG, and loss of the normal reactive tachycardia following a Valsalva manoeuvre. Autonomic dysfunction is also a feature of the localised limb changes accompanying an algodystrophy.

Treatment of autonomic neuropathies is difficult. If cardiovascular symptoms dominate the picture, support tights to aid venous return and fludrocortisone to reduce hypotension may help. Bowel and bladder disturbances can also be aided by symptomatic drug therapy.

FURTHER READING (PNS)

HMSO Handbook. Aids to the Investigation of peripheral nerve injuries

Wakefield G 1979 Entrapment neuropathies. Clinics in Rheumatic Diseases 5(3): 941–956

Walton J N 1975 Essentials of neurology, 4th edn. Pitman Medical, London

16 Other diseases affecting the musculoskeletal system

I Haematological Disease

Blood diseases can affect the joints by several different mechanisms. Disorders of clotting can cause bleeding into muscles and joints, intravascular sludging can cause infarction and ischaemia of the bone-ends and myeloproliferative disorders may result in direct infiltration of joint tissue with neoplastic cells. Secondary gout or joint sepsis can also arise from the high purine turnover or decreased resistance to infection that may accompany some haematological diseases.

Mechanisms by which blood disorders can affect the joints

1. Bleeding into muscles, joints or periarticular tissue
2. Infarction of subchondral bone
3. Infiltration of joint tissues in myeloproliferative disease
4. Decreased resistance to joint infection.
5. Secondary gout

Joint disease is a major manifestation of haemophilia, Christmas disease and sickle-cell anaemia, often occurs in leukaemia and is an occasional feature of lymphomas and other haemoglobinopathies. Polycythaemia rubra vera is one of the commoner causes of secondary gout, and joint sepsis an occasional event in any ill, immunosuppressed or leukopaenic patient with a severe blood disorder. Myelomatosis frequently presents with bone disease, commonly affecting the vertebra, and is an important cause of 'sinister' back pain (see Chapter 22.II).

Haematological disorders which affect the joints

1. Haemophilia A and B
2. Sickle-cell anaemia
3. Myelomatosis
4. Other haemoglobinopathies and myeloproliferative diseases

HAEMOPHILIA

Haemophilia A (Factor VIII deficiency) is a rare, sex-linked, recessive disorder occurring only in men. Most patients have a family history of the disease, but sporadic new cases are also seen due to a relatively high incidence of spontaneous mutations. Haemophilia B (Factor IX deficiency, Christmas disease) is clinically indistinguishable form Haemophilia A, and is also inherited as a sex-linked recessive disorder of men. Both cause major bleeding into muscles and joints, and as patients get older haemophiliac arthropathy often becomes the dominant clinical problem. Von Willebrand's disease (due to an abnormality of Factor-VIII-related protein) is a rare bleeding disorder affecting both sexes; it causes bleeding into the skin and mucous membranes, but rarely affects the joints.

The bleeding manifestations of haemophilia correlate closely with the degree of Factor VII (or IX) deficiency. Excessive bleeding after trauma or surgery occur in patients with levels less than 50% of normal, but spontaneous muscle and joint bleeds are unusual unless the level is less than 5%. The diagnosis is usually made early in childhood because of excessive bruising or bleeding from the tongue, gums or lips, and the family history is often helpful. Occasional cases with only a partial deficiency, and/or no family history may present later, sometimes with joint or muscle bleeds. The diagnosis is made by assaying the blood level of Factors VIII or IX, and management should be co-ordinated by a special haemophilia centre if possible.

There are three major rheumatological manifestations of haemophilia: bleeding into muscles, acute haemarthrosis and chronic haemophiliac arthropathy.

Rheumatological manifestations of haemophilia
1. Muscle bleeds
2. Haemarthroses
3. Muscle and joint contractures
4. Chronic joint destruction

1. Bleeding into muscle

This is commoner in children than in adults, and recurrences at the same site are uncommon, because fibrous healing obliterates the vessels involved. The common sites are the iliopsoas muscle, the flexor muscles of the forearm, the quadriceps and the anterior tibial muscles in the calf. (Note involvement of flexors, not extensors.)

An antecedent injury, often trivial, is common. Haematomas develop slowly, and pain is the main clinical feature. Swelling then develops, and there may be secondary nerve entrapment leading to neurological damage below the lesion. Protective muscle spasm occurs. If left untreated severe contractures may develop, with possible permanent neurological deficits. Early immobilisation and Factor XIII replacement should be followed by passive exercises as soon as the pain subsides. Corrective splinting is sometimes required to treat muscle contractures.

2. Acute haemarthrosis

This is the commonest feature of haemophilia, and is usually spontaneous, no antecedent trauma being apparent. The joint distribution is characteristic and intriguing. The knees, elbows and ankles are by far the commonest sites to be involved, with shoulders, wrists and sterno-clavicular joints being much less common and other sites relatively rare (Fig. 16.1). It may be relevant that the knee, elbow and ankle are all hinge joints. The bleeding is probably initially intracapsular in the majority of cases; blood then escapes into the joint space and a secondary polymorphonuclear inflammatory synovitis occurs.

Many haemophiliacs get warning symptoms of pricking, warmth or a vague 'disquiet' in a joint before the bleed becomes apparent. Pain, probably due to capsular stretching, followed by joint

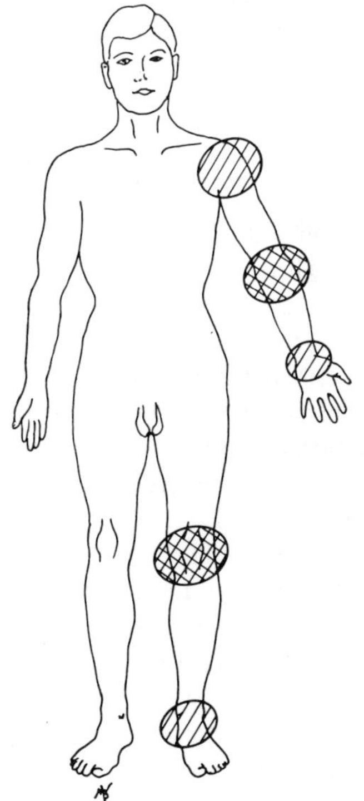

Fig. 16.1 Distribution of joints involved in haemophilia

swelling, then become the major features and rapidly increase in severity over a period of a few hours. The patient presents with a tense, swollen, very painful joint, held in fixed flexion due to protective spasm, with little or no active movement possible. In some acute episodes, pain and muscle spasm are severe but the swelling is minor; this may be due to subarticular rather than intra-articular bleeding.

The diagnosis is usually obvious, but fears of a septic arthritis often arise, and the rare patient presenting later than usual can cause diagnostic difficulty. If the joint is inadvertently aspirated, a thick, blood-stained effusion is obtained, and the differential diagnosis is that of other causes of a haemarthrosis.

Causes of a haemarthrosis

1. Bleeding disorder (e.g. haemophilia)
2. Trauma
3. Villonodular synovitis
4. Charcot joint
5. Pyrophosphate arthropathy
6. Haemangioma
7. Occasional bloodstaining in other destructive or inflammatory arthropathies, (e.g. resolving septic arthritis)

Treatment should begin as soon as possible, and consists of replacing the clotting factor and immobilising the joint. In severe bleeds ice-packs may help, and aspiration may be required if the effusion is very tense or refractory. As soon as the pain subsides, the joint should be mobilised to prevent development of a flexion deformity, and muscles should be exercised to avoid wasting and weakness. With the provision of modern self-treatment at home with cryoprecipitate or freeze-dried clotting factor concentrates, most haemarthroses can be promptly managed, and aspiration or splinting are rarely required.

3. Chronic haemophilic arthropathy

Modern therapy has resulted in dramatic improvement in the life expectancy of severe haemophiliacs. Chronic joint damage is becoming an increasing problem in the survivors, and although it is obviously related to intra-articular bleeding, the mechanisms involved are not clearly understood. Bleeding during childhood causes growth anomalies, with enlargement of the epiphyses, which may contribute to the damage, and subarticular bleeds may also affect the joint surfaces. However, the major contribution to joint destruction probably arises from the secondary synovial changes that result from repeated bleeding. A chronic proliferative synovitis, with the production of a fibrous pannus on the joint surface, occurs. This can be reproduced experimentally by repeated injections of autologous blood into the knees of puppies.

Clinically, chronic haemophilic arthropathy is very characteristic. The distribution is that of acute bleeds (Fig. 16.1), with the knee and elbow taking the brunt of the disease. Flexion contractures, with painful reduction of movement, severe crepitus and bony overgrowth at the joint margin, are usually present. Mild swelling and modest effusions may be present. In addition to flexion deformities, lateral or posterior tibio-femoral subluxation may occur in the knees. Particularly if there has been prior muscle or nerve damage, gross crippling deformities can develop. Acute haemarthroses often become less frequent as the patient gets older, and if the effusion is tapped (under Factor VIII cover), clear yellow synovial fluid, rich in mononuclear cells, may be obtained. In spite of less bleeding, the chronic destructive changes are usually slowly progressive.

Radiology

The radiographic findings include widening of the trabeculae, epiphyseal overgrowth, a very irregular joint surface, subarticular cysts and loss of joint space. The deformities mentioned are seen on the X-ray, and in the knee a widening of the intercondylar notch and condylar squaring are often present (Fig. 16.2). Extensive growth lines and subarticular osteoporosis may be seen, and avas-

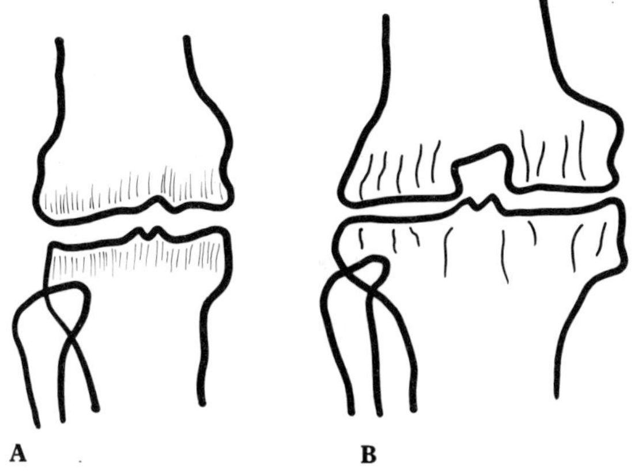

Fig. 16.2 Radiographic changes in haemophilia (AP view of knee). **A**. Normal; **B**. Haemophilia. Note: 1) widening and squaring of intercondylar notch 2) increased width of bone 3) widened, coarse trabeculae 4) narrowing of joint space

cular necrosis occasionally develops in the head of the humerus or femur. Calcification of a subperiosteal haematoma is a rare complication, causing a so-called 'haemophiliac pseudo-tumour'.

Treatment

Treatment is difficult. Physiotherapy to maintain muscle power and a good range of movement helps, and prompt therapy of any acute bleeds is important. Splinting may reduce deformities. If a chronic synovitis is present intra-articular steroid can produce temporary relief and aid the physiotherapy. However, injection carries a high risk of infection, and can only be done under factor VIII cover. Synovectomy (medical or surgical) has been used with some advantage. Reconstructive surgery is occasionally done in severe cases, but can only be considered in specialist units with adequate haematological and surgical expertise present.

HAEMOGLOBINOPATHIES

Alterations in the structure of the two pairs of polypeptide chains which constitute normal haemoglobin causes haemolytic anaemias. The thalassaemias, in which either the α or β chains are defective rarely cause any rheumatological problems, and haemoglobin C disease only affects bones and joints if combined with haemoglobin S disease (sickle-cell disease). Patients with this combination (HbSC) have a high incidence of aseptic necrosis of bone. In pure HbS, musculoskeletal problems are a common major disease manifestation.

Sickle-cell disease (HbS)

This is an inherited disorder, almost entirely confined to Negroes, in which there is a substitution of glutamic acid for valine in the beta chain of haemoglobin. In homozygous patients this renders the red corpuscles vulnerable to hypoxia, which causes them to change shape (sickle) and sludge. They then block small blood-vessels, causing further hypoxia, more sickling and a vicious cycle leading to the 'sickle cell crisis'. Clinical manifestations include haemolytic anaemia, leg ulcers, hepatomegaly, splenic infarction, pulmonary infarcts, haematuria and central nervous system complications. Most patients have a chronic anaemia interrupted by attacks (crises) involving fever, acute abdominal or chest pain and musculoskeletal problems. These may include aching in muscles or joints, acute localised bone or joint pain or acute dactylitis of the hand or foot. Crises may be precipitated by hypoxia, exercise, stress or acidosis, but can occur spontaneously.

The major bone and joint problems in HbS patients are listed below.

Bone and joint problems in sickle-cell anaemia

1. Bone infarcts
2. Aseptic necrosis of bone
3. Joint effusions
4. Hand–foot syndrome
5. Bone and joint infection
6. Hyperuricaemia and gout
7. Changes in bone-marrow space

1. Bone infarction

A crisis often causes blockage of small blood-vessels in bone and thus an infarct. This results in severe bone pain, commonest in the hands. It is followed by periosteal elevation, a common radiological feature of HbS; growth changes of the epiphyses occur in children, and small medullary or articular defects that may look like osteochondritis dissecans.

2. Aseptic necrosis

Occulusion of end-arteries at the articular margin can cause aseptic necrosis. This is commonest in the head of the femur, humeral head and tibial condyles. It may cause very painful, disabling joint problems and is the most severe musculoskeletal complication of HbS. The appearances and natural history are the same as in other cases of aseptic bone necrosis irrespective of the cause.

3. Joint effusions

Crises are often accompanied by warm, painful joints which develop inflammatory effusions, taking about 2 weeks to resolve. The knees and elbows are the commonest sites. Haemarthroses are rare.

4. The 'hand–foot syndrome'

This is dramatic swelling of the hand or foot, with either individual digits (dactylitis) or the whole extremity involved. It occurs principally in childhood during a sickle crisis. The cause is not clear, but is probably related to multiple areas of infarction. The painful swellings slowly resolve over 2–3 weeks.

5. Bone and joint infections

HbS patients have an increased susceptibility to infection. Osteomyelitis is common, and although a variety of organisms may be found, *Salmonella* is particularly frequent. The severe bone pain and constitutional features may be difficult to distinguish from a crisis with a bone infarct. Septic arthritis occasionally occurs.

6. Hyperuricaemia and gout

Due to increased cell turnover, hyperuricaemia is common (40% of patients). Gout is rare but has been reported.

7. Bone changes due to marrow expansion

The haemolysis puts extra demands on bone marrow, leading to expansion, widening and coarsening of bony trabeculae, as in other haemolytic anaemias. These changes are prominent throughout the axial skeleton. In HbS characteristic vertebral changes may develop, a cup like indentation occurring in the abnormal bones (Fig. 16.3).

There is no specific treatment for HbS. Arthralgias, effusions and bone infarcts need no therapy except for rest, analgesia and perhaps oxygen therapy for the sickle crisis. Early avascular necrosis can be treated by avoiding weight-bearing, this may prevent subsequent bone and joint destruction. A high index of suspicion of bone or joint infection, or sepsis elsewhere, is always appropriate.

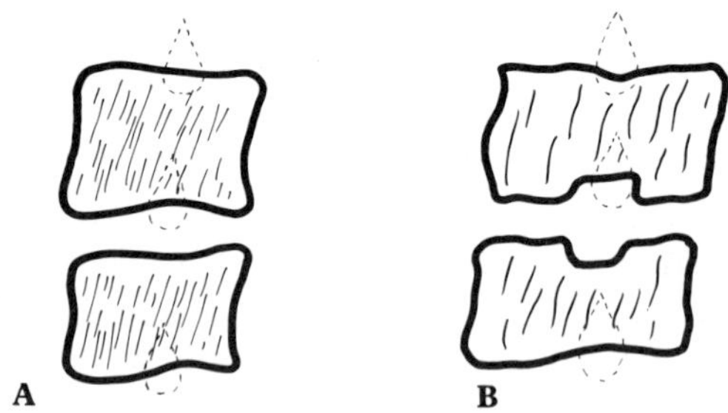

Fig. 16.3 Radiographic changes in the spine in sickle-cell anaemia. **A**. Normal; **B**. Sickle-cell disease. Note the coarsened trabecular pattern and cup-like indentations

MALIGNANT DISEASE

Leukaemias often cause arthralgia or arthritis, which are occasionally the presentation of the disease. Bone involvement with local pain and tenderness is common in lymphomas, but joint disease is not. Myeloma often presents as osteoporosis, as atypical back pain or with a pathological fracture. Arthralgias can occur and occasionally arthritis, especially in hypercalcaemic patients. All myeloproliferative diseases can cause secondary hyperuricaemia, especially when treated, and allopurinol is often given routinely with cytotoxic drug therapy. However, gout is rare in these patients, perhaps because of the relatively short duration of hyperuricaemia or lack of predilection to crystal deposition.

Leukaemia

All leukaemias can cause arthralgias or a mono- or polyarthritis. This is commonest in children with acute leukaemia, and if it is the disease presentation, can cause confusion with other childhood arthritides. Knees and ankles are often involved and the condition is usually asymmetrical. The pain is often very severe, and may be accompanied by modest signs of joint inflammation. A migratory pattern may develop, mimicking rheumatic fever. The condition is attributed to leukaemic infiltration of joints and periarticular tissues. Treatment for the joints is symptomatic, and the pain subsides with treatment of the leukaemia.

HAEMATOLOGICAL THERAPY

Musculoskeletal problems occasionally arise from therapy used for blood disorders. Uric acid levels can rise dramatically during the treatment of myelo-proliferative disorders, and gout or acute precipitation of uric acid in the kidney can result. Allopurinol is given routinely to avoid this. Arthralgia is a common feature of reactions to incompatible blood transfusion, and aching in the muscles or joints may be the first sign of a transfusion reaction. Parenteral iron therapy is particularly dangerous in patients with RA, and should be avoided because of the high risk of anaphylactic reactions. Even oral iron can occasionally exacerbate RA, and it should only be given in patients with unequivocal evidence of true iron deficiency. Anticoagulants very occasionally cause a haemarthrosis, and prolonged heparin therapy (for months, as sometimes used in pregnancy) can cause osteoporosis.

FURTHER READING (HAEMATOLOGICAL DISEASE)

Bywaters E G H 1975 Rheumatological manifestations of systemic disease. Clinics in Rheumatic Diseases 1.

II Malignant Disease

There appear to be three main possibilities for interrelationship between malignancy and rheumatic disease:

1. Malignancy may give rise to a rheumatic disorder (by direct invasion of musculoskeletal structures, by metabolic alteration or by 'non-metastatic' effects).
2. Rheumatic syndromes themselves may predispose to malignancy.
3. Malignancy may occur as a complication of immunosuppressive drugs or radiotherapy used in treatment.

Non-metastatic manifestations occur in up to 15% of patients with malignancy. Ectopic hormone production is the commonest paraneoplastic effect seen, accounting for one-third of those identified, but connective tissue, neuromuscular and haematological manifestations account for the majority of those remaining. A direct causal relationship may be established in some instances where resection of the tumour results in resolution of the syndrome, but in others the possibility remains that both processes share a common, unknown aetiology. Whether or not the relationships between malignancy and rheumatic disease are causal or casual, however, their recognition is important since:

1. Awareness that malignancy may present with musculoskeletal symptoms may allow early recognition of an occult, potentially curable neoplasm.
2. Knowledge that a connective tissue process predisposes to malignancy may permit early recognition of a predictable neoplasm.
3. The association between cancer and rheumatic disease may eventually provide insight into the aetiology and pathogenesis of these disorders.

DISORDERS CAUSED BY MALIGNANCY

Malignancy may give rise to a variety of musculoskeletal disorders, Apart from referred pain most of these conditions are uncommon or rare.

Musculoskeletal disorders caused by malignancy

1. Referred pain
2. Secondary hypertrophic osteoarthropathy
3. Carcinoma polyarthritis
4. Arthritis secondary to carcinoid syndrome
5. Polyarthritis due to skeletal invasion/metastases
6. Dermatomyositis/polymyositis
7. Polymyalgia rheumatica syndrome
8. Secondary gout
9. Opportunist infection

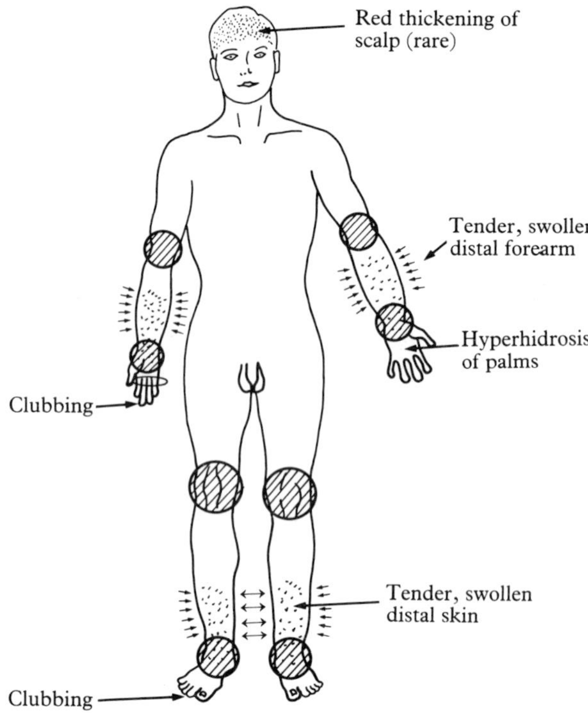

Fig. 16.4 Joint involvement and other features characteristic of hypertrophic osteoarthropathy

Referred pain

Referred pain may be the presenting feature that suggests rheumatic disease; e.g. pain in the shoulder may be the first symptom of bronchial carcinoma, back pain may result from intra-abdominal or intrathoracic malignancy. Careful history and examination should, however, allow distinction from joint disease.

Hypertrophic osteoarthropathy (pachydermoperiostosis)

This uncommon syndrome comprises clubbing, swelling of the distal parts of the limbs, periosteal new bone formation and arthritis. It may rarely present as a primary disorder showing autosomal dominant inheritance and gradual onset around puberty, but more usually is seen secondary to underlying malignancy, being only rarely associated with the other disorders that cause clubbing. It complicates 5% of bronchial carcinoma (the commonest cause) and 50% of mesothelioma or neurilemmoma involving pleura or diaphragm.

The typical patient is a middle-aged man who presents with acute onset of pain, tenderness and swelling affecting the distal portions of all limbs. The pain is aching in nature and characteristically worsened by dependency and relieved by elevation. Warmth and 'burning' of the distal limbs is common, frequently exacerbated by bedclothes at night. Joint stiffness most commonly affects knees, ankles, elbows, wrists and MCPs. Symptoms usually precede other manifestations of malignancy by several months.

Examination (Fig. 16.4) may reveal tenderness, effusion, soft-tissue swelling and reduced range of movement of involved joints, and overlying skin may be dusky red, warm and thickened. Swelling and tenderness, however, are characteristically maximal over the distal ends of long bones, particularly the radius and tibia, where periosteal reaction is most marked. Clubbing is usually present and hyperhidrosis of palms and soles may be an additional diagnostic feature. Thickening of the scalp, telangiectasia and gynaecomastia occasionally occur. Although usually symmetrical, unilateral involvement of one arm may occur with a Pancoast's tumour or intrathoracic aneurysm.

X-rays may show proliferative periosteal changes and overlying soft-tissue swelling along the distal portions of the diaphyses of the forearms and legs as well as in the shafts of the phalanges

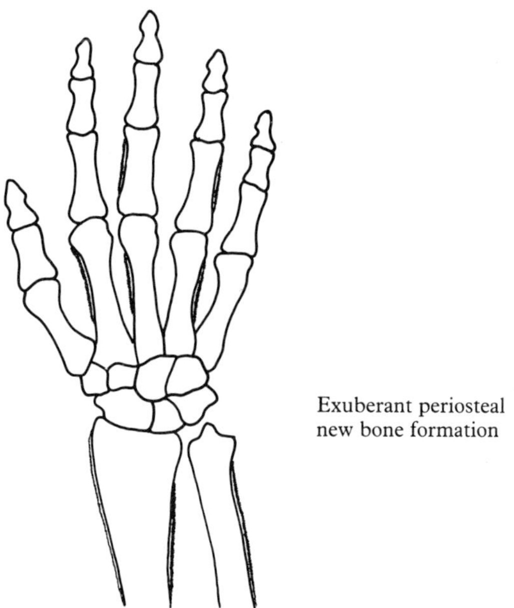

Fig. 16.5 Hypertrophic osteoarthropathy

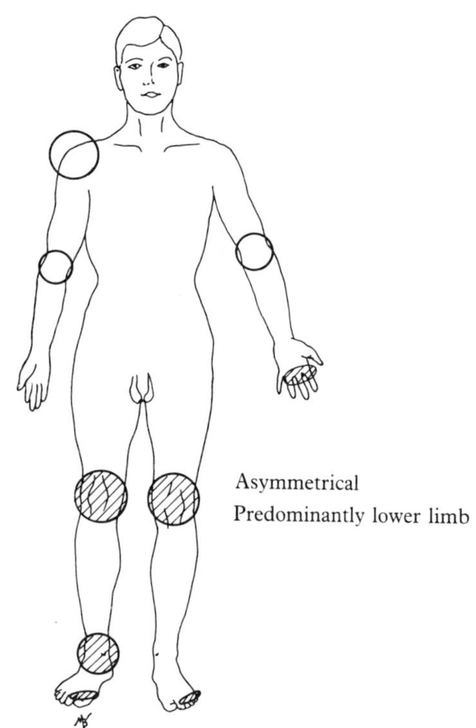

Fig. 16.6 Typical joint distribution in carcinoma polyarthritis

(Fig. 16.5). Later, osteoporosis, cortical thickening and tufting of distal phalanges may also develop. A technetium scan gives a diagnostic pattern of activity even in the absence of radiographic changes. In most cases the chest X-ray will reveal the underlying neoplasm.

The course of the condition follows that of the underlying disease. Improvement follows vagotomy, exploratory thoracotomy and removal of the primary: eradication of the malignancy can effect a cure. Analgesics, NSAIDs, steroids or ACTH may be of help in incurable cases. The pathogenesis of this condition remains unknown. Although increased vascularity secondary to neuronal reflexes or circulating hormones, and circulating immune complexes, have been suggested as causal, supportive evidence in favour of these theories is lacking.

Carcinoma polyarthritis

This uncommon syndrome clinically resembles RA and is particularly associated with carcinoma of the bronchus, prostate and breast. Joint symptoms may precede other manifestations of malignancy by many months. As with hypertrophic osteoarthropathy its pathogenesis is obscure.

Middle-aged and elderly men are particularly affected (M:F 2:1 — peak age 50–65). Onset is characteristically explosive and severe with pain and morning stiffness in many joints (Fig. 16.6), superficially resembling late onset RA (p 45). Distinguishing features, however, include: 1. asymmetrical joint involvement in 50%; 2. predilection for lower limb joints (knees, ankles); 3. sparing of wrist and small joints of hand.

The absence of nodules, persistent seronegativity of rheumatoid factor and minimal X-ray changes are also usual, but differentiation from RA is often clinically difficult. In those cases secondary to carcinoma of the bronchus the CXR is usually abnormal at presentation. The condition must be suspected in any patient with late onset polyarthritis and a CXR always performed. The course of the arthritis tends to follow that of the underlying malignancy.

Arthritis secondary to pancreatic disease

Pancreatic carcinoma may rarely present with a florid, often symmetrical polyarthritis, predominantly affecting ankles, knees and small joints of the hands: mono- or oligoarthritis is less usual. Pain is often severe and joints are usually tender, warm, red and swollen. Nodules may appear synchronously with the arthritis and superficially resemble erythema nodosum except that they predominate over thighs and buttocks and occasionally are widespread. Biopsy shows them to result from fat necrosis. Serum lipase and amylase are inevitably raised and peripheral blood eosinophilia may be marked. The combination of a severely painful polyarthritis, atypical nodules and eosinophilia in an ill patient should suggest the diagnosis. Treatment, including steroids, is frequently ineffective. A similar presentation, which may resolve completely within a few weeks to leave no residua, may occasionally be seen in patients with acute pancreatitis.

Arthritis secondary to carcinoid syndrome

Transient arthritis, presenting as symmetrical pain and swelling of finger interphalangeal joints, may rarely occur during the course of this uncommon syndrome. Persistent flexion contractures may eventually develop which superficially resemble scleroderma. Major features of the syndrome are attacks of facial flushing leading to persistent erythema and telangiectasia, weight-loss, chronic diarrhoea, asthma, hepatomegaly and right-sided heart lesions. The syndrome results from release of 5-hydroxytryptamine and other bioactive amines from carcinoid metastases in the liver (rarely from a lung primary). Markedly increased urinary 5-hydroxyindole acetic acid excretion confirms the diagnosis. The condition is slowly progressive and treatment is frequently disappointing.

Skeletal invasion or metastases

Malignant involvement of bone may rarely cause a 'sympathetic' synovitis in an adjacent joint and present as a monoarthritis or an asymmetrical oligoarthritis. Small bones and joints are rarely involved. Examination reveals local bony tenderness and X-rays confirm the diagnosis.

Polyarthritis may be the presenting symptom of acute leukaemia, particularly in childhood. The child commonly looks ill and complains of pain, predominantly in the back and large joints. Pain is often bilateral, symmetrical and severe and is characteristically disproportionate to any signs present in the joints. Fever and anaemia are common, but 30% have no signs outside the locomotor system. Sternal tenderness and disproportionate anaemia (frequently below 10 g) should always raise suspicion of the diagnosis and lead to marrow aspiration. X-rays are often normal but may show periarticular osteoporosis, periosteal elevation or osteolytic lesions. Response to anti-leukaemic therapy is often dramatic.

In multiple myeloma there are three possible mechanisms for joint pain: 1. deposition of amyloid; 2. involvement of adjacent bone; 3. secondary gout. Such patients, however, more commonly present with back pain than with peripheral joint problems (p 399).

Dermatomyositis/polymyositis

These diseases may occasionally be associated with occult malignancy, particularly of ovary, uterus, lung, breast and stomach. Underlying malignancy should particularly be suspected when presentation is in adults, especially in men over 50. Improvement may follow successful treatment of the carcinoma.

Polymyalgia rheumatica

Polymyalgia rheumatica may rarely be the presenting feature of underlying neoplastic disease, though there is no evidence for association with any particular tumour type (p 219). No association with temporal arteritis has been reported.

Secondary gout

This particularly occurs with myeloproliferative disorders such as leukaemia, lymphoma and myeloma, and complicates 5% of cases of polycythaemia rubra vera, in which it may precede the diagnosis by many years. Disseminated malignancy, especially when treated with cytotoxics, may cause secondary gout, though in the majority of cases the hyperuricaemia causes renal problems rather than gout, thus emphasising the importance of local tissue factors in crystal nucleation (p 158) Allopurinol is usually effective in preventing hyperuricaemia during cytotoxic administration. (Such prophylaxis requires reduction in dosage of 6-mercaptopurine).

Opportunist infection

This particularly occurs with leukaemia and myeloma, and is an important complication of immunosuppressive treatment. Manifestations are those of septic arthritis or osteomyelitis, although atypical sites may be involved (p 190).

RHEUMATIC DISORDERS THAT PREDISPOSE TO MALIGNANCY

Progressive systemic sclerosis

The incidence of alveolar cell carcinoma is increased in patients with progressive systemic sclerosis, particularly in those with long-standing lung disease (p 117). Awareness of this complication is especially important since this particular tumour type is slow growing and early resection can result in a favourable prognosis (50% 5-year survival).

'Scleroderma lung' clinically produces slowly progressive dyspnoea and fine basal rales. The occurrence of pain, productive cough, haemoptysis, large effusion or abrupt respiratory decompensation in a patient with PSS should therefore alert one to an underlying complication, such as opportunist pneumonia, heart failure or alveolar cell carcinoma, and lead to thorough investigation. The reason for predisposition to this particular histological type is unknown, but it is of interest that 10% of all alveolar cell carcinomas occur in a setting of pulmonary fibrosis.

Sjögren's syndrome

Deficiency of immune surveillance has been postulated as the cause of the increased incidence of lymphoma in this condition. Although lymphadenopathy and hepatosplenomegaly are normal features of SS, development of lymphoma should be suspected if there is marked enlargement and asymmetry of nodes, rapid increase in size of a node or regional group, or progressive fall in serum immunoglobulins from previously elevated levels (p 256).

Paget's disease

Osteogenic sarcoma is a dreaded complication of Paget's disease, with survival after diagnosis of usually less than one year. Its development is generally heralded by persistent severe pain (p 343).

Osteomyelitis

Squamous cell carcinoma is a recognised, though rare, complication of chronic osteomyelitis.

FURTHER READING(MALIGNANT DISEASE)

Caldwell D S 1981 Musculoskeletal syndromes associated with malignancy. Seminars on Arthritis and Rheumatism 10 (3): 198–223

III Endocrine Disorders

Almost all hormones have as one or more of their target cells the connective tissue cells, fibroblasts, chondrocytes, osteoblasts and sometimes lymphocytes and plasma cells. It is therefore hardly surprising that many endocrine disorders, of either deficiency or excess, should manifest within the osteoarticular and muscular systems. In many instances rheumatic complaints occur as a minor component of the endocrine syndrome, but occasionally musculoskeletal and articular manifestations dominate the clinical picture and lead to initial consideration of primary rheumatic disease. Articular involvement may result directly from hormonal alteration in joint architecture, or indirectly following subchondral bone disruption with secondary damage to overlying articular structures (both well exemplified in hyperparathyroidism). Although several of the articular syndromes continue to progress after correction of the underlying metabolic abnormality, others do not, and the general reversibility of the endocrine disorders adds special importance to their recognition.

Although the importance of hormone–target-cell interaction on the growth, structure and function of tissues is well recognised, the mechanisms that permit specificity and amplification of the hormone ('first messenger') signal are still but poorly understood. Steroid hormones appear to act via a protracted sequence involving cellular entry, binding to specific protein, attachment to chromatin and eventual direction of specific protein synthesis. In contrast, catecholamines and many polypeptide hormones act rapidly via specific interaction with membrane-bound adenyl cyclase to increase intracellular cyclic AMP ('second messenger') and thus immediately influence a variety of pre-existing enzyme systems. Intracellular calcium and calmodulin (a ubiquitous calcium-binding protein) appear to be important regulators of the cell response, and further elucidation of such cellular mechanisms promises the possibility of pharmacological modification of vital cell functions.

In this chapter the recognised rheumatic manifestations of endocrine disorders will be listed and the more specific conditions described.

THYROID DISEASE

Hyperthyroidism

Hyperthyroidism may produce a florid disease, often accompanied by exophthalmos, in young adults, but in older patients the clinical picture is usually less florid. Rheumatic manifestations associated with this disease are rare.

Clinical features of hyperthyroidism

General

1. Goitre (± bruit, thrill)
2. Heat intolerance
3. Warm, moist skin
4. Weight loss (+ increased appetite)
5. Tiredness, irritability
6. Fine tremor
7. Tachycardia, exertional dyspnoea
8. Atrial fibrillation, heart failure (elderly)
9. Eye signs
   a) Eyelid oedema
   b) Conjunctivitis
   c) Exophthalmos
   d) Lid retraction, lid lag
   e) Opthalmoplegia (superior rectus)
10. Pretibial myxoedema
11. Splenomegaly

Musculoskeletal (all uncommon)

1. Thyroid acropachy
2. Proximal myopathy
3. Periarthritis
4. Osteoporosis
5. (Drug-induced lupus)

Acropachy

This presents insidiously with bilateral, symmetrical soft-tissue swelling of the hands and feet. Pain, warmth and inflammatory features are minimal, and stiffness is usually the only complaint. Onset occurs some years after successful treatment of hyperthyroidism and many patients are in fact hypothyroid. Acropachy only occurs in patients with Grave's disease (1%), and exophthalmos,

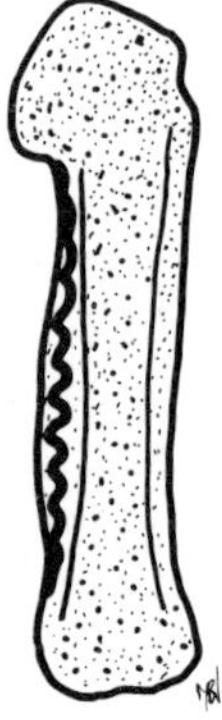

Fig. 16.7 Lacy 'soap-bubble' periostitis in metacarpal bone

pretibial myxoedema and clubbing inevitably co-exist. X-rays may reveal characteristic irregular 'soap-bubbly' subperiosteal new bone formation, particularly involving the radial aspect of the first and second metacarpals, the ulnar aspect of the fifth metacarpal, the metatarsals and phalanges (Fig. 16.7). The pathogenesis of this rare condition is obscure and the significance of elevated LATS levels in most patients is uncertain. No treatment is required and nothing appears to alter its progress.

Periarthritis

Thyrotoxic patients may occasionally develop severe stiffness and limitation of shoulder movement. Capsular thickening with surrounding soft-tissue swelling may be detected both clinically and radiologically but effusions and inflammatory features are absent. Knees, hips and MCP joints are less commonly involved. Standard treatments for bursitis are unsuccessful (p 359), but the condition resolves completely on correction of the hyperthyroidism.

Clinical features of hypothyroidism

General

1. Cold intolerance
2. Weight gain
3. Constipation
4. Hoarse voice
5. Poor memory
6. Depression
7. Menorrhagia
8. Coarse skin
9. Dry hair
10. Hair/eyebrow loss
11. Slow relaxing reflexes
12. Bradycardia
13. Deafness

Rheumatic

1. Major
   a) Carpal tunnel syndrome
   b) Stiffness, muscle cramps
2. Minor
   a) Myopathy
   b) Arthropathy
   c) Epiphyseal dysplasia (cretinism)

Hypothyroidism

Hypothyroidism is a common endocrine disease that particularly affects middle aged women. Musculoskeletal manifestations may be the presenting feature.

Carpal tunnel syndrome

This is a common complication, affecting 10 per cent of patients. It results from a combination of 1. direct pressure from oedematous or pseudomucinous material within the tunnel; and 2. peripheral neuropathy. Similar effects may lead to median plantar nerve compression in the foot. Local steroid injection is less effective than in other causes of carpal tunnel but response to thyroxine replacement is usually dramatic.

Stiffness, cramps

Generalised, diffuse muscle-aching and stiffness are common, particularly affecting shoulders, thighs and calves. Aching is made worse by exercise, and morning stiffness may be so severe as to simulate polymyalgia rheumatica. Nocturnal calf cramps are a frequent accompaniment. Muscles are rarely tender but may appear firm and enlarged. Slow relaxing reflexes and other features of hypothyroidism should suggest the diagnosis. Rapid response usually follows thyroxine replacement.

Myopathy

Hypothyroidism occasionally causes a marked, severely painful proximal myopathy which may be associated with muscle hypertrophy (Hoffman's syndrome) and pseudomyotonia (sustained muscle contraction on direct percussion but without the characteristic EMG changes). Mucinous deposits and a mixed myopathic/neuropathic picture is seen on histology and serum CPK levels may be markedly elevated. Response to thyroxine replacement is usually complete.

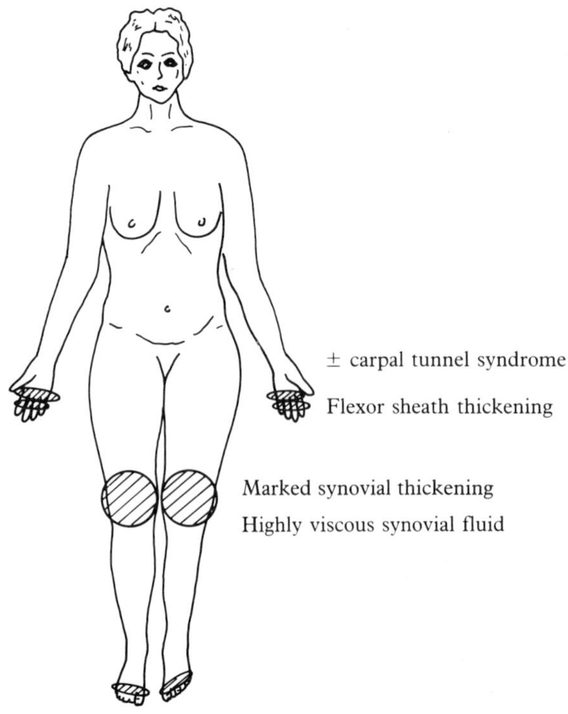

Fig. 16.8 Hypothyroid arthropathy

Arthritis

Florid myxoedema is occasionally associated with a characteristic arthropathy that superficially mimics RA (Fig. 16.8). Presentation is insidious, with pain and swelling of knees and small joints of the hands and feet (MCP, PIP, MTP joints), often accompanied by thickening of the flexor-tendon sheaths of the hand. Morning stiffness, however, is not a feature and joints are rarely warm or tender on examination. Synovial thickening may be marked, and knee effusions are typically difficult to detect because the SF is thick and the fluid wave is slow to appear. Aspiration characteristically reveals SF that is highly viscous due to excess hyaluronate. X-rays show soft-tissue swelling and periarticular osteopenia but no erosions. With the exception of the flexor-tendon sheath thickening, which may be helped by local steroid injection, the condition rapidly resolves with thyroxine replacement.

Chondrocalcinosis due to CPPD crystal deposition (p 175) is more frequent in hypothyroid patients, and thyroxine treatment may precipitate acute attacks of pseudogout. Pyrophosphate arthropathy may be responsible for the increase in tibial plateau collapse reported in hypothyroid patients, but CPPD crystals appear to play no part in the non-inflammatory arthropathy of myxoedema. If pyrophosphate arthropathy has developed it will continue to progress despite thyroxine replacement. Stimulation of membrane-bound adenyl cyclase by excess TSH would theoretically lead to increased production of both hyaluronate and inorganic pyrophosphate and may partly explain some of the effects on synovium seen in hypothyroidism.

PARATHYROID DISEASE

Hyperparathyroidism

This not uncommon disease particularly affects women and often escapes detection for many years because of the non-specific nature of the symptoms. Bone and joint disease are cardinal features of the condition.

Clinical features of hyperparathyroidism

General

1. Diffuse abdominal pain
2. Anorexia, nausea
3. Constipation
4. Lethargy
5. Alteration in personality
6. Polydipsia, polyuria
7. Renal colic, renal stones
8. (peptic ulcer)
9. (pancreatitis)

Musculoskeletal

1. Major
   a) Parathyroid bone disease
   b) Subchondral bone collapse
   c) Chondrocalcinosis and pyrophosphate arthropathy
2. Minor
   Erosive arthritis

Bone disease

Both primary and secondary hyperparathyroidism cause identical bone disease characterised by accelerated removal of both mineral and organic elements (i.e. osteopenia). This histologically results in reduction in number of trabeculae, increase in osteoclasts and a dense fibrovascular marrow. Exuberant osteoclast activity in primary disease in addition may give rise to cysts and 'brown tumours', although such gross 'Von Recklinghausen's disease of bone' is now rare. The overall effect is gross mechanical weakening of bone.

Patients present clinically with bone pain. Localisation of symptoms is characteristically poor and a long-standing history of non-specific, diffuse aches and pains is usual. Back pain is common but again shows no specific features. Symptoms usually appear disproportionate to any physical signs, and other indefinite symptoms of hyperparathyroidism, such as fatigue, weakness, personality change and diffuse abdominal discomfort, often compound to reduce the patient's credibility, resulting in long delays in diagnosis. As bony involvement becomes more pronounced, however, the following radiological changes may appear:

Early

characteristic subperiosteal erosions, best seen in phalanges (Fig. 16.9)

generalised demineralisation with 'ground glass' appearance.

Late

Horizontal radiolucent areas across the middle of vertebral bodies ('rugger-jersey' spine)

Resorption of both ends of clavicles

Loss of lamina dura around teeth

'Wrapping' of patella around femur

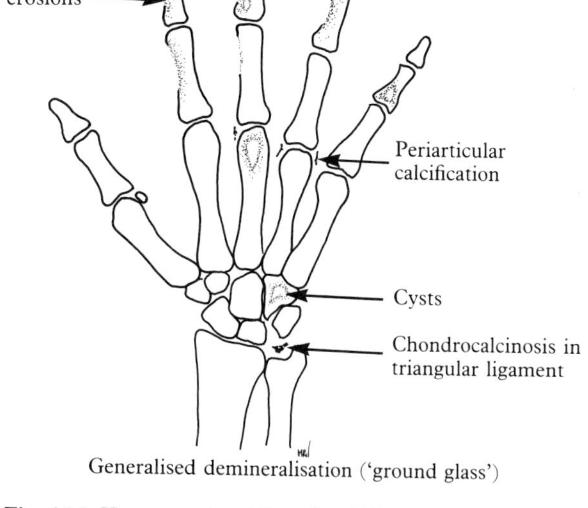

Fig. 16.9 Hyperparathyroidism: hand X-ray changes

Bone cysts, compression fractures, Schmorl's nodes, kyphosis

Nephrolithiasis and nephrocalcinosis

Laboratory findings are summarised in Table 16.1. Patients with primary hyperparathyroidism tend to have a hyperchloraemic acidosis which may be useful in differentiation from other causes of hypercalcaemia (usually associated with hypochloraemic alkalosis): parathormone radioimmunoassay will confirm the diagnosis. Bone disease is included in the criteria for surgical removal of hyperfunctioning parathyroid tissue and successful parathyroidectomy usually results in relief of bone pain and cessation of the abnormal bone resorption. Hypocalcaemia and hypomagnesaemia are common postoperatively and should be treated promptly, and patients with severe bone disease

Table 16.1 Laboratory findings in hyperparathyroidism

	Serum calcium	Serum phosphate	Alkaline phosphatase	Urinary calcium	Urinary hydroxyproline
Primary hyperparathyroidism	↑	↓	N	↑	N
Primary hyperparathyroidism with bone disease	↑	↓	↑	↑	↑
Secondary hyperparathyroidism	N/↓	N/↑	N/↑	↓	N/↑
Secondary hyperparathyroisism with osteomalacia	N/↓	↓	↑	↓	↑

are often given vitamin D supplements until the alkaline phosphatase returns to normal.

Subchondral bone collapse and 'secondary' OA

Bone disease may result in pathological microfracture and collapse of adjacent articular structures. This is particularly seen at the knee, where tibial plateau collapse may follow even minor trauma. Patients complain of sudden onset of pain and swelling around the knee, and on examination there may be localised bony tenderness and a bloodstained effusion. Such traumatic synovitis tends to be recurrent, leading eventually to joint deformity and osteoarthritis. Other joints, particularly the tarsus and carpus, may similarly be involved. Such secondary joint involvement will progress despite correction of the parathyroid bone disease.

Chondrocalcinosis and pyrophosphate arthropathy

Chondrocalcinosis occurs in up to 25% of patients with hyperparathyroidism and acute and chronic disease ('pyrophosphate arthropathy') may occur in a proportion of these (p 175). Acute attacks particularly follow parathyroidectomy when hypocalcaemia is marked, and this observation is used to support the 'crystal-shedding' hypothesis (p 168). Once present, chronic pyrophosphate arthropathy persists, in spite of parathyroidectomy and metabolic correction.

Increased PTH levels, in the absence of parathyroid disease, have been reported in a high proportion of patients with pyrophosphate arthropathy or with OA, but the significance of this is unclear.

Erosive arthritis

Although its pathogenesis is obscure, erosive polyarthritis is a well recognised, though uncommon, feature of hyperparathyroidism. It has been postulated that hypervascularity in the periosteum may induce, via putative connections, increased vascularity in the synovium, but erosive synovitis can occur in the absence of subperiosteal changes and the mechanism of production of the erosions is unclear.

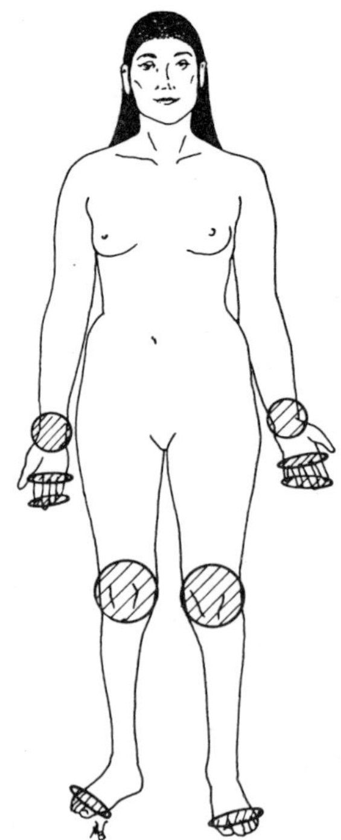

Fig. 16.10 Erosive arthritis in hyperparathyroidism

Patients present with insidious onset of pain and stiffness symmetrically affecting small joints of the hands, wrists, feet and knees (Fig. 16.10). Morning stiffness and malaise may be marked and the finding of radiological juxta-articular erosions may add to the clinical resemblance of this condition to RA, with which it is usually confused. Distinguishing features which suggest the diagnosis, however, include:

1. A 'shaggy' appearance to the erosions, with 'whiskering' at joint margins
2. Predilection for DIP, MCP, radiocarpal and radioulnar involvement with relative sparing of PIPs
3. Rarity of joint space narrowing and juxta-articular osteopenia
4. Other features indicating parathyroid bone disease (see above)

This condition usually responds well to parathyroidectomy and subsequent improvement in radiological changes would seem to support an osteogenic origin for the erosions.

Miscellaneous conditions

Although hyperuricaemia is common, particularly in the presence of nephrocalcinosis and hypercalcaemic tubular nephropathy, there is no firm evidence for an increased incidence of gout. Increased laxity of periarticular structures with tendency to ligamentous rupture and avulsion has been reported, and metastatic calcification due to hydroxyapatite may occur in periarticular structures, especially in those with secondary hyperparathyroidism and renal disease (p 184).

Hypoparathyroidism

All forms of this rare condition may be accompanied by soft tissue calcification. Ectopic apatite deposition occurs because of the high serum phosphate which elevates the calcium phosphate product above a critical level. Affected patients may complain of progressive stiffness and limitation of movement in the spine, hips and shoulder and thus superficially resemble ankylosing spondylitis. Inflammatory features, however, are absent and X-rays show non-marginal syndesmophytes ± extensive peripheral and ligamentous calcification: sacroiliitis and other changes of AS do not occur. Calcium and vitamin D may control symptoms of hypocalcaemia such as cramps, parasthesiae and tetany.

Patients with the rare condition of pseudohypoparathyroidism often have round faces, extensive subcutaneous calcification and shortened metacarpals and metatarsals. A dimple may occur at the normal knuckle location when the patient makes a fist. Treatment is again symptomatic, with calcium and vitamin D.

DIABETES MELLITUS

Osteoarticular disease occasionally occurs as a direct complication of this common endocrine disorder. Coexistant but unrelated rheumatic disease, however, is more usual, and certain conditions are reported to occur with increased incidence.

Clinical features of diabetes mellitus

General

1. Ocular disease
   a) Retinopathy
   b) Cataracts
   c) Glaucoma
2. Neurological disease
   a) Peripheral neuropathy
   b) Mononeuritis multiplex
   c) Autonomic neuropathy
      (i) Impotence
      (ii) Postural hypotension
      (iii) Diarrhoea
   d) Amyotrophy
3. Renal involvement
   a) Pyelonephritis
   b) Glomerulonephritis
4. Premature, widespread atherosclerosis
5. Skin disease
   a) Fat atrophy/hypertrophy
   b) Ulceration, infection
   c) Necrobiosis lipoidica
6. Recurrent infections

Rheumatic

1. Direct complications
   a) Septic arthritis/osteomyelitis
   b) Diabetic osteopathy
   c) Neuropathic joints
2. Associated conditions:
   a) Diabetic stiff hands (cheiroarthropathy)
   b) Periarthritis (especially frozen shoulder)
   c) Forrestier's disease (DISH)
   d) Dupuytren's contracture
   e) Chondrocalcinosis
   f) Osteoarthritis
   g) Gout

Diabetic osteopathy or 'osteolysis'

Forefoot osteolysis appears to be a unique complication of diabetes and may occur when the diabetes is mild or even unrecognised. The usual presenting feature is forefoot pain, exacerbated by

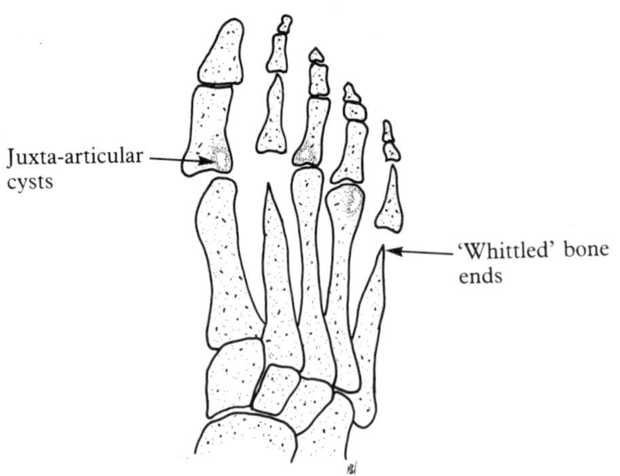

'Spotty' generalised osteopenia
Articular surfaces generally well preserved

Fig. 16.11 Diabetic osteolysis

walking. X-rays show progression from 'spotty', generalised osteopenia of the distal metatarsals and proximal phalanges to complete lysis of bone ends, giving a 'whittled' bone appearance. Well demarcated juxta-articular cysts frequently co-exist but articular-surfaces are well preserved (Fig. 16.11). The lytic process may halt at any stage and be followed by full restoration of structure and function. Such bony dissolution may occur in the absence of infection, neuropathy or angiopathy (indeed such osteolysis implies increased vascularity) and its pathogenesis is not understood.

There is no specific treatment. The usual differential diagnosis is osteomyelitis, but the absence of gross neurological defect, lack of plantar callus, absence of inflammatory features, systemic well-being and characteristic X-ray changes should all suggest osteolysis.

Neuropathic joints

This may develop as a complication of chronic diabetic neuropathy and most frequently involves the tarsal and tarso-metatarsal joints (less commonly the MTP, ankle: rarely the knee, wrist, spine). Radiological and pathological features are common to all types of Charcot joint (p 231).

Diabetic stiff hands (cheiroarthropathy)

This presents as tightening of the skin over the fingers, occasionally with pain, preventing the patient from laying the palms flat. The flexor tendons may be tight, though not necessarily thickened, and fingers show limited extension at MCP and IP joints. It has been reported in up to one fifth of juvenile-onset insulin-dependent diabetics but may also occur in middle-aged diabetics and in first-degree relatives. An association with short stature and increased tendency to vascular complications has been suggested. The condition is not progressive and is rarely troublesome.

Putative associations

Although several studies report an increased incidence of chondrocalcinosis and pyrophosphate arthropathy in patients with maturity-onset diabetes this most probably reflects association between two common age-related phenomena (p 175). Similarly, the interrelationship between gout and diabetes is controversial and clouded by variable definitions of glucose intolerance and by the influence of obesity and hyperlipidaemia (p 164). The higher incidence, more severe involvement and earlier age of onset of primary generalised osteoarthritis in diabetics is better substantiated — both conditions have strong genetic implications and may share a common hereditary pattern (p 145).

ACROMEGALY

This uncommon disorder often escapes detection for many years. Rheumatic symptoms occur in the majority of acromegalics and may be the presenting feature. Early recognition of the underlying disease is important since treatment of the pituitary adenoma is potentially curative.

Back pain and hypermobility

Low back pain, worsened by exercise and unaccompanied by stiffness, is a frequent symptom.

Clinical features of acromegaly

General

1. Leathery, furrowed skin
   a) ± increased sweating
   b) ± seborrhoea
   c) ± hirsutism
2. Large hands, feet
3. Prominent jaw, supra-orbital ridges
4. Splanchnomegaly
5. Large tongue
6. Headache
7. Visual-field defects
8. Hoarse voice, goitre
9. Weakness
10. Impotence
11. Gynaecomastia/galactorrhoea
12. Gonadal atrophy
13. Amenorrhoea
14. Glycosuria
15. Hypertension

Rheumatic (all common)

1. Back pain + hypermobility
2. Carpal tunnel syndrome
3. Acromegalic arthropathy
4. Raynaud's phenomenon

Objective signs are few and lumbar movement is normal or excessive. Lumbar hypermobility is particularly marked in elderly patients in whom spinal movement is normally decreased. Higher in the back the thoracic spine may be more fixed and kyphotic, but neck movements are usually well maintained.

X-rays show kyphosis and vertebral body enlargement — the latter appearing as 'scalloping' or exaggeration of the posterior concavity of the lumbar vertebrae (Fig. 16.12). Osteoporosis is often marked but the precise pathogenesis of the backache is unknown. Symptoms may improve following early correction of the growth hormone excess.

Carpal tunnel syndrome

This affects 50 percent of acromegalics and is usually bilateral. Diurnal variation is less marked than usual and objective sensory or motor signs are rare. Treatment of the pituitary lesion results in rapid recovery, suggesting oedema as a major factor in its causation, although bony and soft tissue overgrowth may also play a part.

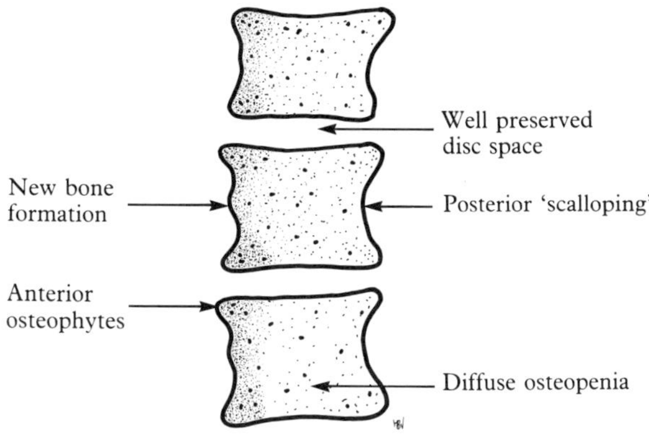

Fig. 16.12 Lumbar spinal changes in acromegaly

Acromegalic arthropathy

Hyperstimulation of chondrocytes, fibroblasts and other connective tissue cells by excess growth hormone results in:

1. Increased production of ground substances, leading to thickened but unduly friable cartilage matrix
2. Fibrous and fatty hyperplasia within synovial villi, grossly leading to hypertrophy
3. Increased growth of bone and soft tissues.

The vulnerability of the thickened cartilage to precocious fissuring and ulceration results in a continuous cycle of cartilage fragmentation, disordered joint mechanics and tissue repair with exuberant remodelling.

50% of acromegalics show evidence of joint disease (Fig. 16.13), though signs are usually more prominent than symptoms. The knees are most commonly involved, the patient developing gradual onset of pain in both knees, worse on weight-bearing. Stiffness and other inflammatory features are notably absent. Shoulders and hips may similarly be affected, but symptoms from

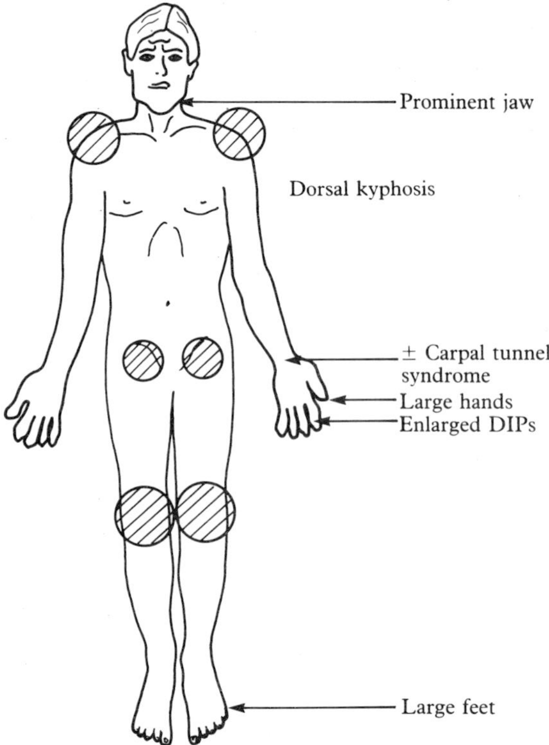

Fig. 16.13 Acromegalic arthropathy

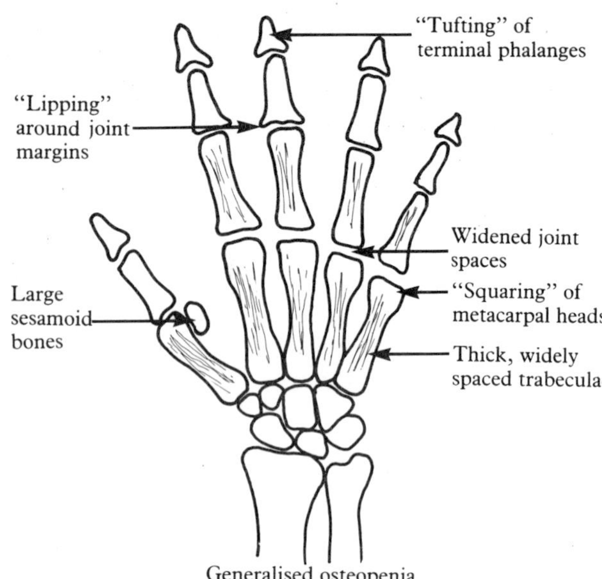

Fig. 16.14 Acromegaly: hand X-ray changes

involvement of small joints in the hands are unusual. Examination of knees typically reveals continuous, coarse crepitus but little restriction in range of movement. The patella often rides well clear of the femoral condyles and is fairly mobile, unlike the 'stuck' patella common in other forms of 'degenerative arthritis' Exuberaut pre-patella bursae, bony overgrowth and soft-tissue swelling may all contribute to joint enlargement, but effusions are rarely marked. Crepitus and effusion may be found in the shoulders, but again mobility is characteristically well-maintained. The hip is the joint most commonly compromised by severe changes. In the hands, objective evidence of arthritis is unusual except at the first CMC joint, and enlarged DIPs are particularly noticeable in showing a wide range of pain-free movement. The coarse, thickened skin, hirsutism, increased sweating and other classical features of acromegaly may readily suggest the diagnosis, but the rheumatological clue is the combination of marked crepitus with non-inflammatory joint swelling and retention or even increase in the range of joint movement.

Radiographic changes are characteristic (Fig. 16.14). Eventually the X-ray appearance of severely involved knees or hips is the same as that

Radiographic changes that may be present in acromegaly

1. Widened joint spaces (due to cartilage hyperplasia)
2. Thickened, widely-spaced bony trabeculae
3. Squaring of metacarpal ends and enlargement of femoral and tibial condyles
4. 'Tufting' of distal phalanges and bony outgrowth ('lipping') around joint margins
5. Increase in size of sesamoid bones
6. Generalised osteoporosis
7. Increase in heel-pad thickness; abnormality of the sella turcica; increase in frontal sinuses

of severe OA from any cause, with the accent on bony hypertrophy and remodelling of ossifying tissue.

Once acromegalic arthropathy has developed it is generally irreversible and treatment of the pituitary lesion is without effect.

Raynaud's phenomenon

This occurs in up to 25% of patients. Involvement is more marked in hands than feet and its cause is unexplained.

ADRENAL DISEASE

Patients with endogenous Cushing's syndrome may develop profound osteoporosis with crush fractures, and aseptic necrosis identical to that seen secondary to high dose corticosteroid therapy. No specific arthropathy, however, has been described.

FURTHER READING (ENDOCRINE DISORDERS)

Bland J H, Frymoyer J W, Newberg A H, Reevers R, Norman R J 1979 Rheumatic syndromes in endocrine disease. Seminars in Arthritis and Rheumatism 9(1): 23–65

Holt P J L 1981 Locomotor abnormalities in acromegaly. Clinics in Rheumatic Diseases 7(3): 689–709

Kyle V, Hazleman B L 1981 The thyroid. Clinics in Rheumatic Diseases 7(3): 711–72

Holt P J L 1981 Rheumatological manifestations of diabetes mellitus. Clinics in Rheumatic Diseases 7(3): 723–746

IV Metabolic Diseases

INTRODUCTION

The diseases discussed in this chapter are all rare in terms of the numbers of patients affected but they are of considerable theoretical importance because of the insight they provide into the mechanisms by which joints can be damaged. In ochronosis, for example, a metabolic defect in amino acid metabolism results in the deposition of abnormal pigments in connective tissues causing accelerated cartilage degeneration and premature severe obsteoarthritis. Ochronosis would not have been so easily distinguished from the mass of osteoarthritis in the population but for the fact that the tissues are stained a striking black colour. Possibly there could be a host of minor defects in amino acid metabolism producing colourless metabolic products resulting in osteoarthritis. The accumulation of a metal such as iron in haemochromatosis may have a direct adverse effect on the joint tissues by acting as a catalyst in the production of superoxide radicals and hence promoting inflammation, but also may have an indirect effect by inhibiting pyrophosphatase enzymes causing deposition of calcium pyrophosphate and leading to chondrocalcinosis and attacks of pseudogout.

OCHRONOSIS

This is a rare disease inherited as an autosomal recessive trait which is also known as *alcaptonuria*. It is due to lack of the enzyme homogentisic acid oxidase and as a result excess homogentisic acid, produced during the metabolism of phenylalanine and tyrosine, accumulates in the serum and is excreted in the urine. A black pigment derived from homogentisic acid is deposited in the connective tissues of the body, particularly in hyaline cartilage of joints, in the annulus fibrosus and nucleus pulposus of the intervertebral disc, in the cartilage of the ears, nose and trachea, in the walls of large arteries, in tympanic membranes and in sclerae. The mechanism by which ochronotic

Clinical features of ochronosis

Extra-articular

1. Pigmented ears and eyes
2. Dark urine on standing
3. Black sweat

Articular

1. Low-back pain
2. Kyphosis
3. Knee effusions
4. Calcified intevertebral discs
5. Vertebral fusion

pigments cause degenerative changes in cartilage is not known but it is postulated that they may either have a direct effect on the cartilage itself or inhibit some of the enzymes involved in cartilage metabolism.

CLINICAL FEATURES (Figs 16.15 and 16.16)

A few cases of ochronosis are diagnosed shortly after birth because the urine leaves black stains on nappies which characteristically become deeper rather than disappear when washed in alkaline detergents. Some patients are detected because they complain of continually passing dark urine, but this is uncommon. The majority are diagnosed when they are investigated in middle age for arthritis, because they are found to have black cartilage at surgery, or because of a false-positive test for diabetes (homogentisic acid is a reducing substance).

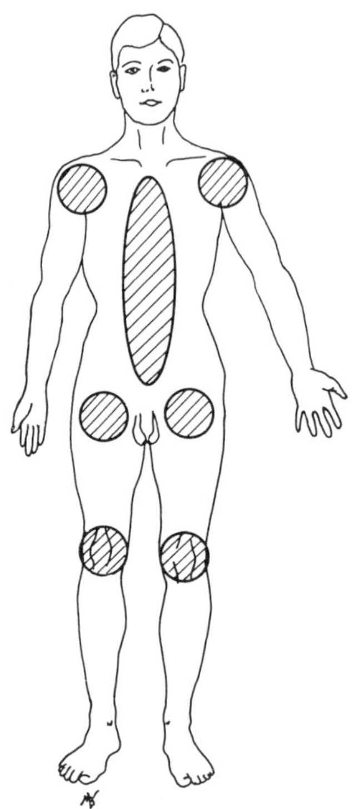

Fig. 16.15 Distribution of joint involvement in ochronosis

The arthritis of ochronosis affects men earlier and more severely than women. Early on the disease resembles rheumatoid arthritis with episodes of pain, swelling and stiffness in the knees, hips and shoulders. Eventually spinal disease dominates the clinical picture, with low back pain and stiffness associated with kyphosis of the thoracic spine, loss of the lumbar lordosis and reduced chest expansion, a clinical picture that may be easily mistaken for ankylosing spondylitis.

Typical pigmentary changes in the ear cartilage and the sclera are very useful in making the diagnosis, but they are only usually present in patients over the age of about 40. Pigments are excreted in the perspiration, staining the skin of the groins and axillae a brownish colour and the ear wax may be black. Classically, urine from a patient with ochronosis will go black if left standing, starting at the top and gradually spreading down through the urine as the homogentisic acid is oxidised by exposure to the air. This is rarely seen in practice unless the urine is left for many hours. The process can be greatly accelerated by alkalinising

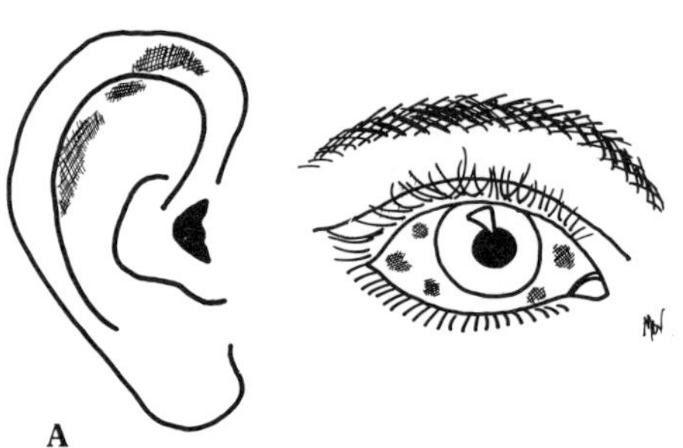

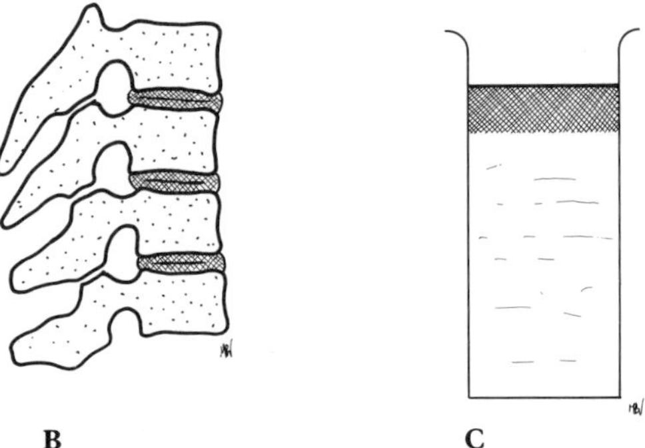

Fig. 16.16 Other features of ochronosis **A**. Black pigment in the ear cartilage and sclera **B**. Intervertebral disc calcification **C**. Exposed surface of urine darkens on standing

the urine. The diagnosis cannot be made on this test alone and should be confirmed by paper chromatography of the urine. Specific enzymatic methods are also available for quantitative measurement.

Radiological features of ochronosis are almost pathognomonic, particularly in the spine. The intervertebral discs of the lumbar spine are narrowed and densely calcified and some of the vertebral bodies may be fused. The sacro-iliac joints are normal and calcification of the interspinous ligaments does not occur. Osteophyte formation is minimal. The peripheral joints show degenerative changes with calcific deposits in the periarticular ligaments and occasionaly osteochondral loose bodies. Unlike OA, the shoulder is commonly affected.

There is as yet no effective way of increasing the levels of homogentisic acid oxidase and dietary restriction of tyrosine and phenylalanine is impractical. Treatment is aimed at relieving the symptoms of the arthritis.

HAEMOCHROMATOSIS

Introduction

This is a disorder of iron metabolism characterised by massive iron overload and deposition of haemosiderin in tissues, particularly liver, pancreas, heart, testes and pituitary and accumulation of melanin in the skin. Family studies indicate that this is a hereditary disorder but the mode of inheritance is not established. It is of interest that over 78% of patients carry HLA-A3. The underlying biochemical defect has not been clearly defined but results in excess absorption of iron from the gut. The exact mechanism by which arthritis occurs is not known but a direct relationship with iron overload is suggested by the finding of excess iron in articular cartilage and synovial lining cells and the development of a similar joint disease in secondary haemosiderosis associated with chronic haemolytic states and in Bantu beer drinkers. The effect of iron on phosphatase enzymes and the possible role this may play in calcium pyrophosphate deposition has already been mentioned in the introduction.

Clinical features of haemochromatosis

Extra-articular

1. Skin pigmentation
2. Loss of body hair
3. Impotence
4. Diabetes (bronzed diabetes)
5. Hepatomegaly
6. Cirrhosis
7. Heart failure

Articular

1. Arthritis 2nd & 3rd MCPJs
2. Pseudogout attacks
3. Chondrocalcinosis

Clinical features (Fig. 16.17)

Men are affected much more frequently than women and this difference may be due to iron loss from the body during menstruation. There is a prolonged asymptomatic prelude before onset of

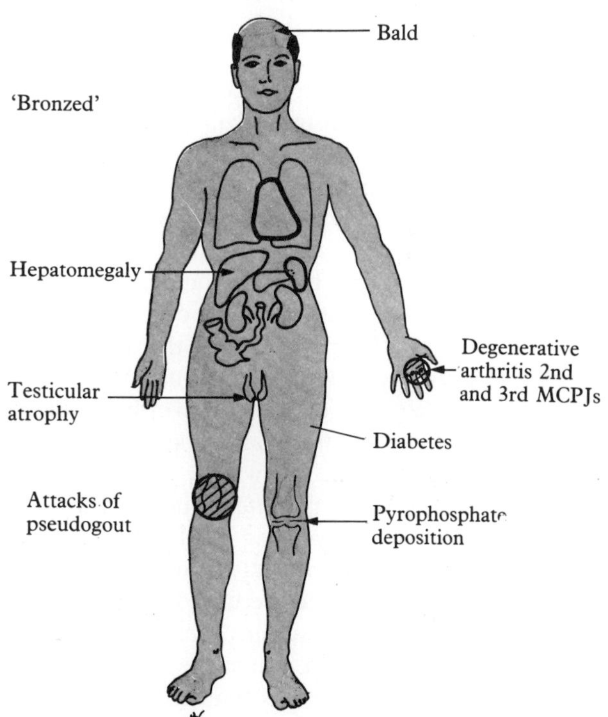

Fig. 16.17 Clinical features of haemochromatosis

clinical features at around the age of 40 years. The classic triad of haemochromatosis is skin pigmentation, cirrhosis and diabetes and the commonest presenting features are weight-loss, malaise and loss of libido. The skin pigmentation is of such gradual onset that it passes unnoticed by the patient or his family or is dismissed as suntan. In late disease, ascites may occur as a complication of cirrhosis and dyspnoea and oedema from cardiac failure. The diabetes of haemochromatosis is usually insulin-dependent and the incidence of diabetic complications such as retinopathy and nephropathy are the same as in non-haemochromatotic diabetics.

About half the patients develop an arthropathy, usually around the age of 50. Early complaints are of a mild generalised arthralgia with pain and stiffness in the fingers, particularly the second and third MCPJs which go on to develop mild destructive changes with bony swelling and loss of joint space on X-ray. The hips and shoulders may also be affected and occasionally hip joint replacement is necessary but generally severe disability and deformity do not occur. 30% of patients have superimposed attacks of pseudogout, usually in the knees and occasionally wrists and when these attacks occur along with the changes in the hands, the patient may be mistakenly diagnosed as having RA.

The earliest changes on X-ray are similar to OA, with joint-space narrowing, sclerosis and sub-articular cysts but particularly effect the second and third MCPJs, carpal bones, shoulder, knees and hips. In contradistinction to OA, cyst formation is more prominent particularly in the carpus and there is a relative lack of osteophytes. Widespread chondrocalcinosis is present in two-thirds of patients, usually in the fibro- and hyaline cartilage of the knee and also in the wrists, hip, symphysis pubis and annulus of the intervertebral disc.

The diagnosis is suggested by the presence of a raised serum iron and saturation of the iron binding capacity. The serum ferritin is also elevated and is a more sensitive marker and correlates well with the total iron stores. A liver biopsy to assess iron deposition is the definitive test and should be carried out if the blood coagulation tests are normal. Iron stores can be estimated by measuring urinary iron excretion following chelation with desferrioxamine.

Regular weekly venesection of 500–1000 ml of blood to remove excess iron will improve many of the extra-articular features of haemochromatosis, particularly diabetes, but has no effect on the established arthropathy, possibly because by that time the damage is irreversible and progressive. It is possible that early detection and treatment of haemochromatosis may prevent the development of the arthropathy but this has yet to be demonstrated. Family members should be screened to detect the disease in its asymptomatic stage.

WILSON'S DISEASE

Introduction

This rare disorder of copper metabolism is inherited as an autosomal recessive and is characterised by accumulation of copper in the tissues, particularly brain and liver, resulting in a neurological syndrome and cirrhosis of the liver. A characteristic arthropathy such as seen in ochronosis or haemochromatosis does not occur, but nevertheless over 70% have radiological skeletal abnormalities including osteoporosis, osteochondritis dessicans, premature osteoarthritis and recurrent fractures. A renal tubular defect is sometimes present, leading to rickets and osteomalacia. It has been suggested that the joint manifestations are the result of continuous tremor on thin bones.

Clinical features of Wilson's disease

Extra-articular

1. Cirrhosis
2. Mental retardation
3. Tremor
4. Rigidity
5. Chorea
6. Kayser-Fleischer corneal rings

Articular

1. Osteoporosis
2. Fractures
3. Degenerative arthritis
4. Para-articular bone fragments
5. Generalised hypermobility

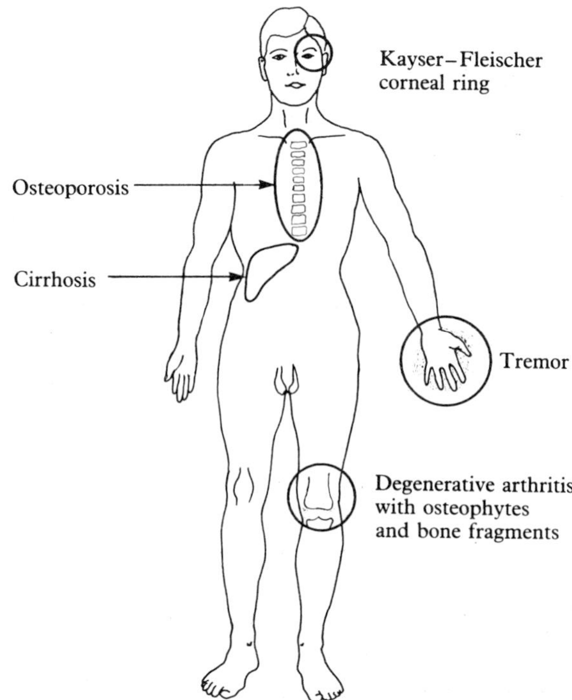

Fig. 16.18 Clinical features of Wilson's disease

Clinical features (Fig. 16.18)

Men and women are affected equally. The presentation is very variable, with hepatic disease dominating in some and the neurological syndrome in others. Intellectual deterioration is often one of the earliest features, starting in adolescence. This may be followed by extrapyramidal features of tremor, ataxia and cog-wheel rigidity. The earliest sign of hepatic involvement is hepatosplenomegaly progressing to a picture of chronic hepatitis and cirrhosis. Greenish-brown Kayser–Fleischer rings around the corneo-scleral junction are pathognomonic of this disease but may appear at any stage or be absent throughout. The joint problems usually begin around the age of 30 and affect mainly the hands, wrists and knees in a symmetrical fashion. Pain and limitation of movement are the main features, accompanied by swelling, tenderness and crepitus but without inflammation. Sometimes the elbows and shoulders are also affected.

Radiological examination shows generalised osteoporosis, and occasional fractures or pseudofractures. Affected joints exhibit degenerative changes with loss of joint-space, sclerosis and osteophyte formation. Small bony fragments are often seen adjacent to the joint margins.

The diagnosis is made by demonstrating an increased urinary copper excretion with a reduced serum copper and caeruloplasmin level. Copper can be shown to be extensively deposited in the liver and brain but has not been demonstrated in the synovium.

Untreated Wilson's disease is invariably fatal. The aim of treatment is to reduce dietary copper and remove excess copper from the tissues with chelating agents. D-penicillamine is the drug of choice given in a dose of 1 g a day. After several months' treatment, clinical improvement is usually observed. The earlier treatment is started the better the outcome and clinical manifestations can be entirely prevented if treatment is started in the asymptomatic stage. For this reason it is particularly important to screen family members. These patients remain on penicillamine for many years and may develop the same complications as seen in RA, including a drug-induced lupus-syndrome, thrombocytopenia and rash.

HOMOCYSTINURIA

Introduction

This disease is caused by an inherited deficiency of the enzyme cystathionine synthetase which causes accumulation of metabolites of homocystine which appear to interfere with the normal cross-linkage of collagen. This results in a characteristic disorder of connective tissue complicated by a marked tendency to vascular thrombosis.

Clinical features of homocytinuria

1. Marfanoid habitus
2. Stiff joints
3. Dislocated knees and 'rocker-bottom' feet
4. Mental impairment
5. Osteoporosis and fractures
6. Thrombotic incidents

Clinical features

Superficially these patients are similar to those with Marfan's syndrome. They are tall and thin with myopia and dislocated lenses. However, instead of joint laxity there is stiffness of joints. The skin and bones are thin and fractures common. Knock-knees and flat-feet may result in a shuffling toe-out 'Charlie Chaplin-like' gait. These patients also often have intellectual impairment thought to result from repeated minor cerebral thromboses and pulmonary and renal vascular thromboses which may result in premature death.

The cyanide nitroprusside test is useful for screening the urine for homocystine but the diagnosis must be confirmed by quantitative analysis of urinary amino acids.

Some patients improve with low methionine diets and large doses of pyridoxine. The earlier treatment is begun the better the response. It is now possible to diagnose this condition prenatally.

HYPERLIPOPROTEINAEMIA

Familial hypercholesterolaemia

This is an inherited disorder which results in a deficiency of cellular receptors for apolipoprotein B or low-density lipoproteins and as a consequence, serum levels of cholesterol rise markedly.

Clinical features

The homozygotes are severely affected and present in childhood with cutaneous xanthomas, corneal arcus and ischaemic heart disease. The arthritis, which is unrelated to the development of the skin lesions, takes the form of a large-joint migratory arthritis associated with redness and swelling. The children are often febrile and have cardiac murmurs and a raised ESR, so that the diagnosis is often mistaken for rheumatic fever. The joint disease is transient and does not progress, although the children die young from premature atherosclerosis. The mechanism of the joint inflammation is ill-understood. Cholesterol crystals have not been demonstrated in the joint fluid and radioisotope scans suggest that the inflammation may be peri- rather than intra-articular.

The heterozygotes present in adolescence with acute episodes of Achilles tendinitis or arthritis of the knees which last 2–3 days and recur two or three times a year. Cutaneous lesions of hypercholesterolaemia are often, but not always present.

X-rays are normal despite recurrent episodes. The diagnosis is confirmed by measuring the serum lipids. Dietary restriction, lipid lowering drugs, plasma exchange and intestinal bypass surgery are used to lower the cholesterol level, depending on severity.

Type IV hyperlipidaemia

This is an acquired abnormality in which serum triglycerides are elevated. It may be associated with other metabolic disorders such as diabetes mellitus, alcoholism and obesity and there is a strikingly high incidence in men with gout.

Clinical features

The patients are middle-aged and older and men and women are affected equally. There is no one clear-cut clinical pattern. Some patients have a persistent mild oligoarthritis affecting the hands and feet with periodic exacerbations. Others have episodic arthritis of a few days duration.

X-rays of affected joints often show mild juxta-articular osteoporosis without erosions, but occasionally in association with metaphyseal cysts. The diagnosis may be confirmed by finding elevated triglycerides. The glucose tolerance test is also often abnormal. The lipaemic serum may cause a false positive latex test.

Many of the articular features improve with lowering of the serum triglycerides by dietary means.

FURTHER READING (METABOLIC DISEASES)

Stanbury J B, Wyngaarden J B, Fredrickson D S 1978 The metabolic basis of inherited disease. McGraw-Hill, New York

O'Brien W M, La Du B N, Bunim J J 1963 Biochemical, pathological and clinical aspects of alcaptonuria, ochronosis, and ochronotic arthropathy. American Journal of Medicine 34: 813

Hamilton E, Williams R, Barlow K A, Smith P M 1968 The arthropathy of idiopathic haemochromatosis. Quarterly Journal of Medicine 37: 171–182

Schumacher H R Articular cartilage in the degenerative arthropathy of haemochromatosis. Arthritis and Rheumatism 5: 1460–1468

V Storage Diseases

LYSOSOMAL STORAGE DISEASES

These are a group of rare, genetically determined diseases usually presenting in infancy. Bone and joint abnormalities form only a small part of the clinical picture which is dominated by a mixture of features including striking visceral involvement, mental impairment, stunted growth and skeletal deformity. These children are not generally seen by rheumatologists because they die at an early age.

The Mucopolysaccharidoses

These are inter-related disorders in which one of the mucopolysaccharides (or *glycosaminoglycans* as they are now called) accumulates inside cells due to a deficiency of a lysosomal enzyme necessary for its degradation. The abnormal gene coding for the enzyme is recessively inherited and there is often consanguinity in affected families. Table 16.2 summarises the clinical and biochemical features of the major mucopolysaccharidoses.

Hurler's syndrome is the classic disease. The child usually appears normal at birth, although umbilical hernia and rhinitis are common. Within a year the features become coarse and ugly with enlargement of the head, wide-set protruding eyes, depressed nose, bulging cheeks and thick lips. The child is hirsute with a low hairline and bushy eyebrows. There is progressive blindness, deafness and intellectual impairment and visceral enlargement due to accumulation of mucopolysaccharide (Fig. 16.19).

The characteristic skeletal abnormalities are known collectively as *dysostosis multiplex*. The bones fail to grow and develop properly, so there is short stature, bowing of long bones, kyphosis, stubby fingers, clawed hands, knock knees and flat feet. On X-ray the calvarium is distorted and the base of the skull elongated, producing a J-shaped

Table 16.2 Classification of the major mucopolysaccharidoses. A–R, X–R = autosomal or X-linked recessive mode of inheritance; DS, HS, KS = dermatan sulphate, heparan sulphate, keratan sulphate

Name	Clinical features	MPS	Enzyme
Hurler	Skeletal, visceral Corneal clouding Mental retardation Death by 10 A–R	DS, HS	α-L-Iduronidase
Hunter	Milder than Hurler No corneal clouding Death by 15 X–R	DS, HS	Iduronate sulphatase
Scheie	Mild, with normal life span A–R	DS, HS	α-L-Iduronidase
Sanfilippo	Mild visceral Severe mental A–R	HS	Acetyl-co-A-glucosamine-N-acetyltransferase
Morquio	Severe skeletal Normal mental A–R	KS	N-Acetyl-galactosamine-6-sulphatase
Maroteaux-Lamy	Severe skeletal Corneal clouding Normal mental Death by 20 A–R	DS	N-acetyl-galactosamine-4-sulphatase

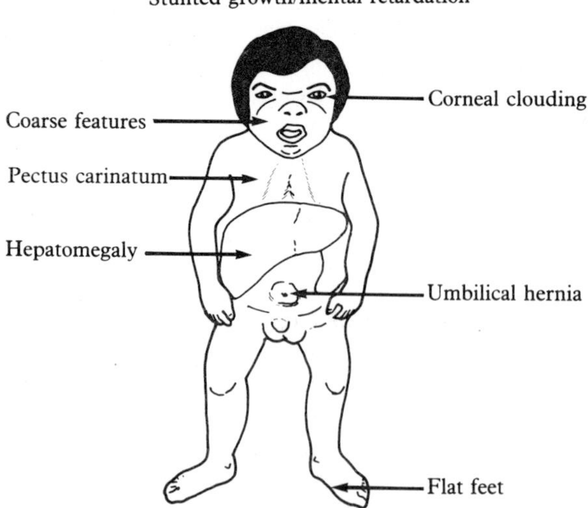

Fig. 16.19 Clinical features of Hurler's syndrome

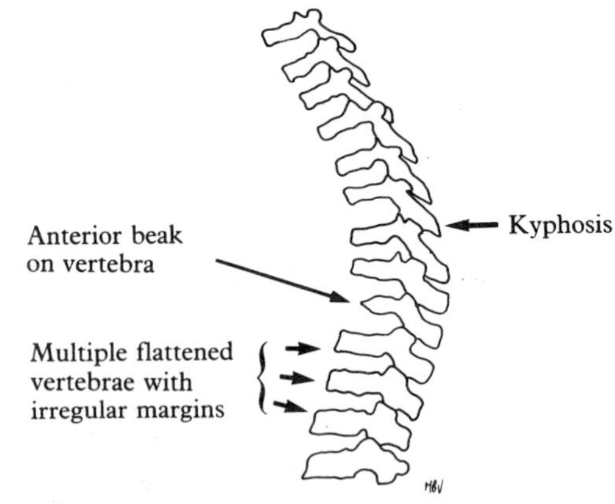

Fig. 16.20 Typical radiological features of the spine in Morquio's disease

sella turcica. Widening of the shafts of bones, particularly the clavicle and ribs, gives an 'oar-like' appearance. Anterior portions of the vertebral bodies fail to ossify, particularly in the lower thoracic and upper lumbar region and may collapse forming a gibbus. The hands show a claw-like deformity with delayed carpal ossification, points on the proximal ends of the metacarpal bones and 'bullet-shaped' phalanges. Odontoid hypoplasia and atlanto-axial subluxation are common.

The diagnosis is best made on the typical clinical and radiological features and can be confirmed by a simple urine test for detecting excess mucopolysaccharide. The specific type can then be characterised by column chromatography.

There is no effective therapy and death usually occurs before the tenth year of life from hydrocephalus and cardiac disease. Recently, attempts to replace the deficient enzyme by injecting normal plasma or white cells have been shown to be of some benefit, but only in the short term.

Hunter's syndrome is a milder form of Hurler's syndrome. These patients can survive into adulthood and may be prone to premature osteoarthritis of the hip.

Patients with Morquio's syndrome also have a better prognosis and frequently survive into middle life. There is a high incidence of atlanto-axial subluxation which may lead to cervical-cord compression and prophylactic surgery is indicated although not always successful. People with truncal dwarfism and a dysplastic appearance to the vertebral bodies on X-ray have tended to be labelled as *forme fruste* Morquio's syndrome, but probably represent types of spondyloepiphyseal dysplasia (Fig. 16.20).

Ganglioside storage diseases

These conditions are characterised by the accumulation of ganglioside in liposomes due to an inherited enzyme defect. Tay–Sachs disease is the best studied example in which there is an absence or deficiency of the enzyme hexosamide A and abnormal lipid storage in the nervous system. There is progressive mental deterioration, blindness and a characteristic cherry-red macular spot. The locomotor system is not a target for this disease.

One very rare type of ganglioside storage disease, Faber's disease (*diseminated lipogranulomatosis*) has arthritis as a prominent feature. Affected babies appear normal at birth but within a few weeks develop swollen, painful limbs. The joints are affected by an aggressive, erosive arthritis, associated with pigmented nodular swellings in the periarticular tissues. Death usually occurs by the age of 2.

Fabrey's disease (angiokeratoma corporis diffusum) is an X-linked deficiency of the enzyme ceramide trihexosidase. It is characterised by episodes of fever, lightening limb and abdominal pains, proteinuria and haematuria. Some patients also develop a painful arthritis of the fingers, particularly of the distal interphalangeal joints, elbows and knees. Avascular necrosis of the femoral head is common. Clusters of red papular skin lesions about 4 mm in diameter occur around the pelvic region. Death usually supervenes around middle age from hypertension and renal failure but there are reports of prolonged survival following renal transplantation.

Gauchers disease is due to an inherited defect of glucocerebrosidase which results in accumulation of Gaucher's cells in tissues through the body and particularly in the bones. It presents as either a severe progressive neurological disorder in childhood or as a relatively benign musculoskeletal disorder of teenagers and adults. Episodes of pain in the hips, knees and shoulders are often accompanied by low-grade fever so that it is easily mistaken for osteomyelitis. Pathological fractures and avascular necrosis of the femoral head are common. Occasionally, patients also have a flitting polyarthritis which may lead to joint destruction. On X-ray the bones show areas of rarefaction interspersed with sclerosis and cortical thinning. The distal end of the femur is characteristically enlarged — the 'Ehrlenmeyer flask' appearance. The serum acid phosphatase is very high and there is often a monoclonal increase in immunoglobulin. The diagnosis is confirmed by demonstrating Gaucher cells on biopsy of affected tissue. There is no effective treatment. Bone pain can be relieved by corticosteroids. Splenectomy, which is often performed to correct haematological manifestations, frequently makes the musculoskeletal symptoms worse.

MISCELLANEOUS

Histiocytosis X group

This group of diseases includes Hand–Schüller–Christian (HSC), Letterer–Siwe (LS), and eosiniphilic granuloma of bone (EGB). Histologically these conditions are all characterised by the development of granulomas which contain eosinophils, lipid-filled macrophages and multinucleated giant cells. There is still debate as to whether they represent different ends of the spectrum of the same disease or are separate entities. LS presents below the age of 3 with fever, recurrent infection, hepatosplenomegaly and lymphadenopathy with multiple punched-out lesions in rarefied bone. Older children have multiple cranial deposits at the base of the skull, exophthalmos and diabetes insipidus — the *Christian triad*. EGB are usually solitary, but occasionally multiple, lytic lesions of bone occuring in the skull, vertebrae and long bones of children and young adults (Fig. 16.21). The lesions usually heal spontaneously but progression to HSC has been reported. Isolated lesions in vertebral bodies may cause collapse and EGB is now thought to be the underlying pathological process in Calvé's disease (Fig. 16.22). The prognosis of LS and HSC is bad since both diseases are usually fatal, whereas EGB is self limiting.

Glycogen storage disease

Classical glycogen storage disease is due to deficiency of glucose-6-phosphatase, which releases free glucose from the liver. Multiple metabolic consequences result, including hypoglycaemia,

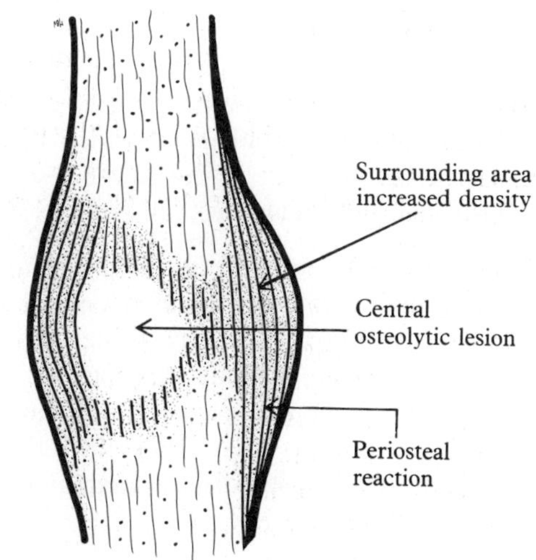

Fig. 16.21 Eosinophilic granuloma of bone

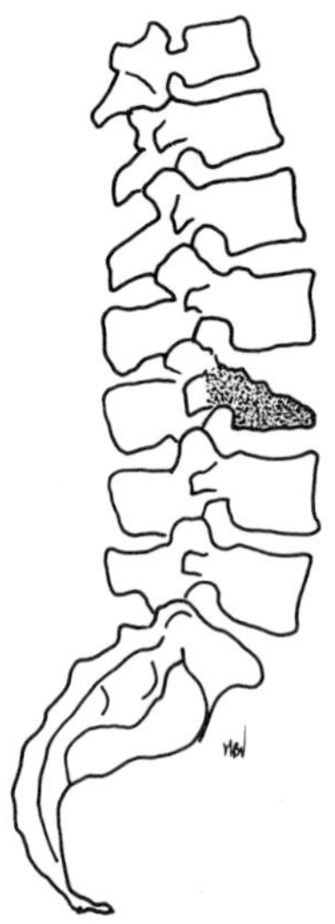

Fig. 16.22 Vertebra plana (Calvé's disease)

hyperlipidaemia and severe episodes of metabolic acidosis with elevated pyruvate and lactate levels. Occasionally, this can lead to functional impairment of tubular transport of uric acid, resulting in hyperuricaemia and attacks of gout.

FURTHER READING (STORAGE DISEASE)

Wyngaarden J B, Fredrickson D S 1978 The metabolic basis of inherited disease. McGraw-Hill, New York

VI Sarcoidosis

Sarcoidosis is a multi-system granulomatous disorder of unknown aetiology in which the principal site of involvement is the lower respiratory tree. Two main forms are recognised:

1. *Acute, transient sarcoidosis* (common): acute presentation with erythema nodosum often heralds this limited form that undergoes spontaneous resolution without sequelae.
2. *Chronic, persistent sarcoidosis* (rare): insidious onset of symptoms may lead into this less favourable, generalised disease characterised by progressive fibrosis.

Polyarthritis may be a prominent, and even presenting, feature of both types, and in chronic sarcoid there may additionally be involvement of bone or muscle.

PATHOGENESIS

Histologically, sarcoidosis is characterised by the widespread presence of non-caseating epithelioid cell granulomata. Such 'sarcoid granulomata' are not specific, however, and are seen in several other idiopathic conditions associated with altered immunity (e.g. primary biliary cirrhosis, Crohn's disease, hypogammaglobulinaemia, SLE, neoplasia), and may be produced in response to a wide variety of extrinsic agents including infections, chemicals and dusts.

Immunological abnormalities are a consistent finding but differ in acute and chronic forms. In acute sarcoid delayed hypersensitivity is suppressed and circulating immune complexes and complement activation products are frequently demonstrated, supporting an immune complex pathogenesis for the early transient skin and joint lesions. In chronic disease, however, lymphoproliferation with B-cell overactivity is more pronounced, delayed hypersensitivity may be normal and immune complexes are infrequent. In this situation tissue damage appears to be caused predominantly by compression and fibrosis from persistent and widespread granuloma formation.

No tissue type predisposes to sarcoidosis but there is some evidence that HLA-A1, B8 individuals are more likely to express their disease in the form of acute arthritis, erythema nodosum and anterior uveitis, while HLA-B13 individuals are more prone to develop persistent chronic disease. This differs from the normal situation, where acute iritis shows strong association with HLA-B27 (p 66).

CLINICAL PRESENTATION

Patients with sarcoidosis present in one of four ways:

1. With symptomatic thoracic involvement (dyspnoea, cough, chest pain, haemoptysis)

2. With extrathoracic involvement of skin, joints, eyes or CNS
3. With constitutional symptoms of fever, malaise, weight loss
4. With asymptomatic hilar lymphadenopathy detected on routine CXR

Arthritis is a common manifestation occurring in up to 40% of patients. Although sarcoid shows an equal sex incidence, arthritis is two to three times more common in women. Two distinct patterns are recognised.

Acute, early arthritis

This usually occurs at the onset of the disease, often as the presenting feature, with symmetrical polyarthralgia, erythema nodosum and bilateral hilar lymphadenopathy (Löfgren's syndrome). Onset during pregnancy or lactation is classical but infrequent.

> **Clinical features of acute sarcoid**
> *General*
> 1. Fever
> 2. Malaise
> 3. Erythema nodosum
> 4. Acute iritis/conjunctivitis
> 5. Lymphadenopahty/splenomegaly
> 6. (Hilar lymphadenopathy on CXR)
>
> *Musculoskeletal*
> Acute self-limiting arthritis

The typical patient is a young, fit woman who complains of rapid onset of stiffness and pain in one or more large joints, usually the ankles or knees. Symptoms characteristically reach maximum intensity within 2–3 days and move from one region to another in additive fashion to involve both ankles and knees, and commonly wrists, elbows, shoulders, MCPs and finger PIPs. Distribution is eventually symmetrical in most cases (Fig. 16.23). Much of the inflammation is periarticular, there typically being marked swelling, tenderness and occasional erythema, but only minimal joint effusion and a surprisingly good range of joint movement. Although initially severe, symptoms usually improve within days or weeks and the arthritis and periarticular inflammation resolve spontaneously without residua in 4–6 months or less.

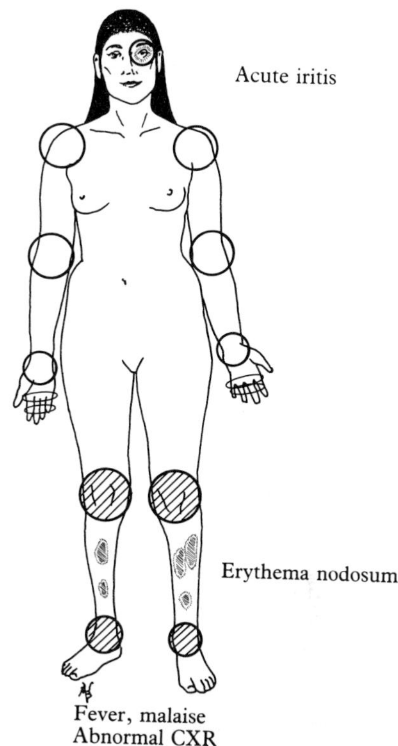

Fig. 16.23 Acute sarcoid arthritis: joint distribution and commonly associated features

Erythema nodosum commonly appears synchronously with joint symptoms, or follows them after 4 weeks. Skin lesions typically present as crops of tender, raised nodules on the anterior aspect of the lower legs, at first bright red but then becoming darker and eventually fading like a bruise over 2–6 weeks: recurrence of nodules occasionally occurs.

Other common features include fever, general malaise, acute iritis or conjunctivitis. Examination may additionally reveal lymphadenopathy and splenomegaly, but these are usually unimpressive and temporary.

Chronic, late arthritis

Although this may occur early, it typically follows other manifestations of sarcoid by months or years and generally involves an older population than the acute form.

Patients, often in middle age, most commonly present with recurring, episodic pain and stiffness affecting the same joints as the acute syndrome (ankles, knees, wrists, small joints of the hand) but differing in being more persistent. Acute inflammatory exacerbations are characteristic and may be sufficiently severe as to mimic acute gout. Tenosynovitis of fingers of wrists may also occur, occasionally leading to flexion contractures of the fingers and carpal tunnel syndrome. Symmetrical joint involvement is most usual resulting in a picture that clinically resembles RA (Fig. 16.24); chronic oligo- or monoarthritis may also occur, and produce destructive changes that suggest chronic joint sepsis.

Parenchymal lung disease is usually present and 50% have chronic skin lesions. Chronic iritis, with or without secondary glaucoma or cataract, is present in another third, but other features of chronic disease are less commonly present.

Osseous sarcoid affects 10% of patients with chronic disease and is particularly seen in those with prominent skin lesions and progressive systemic involvement. Bone cysts form, particularly in phalanges and metacarpals, producing asymmetrical finger swellings which are occasionally painful ('sarcoid dactylitis'). Destructive

Clinical features of chronic sarcoid

General

1. Skin lesions
   a) Plaques
   b) Keloids
   c) Lupus pernio (chronic violaceous, disfiguring)
2. Eye lesions
   a) Chronic iridocyclitis
   b) Chorioretinitis
   c) Cataracts
   d) Glaucoma
   e) Keratoconjunctivitis sicca (with salivary gland enlargement)
3. Lymphadenopathy
4. Hepatosplenomegaly
5. Pulmonary fibrosis ± cor pulmonale
6. CNS disease
   a) cranial nerve palsy (VII, II, X, XII)
   b) Basal meningitis
   c) Hypopituitarism
   d) Diabetes insipidus
7. Peripheral polyneuropathy, mononeuritis multiplex
8. Pericarditis, arrythmias (secondary to granulomata)
9. Fever, malaise
10. (Infiltrates/fibrosis on CXR)

Musculoskeletal

1. Chronic arthritis
2. Tenosynovitis
3. Carpal tunnel syndrome

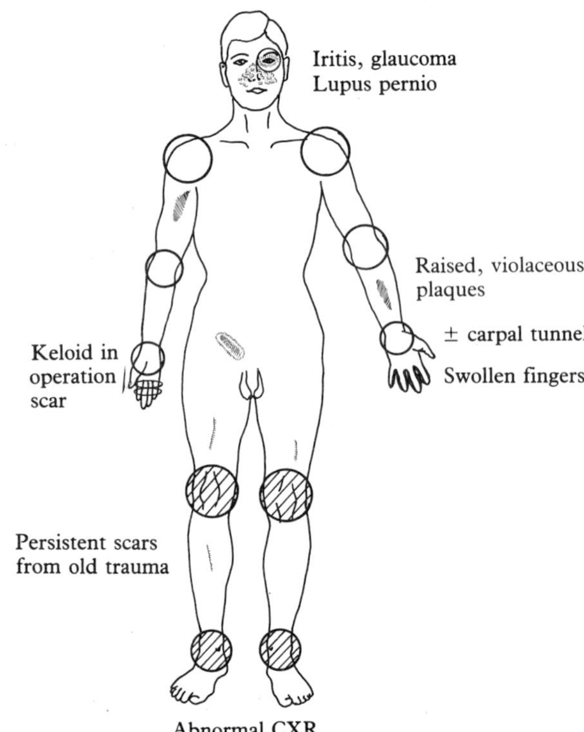

Fig. 16.24 Chronic sarcoid arthritis: joint distribution and common associated features

lesions may, however, occur elsewhere and lead to erosion of nasal bones with subsequent 'saddle-nose' deformity or to multiple fractures of long bones with secondary joint involvement.

Muscle involvement may produce ill-defined, asymmetrical muscle pains, rarely associated with palpable tender nodules. Symmetrical weakness and wasting of proximal muscles may occasionally result from a diffuse myopathy.

INVESTIGATIONS

A raised plasma viscosity or ESR, mild anaemia, diffuse hypergammaglobulinaemia and weakly-positive rheumatoid factor or ANF are common in both acute and chronic disease, and hypercalcaemia with hypercalciuria is an occasional finding.

Joint X-rays in the acute syndrome show only soft-tissue swelling, but bilateral hilar lymph-adenopathy is usually present on CXR. In chronic disease joint changes may be pronounced and characteristic, largely due to bone involvement (Fig. 16.25), and the CXR commonly shows parenchymal infiltration/fibrosis.

Synovial biopsy in acute arthritis shows only non-specific changes. In chronic arthritis, however, typical sarcoid granulomata may be found.

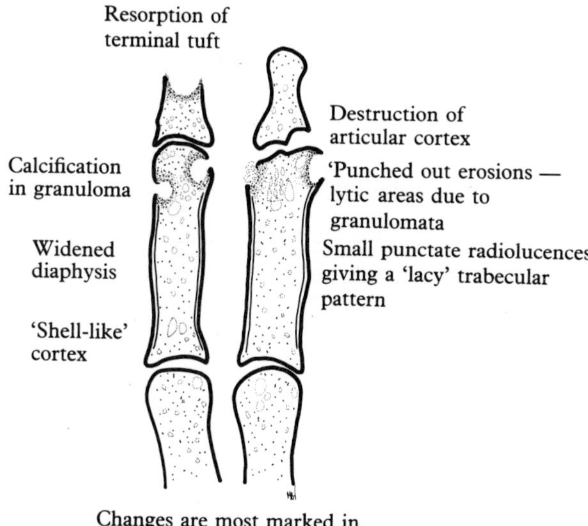

Fig. 16.25 Characteristic X-ray changes of chronic sarcoid

The Kveim–Siltzbach test is positive in the majority of patients with acute sarcoidosis but may be negative in chronic disease. Other abnormalities commonly occur which although supportive of the diagnosis are of more value in monitoring disease activity, e.g.:

1. Cutaneous anergy (shown by absent tuberculin test) and decreased *in vitro* T-cell proliferation in response to mitogens are characteristic of acute, active disease.
2. Serum angiotensin converting enzyme (SACE) and lysozyme levels are raised in patients with active pulmonary disease but fall to normal in remission, in chronic disease and during treatment with steroids.
3. Urinary hydroxyproline excretion is raised in active disease.

DIAGNOSIS

No single test for sarcoidosis is conclusive and the diagnosis usually rests on several supportive findings (principally typical CXR changes) in the appropriate clinical setting.

Acute presentation with Löfgren's syndrome is characteristic and should always suggest the diagnosis. Erythema nodosum alone may occur in a number of other conditions. In some of these

Causes of erythema nodosum

Common

1. Idiopathic (25–50%)
2. Sarcoidosis
3. Streptococcal infection

Less common

1. TB
2. Drugs — especially sulphonamides, oral contraceptives,
aspirin, iodides, bromides
3. Crohn's disease, ulcerative colitis
4. Other infections — especially leprosy, disseminated fungal disease
5. Mycoplasma pneumoniae
6. Toxoplasmosis
7. Lymphogranuloma venereum

conditions, particularly TB, chest X-ray changes may co-exist and cause confusion. TB can usually be differentiated, however, since: 1. Hilar adenopathy is usually unilateral; 2. If arthritis is present it is insidious in onset, persistent, asymmetrical, and commonly mono- or oligo-articular; 3. Cutaneous anergy and non-caseating granulomata are uncommon. In the absence of erythema nodosum, diagnosis of acute sarcoid arthritis is more difficult, but should be suggested by the additive joint involvement and marked periarthritis, particularly of the ankle. In the appropriate clinical setting, CXR should be repeated if initially negative.

Diagnosis of chronic sarcoid arthritis rests on recognition of multisystem involvement with examination for lung, skin and eye disease. Biopsy confirmation is often required, especially if presentation is with chronic persistent monoarthritis (p 393).

TREATMENT

Simple physical measures and NSAIDs usually afford adequate symptomatic control of acute arthritis, but if joint symptoms or fatigue are severe, ACTH, or steroids in low doses, have an abortive effect on the acute syndrome and often lead to rapid improvement For chronic arthritis steroids are usually given if there is progressive joint destruction and severe systemic involvement, but response may be disappointing, especially with major CNS, cardiac or bone disease. The case for cytotoxic or immunosuppressive agents remains unproven.

PROGNOSIS

The acute arthritis is always self-limiting, but the prognosis for chronic disease is generally poor. Death is mainly from pulmonary insufficiency, aspergillosis (with massive haemoptysis) or myocardial infiltration. Irrespective of the presenting features over 90% of patients have an abnormal chest X-ray and staging at presentation has proved to be of prognostic value.

Further reading (SARCOIDOSIS)

Weisenhutter C W, Sharma O P (1979) Is Sarcoidosis an autoimmune disease? Report of 4 cases and a review of the literature. Seminars in Arthritis and Rheumatism 9(2): 124–144

Jones D G, Neville E, Siltzbach L E et al 1976 A worldwide review of sarcoidoses. Annals of the New York Academy of Science 278: 321

Blomgren S E 1974 Erythema nodosum. Seminars in Arthritis and Rheumatism 4(1): 1–24

VII Amyloidosis

INTRODUCTION

Amyloidosis is a rare, life-threatening condition in which an insoluble fibrillar proteinaceous material accumulates extracellularly in tissues, gradually replacing the affected organs and causing severe functional impairment. It may be inherited, acquired, generalised or localised. Several of the acquired forms are relevant to the rheumatic diseases. Primary amyloidosis and that occurring with immunocytic dyscrasias such as myelomatosis may present with an arthropathy mimicking rheumatoid arthritis. A secondary form, called *reactive systemic amyloidosis*, may occur as a complication of chronic inflammatory arthritis, particularly RA, AS and JCA. In the UK approximately 5% of patients with RA develop amyloidosis in life and many more are found to have it as an incidental finding at post-mortem. These figures are much higher than those reported from other countries, such as the USA but the reasons for such geographical variation are unknown.

Frequency of AA amyloidosis in the rheumatic diseases

Disease	Frequency
Rheumatoid arthritis	5%
Juvenile chronic arthritis	4%
Ankylosing spondylitis	3%
Psoriatic arthropathy	Uncommon
Reiter's syndrome	Uncommon
Scleroderma	Uncommon
Dermatomyositis	Uncommon
Systemic lupus erythematosus	Very rare

AETIOLOGY AND PATHOGENESIS

90% of an amyloid deposit is composed of rigid, non-branching fibrils with a hollow central core, which are wrapped together in a unique, anti-parallel twisted, beta-pleated sheet configuration which is not normally found in mammalian proteins but is common in the invertebrate kingdom. Silk is an example of such a fibril. This abnormal configuration renders the protein resistant to digestion by most mammalian proteolytic enzymes. Deposits of amyloid fibrils are always associated with small amounts of another protein called *P component*. This is similar in structure to CRP and is found as a normal constituent of many tissues which are preferred sites for amyloid deposition. Its role is not understood but it may be important in determining the localisation of the amyloid deposits. It is now known that several different proteins can be converted into amyloid fibrils (Table 16.3), and that the underlying pathology of amyloid disease lies in aberrant handling of excess protein material derived from many different sources. In reactive systemic amyloidosis complicating the rheumatic diseases, the precursor portein is antigenically related to the acute-phase reactant serum amyloid A (SAA) which is produced by the liver in response to a factor, interleukin I, released from activated macrophages at sites of inflammation. This type of amyloidosis is called *type AA*. Most patients with inflammatory arthritis have high levels of SAA for prolonged periods, but only a small proportion go on to develop AA amyloidosis, suggesting that other factors are important in determining who will and who will not develop amyloidosis. It may be that certain genetically-determined polymorphic forms of SAA are more amyloidogenic.

Multiple myeloma and other immunocytic dyscrasia, in which there is abnormal production of immunoglobulin, are occasionally complicated by amyloidosis (approximately 6–15%). The precursor protein in these cases is derived from immunoglobulin light chains and is called *AL amyloid*. AL amyloid also occurs in the absence of any obvious underlying disease. Peptic degradation of immunoglobulin light chains *in vitro* from patients with AL amyloid results in the production of fibrillar material resembling amyloid under the electron microscope and it may be that the defect in amyloid disease is abnormal degradation of the precursor protein which produces the aberrant protein fibril. This degrading activity has been shown to be present in the serum and at cell

Table 16.3 Clinical amyloidosis syndromes and associated precursor protein

Clinical syndrome	Amyloid fibril type	Precursor protein
Generalised		
Primary amyloidosis	AL	Immunoglobulin light chain
Immunocyte derived — Multiple myeloma — Waldenstrom's — Plasmacytoma	AL	Immunoglobulin light chain
Monoclonal gammopathy		
Heavy chain disease		
Reactive systemic amyloidosis — Rheumatic (RA, AS, JCA) — Infectious (TB, leprosy, suppuration) — Inflammatory (Crohn's, FMF)	AA	Serum amyloid A
Familial Portuguese neuropathy	A_{fap}	Pre-albumin
Localised		
Cutaneous amyloidosis		Unknown
Medullary carcinoma thyroid	A_{mct}	Calcitonin
Senile cardiac amyloidosis	A_{sca}	Unknown

surfaces and is probably due to the activity of a serine esterase. In RA patients with amyloidosis there is a marked reduction in the degrading factor activity of serum compared to patients with RA without amyloidosis and controls (Fig. 16.26).

The distribution of amyloid throughout the body is quite different in the various forms. AA amyloid accumulates primarily in the liver, spleen, kidneys and gastrointestinal tract (Fig. 16.27) whereas AL amyloid tends to favour the heart,

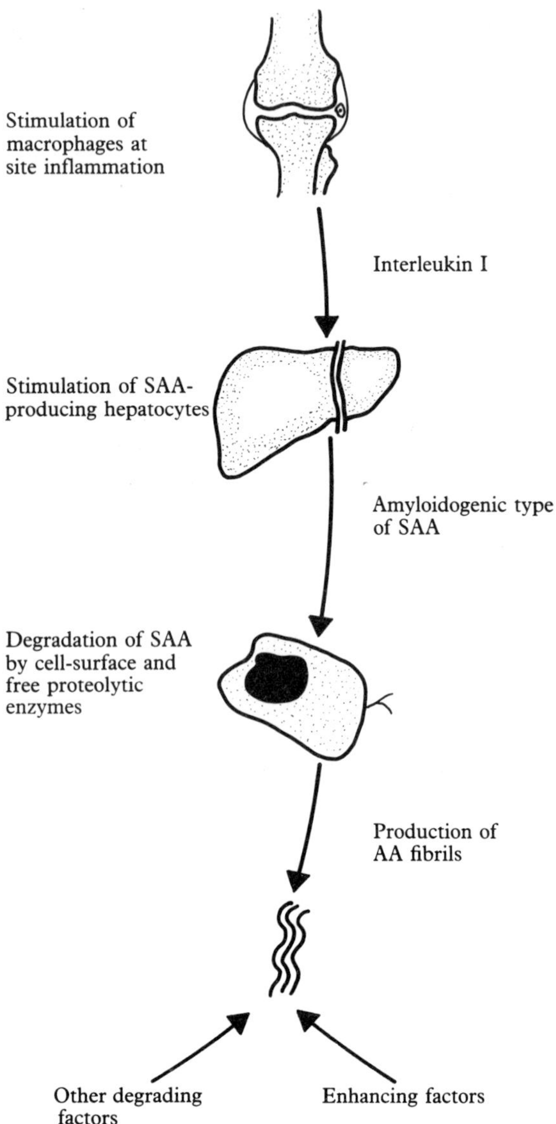

Fig. 16.26 Current hypothesis on the pathogenesis of AA amyloidosis

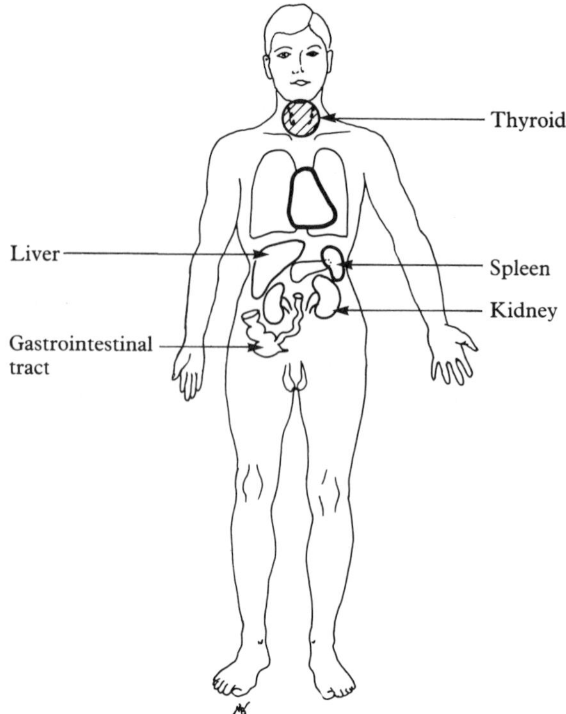

Fig. 16.27 Distribution of AA amyloidosis

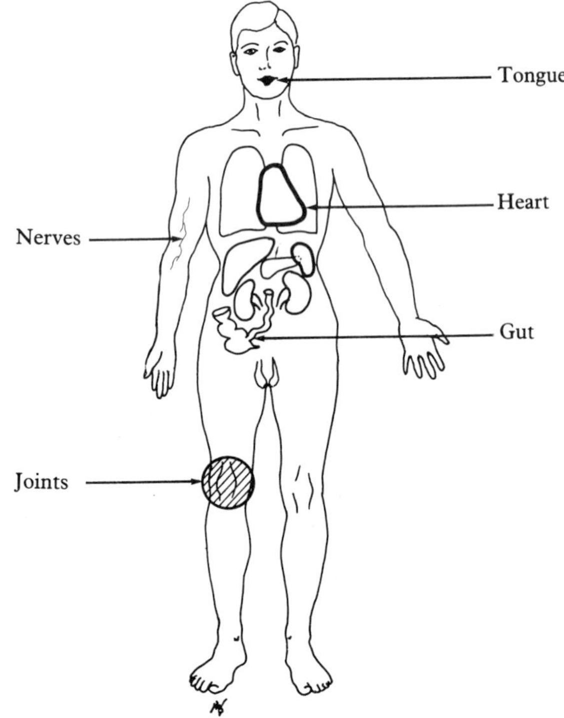

Fig. 16.28 Distribution of AL amyloid

tongue and blood-vessels, particularly the vasa-vasorum and the gastrointestinal tract (Fig. 16.28). Macroscopically, involved organs are characteristically enlarged, pale and firm. The amyloid fibrils can be detected by staining tissue sections with Congo Red, followed by polarised-light microscopy. Amyloid gives a characteristic green birefigrence. AA and AL amyloid can be distinguished by pretreatment of the section with potassium permanganate PP which abolishes the Congo Red reaction in AA amyloid. The staining techniques are not entirely reliable and confirmation should be obtained by electron microscopy (Table 16.4).

Table 16.4 Characteristics of the main amyloid syndromes

	Primary	*Secondary*
Cell source:	Plasma cell	Hepatocyte
Site:	Bone marrow	Liver
Product:	Light chains and fragments	apo–SAA
Distribution:	Focal Disseminated	Disseminated
Differentiation:	PP sensitive	PP resistant

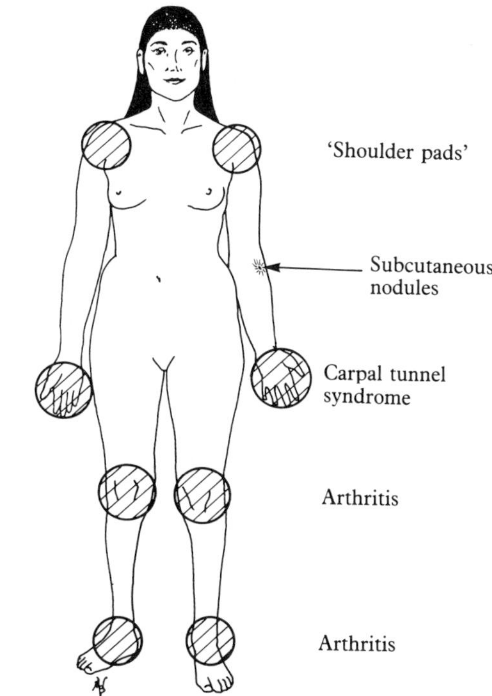

Fig. 16.29 Features of amyloid arthropathy

CLINICAL FEATURES

AA amyloidosis typically presents as proteinuria in a patient with a rheumatic disease, usually long-standing rheumatoid arthritis. The clinical picture is dominated by renal involvement with the proteinuria progressing to frank nephrotic syndrome and ultimately renal failure. If the gastrointestinal tract is extensively infiltrated, diarrhoea and weight-loss from malabsorption may also be features. Although the liver and spleen are frequently enlarged, these organs do not show functional impairment. Renal vein thrombosis is an occasional complication causing massive proteinuria, haematuria and sudden sharp decline in renal function. The course of AA amyloidosis is one of relentless progression culminating in death from renal failure within a year of two of onset although the natural history is variable with the occasional patient following a more benign course.

The clinical picture of AL amyloid and several of the other heredofamilial types is quite different. The heart, tongue and nervous system are prime targets so the features such as cardiac arrhythmias, postural hypotension, dysphagia, peripheral and autonomic neuropathy dominate the picture. This type of amyloid may affect the locomotor system causing an amyloid arthropathy (Fig. 16.29). This can involve any joint but frequently has a similar distribution to RA. The joints are swollen, firm, painful and stiff but inflammation is less marked than in RA and erosions do not occur. Subcutaneous nodules are found in nearly half the cases and occasionally infiltration around the gleno-humeral joint produces a characteristic 'shoulder-pad' sign. Carpal tunnel syndrome is also common. AL amyloid has a very grim prognosis, particularly when it is the result of multiple myeloma. Death occurs within a few months and is usually due to cardiac disease.

DIAGNOSIS

The diagnosis of amyloidosis is made by biopsy and histological examination with the appropriate stains of the clinically-affected tissues. A rectal biopsy is also useful, since it is positive in the majority of patients with AA amyloidosis, but a renal biopsy is also necessary to assess the extent of involvement. There are no useful serological tests in the diagnosis of AA amyloid. The SAA is usually only mildly elevated in established cases. Skeletal survey, bone-marrow aspiration, immunoglobulin estimation and serum and protein electrophoresis are indicated to detect an immune dyscrasia in the case of AL amyloid. The diagnosis of amyloid arthropathy may be confirmed by demonstrating fibrils in synovial biopsy or synovial fluid, in a subcutaneous nodule or in tissue taken during a carpal tunnel decompression.

MANAGEMENT

There is no conventional treatment for amyloidosis. It seems sensible to surpress the underlying disease process, such as RA or multiple myeloma, with specific therapy where possible, but the evidence that this beneficially affects the outcome is not strong. As AA amyloid progresses, the problems are ones of fluid balance, blood-pressure control and treatment of uraemia and they are best handled by a nephrologist. Younger patients are being taken on to renal dialysis and transplant programmes, with some success since the amyloid does not necessarily recur in the transplanted kindey.

The use of colchine to suppress episodes of fever and serositis in FMF has been shown to delay or halt the development of amyloidosis but it is not effective in established disease. Drug therapy aimed at dissolving deposits has been largely disappointing, with the possible exception of dimethylsulphoxide which has been shown to increase urinary excretion of amyloid fibrils and perhaps to slow progression. Unfortunately it is badly tolerated by most patients, since it makes them smell of rotting garlic and few can persist with it for any length of time. Chlorambucil is being used in young children with severe JCA complicated by AA amyloidosis, but no conclusive results are yet available.

REFERENCES (AMYLOIDOSIS)

Glenner G G 1980 Amyloid and amyloidosis — the β-fibrilloses. I and II. New England Journal of Medicine 302: 1283–1292; 1333–1343

Glenner G G, Costa P, de Freitas F (eds) 1980 Amyloid and amyloidosis. Excerpta Medica, Amsterdam

VIII Familial Mediterranean Fever (*Synonyms: Periodic Disease; Benign Paroxysmal Peritonitis*)

Familial Mediterranean fever (FMF) is a disorder inherited as an autosomal recessive and is mainly confined to populations originating on the south and east shores of the Mediterranean. It is characterized by acute self-limited attacks of fever accompanied by peritonitis, pleuritis and arthritis, which first develop in childhood or adolescence and occur intermittently throughout life.

FMF occurs predominantly in Sephardic and Iraqui Jews, Turks, Armenians and Levantine Arabs, although sporadic cases are rarely seen in Anglo-Saxons and the European races. It appears to be inherited as a single autosomal recessive, and in Israel the prevalence of homozygotes is approximately 1/2000.

AETIOLOGY AND PATHOLOGY

The underlying cause and the factors which trigger the acute attacks are unknown. The pathological changes are non-specific and are those of acute inflammation. These changes are transient, but peritoneal adhesions sometimes develop which can lead to intestinal obstruction. The major complication in a proportion of cases is amyloidosis. Amyloid fibres are composed of amyloid A protein and the distribution is that of secondary amyloidosis with major involvement of the renal glomeruli.

CLINICAL FEATURES

Attacks first develop in childhood or adolescence and recur intermittently throughout life, often once a month or more with occasional remissions lasting a few months. Rarely the onset of the attacks is in infancy or in middle age. The duration and frequency of attacks varies enormously not only from patient to patient but also in the same patient. During periods of freedom the patient is normal unless amyloidosis develops.

Acute attacks last 24–48 hours and fever with temperatures reaching 38–40 °C accompanies virtually every attack. This may be the only manifestation but usually fever is accompanied by any of the manifestations shown below.

Clinical features of FMF
1. Fever
2. Abdominal pain: peritonitis lasting 12–24 hours
3. Chest pain: usually pleurisy; occasionally pericarditis
4. Synovitis: monoarticular or oligoarticular
5. Skin changes: erysipelas-like erythema on ankles

Peritonitis occurs in most cases, producing pain accompanied by features such as distention, abdominal rigidity and rebound, and ileus which may mimic acute abdominal emergencies.

Pleurisy is also a common manifestation, causing pleuritic pain. This is usually unilateral and accompanied by reduced breath sounds and a small pleural effusion.

Joint Manifestations

Synovitis occurs in 70% and may occur in the absence of other features. Sometimes it is accompanied by a characteristic, sharply-defined, erysipelas-like skin lesion above the ankle. Typically there is a monoarthritis or an asymmetrical oligoarthritis, with severe pain and tenderness out of proportion to the degree of swelling, warmth and redness, which lasts 1–2 days. Knees are most commonly affected, but any joint can be involved, including the sacro-iliac joints. When effusions occur they tend to become chronic with the development of periarticular osteoporosis. Joint damage is unusual and complete functional recovery is the rule.

Amyloidosis

This complication leads to proteinuria and subsequently to death from renal failure. It occurs in 40% of Sephardic Jews or Turks but more rarely in other patients with FMF.

LABORATORY FINDINGS AND DIAGNOSIS

An acute attack is accompanied by a raised ESR, elevated levels of acute phase proteins such as CRP, SAA and haptoglobin, and a marked leukocytosis. Persistent proteinuria and abnormalities of renal function indicate the presence of amyloid which can be confirmed by renal biopsy.

The diagnosis is entirely a clinical one and is suggested by recurrent self-limited attacks in a patient with an appropriate ethnic background or a positive family history.

Disorders commonly considered in the differential diagnosis are listed below. In particular, FMF often mimics acute abdominal emergencies and many patients undergo laparotomy.

Differential diagnosis of FMF
1. Fever of unknown origin
2. Acute abdominal emergencies — include:
   Appendicitis
   Pancreatitis
   Cholecystitis
   Intestinal obstruction
3. Oligoarthritic form of JCA

TREATMENT AND PROGNOSIS

Colchicine, if taken regularly, reduces the frequency of attacks in most but not all patients. It is also reported to prolong the course of renal amyloidosis.

The prognosis is determined by the development of amyloidosis leading to renal failure. It is poorest in the Middle East where amyloidosis may cause death in adolescence.

FURTHER READING (FMF)

Sohar E, Gafni J, Pras M, Heller H 1967 Familial Mediterranean fever. A survey of 470 cases and review of the literature. American Journal of Medicine 43: 227–253
Sohar E, Pras M, Gafni J 1975 Familial Mediterranean fever and its articular manifestations. Clinics in Rheumatic Diseases 1(1): 195–209

IX Whipple's Disease

This is a rare, multi-system disorder in which PAS-staining macrophages laden with poorly-characterised material are found in many tissues, but particularly the small bowel and draining lymph nodes. Arthritis or arthralgia is the commonest manifestation (90%) and characteristically predates the other cardinal signs (abdominal pain, diarrhoea and weight-loss) by many years, being the presenting feature in over half the cases.

Aetiology

Although the precise cause of Whipple's disease is unknown, there is good circumstantial evidence to favour an infective, probably bacterial, aetiology:

1. The glycoprotein granules within the 'foamy' PAS-positive macrophages consist of closely-packed membranes, vesicles and granules that appear to be partially-digested bacterial products.
2. Cell-wall-deficient streptococci have been isolated from prolonged monolayer culture of involved lymph-node tissue.
3. Antimicrobial therapy readily reverses the clinical and pathological features of the disease.

Other factors, however, such as the male predominance, inability to isolate a specific organism and unique cellular response, suggest that impairment of host factors plays a vital part in pathogenesis. Impaired cell-mediated immunity is common in patients with active disease and may persist even after effective antibiotic therapy. Incomplete lysis of phagocytosed bacteria suggests a possible defect in macrophage function, and the fact that many of these patients are farmers has led to speculation on the aetiological relevance of chronic exposure to animal and bird products. Although Whipple's disease is still included by some within the seronegative spondarthritides, the demonstration of bacterial agents within involved joints and resolution of arthritis following antibiotic therapy argues against there being any 'reactive' component to the arthritis (p 66).

CLINICAL FEATURES

Caucasians aged 25–50 are particularly affected with a male predominance of 6: 1.

Periodic attacks of peripheral arthritis commonly dominate the clinical picture for many years. Several joints are usually affected, often in migratory fashion. Knees and ankles are most commonly involved, followed by wrists, shoulders, elbows and small joints of the hand (Fig. 16.30). Attacks

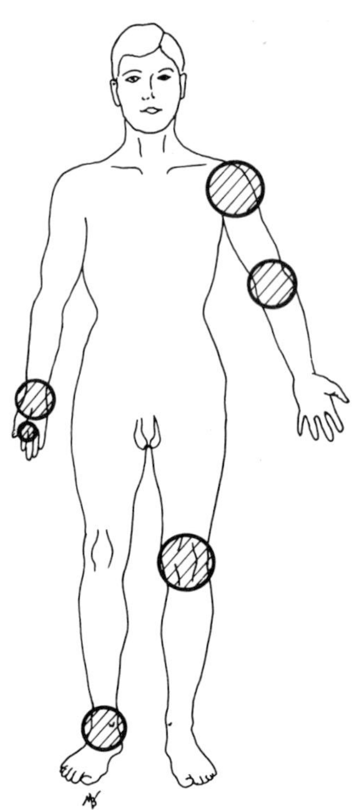

Fig. 16.30 Sites of involvement in Whipple's disease

are typically dramatic but self-limiting, lasting from only several hours to a few weeks. Signs of synovitis may be present during attacks but complete resolution without residua is the rule. Unlike the situation with inflammatory bowel disease, the peripheral arthritis shows no relationship to the severity of bowel symptoms.

Axial involvement in this condition is controversial. Back stiffness is a common complaint, but objective sacroiliitis or spondylitis occurs perhaps in only 7% and 4% of patients.

Non-articular features are protean but usually take many years to develop. Apart from Whipple's triad of malabsorption, diarrhoea and weight-loss, patients may experience repeated inflammatory episodes affecting lung, pleura, pericardium and thyroid. Intermittent fever and general malaise are common, and progressive, often subtle, CNS disturbance is well recognised. Physical findings may include emaciation, lymphadenopathy, hyperpigmentation, clubbing, hepatosplenomegaly, oedema, hypotension and anaemia.

Diagnosis and management

A high index of suspicion is required if the diagnosis is to be made early in the course of the disease. The peripheral arthritis usually resembles other periodic syndromes such as gout or palindromic rheumatism but is commonly misdiagnosed as atypical, mild rheumatoid disease in a young to middle-aged man. X-rays show only mild juxta-articular porosis, and the synovial fluid is usually unremarkable. The chronic, but mild, course of the arthritis and its lack of specific features usually results in delay in correct diagnosis until gut symptoms, pleurisy, CNS or hormonal problems have developed. Even at this multisystem stage, confusion with sarcoidosis or SLE is frequent.

Inappropriate anaemia and low serum folate usually lead to investigation of the bowel and to the correct diagnosis. Confirmation is by demonstration of PAS positive inclusions in jejunal biopsy material (multiple biopsies are preferable since involvement may be patchy). Positive histology may also be obtained from other involved sites including synovium, and synovial fluid smears stained with PAS may demonstrate similar material within PMNs and synovial cells. Bacterial culture of involved tissue is inevitably disappointing.

Whipple's disease is uniformly responsive to prolonged antibiotic therapy (tetracycline 1 g daily for 12 months, following an initial 10 days treatment with parenteral penicillin and streptomycin). Joint symptoms should abate progressively, and persistence or recurrence of synovitis should lead to reappraisal of the drug regime and a trial of erythromycin. Patients should be followed up for life.

FURTHER READING (WHIPPLE'S DISEASE)

Le Vine M E, Dobbins W O 1973 Joint changes in Whipple's disease. Seminars in Arthritis and Rheumatism 3: 79

Kelly J J, Weisiger B B 1963 The arthritis of Whipple's disease. Arthritis and Rheumatism 6: 615

Khan M A Axial arthropathy in Whipple's disease. Journal of Rheumatology 9: 928–929

Rubirow A, Canoso J J, Goldenberg D L, Cohen A S 1976 Synovial fluid and synovial membrane pathology in Whipple's disease. Arthritis and Rheumatism 19: 820

X Multicentric reticulohistiocytosis

INTRODUCTION

This is a very rare disease of unknown aetiology, characterised by skin nodules and a destructive arthritis. There are less than 100 cases in the world literature. The underlying pathological process is accummulation of cells full of PAS-positive material in the skin, in and around the joints and, less commonly, in other sites, particularly muscle, pleura and pericardium. The significance of this disease is that, although so rare, it can superficially bear a close resemblance to RA.

CLINICAL FEATURES

White races appear particularly susceptible with a 3:1 female predominance. The mean age of onset is 43 although it has been described in a child of 10. Over half of the patients present with a symmetrical, peripheral polyarthritis followed

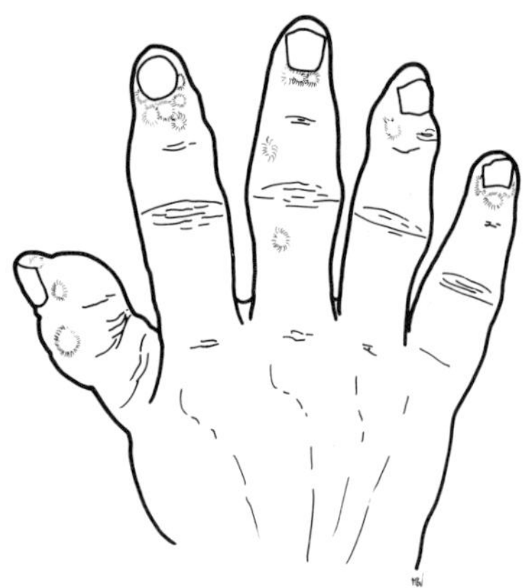

Fig. 16.31 The hand in multicentric reticulohistiocytosis showing distribution of nodules and arthritis mutilans

some months or even years later by the skin lesions. The arthritis commonly involves the distal interphalangeal joints of the hands, followed in frequency, by the knees, elbows and shoulders. There is often marked morning stiffness and the joints are tender, swollen and warm. Three-quarters of patients develop articular and periarticular erosions and in 40% severe joint destruction results in arthritis mutilans. Atlanto-axial subluxation, tenosynovitis and protrusio acetabuli may also occur. The reddish-brown nodular skin lesions vary in size from a few millimetres to several centimetres and may be painful or itchy. They are found around the nose and ears, the neck, trunk and over the dorsum of the hands, particularly around the nails (Fig. 16.31). Large nodules over the elbows may be clinically indistinguishable from rheumatoid nodules. Nodules also develop in the mucosa of the nose and mouth, the subcutaneous tissues, synovium and periosteum. The facial lesions may become massive and confluent, producing leonine facies and gross disfigurement. Xanthelasma palpebrarum are present in about 40%. Cases have been reported with evidence of multi-system involvement including myositis, pleural effusions, gastric ulcers, pericarditis, lymphadenopathy, pathological fractures, epilepsy and primary biliary cirrhosis. A significant number of patients go on to develop a terminal haematological malignancy and cases have been described with paraproteinaemias.

DIAGNOSIS AND TREATMENT

The differential diagnosis includes RA, lepromatous leprosy, sarcoidosis, xanthomatosis, generalised eruptive histiocytosis or histiocytosis X. The diagnosis is confirmed by biopsy of a lesion from skin or synovium which shows characteristic aggregations of multi-nucleated giant cells with a granular ground-glass cytoplasm, containing accumulations of PAS-positive material thought to be a muco- or glycoprotein, together with a lipid material.

There are no specific laboratory tests. There is usually a mild anaemia and slight elevation of the ESR and 30% have raised serum cholesterol. The latex test is negative.

The X-rays show circumscribed articular and para-articular erosions, particularly around the interphalangeal joints of the hands. Juxta-articular osteoporosis is mild or absent. The joint lesions are very destructive but the joint space is sometimes paradoxically increased due to accumulation of abnormal nodules of tissue in the synovium.

There is no conventional specific treatment. Spontaneous remissions have been reported but the majority progress to disability and disfigurement. Attempts have been made to treat this disease with immunosuppressive agents, such as cyclophosphamide and azathioprine, with variable success.

FURTHER READING

Barrow M V, Holubar K 1969 Multicentric reticulohistiocytosis: a review of 33 patients. Medicine 48: 287

XI Disorders Caused by Diet, Drugs and Toxins

The association between dietary factors and the development of arthritis is very strong in folklore and a multitude of exclusion diets have been put forward as cures of chronic forms of arthritis such as RA. In most cases there is as yet no experimental evidence to support these and studies of dietary habits of patients with RA, for example, have in general found no single abnormality. In a few cases, however, dietary factors and the ingestion of certain drugs and toxins have been implicated in the aetiology of certain rheumatic diseases.

DIET

1. Dietary factors in hyperuricaema and gout

Certain dietary factors listed below may elevate uric acid levels, either by increasing the production or by reducing the renal clearance of uric acid. In suspectible individuals these factors may have a role in precipitating gout. There is a positive association between serum uric acid levels and body bulk and there is considerable evidence that obesity is a factor in hyperuricaemia. Purine-rich diets and regular ingestion of alcohol, including beer, may elevate uric acid levels by increasing the purine load. On the other hand, short-term alteration in diet such as starvation and ingestion of large amounts of fat or alcohol may cause hyperuricaemia by reducing renal clearance of uric acid through hyperlactacidaemia.

Dietary factors in hyperuricaemia and gout

1. Obesity
2. Purine-rich diets (meat extracts, offal, fish, game)
3. Regular alcohol consumption including beer
4. Starvation
5. High fat diet
6. Consumption of large quantities of alcohol

2. Obesity and osteoarthritis

Some surveys have shown a correlation between obesity and both the prevalence and severity of osteoarthritis. Interestingly, this involves not only the weight-bearing joints but also the peripheral non-weight-bearing joints such as the fingers. This association is controversial, however, and has not been demonstrated in all studies.

3. Scurvy

Scurvy is the only vitamin deficiency associated with joint manifestations, which take the form of recurrent haemarthroses.

DRUGS

A wide variety of drugs may induce musculoskeletal symptoms. Some of these reactions are summarised below.

Drug reactions affecting the musculoskeletal system

1. Acute gout
2. SLE-like syndromes
3. Serum-sickness reactions and vasculitis
4. Arthralgias or arthritis
5. Aseptic necrosis
6. Muscle pain or cramps
7. Myositis
8. Myaesthenia gravis
9. Metabolic bone disease: osteoporosis and osteomalacia

1. Acute gout

Thiazide diuretics increase serum uric acid levels and may precipitate acute gout in predisposed individuals. Gout may be precipitated by other drugs which cause a transient hyperuricaemia. These include cytotoxic agents in patients with leukaemia or lymphoma, producing increased breakdown of nucleic acids and urate overproduction, vitamin B_{12} administration to patients with untreated pernicious anaemia, radioactive phosphorus in polycythaemia, and pyrazinamide. Gout may also occur during the early stages of therapy with allopurinol or uricosuric agents. In rare cases it is precipitated by penicillin or insulin, as an idiosyncratic reaction, without apparent alteration in urate levels.

Drugs that may precipitate acute gout

1. Elevation of serum uric acid
   a) Diuretics
   b) Cytotoxic drugs
   c) Pyrazinamide
2. Serum uric-acid-lowering agents
   a) Allopurinol
   b) Uricosuric agents
3. Idiosyncratic reactions
   a) Penicillin
   b) Insulin

2. Drug-induced SLE

A lupus-like syndrome can develop after ingestion of certain drugs. Associations are best documented with procainamide and hydralazine, and to a lesser extent with isoniazid and certain anti-convulsants. Anti-nuclear antibodies develop in 50–75% of patients taking procainamide or hydralazine in sufficient doses for 9–12 months. Of these, 20–50% develop clinical features. Drug-induced lupus occurs more readily in slow-acetylators, and hydralazine-induced lupus shows a close association with HLA-DR4. It is possible that drugs such as procainamide, hydralazine and isoniazid combine with nuclear macromolecules with the stimulation of an immune response in susceptible individuals. The primary amino group common to these compounds appears to be important, since the acetylated product of procainamide (acetylprocainamide) is much less effective in inducing anti-nuclear antibodies. A large number of other drugs may cause an SLE-like illness on rare occasions which probably represents an allergic reaction.

Drug-induced lupus occurs more often in the elderly and the clinical picture is very similar to idopathic lupus in this age group, with prominent cutaneous, joint, pericardial, pleural and pulmonary manifestations but rare renal involvement.

ANA are present in high titres. These can be shown to react predominantly with histones, especially the H_2 fraction. Antibodies characteristic of idiopathic lupus, such as anti-native DNA, are only rarely present, and serum complement levels usually remain normal. Discontinuation of the offending drug usually results in rapid resolution of the symptoms, although anti-nuclear antibodies may persist for several months.

Drugs reported to induce SLE

Frequent association

1. Procainamide
2. Hydralazine
3. Isoniazid
4. Anti-convulsants
5. Chlorpromazine

Rare association

1. Oral contraceptives
2. Chlorthalidone
3. Griseofulvin
4. Levodopa
5. Methyl Dopa
6. Methysergide
7. Penicillin
8. Penicillamine
9. Prazosin
10. Propylthiouracil
11. Quinidine
12. Reserpine
13. Streptomycin
14. Sulphonamides
15. Tetracycline

3. Serum-sickness reactions and vasculitis

Serum-sickness reactions are a well-known complication of drug therapy. Most antibiotics, but especially penicillin, can induce such a reaction by acting as a hapten, as can drugs such as hydralazine, griseofulvin and propylthiouracil. On occasions these and other drugs such as thiazide diuretics and amphetamines may cause cutaneous vasculitis with or without systemic complications.

4. Arthralgias or arthritis

Arthralgias are a prominent feature of the 'steroid-withdrawal syndrome' which may complicate dose reduction in patients on long-term corticosteroid therapy. In severe cases arthralgias and myalgias are associated with anorexia, nausea, lethargy and weakness, but not necessarily with biochemical evidence of hypo-adrenocorticism.

Arthritis or arthralgias occasionally accompany administration of a variety of drugs such as glibenclamide, α-methyl dopa, propranolol, and isoniazid. *Rheumatisme barbiturique* is a term used to describe rare cases of arthralgia, sometimes accompanied by contractures, attributed to barbiturates, usually in high doses. Arthralgias and myalgias are commonly reported by women on oral contraceptives. Myalgias especially affect the calf on walking and must be distinguished from a deep venous thrombosis. Both smallpox vaccination and rubella immunisation may be followed by acute arthritis.

Drug-induced arthralgias or arthritis

1. Steroid withdrawal syndrome
2. Glibenclamide
3. α-methyl dopa
4. Propranolol
5. Isoniazid
6. Barbiturates
7. Oral contraceptives
8. Immunisation against smallpox and rubella

5. Aseptic necrosis and corticosteroids

Aseptic necrosis, usually of the femoral head but also of other sites such as the humeral head, may be caused by corticosteroids. This side-effect is unpredictable but usually occurs after prolonged or high doses of steroid.

6. Muscle abnormalities induced by drugs

Myalgias are common following reduction in the steroid dose, and have been described in association with stiffness and weakness in patients on large doses of clofibrate. Cramps may be caused by agents which retain fluid or cause sodium- or potassium depletion. Myopathy is a well known complication of corticosteroids, particularly of fluorinated compounds such as triamcinolone. Polymyositis and a myaesthenia gravis-like reaction are rare complications of penicillamine therapy.

Drug-induced muscle conditions

1. Myalgias:	Steroid withdrawal Clofibrate
2. Cramps:	Corticosteroid ACTH Oral contraceptive Diuretics Carbenoxolone
3. Myopathy (Type 2 fibres):	Corticosteroids Chloroquine
4. Myositis:	Penicillamine
5. Myaesthenia gravis:	Penicillamine
6. Local fibrosis:	IM Pentazocine

Local destruction of muscle tissue may occur at sites of drug injection. This can be particularly marked in patients with chronic pain who give themselves IM pentazocine, which can cause fibrosis and contracture with ulceration of overlying skin.

7. Metabolic bone disease

Osteoporosis resulting in vertebral crush fractures may complicate long-term corticosteroid therapy, particularly in post-menopausal women. It has also been reported after long-term heparin therapy, and in children with leukaemia where a remission is being maintained by long-term methotrexate.

Prolonged anticonvulsant therapy, especially a combination of phenytoin and phenobarbitone has caused osteomalacia in institutionalised children.

Drug-induced metabolic bone disease

Osteoporosis

1. Corticosteroids
2. Long-term heparin therapy
3. Long-term methotrexate

Osteomalacia

1. Long-term therapy with aluminium or magnesium hydroxide
2. Prolonged anti-convulsant therapy
3. Diphosphonates

Osteomalacia may also be produced on rare occasions by long-term treatment with non-absorbable antacids to reduce phosphate absorption in chronic renal failure.

TOXINS

1. Saturnine gout

The association between gout and lead poisoning has been well known for many years, and is the result of the toxic effect on renal tubules with reduced urinary excretion of uric acid and precipitation of gout in susceptible individuals. Cases were reported as a result of contact with lead-containing paint, and in the USA it has been related to regular consumption of moonshine alcohol with a high lead content.

2. Kashin–Beck disease

This curious condition was described towards the end of the nineteenth century as endemic in Eastern Siberia, Manchuria and Northern Korea. It is characterized by defective growth and maturation of the epiphyses leading to growth defects and premature osteoarthritis. It is now said to have been eradicated by importing cereals grown outside the endemic area.

Hypotheses on the aetiology include toxic effects of a fungus, *Fusarium sporotrichiella*, which was known to infest cereals grown in those areas.

3. Vinyl chloride disease

A proportion of workers who are exposed to vinyl chloride monomer during polyvinyl chloride (PVC) production develop a syndrome with features of scleroderma. The syndrome is characterised by sclerotic changes in the skin, Raynaud's phenomenon, clubbing of the fingers and osteolysis of the distal phalanges. Some cases develop thrombocytopenia, portal fibrosis and impaired hepatic function and pulmonary fibrosis. Constitutional symptoms are often marked with fatigue, malaise, and muscle and joint pains. Why some (approximately 20%) but not others develop symptoms after exposure to the chemical is intriguing and may involve genetic factors which affect susceptibility.

4. Spanish oil disease

In 1981 a striking new syndrome was described in Spain. It occurred in epidemic proportions and was linked to the ingestion of contaminated rapeseed oil. Acute manifestations were dominated by an allergic pneumonitis with respiratory distress which was accompanied by features such as headache, nausea, muscular and abdominal pain, rash and hepatosplenomegaly. Some cases showed chronic progression, with the development of scleroderma-like changes affecting the limbs and face, pulmonary fibrosis, pulmonary hypertension and neurological manifestations. Widespread vascular changes were demonstrated histologically. The precise nature of the toxic agent is not known, but hypotheses include acetanilide contamination of the oil which reacted with fatty acids to produce toxic oleoanilides, and vinyl chloride contamination from the plastic containers.

REFERENCES (DIET, DRUGS AND TOXINS)

Davies D M 1977 Textbook of adverse drug reactions. Oxford

Harmon C E, Portanova J P 1982 Drug-induced lupus: clinical and serological studies. Clinics in Rheumatic Diseases 3(1): 121–135

Hart F D 1976 Rheumatic disorders. In: Every G S (ed) Drug treatment — rheumatic diseases. pp 654–660

SECTION FOUR

Disorders of bone, collagen and periarticular tissue

17 Bone disease

INTRODUCTION

The formation and resorption of bone is a complex process controlled by the hormones calcitonin, parathormone and vitamin D (Figs 17.1 and 17.2). Normally a fine balance is maintained between the opposing actions of these hormones but there are two major metabolic disorders which result in weakness of the skeleton: osteoporosis and osteomalacia. In osteoporosis there is a reduction in the total mass of bone, but what remains is normally mineralised. In osteomalacia there is failure of mineralisation of the collagen matrix of the bone, the osteoid, so that the bone is structurally abnormal and soft. Sometimes, particularly in elderly people, the two conditions co-exist (Fig. 17.3).

OSTEOPOROSIS

Loss of bone is part of the normal process of ageing in both men and women but occurs more severely in postmenopausal women. Men lose only about 0.15% of their bone mass per year compared to 1% per year for women. As a consequence of this rarefaction of the skeleton, many older women develop fractures, particularly of the wrist, femur and vertebrae. The incidence of distal forearm fractures rises rapidly after the menopause and is thought to represent trabecular bone-loss, whereas the incidence of femoral neck fractures increases steadily after the age of 70, reflecting cortical bone-loss (Fig. 17.4).

Although postmenopausal osteoporosis is by far the commonest form of osteoporosis, there are a number of conditions which produce bone-loss. Long-term steroid therapy is the most frequently encountered of this group in practice.

Causes of secondary osteoporosis

1. Chronic steroid administration
2. Cushing's syndrome
3. Hypogonadism
4. Rheumatoid arthritis
5. Secondary carcinoma
6. Haematological malignancy/myelomatosis
7. Heparin therapy
8. Subtotal gastrectomy
9. Immobilisation
10. Renal failure
11. Thyrotoxicosis
12. Hyperparathyroidism
13. Chronic alcholism

Postmenopausal osteoporosis

Aetiology

There are three theories about the causation of postmenopausal osteoporosis: oestrogen deficiency, dietary calcium deficiency and lack of physical exercise.

Oestrogen deficiency. Histological examination of bone shows osteoclast excess with a relative deficiency in osteoblastic formation surfaces. This

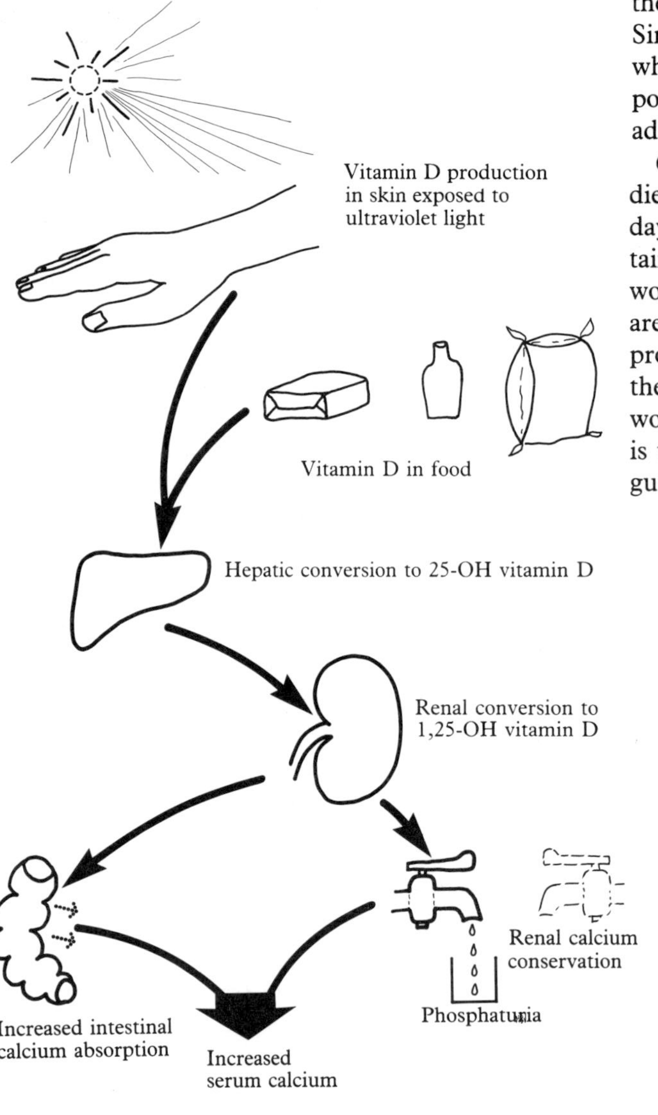

Fig. 17.1 Vitamin D metabolism

negative bone balance is thought to be due to the loss of oestrogens which normally antagonise the bone-resorbing effects of parathormone. Although individually postmenopausal women have normal calcium biochemistry, subtle differences can be detected in groups of women before and after the menopause. The serum calcium, fasting urinary calcium and urinary hydroxyproline levels are all significantly higher in postmenopausal women, although not outside the normal range and reflect the gradual loss of calcium from the skeleton. Since this process occurs in all such women, those who go on to develop clinically-significant osteoporosis must be faster 'bone-losers' because of additional factors.

Calcium deficiency. It has been shown that dietary calcium requirements increase from 1 g per day to 1.4 g per day after the menopause to maintain a neutral calcium balance. Many elderly women only achieve half this amount. Those who are alcoholic, on low sodium diet or avoid dairy products either for economic reasons or because they have acquired lactase deficiency fare even worse. Part of this increased calcium requirement is the result of impaired calcium absorption in the gut.

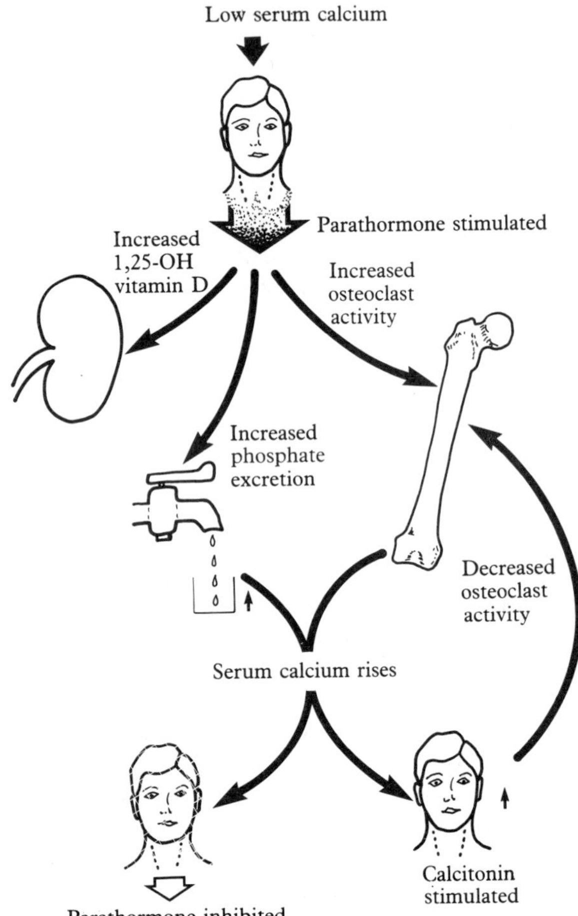

Fig. 17.2 Parathormone and calcitonin metabolism

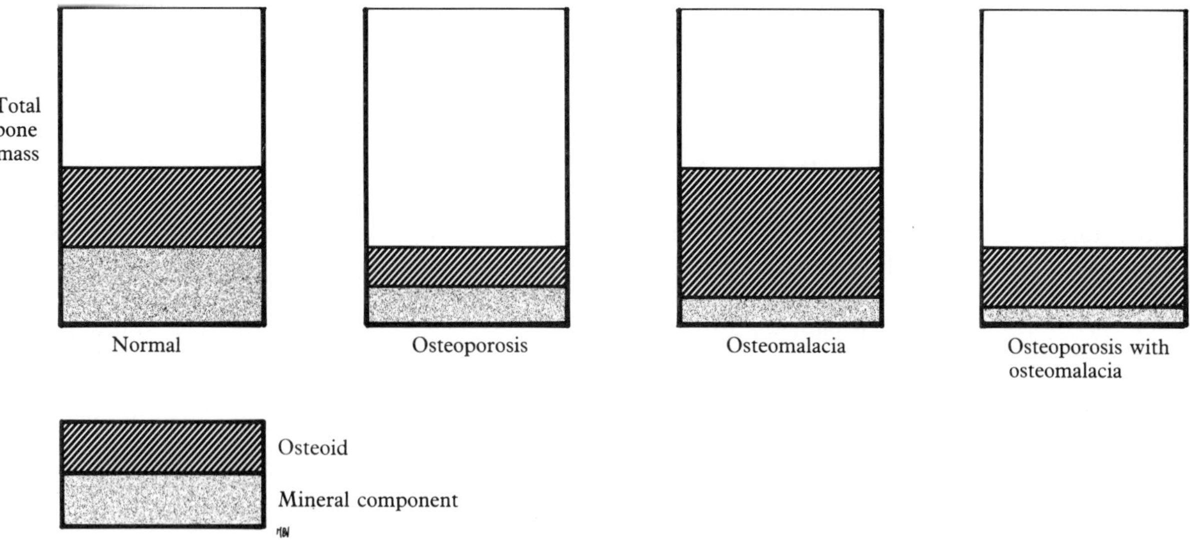

Fig. 17.3 Bone changes in osteoporosis and osteomalacia

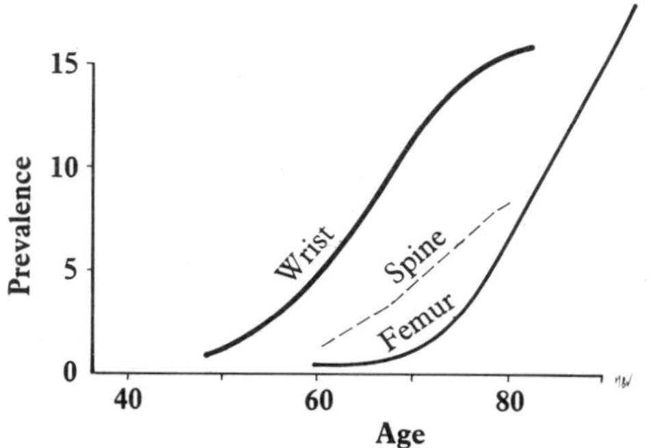

Fig. 17.4 Prevalence of fractures with increasing age in women

Inactivity. The rapid development of osteoporosis in weightless conditions has demonstrated the importance of mechanical factors in maintaining the strength of the skeleton. It has also been shown that bone mass parallels muscle mass so that osteoporosis can be regarded as a form of disuse atrophy of bone. This may also explain why obese women are less prone to osteoporosis since their excess weight places beneficial physical strain on the bones. Adrenal hormones are converted to oestrogens in adipose tissue and this may be another reason why obese women are protected against osteoporosis.

Clinical features

Many elderly women have clinical features of osteoporosis without symptoms. These features include gradual loss of height from anterior wedging of the thoracic vertebrae, which also results in kyphosis (dowager's hump) (Fig. 17.5), and over-riding of the lower costal margin on the pelvic rim causing a characteristic crease in the skin of the abdomen. Acute onset of severe localised back pain from a spontaneous crush fracture of the vertebrae is a common occurrence and often heralds a succession of painful episodes as one

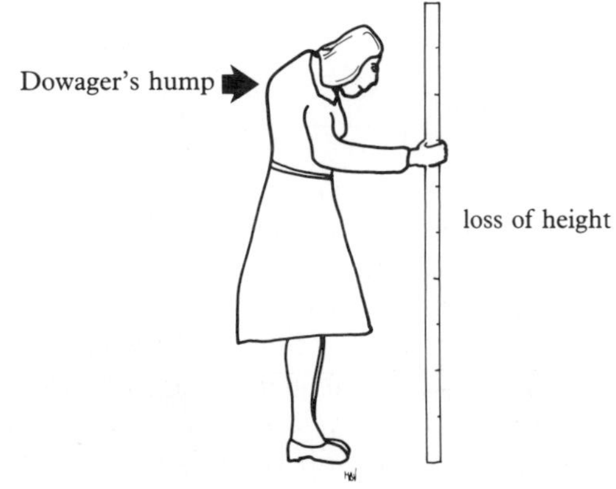

Fig. 17.5 Typical patient with senile osteoporosis

vertebra gives way after another. Root compression is common and causes severe radicular pain in the appropriate dermatome but cord compression virtually never occurs. The pain from a vertebral fracture usually settles after several months as healing takes place but may leave an angulation in the spine. Sometimes, severe chest-wall deformity may result which can cause respiratory difficulties. Other fractures, particularly of the distal forearm (Colles fracture) and femoral neck, occur readily in these patients after trivial trauma. There is some evidence that night sedation predisposes these patients to falls and hence plays a role in generation of osteoporotic fractures.

The differential diagnosis of osteoporosis includes those conditions which cause thin bones and fractures in the older age-group, particularly secondary carcinoma and haematological malignancy such as myelomatosis. Osteomalacia not infrequently co-exists with osteoporosis.

Investigations

The serum calcium and phosphate, and urinary calcium and phosphate are normal. The alkaline phosphatase is also normal but may rise significantly after a fracture. Urinary hydroxyproline may be elevated. Other tests are indicated if a secondary cause is suspected, including full blood-count, ESR, plasma and urinary cortisol, urea, creatinine, thyroid function, protein electrophoresis, immunoglobulin and Bence–Jones protein. Bone biopsy is usually inconclusive and unhelpful in a straightforward case of osteoporosis, but may be useful if osteomalacia is suspected.

Radiological changes are present when over 50% of the skeletal mass is lost. Characteristic features are best seen in a lateral X-ray of the thoracic spine. The vertebrae are less radiodense than normal and may have a density comparable to that of the adjacent lung tissue. There is frequently a paradoxical increase in cortical density which makes the vertebrae appear as if they had a white outline ('white pencil' sign). The trabeculations are frequently coarsened in the line of stress. The nucleus pulposus may balloon into the weakened vertebral end-plate, producing the classic biconcavity which gave rise to the name 'codfish spine'. Herniation of the nucleus throught the bone into the vertebral body produces a Schmorl's node. There may be anterior wedging of some of the vertebrae and old compression fractures (Fig. 17.6). X-rays are useful in the clinical evaluation of patients with osteoporosis but cannot accurately quantify the degree of bone loss or measure its reversal by therapy. Photon densitometry is a technique which does allow fairly precise measurement of bone mineral content of cortical bone — usually measured at the wrist (cortical bone) and lumbar vertebrae (trabecular bone), but this technique is not readily available. Neutron activation analysis measures total body calcium and is probably the most accurate way of assessing osteoporosis but its availability is limited to one or two research centres.

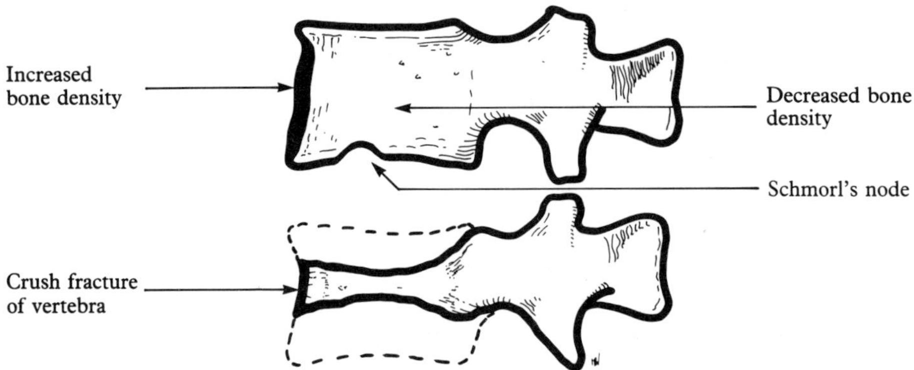

Fig. 17.6 Radiological features of the osteoporotic spine

Treatment

There are three aspects to the management of postmenopausal osteoporosis: treatment of 'end-stage' skeletal failure presenting with fractures, therapeutic measures aimed at recalcifying demineralised bone and prevention of bone loss in 'at risk' women entering the menopause.

Management of osteoporotic fractures. Patients with osteoporotic fractures should ideally be treated by the means which allows the earliest mobilisation, to avoid the often dire consequences that follow a period of bed-rest in elderly people and also to prevent further bone loss. Analgesia and a supportive corset are useful in relieving the pain of a crushed thoracic vertebra. If pain from root compression is intractable, an anaesthetist may be able to help by injecting the involved nerve root. Fractures of weight-bearing long bones are managed where possible by pin and plate fixation or, in the case of femoral neck fractures, by arthroplasty.

Prevention and treatment of bone loss. A major problem in the prevention of osteoporosis is predicting in advance those women who are particularly prone to bone loss. There is no one sure indicator, but factors such as early menopause, low oestrogen status, small skeleton at maturity, calcium malabsorption and lack of physical exercise are pointers. A good diet rich in minerals and protein plus regular exercise are the most useful general measures. Many elderly women lead extremely sedentary lives and would benefit from some form of physical activity such as regular walks or even gentle 'keep-fit' classes.

Many specific treatments are available for the management of osteoporosis which will reverse the negative calcium balance, but less clearly established is their role in preventing fractures in the long term. All depend on a high degree of patient compliance.

Oestrogens have been shown to produce a positive calcium balance with a reduction in recurrence of fractures in established osteoporosis. Their use is justified in women with a natural or artificial menopause before the age of 40 where risk of osteoporosis in high and in those with clinically-significant osteoporosis up to the age of 65. There is an increased incidence of endometrial carcinoma and thromboembolism with this treatment but the risk can be minimised by using a low dose (30 mg ethinyloestradiol) combined contraceptive pill. Absolute contra-indications are: past history of deep venous thrombosis; heart disease; breast cancer; and bad varicose veins. Cyclical menstrual bleeding is resumed on this treatment. In those women in whom oestrogens are contra-indicated, norethisterone (5 mg per day) given alone may also be of benefit. Anabolic steroids have proved disappointing, but further experience with stanazolol is awaited.

Calcium supplements are of value since it has been shown that postmenopausal women have an increased requirement that is often not met by the diet. This is best given as calcium lactate 1.2–1.5 g per day, taken last thing at night since this is when the parathormone exerts its maximal effect on the osteoclasts. Some patients with established osteoporosis have impairment of calcium absorption which can be overcome by giving, in addition to the calcium, a small dose (e.g. 500 units) of vitamin D. This may also be of value in treating co-existing osteomalacia. However, vitamin D also promotes the effect of parathormone on bone, so unless there is a clear indication, calcium salts alone are usually sufficient.

Calcitonin reduces the rate of bone resorption and has been shown to be of short-term benefit, but it has to be given by regular injection, has unpleasant side-effects and resistance often develops. It is not a practical therapy for a disease which requires long-term therapy, but used in short courses in combination with other bone-forming agents, it may prove useful and trials are awaited.

Diphosphonates have a pronounced inhibitory effect on osteoclastic activity and hence on bone resorption, but unfortunately they also inhibit the mineralisation of bone. Further developments with this class of compound may produce something useful.

Sodium fluoride stimulates new bone formation by osteoblasts, but this bone is poorly-mineralised and weak. This defect can be overcome by giving calcium supplements and the beneficial effect is further enhanced by the addition of oestrogens. This triple therapy is most likely to allow recalcification in women with repeated vertebral fractures but should only be attempted where there are facilities to monitor compliance and response.

There are therefore many therapeutic agents in the armamentarium against osteoporosis but which is chosen will depend on the individual case and experience.

Steroid-induced osteoporosis

Osteoporosis is a common complication of steroid therapy and is multifactorial in origin. There is decreased absorption of calcium from the gut and increased loss from the kidney; decreased osteoblastic activity and suppression of oestrogens. Patients with RA are particularly susceptible to these effects, probably because the disease itself causes osteoporosis and also results in reduced physical activity. The effect of steroids on bone becomes significant at doses above 10 mg/day and is less marked with ACTH. A once-daily dose of steroid or, where feasible, alternate-day therapy may reduce the risk and there is a small amount of evidence that calcium supplements, used in the same way as described for postmenopausal osteoporosis, may exert a protective effect.

Juvenile osteoporosis

This is a rare disease which affects children in the prepubertal period, around the age of 8–14 years. It presents with sudden onset of pain, usually in the long bones, and is associated with fractures and profound generalised skeletal osteoporosis. It needs to be differentiated from osteogenesis imperfecta and the childhood leukaemia syndromes. The serum calcium and phosphate are at the upper limit of normal and the alkaline phosphatase may be higher than would be expected for the child's age. There is no specific therapy, but immobilisation and vigorous exercise must both be avoided. Fortunately, the condition is self-limiting, but it may take several years to resolve.

OSTEOMALACIA

Osteomalacia is the end result of a number of different disorders and is characterised by delay or failure of calcification of bone, due either to deficiency or abnormal metabolism of vitamin D, or hypophosphataemia. Rickets is the same condition in children (see p 417). The main causes of osteomalacia are shown below. In practice the commonly encountered causes are dietary deficiency and anticonvulsant therapy.

Causes of osteomalacia

1. Vitamin D deficiency
   a) Dietary
   b) Malabsorption
   c) Lack of sunshine
2. 25OH vitamin D deficiency
   Liver disease
3. 1,25 $(OH)_2$ D deficiency
   Renal failure
4. Hypophosphataemia
   a) Fanconi syndrome
   b) Familial (hypophosphataemic ricketts)
   c) Renal tubular acidosis
5. Increased hepatic metabolism of vitamin D
   Anticonvulsant therapy

Aetiology

Vitamin D is a fat-soluble vitamin, chemically related to cholesterol, which is present in fatty fish and their oils and many other animal products. Its absorption is dependent on bile and fatty acids and is impaired in malabsorption. Vitamin D is also produced in the epidermis on exposure to sunlight and this is the major source of body stores. Vitamin D undergoes hydroxylation first in the liver and then the kidney to its active form, 1–25 $(OH)_2D$, whose major function is to stimulate calcium absorption from the gut and kidney and to mobilise calcium from the bone, thus maintaining the serum calcium at a level necessary for proper mineralisation of bone and normal neuromuscular function. Vitamin D deficiency is endemic in the elderly, particularly those who are disabled or living in adverse social circumstances, and in dark-skinned races living in northern climates while maintaining their native dietary and cultural habits. The difference between those who do and do not develop osteomalacia may be a matter of duration of deficiency and the parathyroid response. In renal failure, the plasma 1–25 $(OH)_2D$ is low due to the inability of the diseased kidney to convert 25 OH D to the active metabolite. There is often marked parathyroid response and the bone disease is therefore a mixture of osteomalacia and hyperparothyroidism. In hypophosphataemia, calcification of osteoid does not occur because the Ca × PO_4 product is too low at the growing points of bone. The osteomalacia is severe but secondary hyperparpthyroidism does not occur.

Clinical features

The typical patient with osteomalacia due to dietary deficiency is a youngish woman who has emigrated from the Indian subcontinent to a country with a cold climate, such as the United Kingdom, several years before onset and is often a vegetarian who maintains her native dress and rarely goes out of the house. She complains of non-specific aches and pains around the shoulders, rib-cage, back and upper thighs. The symptoms have usually been present for a considerable time and the patient has often been told she has 'arthritis' or 'rheumatism' or has been dismissed as neurotic. Another high-risk group comprises the housebound old and disabled living on low incomes and often on a diet of bread and tea. They may present with pathological fractures or non-specific aches and pains, or be detected on a routine X-ray by the 'fuzzy' appearance of their bone.

In addition to bone involvement there is often proximal muscle weakness which may be very subtle but cause difficulty with rising from a chair or going upstairs and patients cannot run. A 'duck-like' waddling gait is often seen in established cases.

On examination, pain may be elicited by pressing over affected long bones or stressing the rib-cage. Signs of neuromuscular hypersensitivity and Chvostek's and Trousseau's signs may occasionally be elicited, but frank tetany is rare. The muscles are not tender and the tendon reflexes are preserved.

Investigations

Biochemical tests are useful in making the diagnosis. The serum calcium is often low, the alkaline phosphatase raised and the 24-hour urinary calcium excretion decreased. The biochemical findings are also affected by the degree of parathyroid response to hypocalcaemia and the different combination of findings are shown in Table 17.1. It is also important to note that significant osteomalacia may be present despite normal calcium biochemistry. The vegetarian patients with osteomalacia are also frequently anaemic due to a combination of iron and folate deficiency.

The classic radiological feature of osteomalacia

Table 17.1 Biochemical findings in osteomalacia

	Nutritional		Tubular defect	Renal failure
	Without 2°Hp	With 2°HP		
Ca	↓	N or ↓	N	↓
PO_4	N	↓	↓	↑ ↑
Alkaline phosphatase	↑	↑	N or ↑	↑
PTH	N or ↑	↑ ↑	N	↑ ↑
Vitamin D	↓	↓	N	↓*
Urinary Ca	↓	↑	N	↓
Urinary PO_4	N	↑	↑ ↑	N or ↑

*$1,25(OH)_2D$

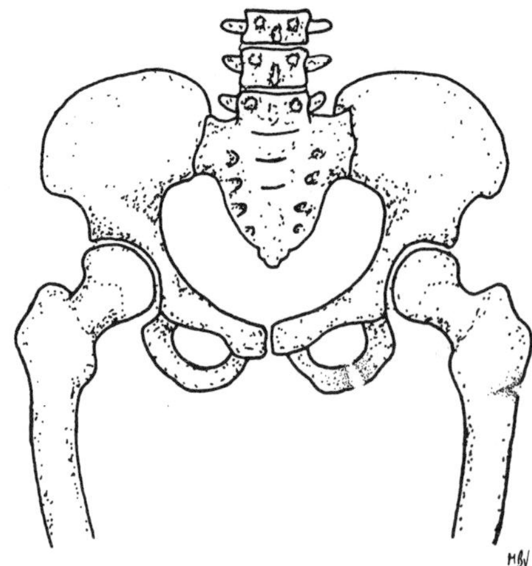

Fig. 17.7 Typical Looser's zone (pseudofracture) in osteomalacia

is the Looser's zones or pseudofractures, which are symmetrical translucent bands occuring at sites of compression stress, particularly in the ribs, axillary borders of the scapulae, pubic rami and lateral cortex of the upper femur. (Fig. 17.7) These pseudofractures are not always present and a widespread loss of bone density with a smudged trabecular pattern should be regarded with suspicion. A bone scan will often show a Looser's zone despite a normal plain X-ray.

A bone biopsy is not necessary in a straightforward case but where the diagnosis is less clear-cut, a plug of bone is obtained with a trephine from the iliac crest under local anaesthetic. The diagnosis of osteomalacia is confirmed if more than 25% of the total bone surface is covered with osteoid or there is less than 60% calcification of the total osteoid-covered surface.

Differential diagnosis

The symptoms of osteomalacia may need to be distinguished from other caused of muscle pain and weakness, particularly PMR, early RA, myositis and hypothyroidism. A search for an underlying cause such as malabsorption may be indicated.

Treatment

When present, an underlying cause should be remedied, e.g. a gluten free diet for malabsorption due to coeliac disease, or alteration of anticonvulsant therapy. Established nutritional osteomalacia is best treated with calcium and vitamin D tablets (300 mg calcium lactate and 500 units or 120 μg vitamin D) in a dose of two twice a day supplying a total daily therapeutic dose of 1000 units per day. After 2–3 months, when the bones have healed, the dose is reduced to 500 units per day, the normal requirement. There is no place in the management of this form of osteomalacia for the more potent forms of vitamin D. Dietary re-education and advice about sun-exposure should also be given. Hypophosphataemic osteomalacia will respond to phosphate supplements plus vitamin D (1–1.5 g per day of phosphate and 50 000 units of vitamin D). In patients with malabsorption, high oral doses of vitamin D, e.g. strong calciferol tablets, containing 50 000 units, or monthly intramuscular calciferol 300 000 units, may be needed. Osteomalacia associated with renal tubular acidosis is treated by correction of the acidosis with oral sodium bicarbonate and calciferol supplements as required.

The therapeutic response of osteomalacia is gratifying, with bone pain and muscle weakness disappearing within 4–8 weeks. Serum calcium may fall initially and then gradually return to normal levels after a few months. The serum alkaline phosphatase rises initially and then falls again as the bones heal. Pseudofractures take on average 2–3 months to disappear from the plain X-ray. Patients treated with vitamin D, particularly the more potent forms, may develop hypercalcaemia and irreversible renal failure and must have their serum calcium measured frequently. Occasionally, patients with long-standing osteomalacia develop hypercalcaemia due to autonomous hyperparathyroidism when the bones have healed on treatment.

Renal bone disease

Impaired renal function causes acidosis, phosphate retention and hypocalcaemia. This combination of factors results in marked secondary hyperparathyroidism. Crippling bone disease and deformity may develop due to a combination of osteomalacia and osteitis fibrosa cystica. Ectopic calcification, particularly of the blood vessels, joint capsule, cornea and kidney is a common complication and may lead to further impairment of renal function.

The biochemical findings vary (Table 17.1) depending on the relative effect of impaired calcium absorption and hyperparathyroidism. Radiological features are a mixture of hyperparathyroidism, osteomalacia and patchy sclerosis. Autonomous hyperparathyroidism is frequently present and is unmasked either during dialysis or following renal transplantation. Parathryoidectomy is often necessary.

Radiological features of renal bone disease

1. Hyperparthyroidism
   a) Cortical thinning
   b) Subperiosteal erosions
   c) Bone cysts
   d) Ground-glass appearance of bone
   e) Ectopic calcification
2. Osteomalacia
   a) Looser's zones
   b) Rarefaction
3. Patchy sclerosis
   'Rugger jersey' spine

REFERENCES (METABOLIC BONE DISEASE)

Avioli L V, Krane S M 1977 Metabolic bone disease, vol 1. Academic Press, New York

Menczel J, Robin G C, Makin M, Steinberg R 1982 Osteoporosis John Wiley, New York

II Paget's disease

INTRODUCTION

Osteitis deformans is a disease of older people in which there is enlargement, softening and deformity of bone. Studies of archaeological skeletal remains reveal that it is an ancient disease. The original skull of Neanderthal man probably contained pagetic bone, which accounted for the erroneous belief that these early people were thickset with heavy overhanging brows, and Ludwig van Beethoven's deafness has also been ascribed to Paget's disease. The classic description was that of Sir James Paget in 1876, and although he called it 'osteitis deformans' believing that it had an inflammatory origin, the disease now bears his name in English-speaking countries.

EPIDEMIOLOGY

The overall prevalence of Paget's disease in the UK is 3%. It is a disease of older people with a less than 0.3% incidence in those under 40, rising to 10% in those over 85. In most series men are more commonly affected than women, in a ratio of 4 : 3, and a family history is found in 16% of patients. Despite the high prevalence in the population, only about 5% of those affected present with symptoms of their disease, the vast majority being discovered accidently on an X-ray, by a raised alkaline phosphatase or following physical examination for an unrelated condition.

There is a great variation in the prevalence of Paget's disease throughout the world: it is common in countries with a predominantly Anglo-Saxon population, particularly the UK, USA and Australia, but is rare in Africa, India, China, the Middle East and, oddly, Scandinavia. The prevalence in American Blacks is similar to that in the white population, suggesting a role for environmental factors. There is also geographical variation within countries: there is a striking clustering of Paget's disease around the Lancashire mill towns in the UK, where nearly 8% of the population over 55 are affected.

PATHOLOGY

Paget's disease is thought to be a primary disorder of the osteoclasts which results in a disturbance in the balance between formation and resorption of bone. In early active disease osteoclasts resorb bone at a rapid rate and the osteoblasts respond by laying down lamellar bone at an equally rapid rate. Cycles of destruction and formation recur so that bone turnover is greatly increased — as much as twenty-fold. Histologically, the bone formed is abnormal, coarse and disorganised. Many hyper-nucleated osteoclasts are present, lying in scalloped-out lacunae surrounded by a mosaic pattern of cement lines indicating previous phases of activity. Active pagetic lesions are highly vascular with a marked increase in blood-flow through them. The bone produced during this phase of disease is light and liable to fracture and deform. In the later phase of the disease osteoclast activity subsides while osteoblast activity continues unchecked, forming dense ivory-hard bone which is heavy and difficult to cut but still weak due to its abnormal structure.

In the monostotic form of the disease (about 10%) a single isolated bone is affected, usually in the pelvis, sacrum or vertebrae. More commonly the disease is polyostotic, affecting primarily weight-bearing bones and the axial skeleton (Fig. 17.8). This distribution suggests that mechanical stress and the presence of red marrow may play a role in localisation of disease.

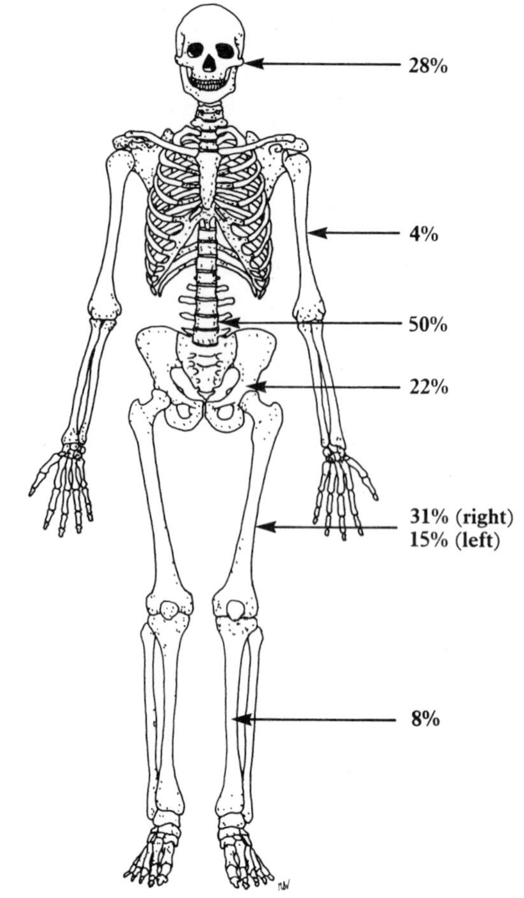

Fig. 17.8 Distribution of Paget's disease

AETIOLOGY

Many factors have been proposed as the cause of Paget's disease, including infection, neoplasia and a hereditable defect. There is strong evidence to support a viral aetiology, possibly of the slow-virus type. Histologically the giant multi-nucleated osteoclasts of Paget's resemble the multi-nucleated syncytial cells characteristic of viral infection. Furthermore, inclusion bodies have been identified in the nuclei of the osteoclasts similar to those seen in subacute sclerosing panencephalitis. A slow virus also takes many years to produce disease, which may explain the prevalence of Paget's disease in the older age-groups.

CLINICAL FEATURES

Paget's disease is usually asymptomatic — the symptoms and signs that do occur depend on the site and extent of skeletal involvement.

Clinical features of Paget's disease

1. Pain — back, hip, bone
2. Fracture
3. Deformity, skull, spine, long bones.
4. Complications
   a) Neurological
      Tinnitus, vertigo, hearing loss, spinal-cord compression, hydrocephalus
   b) Cardiovascular
      High-output failure
      Steal syndromes
   c) Osteosarcoma

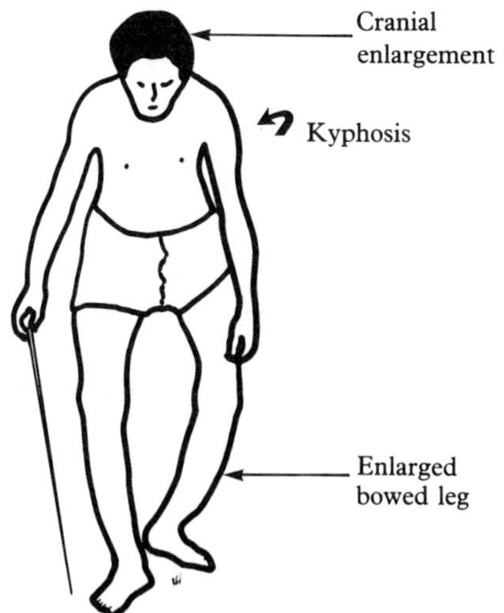

Fig. 17.9 Typical skeletal deformities in Paget's disease

Pain is the commonest symptom, particularly when weight bearing bones are affected. Pagetic bone pain is characteristically burning, hot, deep-seated, not relieved by rest and particularly bad at night. There may be local warmth of the overlying skin and periosteal tenderness along the affected bone. The abnormal shape, size and quality of the bone results in a number of typical skeletal deformities (Fig. 17.9).

Involvement of the skull and spine can cause serious neurological problems. The cranial nerves may be compressed as they pass through the bony foramina in the skull. Hearing loss results either from compression of the eighth nerve in the petrosal ridge or from involvement of the ossicles of the middle ear. The enlarged, heavy, soft skull may sink down over the top of the neck, resulting in basilar invagination. This may cause tinnitus, vertigo and falls from vertobrobasilar insufficiency, brain-stem and cerebellar compression and dementia from internal hydrocephalus. Spinal involvement, particularly above the second lumbar vertabra, may cause cord compression with paraesthesiae, weakness in the legs and impaired bowel and bladder control. Enlargement of the facial bones is rare but can cause a grotesque leonine appearance. The increased vascularity of pagetic bone may occasionally lead to high-output cardiac failure and shunting of blood to highly vascular bone may deprive other tissues of their share of the cardiac output, resulting in 'steal' syndromes.

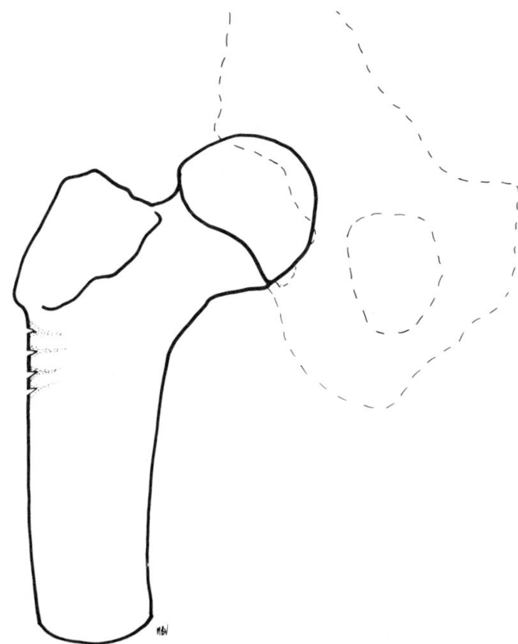

Fig. 17.10 Multiple pseudofractures along the bowed surface of a deformed pagetic femur

Pathological fractures of the long bones are one of the commonest complications of Paget's disease, particularly during the active osteoclastic stage. Most fractures are heralded by a localised increase in pain due to transverse pseudofractures that develop on the convex border of the curved weight-bearing bones (Fig. 17.10).

Osteoscaroma is 40 times more common in pagetic than in normal bone — but the incidence of malignant transformation is only about 1%. The femur is the commonest site but any pagetic bone may be affected. Sudden marked increase in pain or deformity in a previously affected bone should suggest this possibility, particularly if the pain is not relieved by analgesics and is associated with a soft-tissue mass. The prognosis is very poor, with survival of only about 7 months from diagnosis.

INVESTIGATIONS

Useful tests in Paget's disease are shown overleaf.

Investigations in Paget's
1. X-ray
2. Bone scan
3. Biochemical tests
   — serum alkaline phosphatase
   — urinary hydroxyproline
4. Bone biopsy

Radiographs are the most helpful. The affected bones are usually enlarged, deformed and have lost their clear-cut outline. The normal trabecular pattern is replaced by a disorganised, coarse one. In early, active disease, lytic lesions predominate so that the texture is porotic and transparent — like cotton wool. In later disease dense sclerotic bone is seen but usually there is a mixed lytic/sclerotic picture. Multiple hair-line fractures may be seen along the convex side of a bowed long bone. A typical pagetic pelvis shows widespread involvement with obliteration of one hip-joint space. Sometimes only a small area of pelvis is affected, not anatomically confined to one pelvic bone.

Osteoporosis circumscripta describes an early classic X-ray finding of large lytic areas in a portion of the skull. A single vertebra may be dense and sclerotic (*ivory vertebra*), or enlarged and fluffy.

Radioactive technetium bone scanning is a useful tool for delineating the extent of Paget's disease without recourse to multiple X-rays. The scan and plain radiograph agree in 70% of cases. About 15% of lesions are shown on bone scan alone — these are usually active early symptomatic lesions. In another 15% the lesion is visible only on X-ray — these are usually inactive sclerotic lesions. Thus scans are generally more helpful in assessing overall disease activity. Scans are also helpful in suspected sarcomatous transformation, since such lesions are necrotic and therefore less active on a bone scan than would be expected from the appearance on X-ray.

Urinary hydroxyproline is derived from bone collagen and is the best marker of osteoclastic activity and bone turnover. Alkaline phosphatase reflects the osteoblastic activity. Both correlate well with the extent and activity of Paget's disease. Sometimes a sharp rise in alkaline phosphatase is observed which is not accompanied by a parallel rise in hydroxyproline and this should suggest the possibility that a lesion has undergone malignant transformation.

Calcium, phosphate and parathormone levels are usually normal but significant hypercalcaemia and hypercalciuria may result if the patient with Paget's disease is immobilised, e.g. following a fracture. The serum uric acid may be elevated due to increased cell turnover and the incidence of gouty arthritis has been reported to be increased in some series.

Bone biopsy is rarely needed in the diagnosis of Paget's disease, except perhaps in the case of a single lesion. In established disease it may be required to rule out osetosarcoma, particularly if there is an area of increased pain and a soft-tissue mass accompanied by an area of lysis on X-ray.

MANAGEMENT

Treatment is only required for patients with significant symptoms. Pain can often be controlled with reassurance, analgesia and anti-inflammatory drugs. Patients with severe pain uncontrolled by these measures, neurological complications or fractures warrant treatment with specific therapy which is also indicated in patients with active disease at the skull base or a vertebra above L2, in those with softening of the pelvic bones and protursio actabuli and prior to surgery. Three specific drugs are available which act primarily by inhibiting bone resorption; these are calcitonin, diphosphonates and mithramycin. Calcitonin is a hormone obtained from the thyroid glands of salmon or pigs, which is given by subcutaneous injection. The usual regimen is 50–100 MRC units daily for 1 month, reduced to three times a week for another month and then weekly thereafter. It has been shown to speed healing of pathological fractures and ameliorate neurological symptoms as well as relieve pain. It is not always successful and if no pain relief is apparent after 8 weeks it should be stopped. If pain is relieved it is usually continued for a year and then stopped. Rebound is inevitable with time, but a second course can be successful. The activity of the disease and response to therapy can be monitored by measuring the alkaline phosphatase and urinary hydroxyproline. The levels fall to about 50% of the starting level after about 6 months' treatment but after that time there is little further reduction. Radiological improvement is not, as a rule, observed. Apart from the necessity of regular injections, other drawbacks of calcitonin are the expense, the high incidence of side-effects such as facial flushing and nausea and the development of antibodies which reduce its effectiveness.

The introduction of the diphosphonate group of drugs is the latest promising line of treatment. These are analogues of calcium pyrophosphate which decrease bone turnover by inhibiting both osteoblastic and osteoclastic activity and calcification. Etiodronate is the analogue currently in use and it is administered by mouth in a dose of 5 mg/kg for a period of 6 months. Response depends partly on the initial disease activity but up to 60% of patients have relief of pain after 6 months treatment. The benefit often lasts up to 2–3 years after the drug is stopped and control is regained following relapse by a further 6-month course. Diarrhoea and an increase in bone pain are the commonest side effects at onset of treatment. If the dose is kept at about 5 mg/kg and the number of courses limited, osteomalacia is not produced. Good results are being reported using a combined regimen of calcitonin and etiodronate.

Mithramycin is a very toxic but effective drug. Its use is not justified except in an acute emergency situation, e.g. cord compression. It has to be given by intravenous infusion and has the additional useful property of rapidly abolishing pain.

Surgery is not contra-indicated in Paget's disease and joint replacement, osteotomy and internal fixation of fractures are usually successful. For elective surgery it is a good idea to give the patient a period of pre-operative medical treatment which reduces the vascularity of the bone and makes the surgeon's job easier.

RHEUMATOLOGICAL ASPECTS OF PAGET'S DISEASE

The articular surface is not usually involved in Paget's disease but arthritis may occur secondary to the deformity of bones which places abnormal mechanical stresses on weight-bearing joints. A very common rheumatological problem is the elderly patient with pain around the hips who has widespread Paget's disease of the pelvis and head of femur, with joint-space narrowing. The question is to decide if the pain is due to the Paget's disease or to osteoarthritis. The quality of the pain may help. Osteoarthritic pain is aggravated by use, relieved by rest and rarely disturbs sleep, whereas pagetic pain persists day and night. In both diseases examination of the hip may show a painful decreased range of motion. Radiology is unhelpful in deciding the issue except that occasionally Paget's disease appears to narrow the joint-space medially whereas superior-pole narrowing is more common in OA, osteophytes are less prominent in Paget's and there may be protrusio acetabuli due to the softness of the pelvic bones. Two useful clinical manoeuvres can help to sort these out. If the hip joint in injected with lignocaine this will often abolish the pain of OA but not of Paget's, and conversely one injection of mithramycin will relieve pagetic pain but not that of OA.

Patients with Paget's disease also often develop OA of the knee on the unaffected side of the body by favouring the leg opposite to the one which is the site of Paget's disease.

REFERENCES (PAGET'S)

Hamdy R C 1981 Paget's disease of bone. Endocrinology and metabolism 1. Praeger Scientific, Eastbourne

Hosking D J 1981 Paget's disease of bone. British Medical Journal 283: 686–688

III Osteonecrosis

INTRODUCTION

Osteonecrosis means 'death of bone cells', and is a pathological description for a condition which

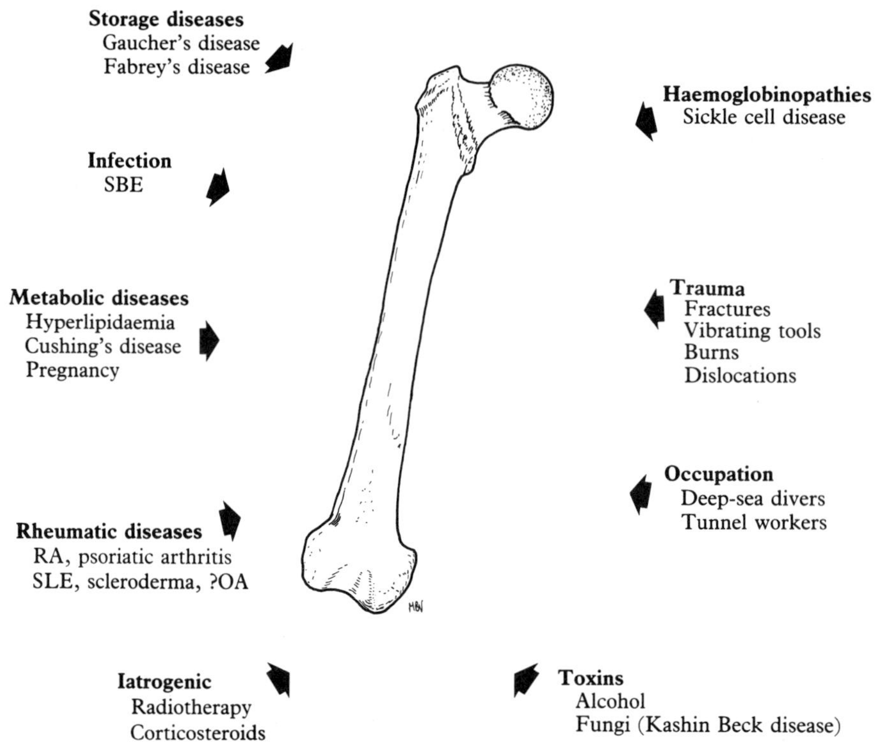

Fig. 17.11 Factors implicated in the aetiology of osteonecrosis

may have many causes (Fig. 17.11). It may occur following trauma in which the blood-supply of bone is interrupted, and is then referred to as *avasular necrosis*. This is a common occurence after a subcapital fracture of the femur, posterior dislocation of the hip or fracture of the scaphoid. Recurrent trauma from the use of tools such as pneumatic drills is thought to account for the high incidence of osteonecrosis of the lunate bone of the hand in some workmen (also called Kienböch's disease). In some of the general conditions associated with osteonecrosis the underlying pathological mechanism is apparent, e.g. thrombosis in blood vessels in sickle-cell disease, nitrogen bubbles in decompression sickness and increased interosseous pressure due to accumulation of abnormal fat-filled cells in Gaucher's disease. In others the mechanism is not so obvious. Alcohol and corticosteroids may have a direct toxic effect on the bone cells without interfering with the blood supply. There remain a substantial group of patients who develop osteonecrosis, commonly of the head of the femur (young men) and medial femoral condyle (middle-aged and elderly women), without any apparent cause.

PATHOLOGY

The cycle of pathological changes in the dead bone varies slightly depending on the cause, but most studies have been done following trauma (Fig. 17.12). The marrow cells disappear first followed later by the osteocytes and fat cells and a clear demarcation develops between the dead and living bone. Repair starts along this line and gradually advances foward. The dead cells are replaced by undifferentiated mesenchymal cells and capillary buds. New osteoblasts form on the surface of the dead trabeculae encasing them in new bone, which causes them to become greatly enlarged and hence more dense on X-ray. Other areas are filled

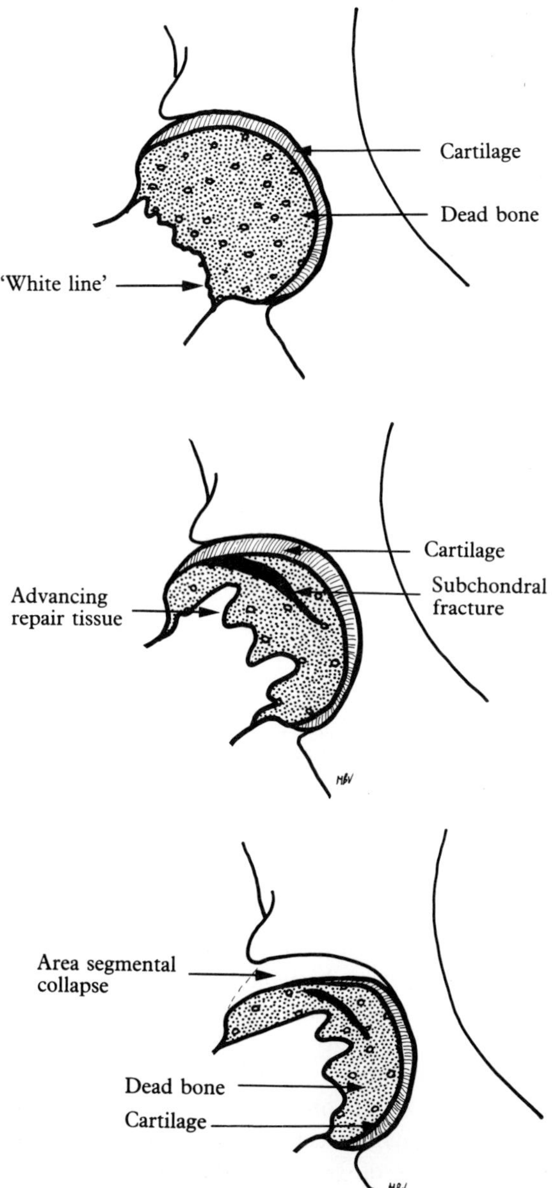

Fig. 17.12 Sequence of changes in osteonecrosis of the femoral head

with fibrous tissue and fibrocartilage. The whole process tends to be patchy throughout the affected bone but reaches the subchondral bone last. Multiple microfractures tend to develop in this region furthest away from the advancing repair tissue and these gradually coalesce into large macrofractures which may cause collapse of segments of dead bone. Consequently, the adjacent joint surfaces become misshapen and incongruous and this leads to secondary destruction of the overlying cartilage. The extent of osteonecrosis is always much greater on histological examination than is suggested by the findings on X-ray.

CLINICAL FEATURES

Idiopathic osteonecrosis presents with pain in the affected joint which is usually low-grade, intermittent and exacerbated by joint movement. The hips, knees and shoulders are most often affected, in that order. Night pain is rare except in medial femoral condyle osteonecrosis. In the early stage there is often a good range of joint movement. Precise diagnosis at this early stage is difficult. The plain X-ray is usually normal until many months from onset. A bone scan done early, i.e. in the first 6 months, will often show decreased uptake of bone-seeking isotope but once repair has started there may be increased uptake. A core biopsy of affected bone will usually confirm the diagnosis. With the passage of time characteristic changes appear on the X-ray. The first sign is a dense white line below the dead segment with a normal joint contour and joint space. Patchy increase in radiodensity appears as repair begins. Later a subchondral lucency or *crescent sign* can be seen at the site of subchondral fracture. As segments of dead bone collapse there is further increase in density accompanied by irregular 'steps' on the articulating surface, abnormal contour to the bone and finally loss of joint space as the cartilage is destroyed. Osteonecrosis is not necessarily progressive and many patients make a complete recovery, particularly medial condyle of the knee osteonecrosis of the knee where the outcome appears to correlate to the area of joint surface involved. The appearance of the crescent sign indicates that progression to joint destruction is likely.

MANAGEMENT

Avascular necrosis following trauma is the province of the orthopaedic surgeon. Speedy reduction and meticulous fixation of fractures will help to reduce the incidence but sometimes it is unavoidable.

Once the diagnosis of idiopathic osteonecrosis has been confirmed either on X-ray or by biopsy, most physicians adopt a 'wait-and-see' policy. The patient is given appropriate analgesia and protected ambulation by the use of a stick and is followed up and X-rayed every few months. Many will heal with this regime. Should further radiological deterioration occur, such as the appearance of a crescent sign, segmental collapse can be predicted, but it is still worth trying to reduce weight-bearing even further by a period of bed-rest or use of crutches. Once severe distortion of the joint has occured arthroplasty is usually the only treatment that will relieve pain and maintain mobility. Some orthopaedic surgeons advocate a more aggressive approach in the early stage. They perform a core biopsy to confirm the diagnosis and also to relieve venous hypertension, arguing that decompression may permit revascularisation healing of early lesions without collapse. Some good results have also been reported from coring out dead bone and packing the area with bone grafts, but these procedures are still experimental.

Efforts should be directed to looking for an underlying cause in cases of idiopathic osteonecrosis and attempting to treat any that are uncovered. It is common in alcoholics, for example, for several joints in succesion to be destroyed, and it may be possible to prevent this by abstinence. Corticosteroids should be stopped where possible, or reduced, or changed to an alternate-day regime.

RHEUMATOLOGICAL ASPECTS OF OSTEONECROSIS

Patients with RA and SLE are prone to develop osteonecrosis particularly of the femoral head. This is probably a direct consequence of continuous steroid therapy in SLE rather than, as was earlier believed, part of the disease itself. In RA the picture is less clear, for although there is a high incidence of osteonecrosis in RA it occurs quite frequently in patients who have never been on steroid. Possibly NSAIDs play a role by suppressing pain, thus permitting a patient to carry on weight-bearing on a compromised hip joint. Sudden severe increase in pain in a hip should suggest the possibility of osteonecrosis rather than just an exacerbation of the underlying disease in these patients.

Patients on chronic steroid therapy for non-rheumatological conditions, for example asthma, may present with a painful hip and it is useful, though not always possible, to distinguish between osteonecrosis and osteoarthritis. The plain X-ray appearance may help, since there is often less marked osteophyte formation or butressing of the femoral neck in osteonecrosis and irregular 'step-like' defects may be present on the articular surface. Once the femoral head has undergone sgemental collapse it can be difficult to distinguish these two conditions.

REFERENCES (OSTEONECROSIS)

Davidson J K 1976 Aseptic necrosis of bone. Excerpta Medica, Amsterdam

Ficat RP, Arlet J 1980 Ischaemia and necrosis of bone. Williams & Wilkins, Baltimore

IV Osteochondritis

There are a group of conditions, grouped together as *osteochondritis*, which are known by many esoteric, usually German, eponyms. Their main claim to homogeneity is a similar radiological appearance and many were in fact described by radiologists. Osteochondritis is defined as a non-inflammatory non-infectious derangement of the normal process of bone growth, occurring at a variety of ossification centres at their time of greatest activity. A cycle of changes affects the portion of growing bone in a similar way to that seen in osteonecrosis. The bone becomes painful, and dense on X-ray and starts to crumble and collapse. Revascularisation follows and the bone recalcifies but there is often subsequent distortion of the bone. Osteochondritis occurs in a number of characteristic sites in the skeleton which are shown with their eponyms in Figure 17.13. All tend to be associated with activity and trauma and

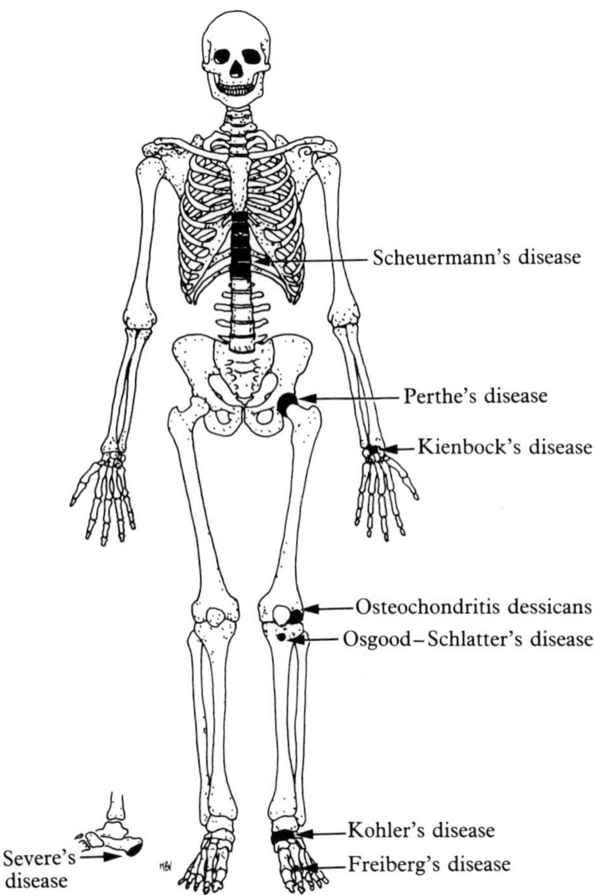

Fig. 17.13 Some common sites of osteochondritis

are generally best managed by rest and, where necessary, avoidance of weight-bearing. There is an increased risk of osteoarthritis developing in the adjacent joint in later life.

SCHEUERMANN'S DISEASE

This is osteonecrosis of the ring epiphysis of the vertebrae and tends to affect adolescent males who present with thoracic back pain and develop a dorsal kyphosis, rounded shoulders and a flat chest. X-rays show anterior wedging of the vertebral bodies, irregularity of the vertebral surface and multiple Schmorl's nodes (Fig. 17.14). This condition is treated with physiotherapy to maintain a good posture but the patient is usually left with a slightly deformed back and residual changes on X-ray.

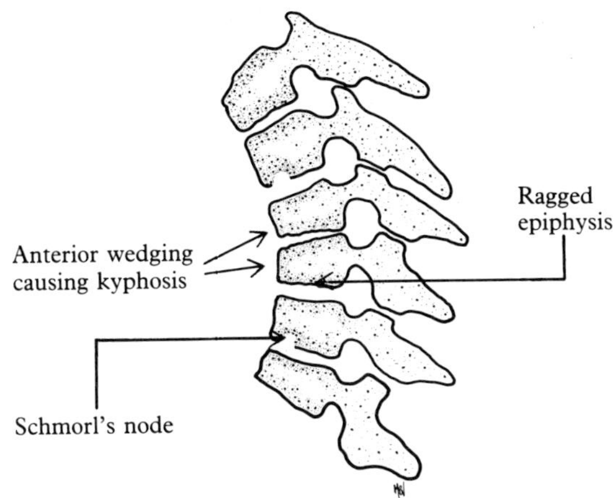

Fig. 17.14 Typical radiological appearance of Scheuermann's disease

PERTHES' DISEASE

This is osteonecrosis occurring in the femoral epiphysis and affects children between the ages of 2–18 with a peak between 4 and 9 years. Boys are affected four times more commonly than girls and the disease is bilateral in 15% of cases. The exact cause in not established but experimentally, prolonged induced effusions in animals produce similar iscaemic changes in the epiphysis.

Perthes' disease classically presents as a limp in an otherwise healthy child associated with some limitation of hip movement. There are no other signs and all blood tests are normal. Antero-posterior and lateral X-rays of the hip are essential in making the diagnosis. The earliest sign is widening of the joint space, followed by increased density in the affected segment of the femoral head. The epiphysis becomes flattened and the neck widens to support the spreading epiphysis. With time the femoral head remodels either back to normal or to a deformed shape. The outcome is determined by the size of the area affected and the amount of collapse of bone that has occurred. The whole process may take up to 4 years to resolve. The management is controversial but generally bed-rest is advised followed by a procedure, either medical with splints or surgical, designed to keep the femoral head contained within the acetabulum. Surgical intervention is absolutely indicated if the epiphysis is subluxed outside the acetabulum. The short-term outlook is good but there is a high incidence of premature osteoarthritis of the hip.

OSGOOD–SCHLATTER'S DISEASE

This condition is thought to be due to interference with the blood supply of the epiphysis overlying the tibial tubercle into which the patello-femoral ligament is inserted. It usually affects boys around puberty who play a lot of sport and presents with pain below the knee which is aggrevated by exercise. There is local tenderness over the tibial tubercle. A lateral X-ray of the knee will show roughening and widening of the tendon insertion. This condition is managed by reassurance and curtailment of sporting activity. If this is insufficient, the knee can be immobilised in a plaster cylinder for 4 weeks. It resolves spontaneously over several years.

OSTEOCHONDRITIS DESSICANS

This is a characteristic form of subarticular osteonecrosis occurring particularly in young men towards the end of the growing period. It most commonly affects the medial femoral condyle near the intracondylar notch, although a similar process occassionally occurs in the capitulum of the humerus in the elbow. A segment of articular surface becomes necrotic and may separate to form a loose osteochondral fragment in the joint cavity.

The patient presents with a history of intermittent pain in the knee aggravated by exercise and associated with a feeling of insecurity when walking. The presence of a loose body is suggested by episodes of intermittent locking or sudden giving way of the joint. There is often a small effusion in the knee and sometimes the fragment can be palpated in the suprapatellar pouch. A tunnel view of the knee must be requested since the affected area may not show on an AP or lateral.

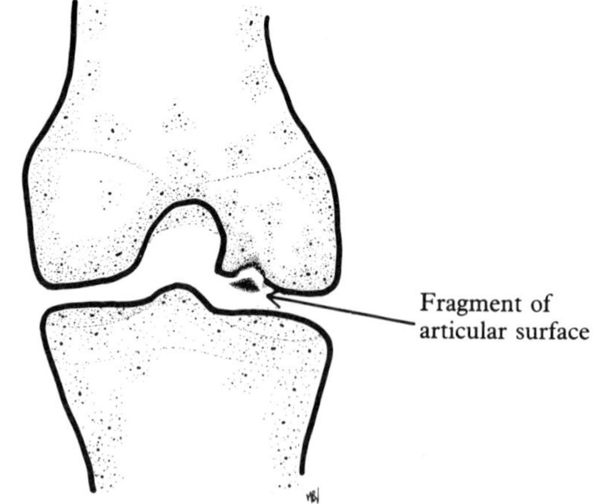

Fig. 17.15 Intracondylar radiograph ('tunnel view') showing osteochondritis dessicans

Before separation, a dense segment may be seen in the intercondylar notch, often surrounded by a clear halo (Fig. 17.15). Later a free sclerotic fragment may be visible plus the crater from which it came. If the detached fragment is composed only of uncalcified cartilage it will not be visible on a plain X-ray and arthrography or arthroscopy may be required. Surgery is indicated to pin a large fragment in place before separation has occurred and to remove a troublesome loose body. About 50% of such men develop premature osteoarthritis of the affected knee.

FREIBERG'S DISEASE

This may occur at any age, but is particularly common in girls in the second decade. It is a form of subarticular osteonecrosis affecting the head of the second or third metatarsal bone of the foot often after an episode of trauma. It presents with persistent metatarsalgia associated with localised pain, stiffness and swelling. The X-ray initially shows a diffuse increase of density with subarticular translucency. Later, a portion of the articular surface may develop a frank osteochondral fracture and sometimes this may separate as in osteochondritis dessicans. More usually, the head of the affected metatarsal becomes flattened and collapsed with secondary osteoarthritic change.

Resection of the metatarsal head may be required later.

KOHLER'S DISEASE

This is osteonecrosis of the navicular bone commonly occurring in young boys between the ages of 3 and 5 years. It presents with pain and swelling aggravated by weight-bearing and associated with restricted movement and tenderness over the navicular. Early on, X-rays show a flattened dense ossification centre which later becomes absorbed and fragmented. Over the next 18 months or so there is revascularisation and restoration of the bone. Rest and protection in a plaster cast is usually all the treatment that is required for this benign, self-limiting condition.

REFERENCES (OSTEOCHONDRITIS)

Adams J C 1981 Outline of orthopaedics, 9th edn. Churchill Livingstone, Edinburgh

Siffert R F 1981 The osteochondroses. Clinical Orthopaedics and Related Research 158

Steel W M 1974 Osteochondritis. Hospital Update 769–777

V Acro-osteolysis

Primary acro-osteolyis is an ill-understood condition in which there is destruction and eventual disappearance of entire bones without any obvious underlying cause such as neoplasia. Two inherited forms have been reported which usually present in childhood or early adolesence with pain and swelling of the affected bone. A proximal form affects young children from the age of 3 years and results in disappearance of the tarsal and carpal bones; and a distal form occurs in older children and young adults causing disappearance of the phalanges, metatarsal and metacarpal bones. The overlying soft tissues can ulcerate and whole fingers may drop off. There is a tendency to spontaneous remission with varying degrees of residual deformity.

Gorham's disease (*disappearing bone disease*) is a form of acro-osteolysis associated with mild trauma. It can affect multiple sites and may result in a boneless limb. The affected bone often lies adjacent to a collection of haemangiomatous material whose role is not clear.

Another non-inherited form of osteolysis, which otherwise resembles the proximal inherited form in all respects, can occur in childhood in association with a severe glomerulonephritis which is frequently fatal.

Secondary osteolysis of the distal phalanges of the hands and feet is seen in Raynaud's disease, PPS, leprosy, peripheral arterial obstruction and vinyl chloride disease.

FURTHER READING (ACRO-OSTEOLYSIS)

Gorham L W, Stout A P 1955 Massive osteolysis (acute spontaneous absorption of bone, phantom bone, disappearing bone); its relation to haemangiomatosis. Journal of Bone and Joint Surgery 37A: 985

Harris D K, Adams W G V 1976 Acro-osteolysis in men engaged in the polymerisation of vinyl chloride. British Medical Journal iii: 712

18 Collagen diseases

The term 'collagen disease' is properly restricted to a small number of genetic conditions in which there is a putative or proven molecular defect in the structural components of connective tissue, i.e. collagen or elastin (p 5). Although collagen defects relate primarily to type I collagen, similar genetic abnormalities of type II may also exist and play a part in other rheumatic diseases such as osteoarthritis.

Collagen diseases are rare and affected individuals usually present to non-rheumatological specialities with major skeletal, ocular or cardiovascular disease. Appreciation of their salient features, however, is relevant to rheumatologists since:

1. Involvement of connective tissue of ligaments, cartilage and bone can result in rheumatic disease
2. *Formes frustes* of the complete syndromes may escape notice and allow initial presentation with rheumatic complaints alone
3. Study of affected patients may allow insight into the mechanisms of joint damage and repair.

Hypermobility is common to many of these heritable disorders and will therefore be considered first, together with the 'benign hypermobility syndrome'.

Hypermobility

Recognition of generalised joint hypermobility first requires definition of a normal range. Such a definition is necessarily imprecise because of the many physiological, racial and social factors which are known to influence joint mobility, e.g.:

1. Mobility decreases from the age of 5–11, undergoes little change during adolescence, but then further declines during adult life
2. Negroes and Indians are more 'loose-jointed' than whites
3. Females tend to be more mobile than males at all ages
4. Joint laxity increases during pregnancy (maximally in the second)
5. Social or occupational customs (e.g. squatting, gymnastics, ballet) may further exert an influence.

In practice, however, individuals with exceptional joint laxity may clinically be recognised by their ability to perform certain passive movements (Fig. 18.1). According to these criteria,5–10% of whites and a higher percentage of Negroes or Indians, will be found to have 'hypermobility', implying merely that they fall at one end of a spectrum of mobility. The majority show no underlying structural or metabolic abnormality and the cause of their hypermobility is presumably constitutional, reflecting normal variation within a population. Only a very small number will owe their joint laxity to a recognised heritable condition.

Benign hypermobility syndrome

Generalised hypermobility may occasionally be advantageous (e.g. ballet dancers, gymnasts), but

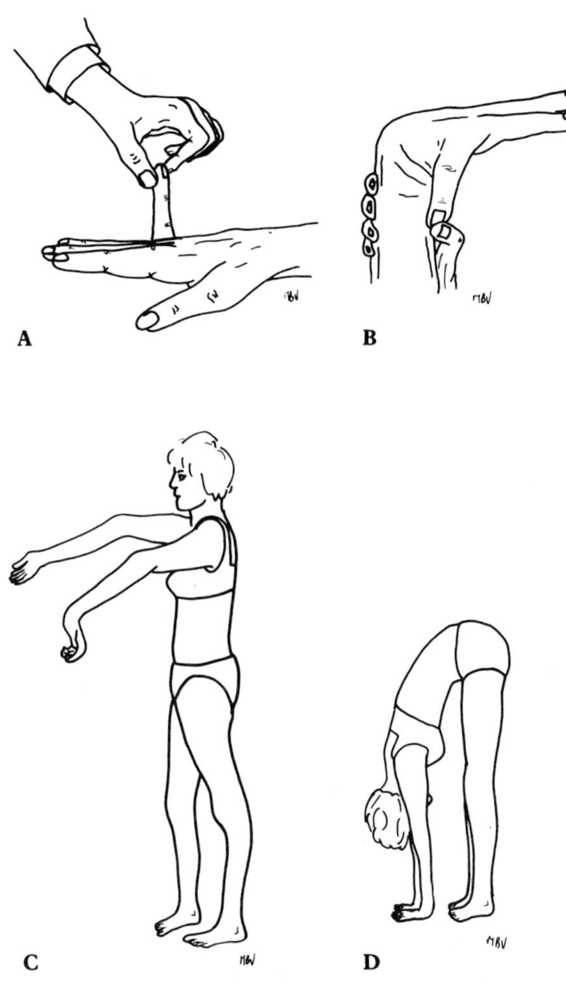

Fig. 18.1 Recognition of hypermobility **A**. Passive dorsiflexion of 5th MCP to 90 ° (score 1 on each side) **B**. Apposition of thumb to volar aspect of forearm (score 1 on each side) **C**. Hyperextension of elbow to beyond 10 ° (score 1 on each side); hyperextension of knee to beyond 10 ° (score 1 on each side) **D**. Ability to place hands flat on floor with knees extended (score 1) Hypermobility = total score of 5 or more

> **Rare causes of generalised hypermobility**
> 1. Marfan's syndrome
> 1. Ehlers–Danlos syndrome
> 3. Osteogenesis imperfecta
> 4. Hyperlysinaemia
> 5. Homocystinuria
> 6. Wilson's disease

some hypermobile but otherwise normal individuals appear to develop musculoskeletal complaints for which no cause other than their joint laxity can be found. Such symptomatic joint laxity, unassociated with arthritis, is termed 'benign hypermobility syndrome'.

The typical patient is a young woman in her late teens or early twenties who complains of knee and ankle pains and low backache of mechanical type (*loose back syndrome*). Occasionally a history of shoulder dislocation may additionally be obtained. Examination is unremarkable except for the finding of generalised hypermobility and occasional small to moderate effusions in the knees. Familial predisposition is common and one or more relatives have usually suffered similar problems. Symptoms generally improve with age, as the joints become less mobile, and nothing apart from full explanation is usually required.

Prolapsed mitral leaflet, diagnosed clinically by a non-ejection systolic click with or without a late systolic murmur, is reported to be associated with generalised joint hypermobility, but despite familial predisposition (with evidence for both autosomal dominant and recessive inheritance) there is no evidence that patients with hypermobility syndrome represent *formes frustes* of a collagen disorder. Generalised, as well as localised, joint laxity has been reported to predispose to pyrophosphate arthropathy (p 178), but its relation to premature OA remains unclear (p 145).

Marfan's syndrome

This is the commonest heritable connective tissue disease, with a prevalence of 1.5/100 000. Its cause is unknown, though abnormalities in nonreducible collagen cross-links, increased collagen turn-over (reflected by high urinary hydroxyproline) and similarities to experimental lathyrism (i.e. interference with cross-linking) suggest a nonenzymatic defect in collagen and elastin maturation and organisation that results in reduced tensile strength of supporting tissues. Autosomal dominant inheritance is usual, affecting both sexes equally, but phenotypic expression is extremely variable. New mutations are uncommon, so a family history is commonly obtained.

The abnormality of structural protein may result in major manifestations in skeletal, cardiovascular and ocular systems.

Skeletal features

The 'Marfanoid habitus' is characteristic (Fig. 18.2). Body proportions are irregular, with arm span exceeding height, and the lower segment measurement (sole to pubis) exceeding the upper (pubis to vertex). Rib elongation may cause chest-wall deformity, and kyphoscoliosis is frequent.

Ligamentous laxity may be striking and lead to genu valgum or recurvatum, pes planus with valgus of the heels, or recurrent joint dislocation (particularly patella, hip or mandible). The combination of generalised hypermobility and long extremities may allow characteristic manoeuvres to be performed (Fig. 18.3). Such gross joint laxity may result in arthralgia typical of hypermobility syndrome, but although joint effusions may be present there is no evidence for predisposition to premature OA.

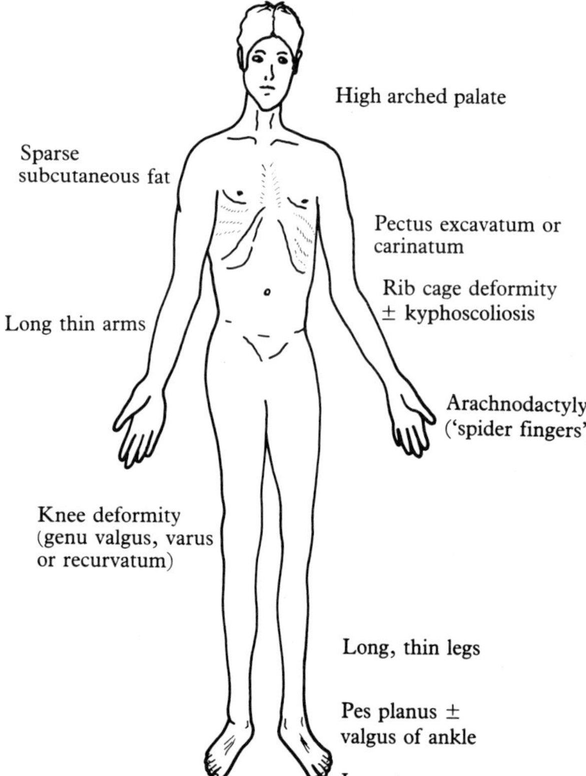

Fig. 18.2 Marfanoid habitus

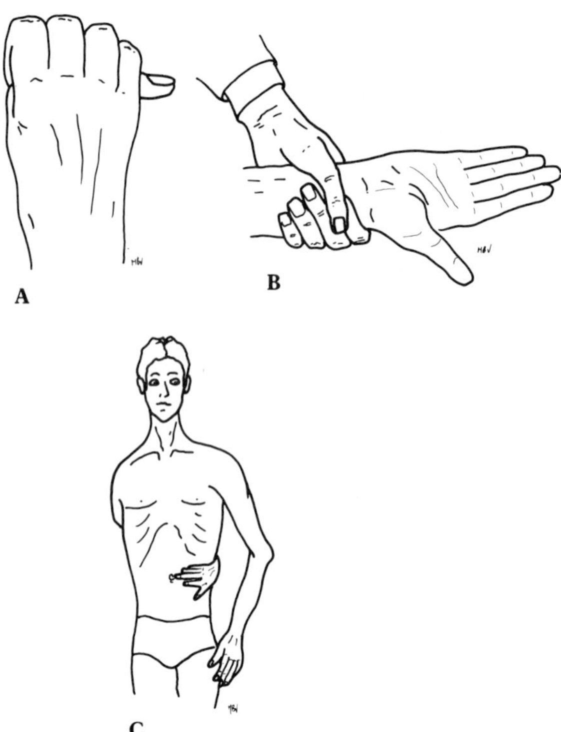

Fig. 18.3 Classic signs in Marfan's syndrome **A**. Steinberg 'thumb sign' — thumb protrudes on ulnar side of clenched fist **B**. 'Wrist sign' — thumb and fingers considerably overlap around opposite wrist **C** . 'Umbilicus sign' — ability to touch umbilicus from behind

Cardiovascular features

The extent of cardiovascular involvement is the principal determinant of life expectancy. Early degeneration of the elastica of the media may result in aneurysmal dilation of the ascending aorta, sinuses of Valsalva and the aortic valve annulus, thus predisposing to aortic dissection and aortic incompetence. Mitral incompetence, involving dilation of the annulus, distortion of leaflets and abnormal chordae, may also occur, and pulmonary artery dilation and rupture, coarctation and other malformations have been reported.

Ocular involvement

This is characterised by ectopia lentis (ectopic lens) which may advance to subluxation or complete dislocation. Myopia is frequent and may predispose to retinal detachment. Eye lesions are usually bilateral.

Other reported abnormalities include peripheral cystic changes in the lungs which predispose to pneumothorax; striae distensae over pectoral and deltoid areas and thighs; small tumours of elastic fibres (elastomas); and camptodactyly (volar contracture of the little finger).

The classical syndrome is easy to recognise, but difficulty may occur with the more frequent *forme fruste*. Only one of the three systems may be involved and there is no single test to establish the diagnosis. Measurement of body proportions, including X-ray metacarpal index, and a positive family history may, however, lend support to the diagnosis, and the pathology of a dissected, replaced aorta may be differentiated from Erdheim's cystic medial necrosis (in the latter normal elastic tissue occurs in areas distant from mucoid pools; in Marfan's elastic fragmentation is severe, widespread and not confined to areas of pooling). Homocystinuric individuals may present a similar morphological appearance, including the lens abnormality, but differ in that they may be mentally retarded and show prominant vasomotor and coagulation problems, and their hands are tight rather than hypermobile (p 309).

Treatment is symptomatic. Anabolic steroids have been used to improve muscle development and ligamentous laxity, and early induction of puberty may hasten epiphyseal closure and reduce final height in girls. Surgical replacement of a dissected ascending aorta may give surprisingly good long-term results.

Ehlers–Danlos syndrome

This is a heterogeneous group of disorders, resulting from interference with normal collagen fibril stability, in which the cardinal features relate to skin and joints. Eight types are currently recognised by differences in clinical expression, mode of inheritance and underlying biochemical defect (Table 18.1),but there is sufficient clinical overlap to justify their inclusion under one title. The diagnosis should be suspected in any individual with joint hypermobility who shows skin hyperelasticity, fragility and easy bruising. The typical clinical picture of the more common Types I and II is described.

Affected infants are often premature, following early rupture of weak fetal membranes ,and show hypotonia, relatively pain-free dislocations, abdominal herniae and delay in motor milestones.

Skin abnormalities

As the 'floppy' child develops, trivial trauma results in lacerations which heal slowly and imperfectly to leave thin 'cigarette-paper' or *papyraceous* scars that show poor retraction ('fishmouth') and pigmentation (from blood products). Small *pseudotumours* consisting largely of fat may be found over elbows or knees, and may occasionally calcify. Easy bruising is characteristic and may be severe due to ease of tracking between the tissue planes: clotting, however, is normal. The skin is soft, velvety and hyperextensible, but unlike cutis laxa shows good recoil. Hyperelasticity is best looked for in palms and soles, where skin is normally firmly bound down: lax tethering over elbows and knees in normal individuals may otherwise be misleading.

Joint abnormalities

Generalised hypermobility may be spectacular especially in young patients, allowing employment as 'India rubber men' or 'human pretzels' (Fig. 18.4). Effusions, foot deformity, spondylolisthesis and kyphoscoliosis, congenital hip dislocation and habitual dislocation of selected joints in later life may all occur and are attributed to this extreme joint laxity. Haemarthrosis is an occasional complication. With increasing age hypermobility becomes less marked and dislocations less troublesome.

Cardiovascular and other features

A feared event is sudden death from rupture of a

Table 18.1 Ehlers–Danlos syndrome

Type		Inheritance	SKIN			JOINT		
			Extensibility	Fragility	Bruising	Hypermobility	Special features	Biochemical defect
I	Gravis	Aut. dom.	+++	+++	++	+++	Classic features — all severe	?
II	Mitis	Aut. dom.	++	++	++	++ (may only affect hands and feet)	Classic features — all moderate	?
III	Benign Hypermobile	Aut. dom.	±	±	±	+++	Contortionism: no skeletal deformity	?
IV	Ecchymotic Sack–Barabas	Aut. dom. or Aut. rec.	±	++	+++	± (mainly digits)	Major vascular and bowel catastrophes	Deficiency of Type II collagen
V	X-Linked	X-Linked	++	±	±	± (mainly digits)	Thin scars	?
VI	Hydroxylysine deficient Ocular	Aut. rec.	+++	++	++	+++	Musculoskeletal deformity May have eye defects	Protocollagen lysyl hydroxylase deficiency
VII	Arthrochalasis multiplex congenita	Aut. rec	++	++	++	+++	Short stature, congenital dislocations	Procollagen peptidase deficiency
VIII	Periodontosis	Aut. dom.		+++	±	++ (mainly digits)	Marked periodontosis with early loss of teeth	?

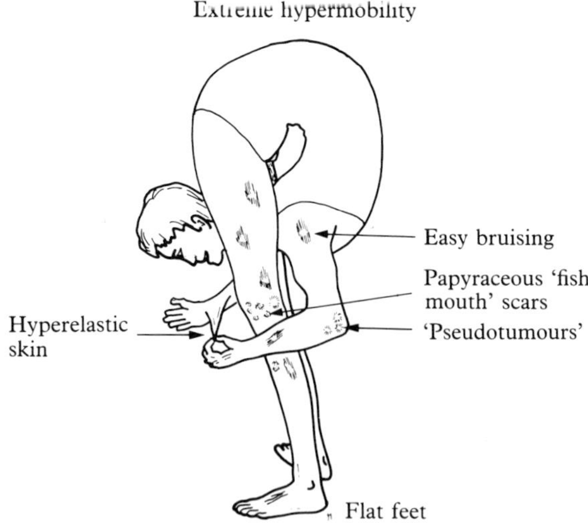

Fig. 18.4 Classic features of Ehlers–Danlos syndrome

major artery or from gut perforation and haemorrhage. Surgery under these conditions is usually disastrous because of thin, easily torn, 'wet blotting-paper' tissues. Pregnancy also carries major risks from perineal lacerations and haematomata, and post-partum uterine prolapse is common.

Epicanthic folds, myopia, microcornea and blue sclera may all be present, and easy eversion of the upper eyelids is a characteristic party trick (Metenier's sign).

Osteogenesis imperfecta (OI)

In this group of generalised disorders bony fragility is the major manifestation. Although abnormalities in synthesis and stability of type I collagen (the major collagen in bone) have been detected in fibroblasts from affected individuals, the precise underlying defect is not known, and the occurrence of woven bone in adult life may be the only characteristic microscopic feature. Four types are distinguished clinically: inheritance is either autosomal dominant or recessive.

In its severest form, OI congenita or Type II, multiple fractures occur *in utero* and during labour, which is usually premature. Characteristic clinical features include beaded ribs, crumpled long bones and multiplex islands in the skull. Those who are not stillborn invariably die as neonates. In milder forms of OI fractures may follow minor stress at any age, though this tendency often diminishes after puberty. Fractures are characteristically transverse and associated with exuberant subperiosteal callus. Severe skeletal deformities such as kyphoscoliosis, short stature and bowed long bones may be crippling and result from generalised osteoporosis and bone softening. Dental abnormalities include hypoplasia, abnormal shape and discoloration (amber to grey).

Generalised joint hypermobility is common and may result in dislocations and tendon ruptures. Thin skin, easy bruising and poor scar formation may also occur. Blue sclera are characteristic and relate to choroidal pigmentation showing through a thin sclera (also seen in Marfan's and Ehlers–Danlos). Pre-senile deafness due to otosclerosis occurs in many families with OI.

Although sodium fluoride or magnesium oxide have both been reported to reduce the fracture rate, there is at present no effective treatment for the bone disease of OI.

Pseudoxanthoma elasticum (PXE)

This is a rare group of disorders resulting from an unknown abnormality that predominantly leads to weakening of elastic tissue. The major clinical manifestations relate to skin, eyes and blood-vessels, and both autosomal dominant and recessive types occur.

Skin lesions

Cutaneous lesions usually appear during late childhood as small, soft yellow papules arranged parallel to the skin lines in flexural areas (Fig. 18.5). Later the skin may thicken, hang in loose, inelastic folds and resemble the skin of a plucked chicken.

Eye lesions

'Angioid streaks',which are breaks in Bruch's membrane, occur in the majority of patients, appearing as nonvascular markings behind the retina and being mainly concentrated around the optic disc. Although highly suggestive of PXE

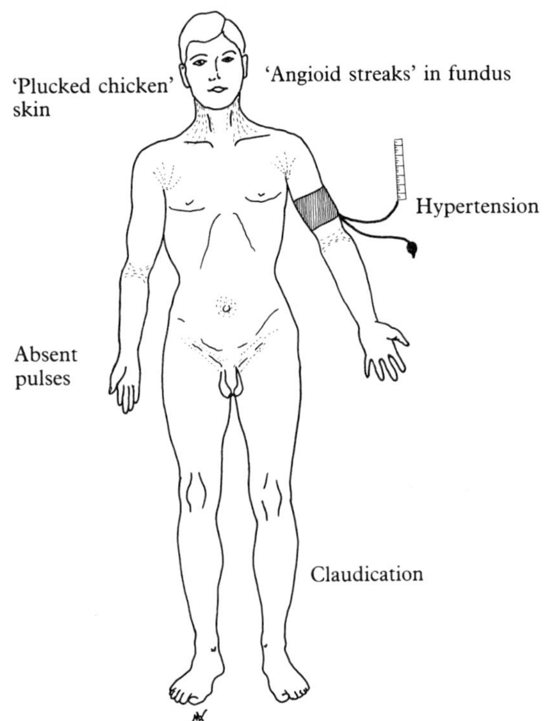

Fig. 18.5 Classic features of PXE

they may also occur in sickle-cell disease and Paget's disease. Choroidoretinitis and retinal haemorrhages occasionally occur to endanger vision.

Vascular lesions

The most serious complication is development of premature and advanced arterial changes indistinguishable from atherosclerosis. Medium-sized vessels are predominantly affected and there is a marked tendency for medial calcification. Peripheral pulses may be obliterated at a young age and result in claudication, gangrene, angina or neurovascular disease. Hypertension co-exists in the majority. Internal haemorrhage is a special feature of this vascular disease, resulting in life-threatening haematemesis or melaena in 10%.

Rheumatological features

Hypermobility occurs in one autosomal dominant form but joint symptoms are generally uncommon. Intermittent ischaemia, cutaneous calcinosis and ulceration, however, place PXE in the differential diagnosis of scleroderma syndromes.

Diagnosis is confirmed by biopsy of affected skin to show granular accumulation of basophilic material with 'dystrophic' calcification in the middle and lower dermis apparently related to degenerate, abnormal elastin. No treatment is available to halt progress of the vascular disease.

Cutis laxa

This rare benign condition is thought to result from an abnormality of dermal collagen. Affected individuals have extensible skin which sags under the influence of gravity, resulting in a characteristic elderly appearance with 'bloodhound' facies. Hooked nose, short columella, everted nostrils and long upper lip may accompany the skin abnormality and laxity of vocal cords may result in a deep voice. Unlike the Ehlers–Danlos syndrome, with which it may be confused, joint hypermobility is uncommon. The diagnosis may be verified by skin biopsy to show marked reduction, clumping and fragmentation of elastic fibres. There is no treatment.

FURTHER READING (COLLAGEN DISEASES)

McKusick V A 1979 Heritable disorders of connective tissue, 5th edn. C V Mosby, St Louis

Prockop D J, Kivirikko K I, Tuderman L, Guzman N A 1979 The biosynthesis of collagen and its disorders. New England Journal of Medicine 301: 23; 77–87

Sandberg L B, Soskel N T, Leslie J G 1981 Elastin structure, biosynthesis, and relation to disease states. New England Journal of Medicine 304: 566–579

Boucek R J, Noble N L, Gurja-Smith Z, Butler W T 1981 The Marfan syndrome: a deficiency in chemically stable collagen cross-links. New England Journal of Medicine 305: 988–991

19 Periarticular, soft-tissue and traumatic disorders

Most rheumatic complaints are caused by disorders of the soft tissues surrounding the joints, rather than by specific arthritic diseases. The majority of these conditions are localised, self-limiting, painful disorders related to trauma, but patients sometimes complain of generalised musculoskeletal pain.

GENERALISED MUSCULOSKELETAL PAIN

Generalised pain without evidence of a specific rheumatic disorder has many possible causes. The history and physical examination should lead to the diagnosis in most cases, investigations being available to confirm a clinical impression of polymyalgia rheumatica, thyroid disease, hypokalaemia or paraproteinaemias, for example.

Influenza and other viral infections are very common causes of transient pain, and Bornholm disease or the prodromal phase of Herpes zoster may cause intense regional pain. Polymyalgia rheumatica (Chapter 12) and the prodromal phase of rheumatoid disease are common rheumatological causes. Systemic disorders which often present to a rheumatologist as generalised musculoskeletal pain include hypothyroidism, early Parkinson's disease, depression and less frequently malignant disease or drug problems such as barbiturate dependence or steroid withdrawal.

Some causes of generalised musculoskeletal pain

1. *Rheumatic diseases*
   a) Polymyalgia rheumatica
   b) Prodromal phase of inflammatory joint and muscle diseases
2. *Infections*
   a) Viral, e.g. influenza, glandular fever etc
   b) Septicaemia
   c) SBE
   d) Others
3. *Drugs*
   a) Contraceptive pill
   b) Chronic barbiturate ingestion (*rheumatisme barbiturique*)
   c) Steroid withdrawal (*steroid pseudorheumatism*)
4. *Miscellaneous*
   a) Hypothyroidism
   b) Parkinson's disease
   c) Malignant disease
   d) Paraproteinaemias
   e) Hypermobility
   f) Osteomalacia
   g) Hypokalaemia
   h) Depression
   i) Psychogenic rheumatism

Young and middle-aged women often present with widespread non-specific pains. Symptoms are usually present at all times of the day, variable in distribution and severity, but tending to centre in or around muscles and joints. They are not made worse by any specific activity, or helped much by drugs or other therapy. Stiffness and exhaustion are common. Physical signs are often absent, although some patients have widespread periarticular tender spots. The disorders tabulated all need careful consideration, although many are suffering from fibrositis, the 'pain amplification syndrome', or simply mild muscle tension and anxiety. Psychogenic rheumatism is difficult and dangerous diagnosis to make.

FIBROSITIS AND PAIN AMPLIFICATION

'Fibrositis' is a term with no clear clinical or pathological definition. Most people use it to refer to the presence of painful tender spots in muscles around the joints. These are common in the muscles of the neck and back of the shoulder, and tender palpable nodules, about 1 cm across, can sometimes be palpated. Histological examinations have indicated that these may sometimes have an inflammatory basis. However, it is also known that deep muscle pain is poorly localised and may arise from pathology some distance away from areas of local tenderness, and there may be no abnormality at the site of the apparent 'fibrositic nodule'. Whatever their cause or pathology, they are common, usually transient, often related to tension, stress or trauma, and generally unimportant. Some patients develop persistent, widespread 'fibrositis' with multiple tender spots and complain bitterly of pain and disability. It has recently been suggested that they may be suffering from an abnormality of pain perception — the *pain-amplification syndrome*. Features of this syndrome include sleep disturbance; widespread, exaggerated periarticular and muscle tenderness; generalised pain, stiffness and exhaustion; and sensitivity of pain to the cold. The syndrome can be reproduced experimentally by deprivation of non-REM (rapid-eye-movement) sleep. Specific sites of point tenderness are described, and help diagnosis (Fig. 19.1). Patients sometimes respond well to low doses of tricylic antidepressants given at night.

The pain-amplification syndrome may exaggerate symptoms and complicate the clinical picture in some patients with established rheumatic disorders, as well as presenting as an isolated disorder.

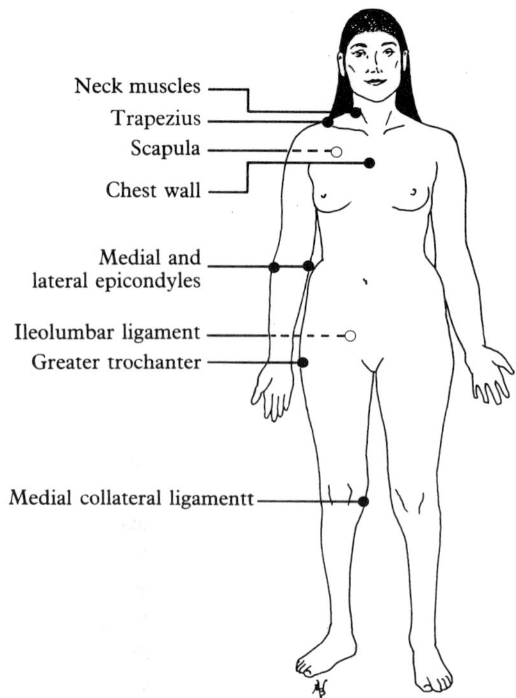

Fig. 19.1 Common sites of tenderness in the 'fibrositis' or 'pain-amplification' syndrome

PSYCHOGENIC RHEUMATISM

Depression often presents with a variety of somatic complaints, including those referrable to the musculoskeletal system. It is widely accepted that other psychiatric disorders can also cause a variety of rheumatic complaints.

The features of psychogenic rheumatism include:

1. 'Atypical' symptoms. The symptoms don't usually fit into an obvious pattern, and patients are polysymptomatic and have numerous aches and pains.

2. Absence of any organic disease. Physical signs are absent and investigations normal. Confusion is often caused by mild 'osteoarthritis' on X-rays, or a weakly-positive antibody test. Patients often cling to this information as proof of a disease which they seem to need.

3. A psychiatric disorder. Depression is commonest and middle-aged women are frequently affected. Anxiety states, hypochondriasis, obsessional neuroses and a variety of other psychiatric states may underly the disorder.

Symptoms are sometimes generalised, although back and neck pain and a variety of other syndromes can be due to psychogenic rheumatism.

The diagnosis should only be made in the presence of all of the above criteria. Management is difficult. Over-investigation and anti-rheumatic therapy are not only unhelpful and unnecessary, but also tend to make matters worse and establish the patients role of exhibiting their psychiatric problem through a rheumatic complaint.

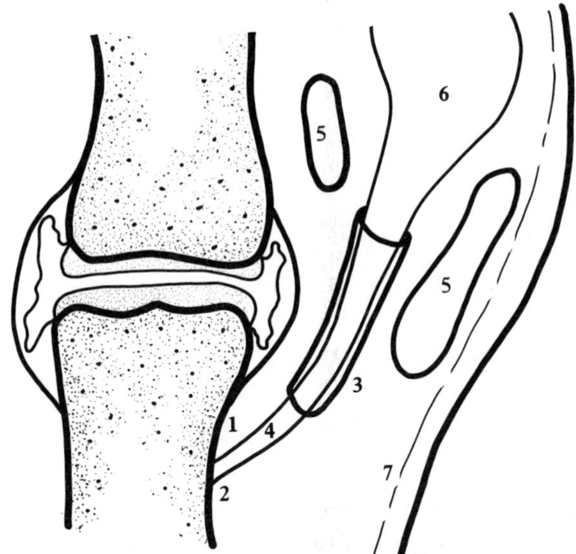

Fig. 19.2 Sites of origin of periarticular pain — 1. Capsule/ligament insertions, 2. Tendon 3. Tendon sheath; 4. Tendon; 5. Bursae; 6. Muscle; 7. Fascia.

LOCALISED SOFT-TISSUE RHEUMATISM

Localised periarticular symptoms can arise from any one of the structures labelled in Figure 19.2. Causes are listed below.

SITES GIVING RISE TO PERIARTICULAR PAIN

Capsules and ligaments

Capsular distension is commonly the main cause of pain in diseases associated with joint effusions.

Causes of periarticular disease

1. *Mechanical*

a) Trauma or overuse

b) Instability of joints

c) Joint deformity

2. *Inflammatory*

a) Sero-negative spondarthritis

b) Other inflammatory joint diseases

3. *Crystal deposition*

Periarticular apatite, pyrophosphate or urate deposits

Ligaments can also give rise to pain if joint disease causes instability.

The richly-innervated capsule and its ligamentous thickenings can also cause pain in the absence of disease of the joint itself. Traumatic strain or tears are the commonest cause. The clinical features include localised pain and tenderness, with exacerbation of symptoms on stressing the involved ligaments. Complete ligament rupture results in instability.

The enthesis

The point of insertion of the capsule, ligaments and tendons into bone is called the enthesis. It is a particularly well innervated area of periarticular tissue, susceptible to traumatic damage and to involvement by rheumatic diseases. Tendon insertions are particularly vulnerable. Disorders of this area are called *enthesopathies*, and common examples include tennis and golfer's elbow and Achilles tendonitis.

The enthesis consists of tendon collagen fibres, which fan out and insert into the bone, interspersed with elastic fibres providing some flexibility to the structure. The bone has an adjacent area of hyaline cartilage through which the tendon fibres pass. The whole area is richly innervated, suggesting a physiological function which may involve control of muscle tone around the joint by monitoring stress on different tendons and ligaments. The vascular supply comes partly from above (muscle), partly from below (bone) (Fig. 19.3). The enthesis is susceptible to trauma,

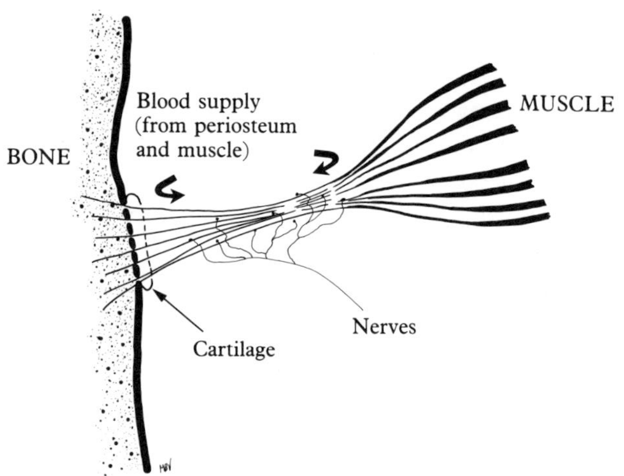

Fig. 19.3 The enthesis

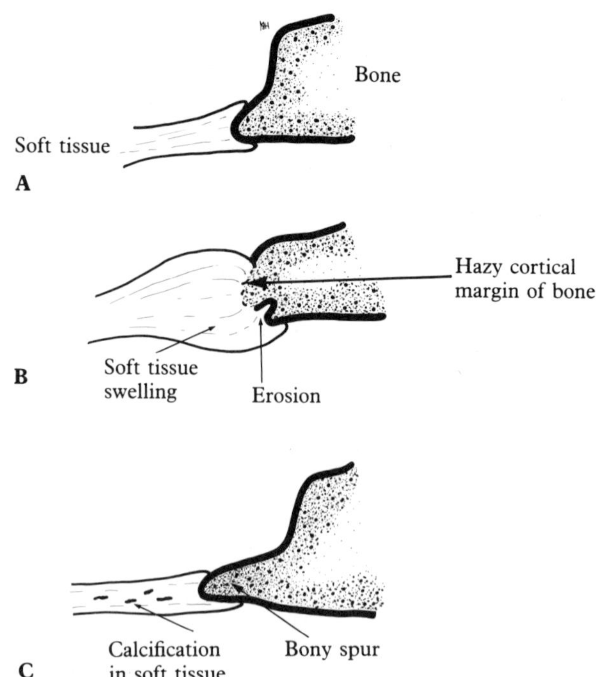

Fig. 19.4 Radiological signs of enthesopathies **A**. Normal **B**. Erosive enthesopathy (e.g. Reiter's syndrome) **C**. Enthesis calcification

to local ischaemia, and to involvement in the sero-negative spondarthritides. The results include acute and chronic inflammatory changes and degeneration; the rich vascular supply helps form granulomatous reactions and the cartilage may calcify and ossify. The radiological changes therefore include soft tissue swelling, erosions, and ossification with 'spur' formation (Fig. 19.4).

Clinical manifestations of an enthesopathy include pain, and highly localised 'point' tenderness. The pain can usually be reproduced by resisted active movement of muscles (e.g. resisted wrist extension in tennis elbow) or by stressing involved ligaments. Slight soft-tissue swelling and signs of inflammation are sometimes present.

Enthesopathies usually respond well to local steroid injections as long as any traumatic cause or overuse is avoided.

Tendons and tendon sheaths

Tendons transmit muscle power to bone via the enthesis. Some are strengthened by bone (sesamoid bones), and others are protected by a lubricating sheath (Fig. 19.5).

Parital or complete rupture of tendons are common. Direct trauma, excessive load (e.g. weight-lifters rupturing the quadriceps tendon) or weakening from ischaemia or infiltration can all cause tendon damage. Steroids may predispose to rupture and infiltration with ochronotic material, urate crystals or calcific deposits can occur.

Sheaths exist where tendons are long, or where movement is great. They form tubes with visceral and parietal surfaces lined by cells similar to synoviocytes, without a basement membrane. Tendon sheaths may become inflamed, infected or stenosed. Minor trauma, overuse, or inflammation as a part of a generalised rheumatic disease (especially rheumatoid arthritis) are the common causes.

Small tumourous swellings of tendon sheaths or tendons may be due to ganglia , localised nodular tenosynovitis, pigmented villonodular tenosynovitis, xanthomata, calcific deposits or rheumatoid nodules. Ganglia are cystic swellings of hyaluronate near to or on a tendon, and have no synovial lining. They are commonest at the wrist, are firm and painless, and can be ruptured (traditionally by a blow from the family Bible). Localised nodular tenosynovitis can occur in young women, and consists of giant cell tumours of

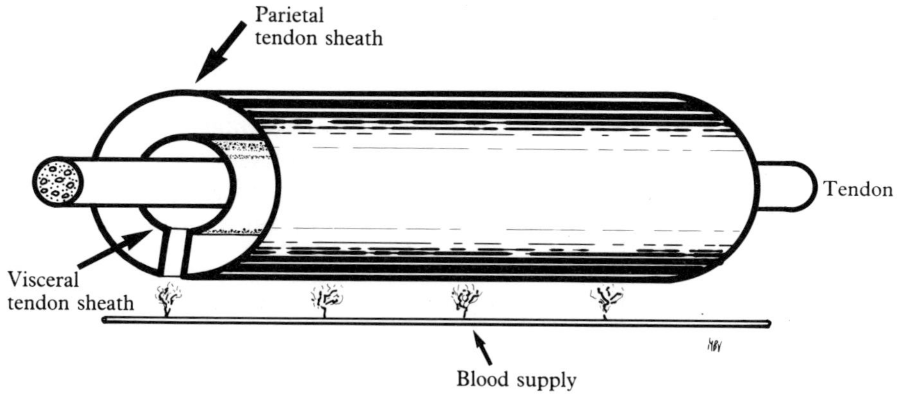

Fig. 19.5 Tendons and tendon sheaths and their disorders

Tenosynovitis

Think of	Trauma
	Rheumatoid disease
Other causes:	SLE
	Reiter's
	Gout
	Amyloidosis
	Sarcoidosis
	TB
	Fungi
	Gonococcal infection
	Other infections
	Hyperlipidaemia

Tendon swellings

Think of:	Ganglia
	Trauma
	Rheumatoid disease
Other causes:	Nodular tenosynovitis
	Pigmented villonodular tenosynovitis
	Xanthomata
	Calcific deposits

tendon sheaths; villonodular synovitis can also affect tendon sheaths as well as joints (see Chapter 13).

The most common and important tendon-sheath lesions include trigger finger, de Quervain's tenosynovitis at the wrist, and the local shoulder lesions such as bicipital tendinitis and rotator-cuff problems.

Bursae

Bursae are similar in structure to tendon sheaths. There are two types — subcutaneous and deep. They become inflamed by trauma or as a part of rheumatic disease and can become infected.

Infection is usually from local spread, and occurs in superficial sites such as the pre-patella bursa. Rheumatoid arthritis usually causes some bursitis — subcutaneous lesions may be obvious (e.g. olecranon bursitis), but deep lesions can give rise to pain which is difficult to localise and diagnose.

Minor repetitive trauma may cause a bursitis, which can become associated with an occupation — housemaid's knee, weaver's bottom, policeman's heel for example. The subacromial bursa and those around the hip, knee and heel are the most important.

Fasciae

Fasciae are connective tissue laminae found subcutaneously or around muscles. In some areas they become thickened and may provide retaining bands, pulleys or mechanical support, as in the wrist, soles of the feet and palm of the hand.

Fascia can become inflamed (fasciitis), or thickened (fibrosis). Fasciitis is not a distinct clinical entity, although a rare form of painful nodular inflammatory fasciitis is described. Fibrosis is very common, and the peculiar miscellaneous group of conditions associated with fascial thickening are shown overleaf.

Muscles

'Muscular rheumatism' is a term used often by patients but rarely by doctors. Tender spots in muscles are common (see fibrositis) as are aching of muscles, myalgia of viral infections and muscle

Fascial diseases (fibrosis)
1. Dupuytren's contracture
2. Peyronie's disease
3. Mediastinal fibrosis
4. Retroperitoneal fibrosis
5. Drug-induced fibrosis
   a) Methysergide
   b) Practolol
6. Vinyl chloride disease
7. Scleroderma
8. Eosinophilic fasciitis } Some inflammation apparent
9. Nodular fasciitis } Some inflammation apparent

cramps. Trauma to muscles is common, causing transient pain and stiffness and more rarely resulting in permanent damage, shortening or calcification (*myositis ossificans*). Myalgia is a feature of polymyalgia rheumatica, although the muscles are not weak or tender in this disorder. Weakness and tenderness suggest one of the rare specific muscle disorders, such as polymyositis.

THE AETIOLOGY OF LOCALISED PERIARTICULAR LESIONS

Trauma

An acute injury may cause strain, partial tears, or complete rupture of capsules, tendons, ligaments and muscles. A secondary inflammatory reaction may then become persistent because of the continued usage of the involved structures.

Periarticular lesions commonly result from repetitive minor trauma, or simple overuse, rather than a single acute injury. Examples include de Quervain's tenosynovitis in young mothers (nappy wrist) and olecranon bursitis in people resting their elbows on the bar (boozer's elbow). Superficial bursae around the knee, elbow, hip and shoulder are particularly susceptible to inflammation from minor repetitive trauma (housemaid's knee, hod-carrier's shoulder, etc).

Seronegative spondarthritides

Enthesopathies are common and may be the presenting feature of these disorders. The heel (Achilles tendonitis and plantar fasciitis) is the commonest site, although lesions in the pelvis and back often contribute significantly to both the clinical and radiological features of these diseases.

Rheumatoid disease

Tenosynovitis and bursitis are almost always present in patients with established rheumatoid arthritis. Hand involvement, particularly of the flexor tendons, extensor carpi ulnaris and synovitis of the dorsal extensor tendon sheath, are common presenting features. Inflammation of these structures is much less common in other inflammatory arthropathies, sometimes helping in the diagnosis of a polyarthritis.

Crystal deposition diseases

Trauma and ischaemia of periarticular tissues may result in deposition of crystals. In patients with gout, peripheral soft tissues (e.g. the helix of the ear) and bursae are often sites of urate deposition, and in pyrophosphate arthropathy crystals are occasionally found in periarticular tendons, ligaments or bursae. Most periarticular crystal deposition involves hydroxyapatite, and tendons are the common site of calcification. Release of crystals into the surrounding soft tissues, bursae or joints may cause acute inflammation (acute calcific periarthritis, see Ch 9.III).

Osteoarthritis

Many of the symptoms of osteoarthritis are due to soft-tissue rheumatism. Changes in the mechanics of a joint cause abnormal stresses to be applied to capsule, ligaments, tendons and entheses, with results identical to those of trauma or overuse. Knee pain in OA is commonly associated with localised tender spots and can be treated in the same way as other periarticular disorders, with a satisfactory outcome.

DIAGNOSIS AND TREATMENT OF LOCALISED SOFT-TISSUE DISORDERS

Localised rheumatic pains need a diagnosis of the anatomical structure involved and of the likely major aetiological factor.

Careful examination of the region should establish the anatomical diagnosis. Localised tenderness and exacerbation of symptoms on stressing the involved structures are the key signs.

The cause can usually be elicited from the history (trauma, overuse, etc) and from a careful search for any signs of a generalised disorder such as a seronegative spondarthropathy.

Investigations are often unnecessary. Radiographs may help exclude significant bone or joint disease, and may confirm the diagnosis of calcific periarthritis. Haematological and biochemical evidence of generalised inflammation is sometimes present and useful. However, the investigations may be misleading. An anatomical diagnosis of a soft-tissue disorder can be made clinically and treated accordingly, irrespective of any associated abnormality. It is a common mistake to follow up the general evidence of inflammation, radiological changes or some other laboratory abnormality without also treating the local lesion. Similarly, the presence of an underlying generalised disorder does not preclude the presence of a localised lesion which needs treatment.

Treatment is usually simple and obvious. If there is a clear aetiological factor such as occupational or recreational trauma, this should be avoided. In some instances mechanical stress on the area can be further protected through splints or appliances. Most lesions respond well to local infiltration of a long-acting corticosteroid preparation and this is usually a simple, safe procedure, giving prolonged relief of symptoms. The precise point of greatest tenderness is isolated and infiltrated. Use of local anaesthetic helps to confirm correct siting of the injection. Avoiding all trauma to the area for a few days after the injection improves the chance of a lasting resolution of symptoms. The physician must beware of possible sepsis (not uncommon in bursae) and have full knowledge of the anatomy of the area so that vital structures such as nerves and vessels are avoided (Fig. 19.6). Tendons must not be injected, as this may result in rupture. Surgical treatment is occasionally required for resistant or severe cases.

OCCUPATIONAL AND TRAUMATIC ARTHROPATHIES

Joint use and rheumatic diseases are interrelated in several ways. The role of trauma and overuse in the generation of soft-tissue lesions has already been mentioned, but repetitive minor trauma can also give rise to localised joint damage of osteoarthritic type, and joint-usage also influences the severity and distribution of established generalised rheumatic diseases, including rheumatoid arthritis and generalised (nodal) osteoarthritis.

Traumatic synovitis

Trauma to a joint may result in a haemarthrosis, damage to intra- or periarticular tissues, or exacerbate an existing arthropathy. A transient synovitis of a normal joint can also occur following direct trauma. This is a monoarticular condition commonest in the knee, wrist or ankle of young adult men. A warm joint effusion develops within hours

Joint trauma and rheumatic diseases
Trauma may cause

1. Haemarthrosis — usually resolves quickly, may need joint aspiration
2. Major structural damage } Predispose to osteoarthritis many years later
3. Joint instability }
4. Exacerbation of a pre-existing rheumatic disease
5. An attack of crystal synovitis in joints with preformed crystal deposits in cartilage or synovium
6. Traumatic synovitis

Contrary to the 'rationalisation' of many patients, there is *no* evidence that trauma 'causes' rheumatoid arthritis and other inflammatory arthropathies.

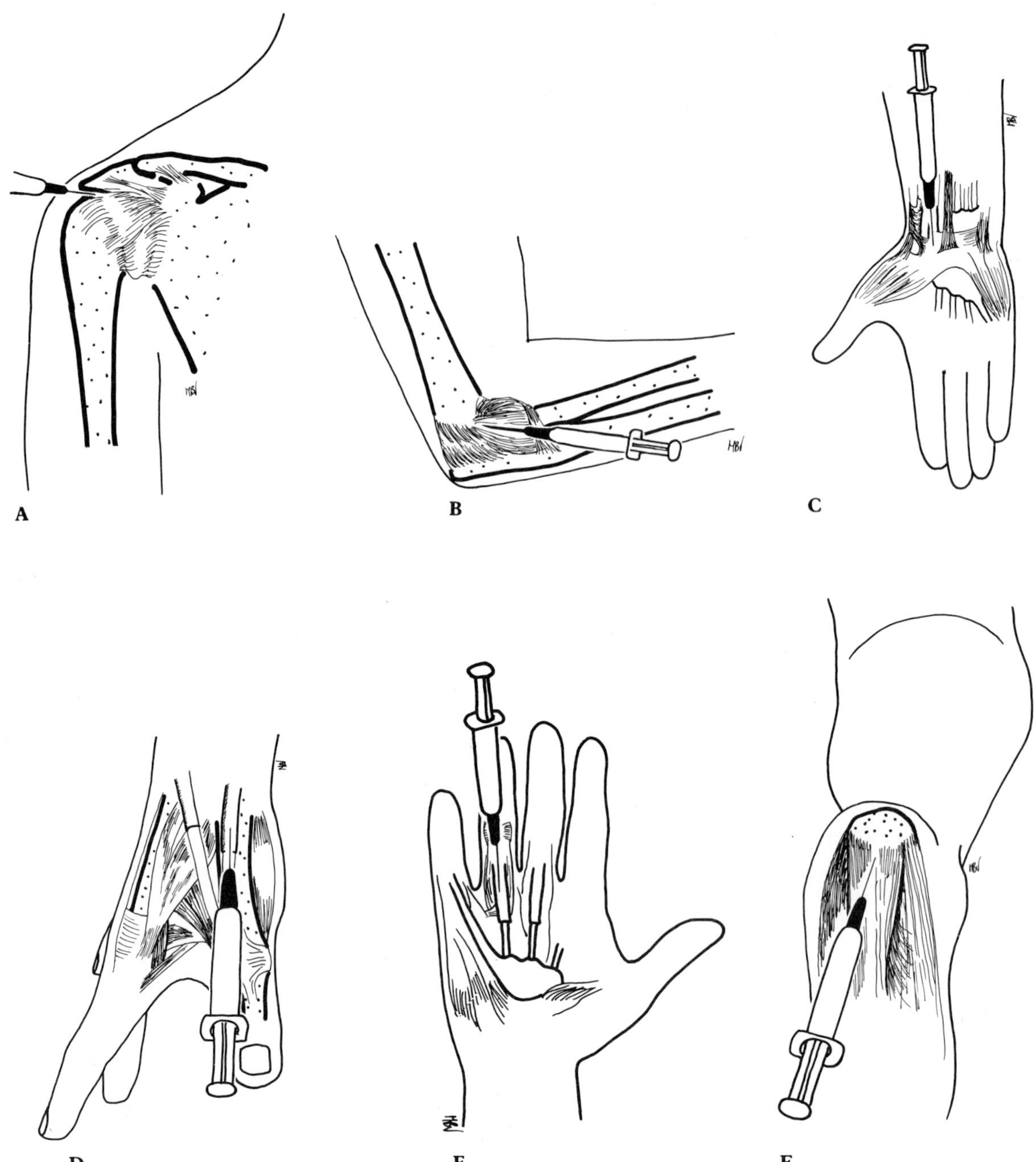

Fig. 19.6 Some sites used in periarticular injection techniques **A**. Around shoulder: subacromial bursa and rotator cuff tendons **B**. Around elbow: lateral epicondyle in 'tennis elbow' **C**. Carpal tunnel **D**. De Quervain's tenosynovitis **E**. Stenosing flexor tenosynovitis **F**. Plantar faciitis

or days of the injury, and slowly resolves over the next few weeks. The synovial fluid is viscous, with a relatively low cell count, and other investigations are normal. No treatment is necessary. The pathophysiology of the condition is not known.

Occupational arthropathies

Several types of occupational arthropathy are recognised with a variety of causes. Where joint disease develops investigations usually reveal radiological evidence of exaggerated local osteoarthritis with extensive osteophyte formation. Periarticular syndromes related to occupation are clinically no different from those of other aetiology. Some of the described lesions are listed below.

Occupation as a cause of rheumatic diseases

1. Acute major trauma (e.g. back injury, traumatic synovitis, limb fracture, etc)
2. Repetitive minor trauma (e.g. bursitis, tenosynovitis)
3. Excessive use of a single joint ('occupational arthritis')
4. Infections (e.g. 'fish-filleter's fingers')
5. Chemical hazards (e.g. Monday morning fever, vinyl chloride disease, etc)

Some occupational arthropathies

1. *'Osteoarthritis'*

Wicket-keeper's hand Goal-keeper's fingers	DIP disease due to hyperextension injuries
Picca-thumper's thumb Bass-player's thumb Ticket-clipper's thumb	CMC disease

   Fast-bowler's foot
   Zulu dancer's hip
   Chauffeur's shoulder
   . . . and many others . . .

2. *Tenosynovitis*
   Hopper's gout (finger tenosynovitis)
   Runner's heel (Achilles tendonitis)
   Nappy wrist (De Quervain's tenosynovitis)
   . . . and many others . . .

3. *Bursitis*

Miner's elbow Beat elbow Student's elbow Boozer's elbow	Olecranon bursitis
Housemaid's knee Nun's knee Carpet-layer's knee	Pre-patella bursitis

   Hod-carrier's shoulder (subacromial bursitis)
   . . . and many others . . .

4. *Enthesopathies*
   Tennis elbow (lateral epicondylitis)
   Golfer's elbow (medial epicondylitis)
   Policeman's heel (plantar fasciitis)
   . . . and many others . . .

5. *Entrapment neuropathies*
   Mother's hand (carpal tunnel syndrome)

6. *Infections*
   Fish-filleter's fingers (erysipeloid infection)
   Beat hand (cellulitis in miners)

7. *Chemicals*

Metal fume fever Polymer fume fever	Arthralgia and fevers after inhalation

   Vinyl chloride disease (acro-osteolysis)
   Saturnine gout (lead damage to renal handling of urate)

BRIEF NOTES ON SOME COMMON PERIARTICULAR DISORDERS

Upper limbs

Subacromial bursitis

1. Inflammation of the subacromial bursa
2. Pain poorly localised, spreads into upper outer part of the arm, exacerbated by passive abduction of the arm

3. Common in adults of both sexes
4. Often related to overuse

'Frozen shoulder'

1. Also called 'capsulitis'. Poorly-characterised pathologically; involves capsular thickening and restriction, with low-grade inflammation.
2. Clinically characterised by a concentric loss of movement of the shoulder, (external rotation is the worst affected movement) and pain felt over the lateral aspect of the arm (C5), often worst at night. Varies in severity. Pain may subside as movements get more restricted.
3. Common in middle-aged and elderly adults F > M. Usually self-limiting but may take months or years to resolve.
4. May be idiopathic, related to overuse, or occur as a secondary complication of any other shoulder syndrome

Tendinitis around the shoulder

1. Damage to the tendons of the rotator cuff, caused by trauma or overuse. May calcify calcific tendonitis).
2. Common in adults of both sexes
3. Poorly-localised shoulder pain
4. Exacerbated by resisted movement of appropriate muscle:
   a) SUPRASPINATUS: Abduction
   b) INFRASPINATUS: External Rotation
   c) SUBSCAPULARIS: Internal Rotation
   d) BICEPS: Supination and flexion of elbow

Tennis elbow

1. Enthesopathy of the common origin of the extensor muscles of the forearm arising from the lateral epicondyle
2. Characterised by local pain and tenderness exacerbated by resisted extension of the wrist
3. Very common in adults of either sex
4. Usually unilateral
5. Often related to overuse

Golfer's elbow

1. Enthesopathy of the origin of the long flexors of the forearm from the medial epicondyle
2. Pain and tenderness exacerbated by resisted wrist flexion
3. Common in adults of either sex

Olecranon bursitis

1. Inflammation of the olecranon bursa producing an uncomfortable swelling over the point of the elbow
2. Common in adults of either sex
3. Causes include trauma (boozer's elbow, student's elbow etc), rheumatoid disease, sepsis and crystal deposition diseases

De Quervain's tenosynovitis

1. Inflammation of tendon sheath of extensor pollucis longus and abductor pollucis brevis as they pass over the head of the radius
2. Painful swelling at wrist, exacerbated by resisted thumb abduction, or forced thumb flexion
3. Often due to overuse (nappy wrist)
4. Common in young adults, F > M

Trigger finger

1. Nodular thickening of flexor tendons causing catching at fibrous stenosis at the level of the MCP joint
2. Common in adults of all ages, F > M
3. Often caused by overuse
4. Common in rheumatoid disease

Camptodactyly

1. Slowly progressive painless flexion of proximal IP joint of little finger
2. F > M: common
3. Develops during first 10 years of life
4. 70% Bilateral
5. Differential diagnosis: Dupuytren's contracture

Dupuytren's contracture

1. Slowly progressive contracture of palmar (and occasionally plantar) fascia resulting in nodular thickening and contracture of the fingers

2. M > F: common
3. Develops after age of 25. Usually bilateral. Ring finger affected most (little and middle finger common, index rare).
4. Associations: liver disease — especially alcoholic; epilepsy; occasionally familial; occasionally associated with other fascial diseases

Garrod's fatty pads (knuckle pad syndrome)

1. Fleshy pads over the dorsum of the interphalangeal joints of the fingers
2. Common, any age, any sex
3. Harmless, symptomless and insignificant
4. Frequently misdiagnosed as arthritis

Chest wall

Teitz's syndrome

1. Recurrent attacks of pain and swelling of the costosternal junction, lasting hours or days at a time
2. Rare condition of adults of either sex
3. Second and third costosternal junctions usually involved

'Precordial catch'

1. Transient attacks of severe chest-wall pain. Often left-sided. Often middle- aged or young men. May be tenderness on 'springing' the chest.
2. Cause unknown
3. Leads to fears of myocardial infarction

Lower limb

Trochanteric syndrome

1. Pain and tenderness over the greater trochanter of the hip, radiating down the lateral aspect of the thigh. Caused by an enthesopathy of hip abductors (in which case resisted abduction causes pain), or trochanteric bursitis.
2. Common in adults of either sex
3. Usually idiopathic. Trochanteric bursitis is a common cause of 'hip' pain in rheumatoid arthritis.

Patella bursitis

1. Inflammation of the pre-patella or infrapatella bursa
2. Causes painful tense swellings in front of the knee
3. Common in adults, F > M
4. Often related to trauma (housemaid's knee, parson's knee, etc), can be caused by crystals, infection or inflammatory arthritis

Anserine bursitis or tendonitis

1. Inflammation of the anserine bursa or associated tendons (sartorius and semi-tendinosus)
2. Causes pain and tenderness over the medial, anterior, border of the upper part of the tibia
3. May be difficult to distinguish structure involved, and from medial ligament syndrome

Medial or lateral ligament syndrome

1. Pain at capsule/ligament insertion of knee into the tibia. Medial > lateral
2. Poorly localised pain around inside or outside of knee
3. Point tenderness over insertion, often exacerbated by stressing the involved tendon
4. Common in adults, F > M
5. Often caused by minor instability. A common cause of 'knee' problems in osteoarthritis.

Achilles tendinitis or bursitis

1. Inflammation of the tendon, its insertion (enthesis) or associated bursa
2. Well-localised heel pain exacerbated by walking, especially stairs and hills
3. Localised tenderness
4. A common overuse injury in adults: M > F
5. Epidemic in long-distance runners
6. Enthesopathy occurs in seronegative disease; bursitis can occur in RA

Plantar fasciitis

1. Inflammation at the insertion of the plantar fascia into the calcaneus

2. Heel pain on weight bearing and walking. Tenderness under the heel.
3. Overuse injury, common in association with flattening of the longitudinal arch ('policeman's heel'). Can also occur in seronegative spondarthritis.

Morton's metatarsalgia

1. Pain in the metatarsal heads radiating into the toes, associated with numbness of the toes
2. Caused by digital neuromas or pressure on interdigital nerves
3. Uncommon. Usually middle-aged women.

FURTHER READING

Dixon A St J 1979 Soft tissue rheumatism. Clinics in Rheumatic Diseases 5(3)
Sheon R P, Moskowitz R W, Goldberg V M 1982 Soft tissue rheumatic pain. Lea & Febiger, Philadelphia

SECTION FIVE

Diagnosis

20 The history and physical examination

Most rheumatic diseases can be diagnosed and assessed from the history and physical examination alone, without the need for special investigations.

Diagnosis depends largely on pattern recognition. The chronological pattern of development of a disease may be pathognomonic — the sequential onset of conjunctivitis, urethritis and arthritis in Reiter's syndrome, or the rapidly worsening night pain in the gouty first MTP are examples. Patterns of disease distribution in the joints and extra-articular tissues may also be diagnostic — examples include the fever, rash, lymphadenopathy and joint disease of systemic JCA ('Still's disease') and the hair loss, skin disease, mouth ulcers, psychiatric disturbance and joint symptoms in active SLE.

The history and examination also allow accurate assessment of the activity of many rheumatic diseases. Active inflammation, for example, is characterised by morning stiffness in the joints, systemic symptoms and local signs in the involved joints. Careful examination of the joints and periarticular tissues will often localise the structures giving rise to pain, and the degree of functional impairment is assessed during both history taking and examination.

These six main features of special note in the clinical assessment of rheumatic diseases are listed below.

Six points to note during the clinical assessment of rheumatic diseases

1. Chronological pattern of disease progression
2. Joint distribution
3. Anatomical structures causing symptoms and signs
4. Pattern of any extra-articular involvement
5. Activity of inflammation or other pathological process
6. Degree of functional impairment

Symptoms of joint disease

Articular

1. Pain
2. Stiffness
3. Deformity
4. Loss of function

Extra-articular

1. Systemic disease (e.g. weight-loss)
2. Local organ involvement (e.g. painful red eye)
3. Psychiatric (e.g. depression)

THE HISTORY

The symptoms of rheumatic diseases include both articular and extra-articular components. Pain, stiffness, or reduced function are the common presenting features.

Pain is a major feature of most joint disorders. Its quality, site and radiation and the factors which change it, need to be assessed. Pain patterns are often diagnostic and the severity and quality of pain often dominate the life of the arthritic patient. Pain thresholds vary and pain is influenced greatly by psychosocial factors; assessment is therefore difficult.

Some pain patterns in rheumatic diseases

1. Mechanical — e.g. unstable joints
   Pain related to joint use only
2. Inflammatory — e.g. Rheumatoid arthritis, ankylosing Spondylitis
   Severe pain and stiffness in joints in the morning and on use
3. Osteoarthritic — e.g. spondylosis, generalised osteoarthritis of peripheral joints
   Pain on joint use, stiffness after inactivity, pain at end of the day
4. Bone pain — e.g. Paget's disease, bony metastases
   Pain at rest and at night
5. Nerve compression — e.g. carpal tunnel syndrome, prolapsed intervertebral disc
   Pain and parasthesiae in dermatome, exacerbated by specific activity

Stiffness is another important symptom. The severity and duration of joint stiffness in the morning often reflects the activity of inflammation, and severe stiffness after immobility is typical of osteoarthritis. Stiffness prevents normal function, and some patients need several hours to get dressed and to work in the morning.

Functional impairment and joint deformity often develop after a presentation with pain or stiffness, but may be early features of rheumatic diseases, and often dominate the symptoms as diseases progress. The functional requirements and aspirations of arthritic patients are essential knowledge: tenosynovitis in the hand is infinitely more important to the concert violinist than it is to a professional footballer, for example.

A good history includes a careful enquiry for symptoms outside the joints: these may include local, systemic or psychiatric disturbances. Malaise, depression and weight loss are often severe in active inflammatory diseases; local symptoms such as pain in the eye or chest may be ignored or dismissed as 'nothing to do with the joints' if patients are not actively asked; and fears and anxiety about rapid progression to a wheelchair are often unspoken but desperate concerns of patients when they first present.

Two aspects of special concern when taking the history are the pattern of the disease (for diagnosis and assessment), and its effect on the life of the patient. *The pattern* with time, and the pattern of distribution can often be presented graphically (Fig. 20.1). A chart of the condition and the effect of various life events and treatments can be very helpful, and can only be drawn after careful, accurate and detailed history taking. *The effect of the disease* can be assessed by asking the patient to describe a typical day, and to compare his or her activity now with that before the onset of the

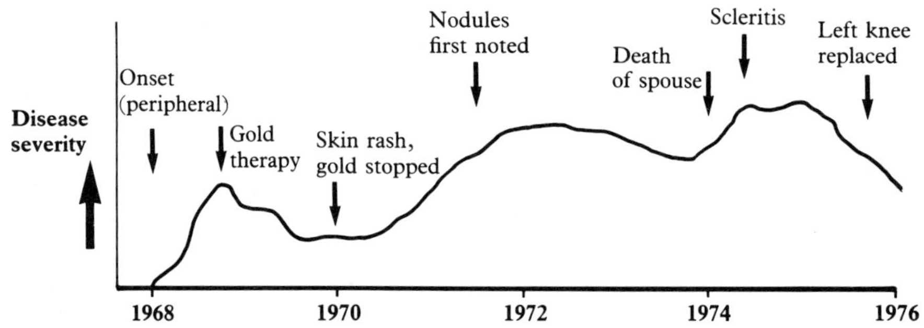

Fig. 20.1 Charting progression of a rheumatic disease. It is often useful to graph disease progression, noting important life events, therapy and complications of the disease. In this example, the progress of a 49-year-old female patient with rheumatoid arthritis is followed.

disease. The history taken by an occupational therapist includes an 'ADL' assessment, which assesses the need and provision of 'Aids to daily living' — appliances to help turn on taps or open doors, for example, or the need for a raised toilet seat. Enquiry into the social and sexual life of the patient and the reaction of friends and relatives is often important as well.

CLINICAL EXAMINATION

The clinical examination involves assessment of general features, the limbs, spine and their function, and other major systems. The order of events varies and is not important, although many clinicians follow the sequence outlined below. After a general assessment of the patient, careful inspection of the hand is a central feature of the examination. The physical signs and functional impairment of the spine and limbs can then be assessed, and finally the other systems can be examined.

Examination of patients with rheumatic diseases

General

1. Gait and function on entering the room
2. Attitude and reaction to the history
3. General appearance
4. Ability to prepare for physical examination

The hand

— 'The patient's calling card'

Assess for signs of:

1. General disease
2. Local joint/periarticular problems
3. Pattern of joint distribution
4. Functional impairment

The limbs and spine

1. Inspection
2. Active movement
3. Simple functional tasks
4. Palpation
5. Passive movement

Systemic

1. Head and neck
2. Chest
3. Abdomen
4. Skin and hair
5. Neurological examination

Joints are examined by inspection, palpation and movement. The chief physical signs are shown below. The muscles and periarticular tissues may be the major sites of disease, and are nearly always affected secondarily by primary joint disorders; exposure and examination of the whole area or limbe is therefore essential. Pain and tenderness can arise from several different structures in and around the joints, but the anatomical site of pathology can usually be revealed by careful examination (Fig. 20.2).

Signs of joint disease

1. Tenderness (joint line or periarticular)
2. Pain on movement
3. Reduced movement
4. Instability
5. Crepitus on movement
6. Heat } Signs of inflammation
7. Redness } Signs of inflammation
8. Fluid swelling } Signs of inflammation
9. Bony or soft-tissue hypertrophy
10. Functional impairment

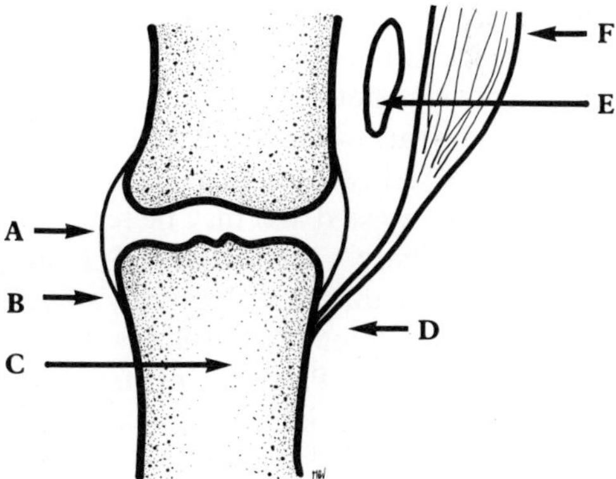

Fig. 20.2 Some possible sites of joint pain and tenderness. It is important to distinguish tenderness all round the joint line (indicating synovitis — **A.**) from tenderness confined to isolated periarticular spots (capsule or ligament insertion — **B.**, tendon insertion — **D.**, bursa – **E.**) Bone (**C**) and muscle (**F.**) tenderness may indicate other disorders such as osteomyelitis or myositis,

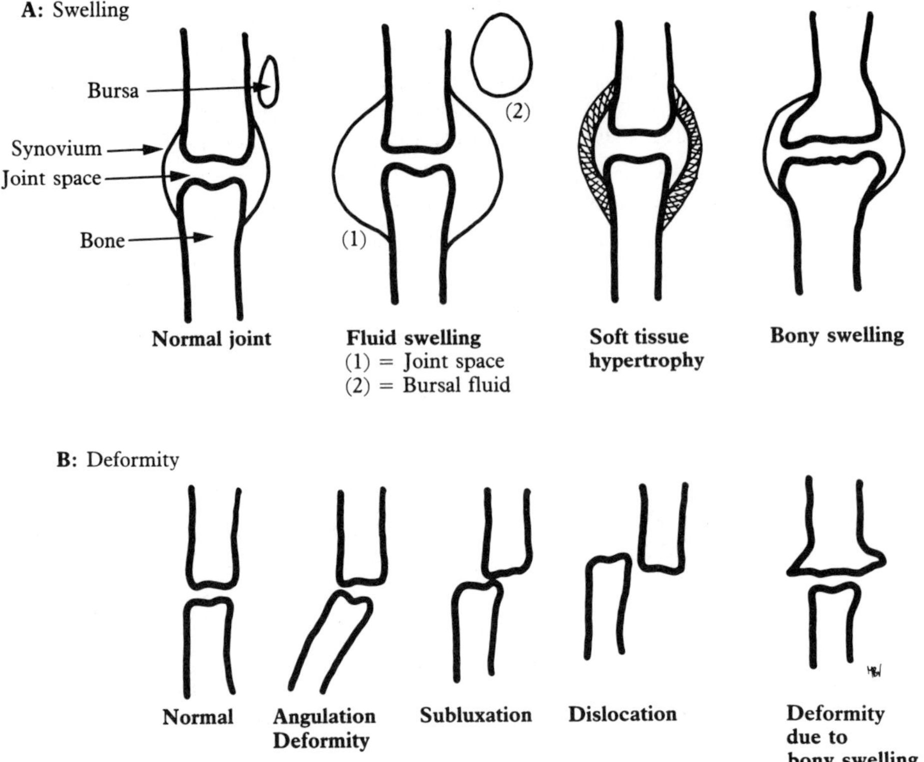

Fig. 20.3 Swelling and deformity of joints **A**. Swelling **B**. Deformity

After inspecting the exposed limb, and comparing the two sides, the patient should be asked to carry out simple tasks which reveal overall function — putting the hands behind the back or head and making a fist, for example. On palpation the skin should be examined first, noting the colour, texture, thickness and temperature over the joints. Muscles acting around damaged joints are usually wasted and may be tender. Swellings may be bony, soft-tissue or fluid-filled. Deformity may be due to dislocation, subluxation or angulation of joints, as well as to a bony deformity (Fig. 20.3). Palpation of the site of tenderness is important: joint line tenderness is a feature of synovitis, but localised periarticular tenderness is often present in soft-tissue disorders (Fig. 20.2). Active movement should be assessed before the examiner moves the joint himself. Crepitus is often felt on movement and instability, fixed deformities and the range of normal and abnormal movements can be recorded.

Three features of special note on examination of patients are the pattern of articular and extra-articular involvement as already mentioned, the activity of the disease, and functional impairment.

Disease activity is of major concern in the management of chronic joint disorders like rheumatoid arthritis. Some idea of the degree of inflammation can be got from examination by recording the presence of classical signs — such as heat, redness and swelling. Temperature differences of less than 1°C can be detected by passing the back of the hand over the involved area, and fluid accumulation is usually due to local inflammation. Redness over the joints only occurs in a few diseases which involve either the skin or periarticular tissue. Several numerical indices have been developed to help assess disease activity further, as mentioned in Chapter 24.I.

The functional assessment of rheumatic disorders involves observing the patient moving his back and limbs and carrying out simple tasks such as

Joint diseases causing redness of the overlying skin

1. Gout (usually severe, causing hot, red, dry skin which later peels)
2. Sepsis
3. Inflamed Heberden's Nodes
4. Rheumatic Fever
5. Palindromic Rheumatism
6. Occasionally in other inflammatory disorders involving periarticular structures

Rashes over joints may also occur in:

1. Dermatomyositis
2. Other connective-tissue disorders
3. Psoriasis

(Beware redness over joints caused by heat lamps or other local therapy)

dressing, undressing, writing or combing the hair. More detailed assessment may be helpful and occupational therapists and physiotherapists may help record the patient's ability to cope with cooking, toilet requirements, and other functions.

FURTHER READING

Polley H F, Hunder G G 1978 Physical examination of the joints. W B Saunders, Philadelphia

21 Regional examination

I The Hand

SITES OF ORIGIN OF MUSCULOSKELETAL PAIN (Fig. 21.1)

Joints

Wrist

1. Radio-ulnar joint. Painful, limited supination and pronation. Tenderness on palpation with pinch grip. Ulnar styloid may be dorsally subluxed, prominant and mobile.

2. Radio-carpal, midcarpal and second to fifth carpo-metacarpal joints. Painful, limited flexion and extension. Tenderness on palpation with thumb on dorsum and fingers supporting volar surface (Fig. 21.2): synovitis may produce dorsal swelling.

3. First carpo-metacarpal joint. Pain on movement. Tenderness on palpation with pinch grip, exacerbated by passive thumb movement.

Metacarpal joints

Pain exacerbated by grip. Tenderness elicited by squeezing across all MCPs (Fig. 21.3) or by

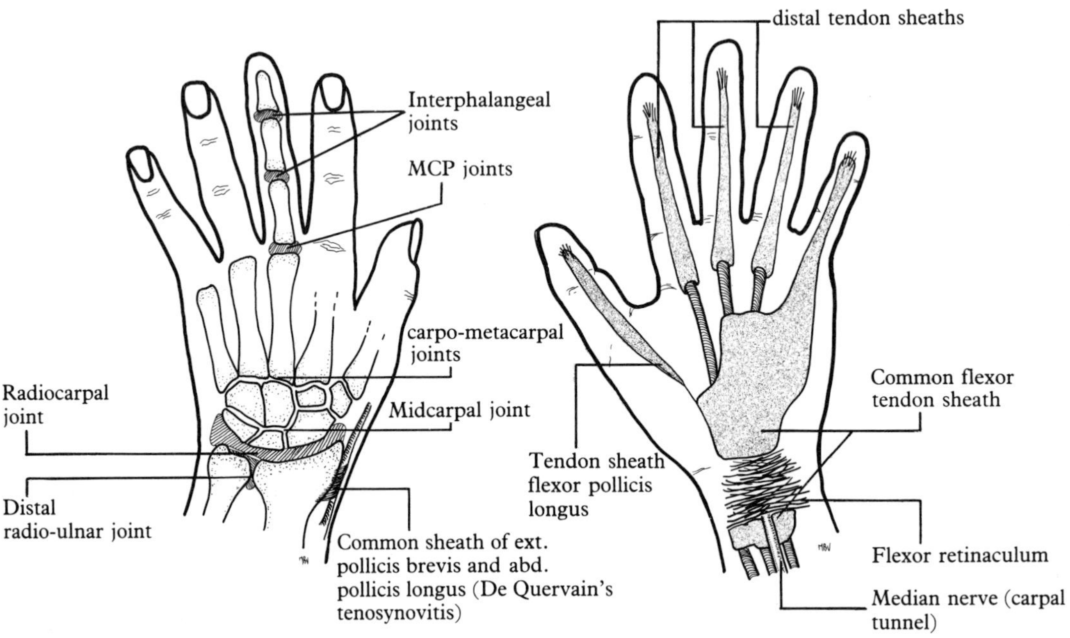

Fig. 21.1 Sites of origin of musculoskeletal pain

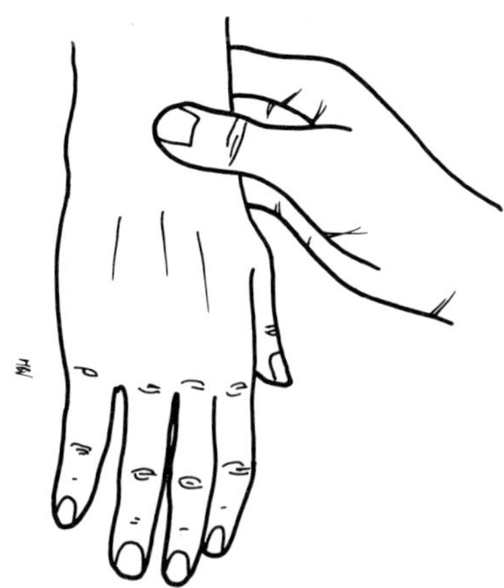

Fig. 21.2 Palpation of wrist joints

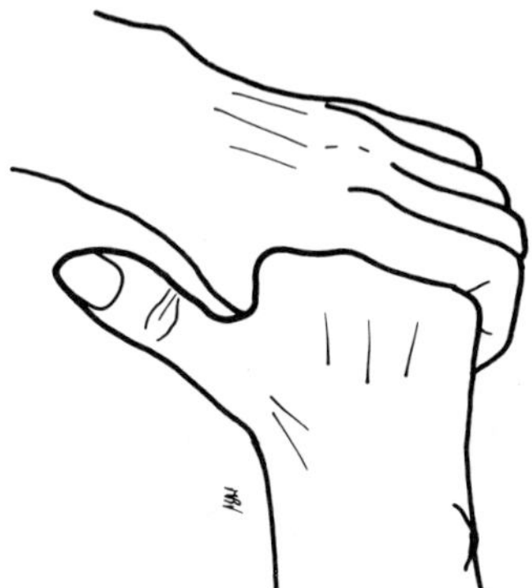

Fig. 21.3 Metacarpal squeeze

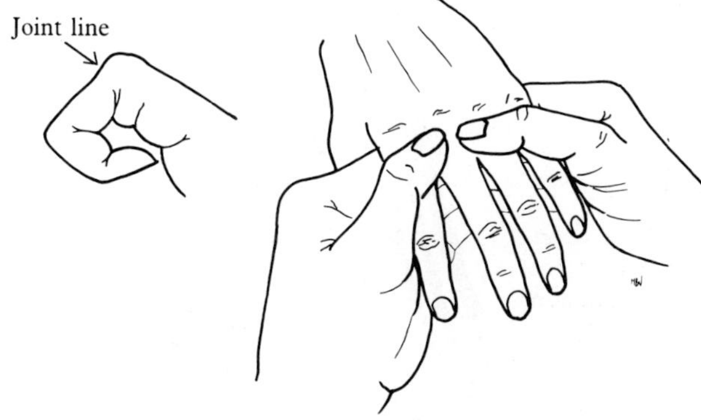

Fig. 21.4 Palpation of MCP joints

palpating over individual joint space about 1 cm distal to apex of flexed knuckles (Fig. 21.4). Synovitis may produce bilateral obliteration of groove between metacarpal heads (Fig. 21.5).

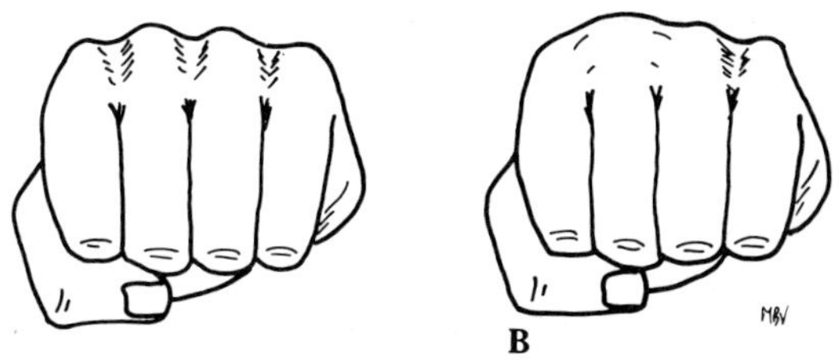

Fig. 21.5 Synovitis of MCP joint **A**. Normal **B**. Synovitis of middle (3rd) MCP

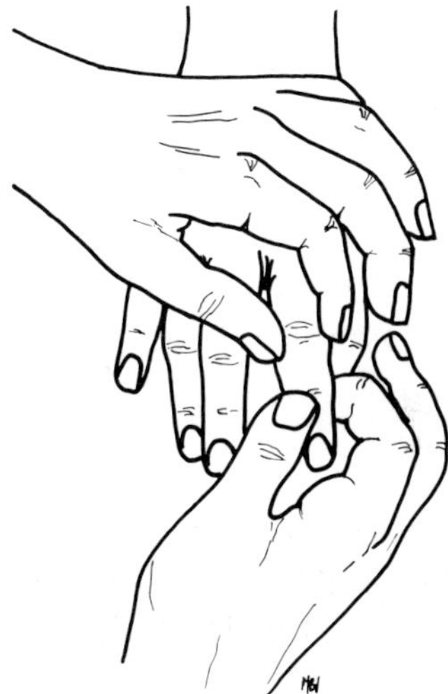

Fig. 21.6 Pressure applied on interphalangeal joint during passive movement

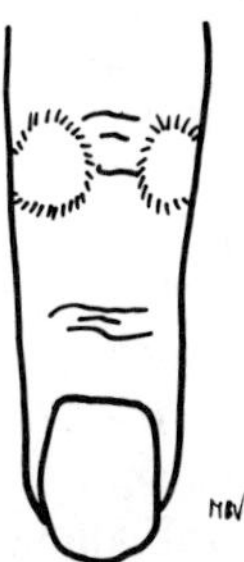

Fig. 21.7 Site of maximal swelling/tenderness in interphalangeal joint synovitis

Interphalangeal joints

Pain, exacerbated by finger movement. Pain elicited by applying pressure (pinch grip) during passive movement (Fig. 21.6). Tenderness and swelling are maximal on dorsolateral and dorsomedial aspects, i.e. either side of dorsal extensor tendon expansion (Fig. 21.7).

Tendon sheaths

Flexor tenosynovitis

Palm and/or finger pain, worse on tight grip. Limited flexion and inability to make tight fist. Crepitus over flexor tendons during passive movement, with or without palpable sausage-shaped swelling along tendon course. 'Triggering' may be associated with palpable nodules within sheath and an area of stenosis at the distal palmar crease, located by palpation along course of tendon. Limitation of movement due to tendon disease may be differentiated from that due to joint disease by examining range of movement when tendons are in maximally relaxed position e.g. for a flexed PIP joint, maximally flex the MCP joint — if PIP now extends the flexion is due to tendon involvement, if not it probably results from joint disease.

Extensor tenosynovitis

Pain over dorsum. Tender, boggy swelling on dorsum with pain on extension during applied pressure. May result in extensor tendon rupture (complete loss of active finger extension) or tendon slip (partial active movement often retained).

De Quervain's tenosynovitis

Non-specific inflammation of common tendon sheath of extensor pollicis brevis and abductor pollicis longus)

Pain and aching over styloid process with radiation into hand or forearm, aggravated by wrist and thumb movement (especially grip). Tenderness over radial styloid, pain on passive thumb movement. Finkelstein's sign is pain on ulnar deviation of wrist with thumb tucked inside flexed fingers (Fig. 21.8). Crepitus may be palpable over course of tendons at wrist.

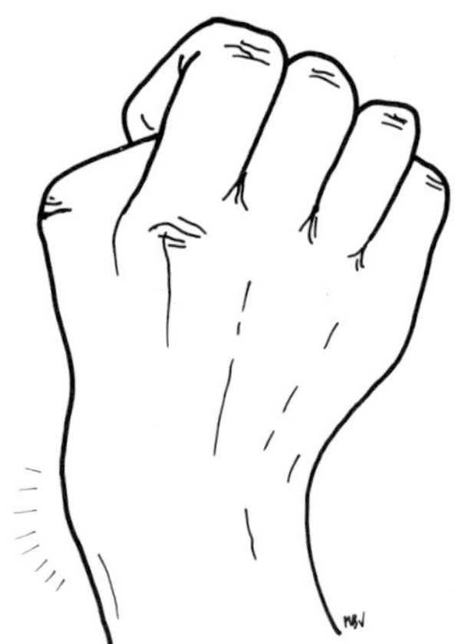

Fig. 21.8 Finkelstein's sign

REFERRED PAIN

Carpal tunnel syndrome

Pain and paraesthesiae in median sensory distribution in hand, worse at night, often with radiation up forearm. Percussion over flexor retinaculum (Tinel's sign) or acute palmar flexion for one minute (Phalen's sign) may reproduce symptoms. Wasting of thenar muscles may be present (p 281).

Ulnar nerve compression

Pain in lateral one and a half fingers and lateral hand: if compression is distal (canal of Guyon) pain affects only volar surface. Tinel's sign may be positive at the site of compression (commonly elbow). Muscle wasting may be present (p 283).

C5, C6, C7, C8 root pressure

Burning pain with or without paraesthesiae in dermatome (Fig. 21.9) and in muscles supplied by

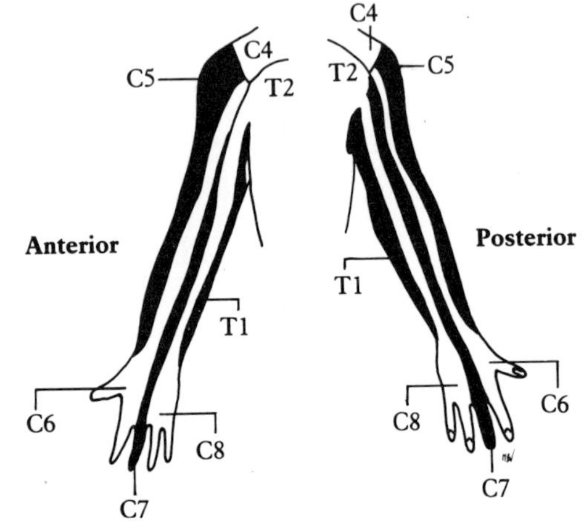

Fig. 21.9 Distribution of sensory spinal roots on surface of arms and hands

homologous motor root, exacerbated by neck movements, coughing or sneezing. Weakness of muscles supplied by roots may also be present.

Causalgia

Unpleasant, burning, persistent pain following peripheral nerve or root injuries (particularly median nerve). Associated with shiny skin and abnormal sweating: extreme tenderness is usual.

TYPICAL DEFORMITIES (Figs 21.10–21.17)

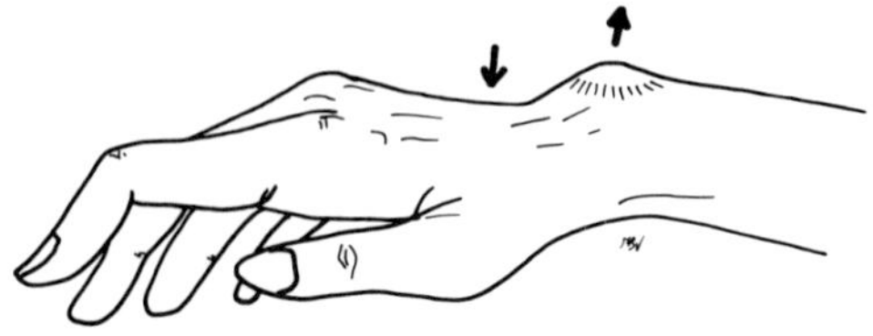

Fig. 21.10 Volar subluxation of the wrist and dorsal subluxation of the ulnar styloid

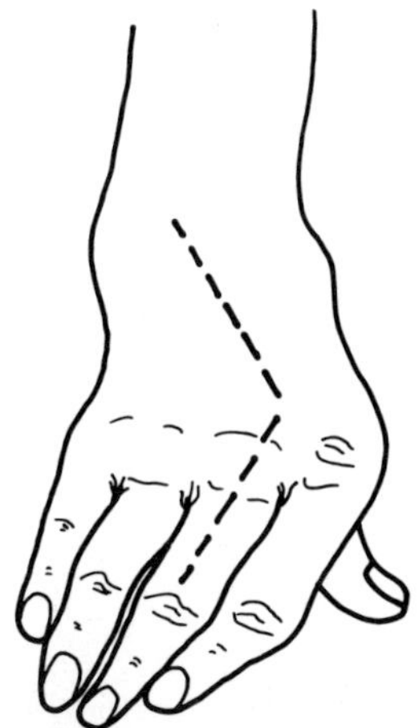

Fig. 21.11 Radial deviation at the wrist and ulnar deviation at the MCP joints

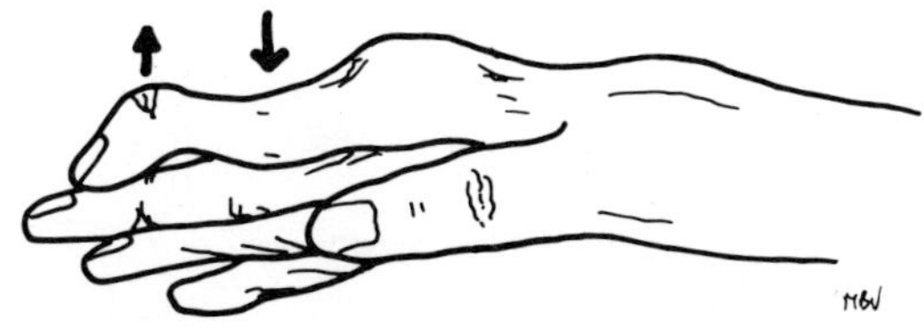

Fig. 21.12 Swan-neck deformity: hyperextension at PIP, flexion at DIP

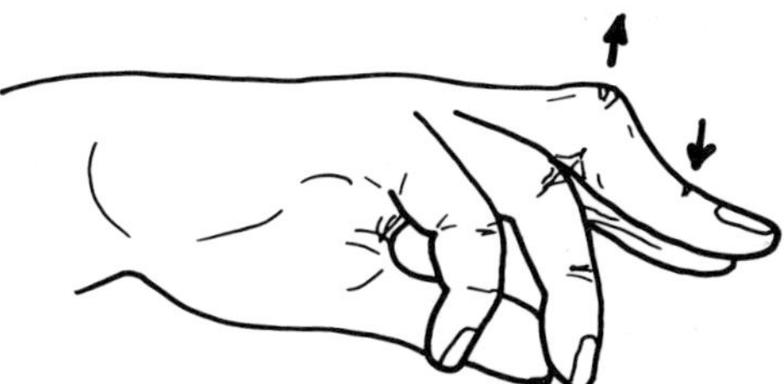

Fig. 21.13 Boutonnière deformity: flexion at PIP, hyperextension at DIP

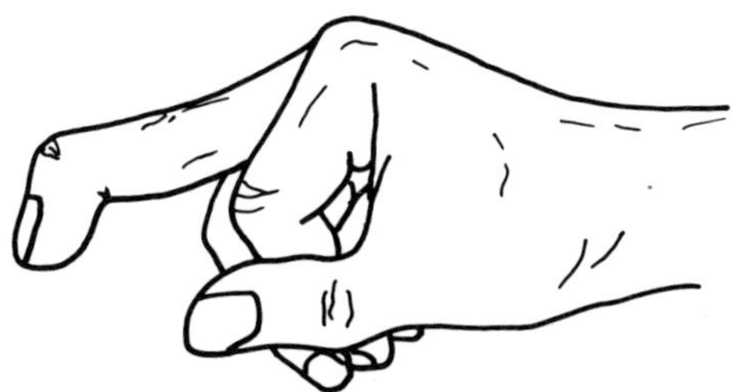

Fig. 21.14 Mallet finger: flexion of DIP with inability to extend terminal phalanx actively

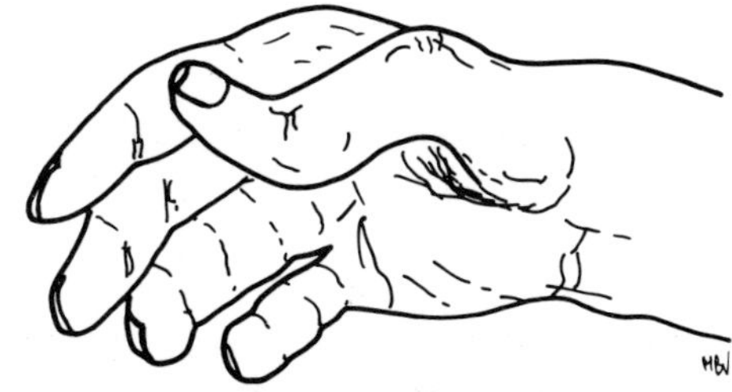

Fig. 21.15 Z-deformity of the thumb

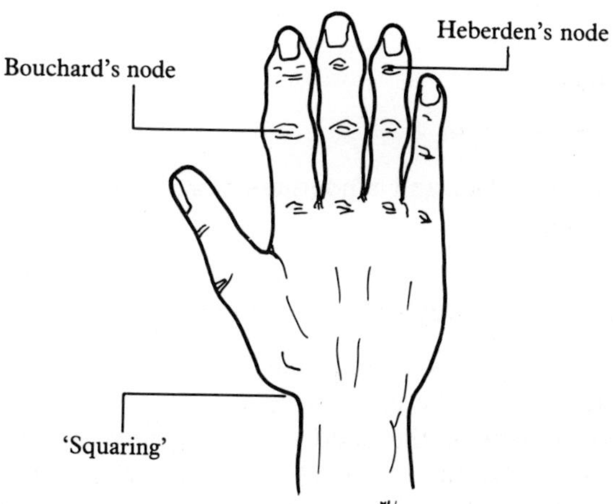

Fig. 21.16 'Squaring' of hand due to 1st carpometacarpal OA

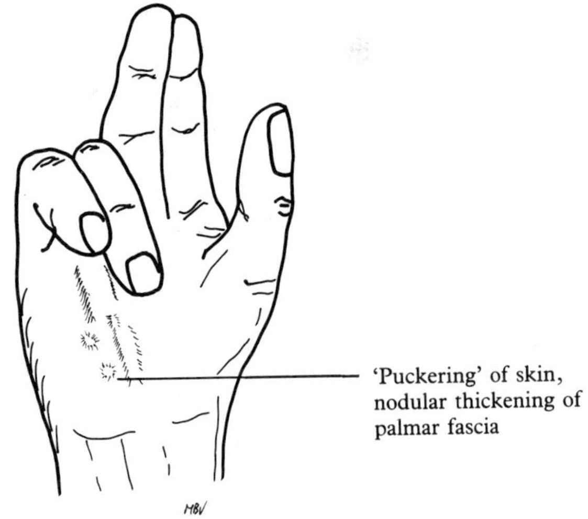

Fig. 21.17 Dupuytren's contracture (severe)

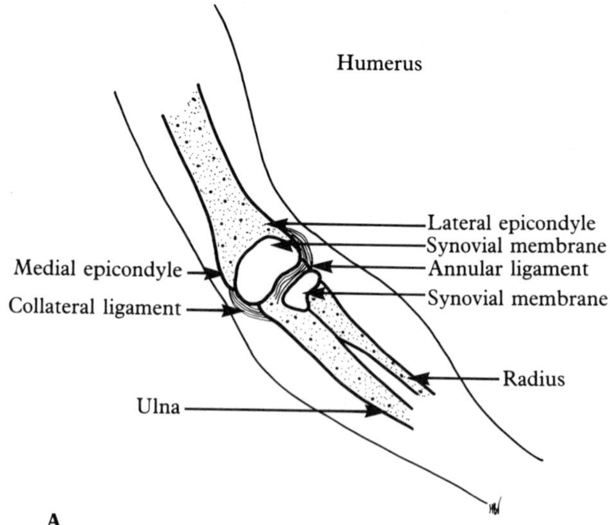

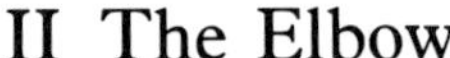

II The Elbow

SITES OF ORIGIN OF MUSCULOSKELETAL PAIN (Fig. 21.18)

The joint

Elbow joint

There is diffuse elbow pain and tenderness of the joint margin. Swelling is first apparent in the para-olecranon grooves. Movements are painful. Flexion deformity occurs early with a reduced range of movements including supination and pronation.

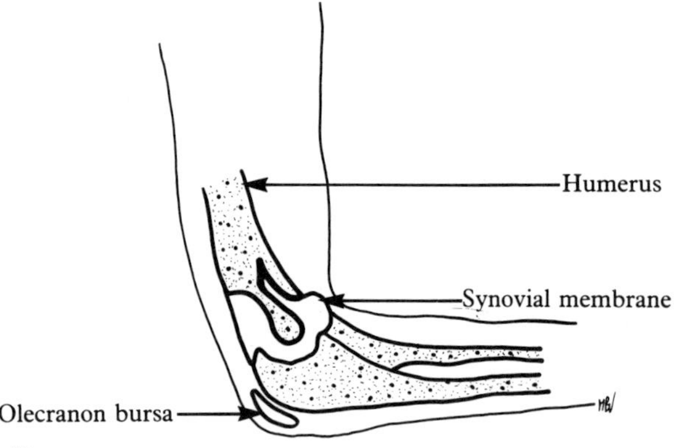

Fig. 21.18 The elbow **A**. Viewed from the front **B**. Lateral view

Bursae

Olecranon bursa

Localised pain and tenderness is accompanied by swelling.

Lateral epicondyle (Tennis elbow) (Fig. 21.19)

Diffuse pain in lateral side of the elbow often radiating into the upper arm and into the forearm and dorsum of the hand is accompanied by tenderness localised to the lateral epicondyle. Pain is aggravated by dorsiflexing the wrist against resistance.

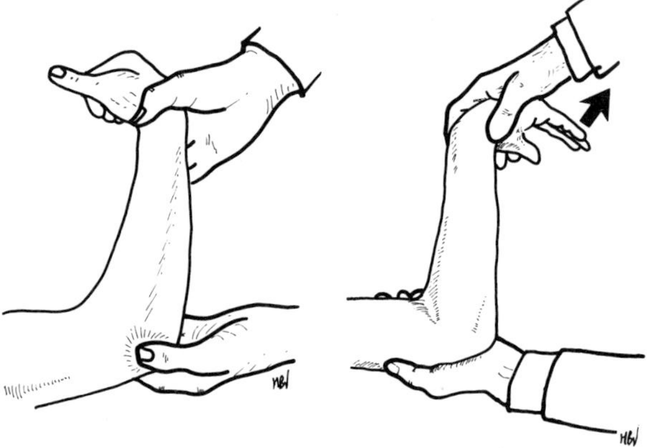

Fig. 21.19 Demonstrating lateral epicondylitis

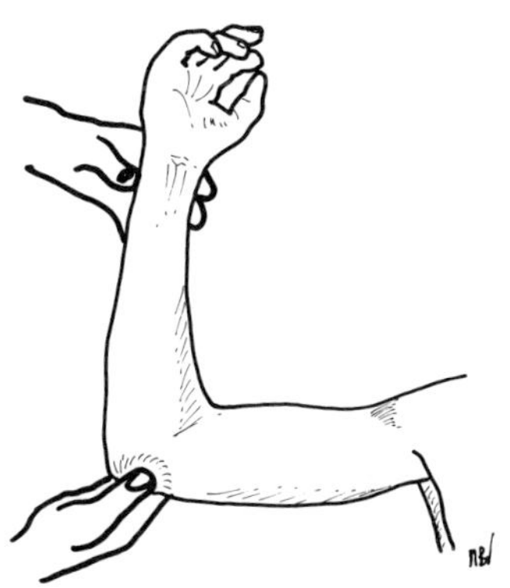

Fig. 21.20 Demonstrating medial epicondylitis

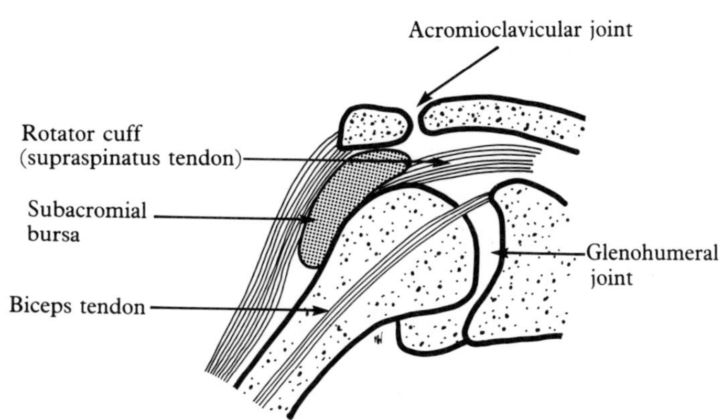

Fig. 21.21 The shoulder

Medial epicondyle (Golfer's elbow) (Fig. 21.20)

Diffuse pain in the medial side of the elbow often radiating into the upper and lower arm is accompanied by tenderness localised to the medial epicondyle. Pain is aggravated by active flexion of the wrist and resisted pronation.

Causes of referred pain in the elbow

From proximal sites

1. Cervical root lesions
2. Thoracic outlet syndromes
3. Brachial plexitis
4. Supraspinatus tendinitis and subacromial bursitis

From distal sites

1. Carpal tunnel syndrome
2. Ulnar nerve entrapment at elbow or wrist

From visceral involvement

Myocardial ischaemia and infarction

III The Shoulder

SITES OF ORIGIN OF MUSCULOSKELETAL PAIN (Fig. 21.21)

The joints

Shoulder joint

Pain, often diffuse, may radiate down the arm into the neck and across the back. Pain and limitation on passive movement of the joint. Tenderness of the joint margin, especially anteriorly below the coracoid process. Movements reduced, especially abduction and external rotation. Test by fixing angle of scapula and compare movement on both sides (Fig. 21.22). If there is an effusion, this is most marked anteriorly.

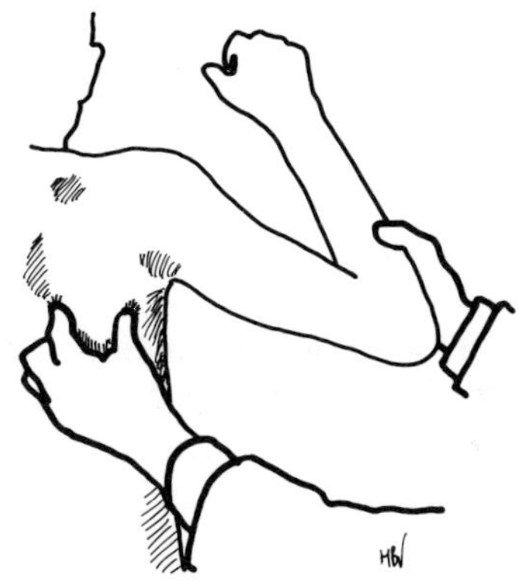

Fig. 21.22 Fixing the scapula to demonstrate glenohumeral movements

Acromioclavicular joint

Localised pain and tenderness; pain aggravated by shrugging of shoulders.

Tendons

Rotator cuff

Pain often localised to the deltoid region. Tenderness in the subacromial space and a painful arc of

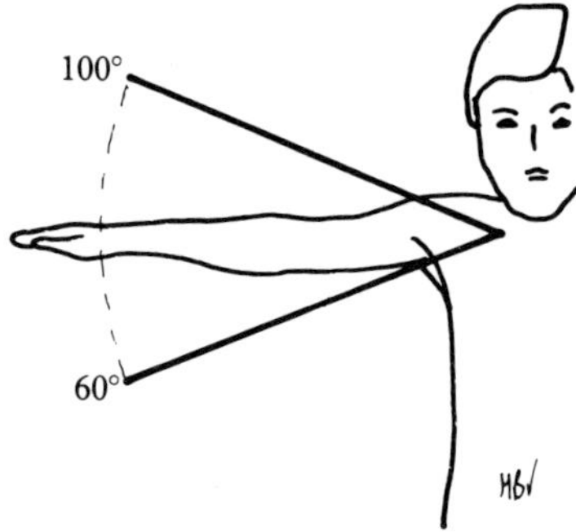

Fig. 21.23 Painful arc due to rotator cuff lesion

abduction (Fig. 21.23). Active movements are reduced, especially abduction and internal rotation. Pain on resisted abduction indicates supraspinatus tendinitis (most common) while pain on resisted external rotation indicates infraspinatus tendinitis; pain on resisted internal rotation indicates subscapularis tendinitis. Passive range of movement is reduced when adhesive capsulitis occurs. Weakness of abduction indicates partial rupture and inability to initiate abduction indicates total rupture of supraspinatus tendon.

Bicipital tendon

Pain radiates from anterior shoulder to forearm, with tenderness in bicipital groove aggravated by rolling the tendon from side to side. Pain is produced by resisted supination when the elbow is flexed (Fig. 21.24).

Bursae

Subacromial bursa

Symptoms and signs are similar to supraspinatus tendinitis, but pain does not occur with resisted movement.

REFERRED PAIN

The commonest cause of referred shoulder pain is cervical spondylosis, but it may be referred from other neck lesions, from visceral involvement and from distant sites.

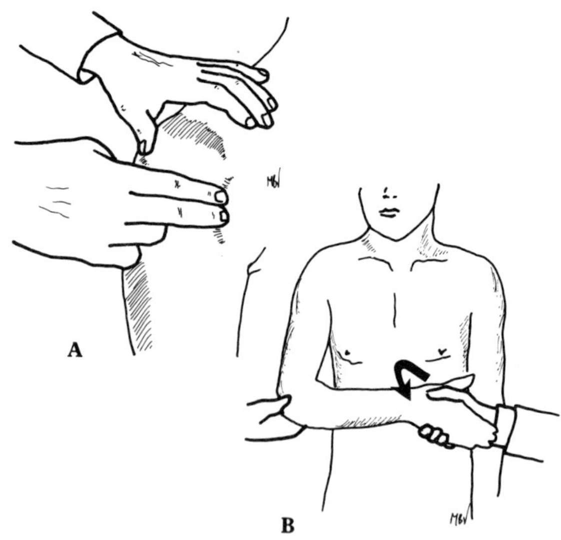

Fig. 21.24 Demonstration of bicipital tendinitis **A**. Tenderness in bicipital groove **B**. Resisted supination when elbow is flexed produces pain

Causes of referred pain in the shoulder

Cervical lesions

1. Cervical spondylosis with root compression
2. Herniated disc
3. Thoracic outlet syndrome
4. Brachial plexitis
5. Herpes zoster
6. Spinal cord tumours

From visceral involvement

1. Myocardial ischaemia and infarction
2. Pleurisy
3. Pulmonary infarction
4. Oesophagitis
5. Gall-bladder disease
6. Perforated viscus
7. Subdiaphragmatic abscess
8. Pericarditis
9. Dissecting aortic aneurysm
10. Pancoast tumour
11. Oesophageal tumour

From distal sites

1. Carpal tunnel syndrome
2. Tennis elbow
3. Nerve entrapment at elbow

IV The hip

SITES OF ORIGIN OF MUSCULOSKELETAL PAIN (Figs. 21.25 and 21.26)

The joint

Hip joint. Pain, often ill-defined, may radiate down anterior aspect of thigh to knee. Pain and limitation on passive movement of the joint. Tenderness anteriorly below mid-point of inguinal ligament. Internal rotation often affected first. Test with patient lying flat, flex knee and hip to 90°, and assess degrees of motion and pain produced by rotation. Always compare movement on both sides.

Tendons

Adductor tendinitis. Anterior and medial pain, worse on exercise. Isolated tenderness over adductor origin. Pain elicited by resisted adduction.

Gluteal tendinitis. Lateral pain exacerbated by resisted abduction.

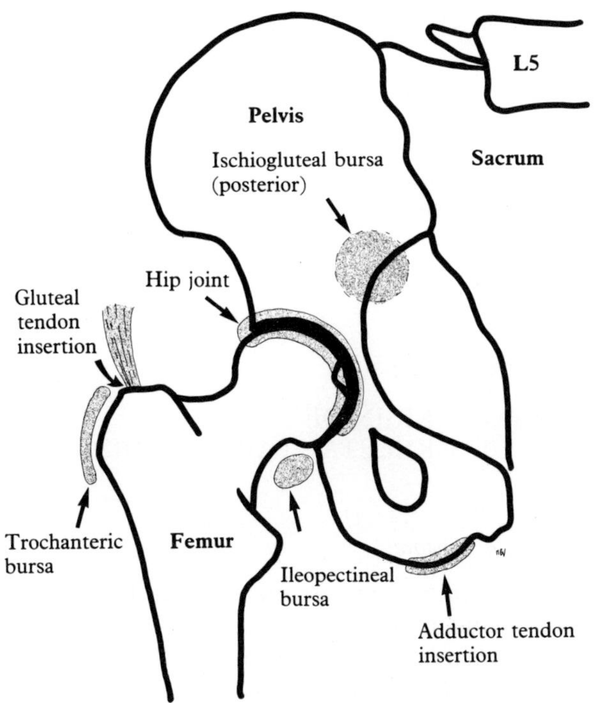

Fig. 21.25 Anatomical sites of pain arising from the hip joint region

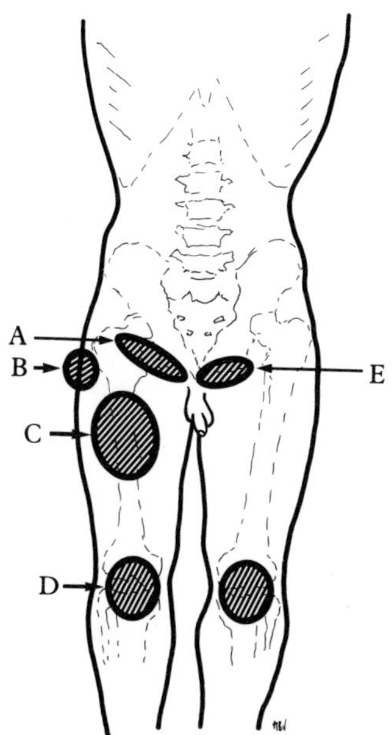

Fig. 21.26 Areas of pain and/or tenderness in disorders arising in or around the hip joint. Hip disease may cause diffuse pain and tenderness in the groin (**A**); pain may radiate to the thight (**C.**) or knee (**D.**). Trochanteric bursitis causes lateral pain and tenderness (**B.**); gluteal tendinitis may cause pain in the same area on resisted abduction. Adductor tendinitis causes pain in the groin on resisted adduction (**E.**). Meralgia paraesthetica causes pain and dysaesthesia in a patch on the front of the thigh (**C.**).

Bursae

Trochanteric bursitis. Lateral, poorly localised 'hip' pain. Point tenderness over greater trochanter. May have pain on resisted abduction.

Ileopectineal bursitis. Anterior pain. Tenderness over the lateral border of the femoral triangle. Pain on forced flexion and extension.

Ischiogluteal bursitis. Posterior pain, may radiate to thigh mimicking sciatica. Tenderness ± swelling over ischial tuberosity; best tested with the hip flexed.

REFERRED PAIN

L3/L3 root pressure

Pain anteriorly on coughing or sneezing, made worse by back movements. Limitation of back movement and scoliosis commonly present. Femoral stretch test positive (Fig. 21.27).

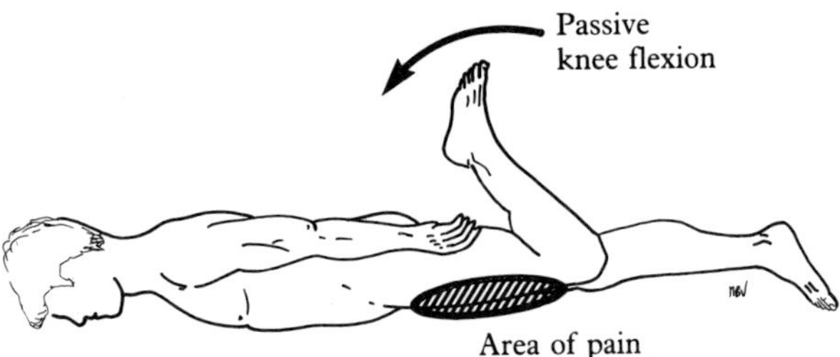

Fig. 21.27 The femoral stretch test. The patient lies prone, the knee is flexed and pain is felt on the front of the thigh if there is pressure on the L2/L3 nerve roots. For the sciatic stretch test see Fig. 22.3)

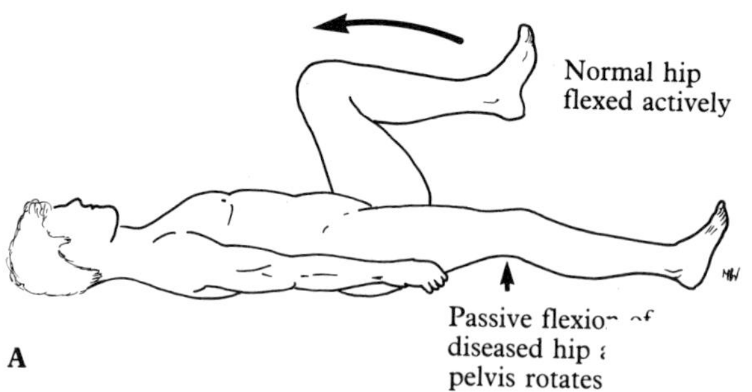

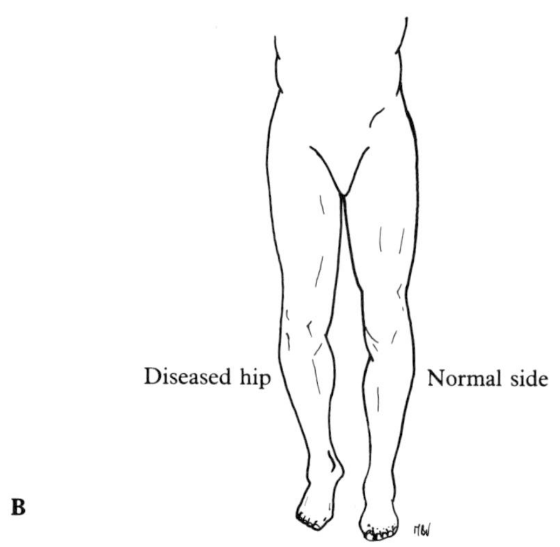

Fig. 21.28 Hip deformities **A**. Flexion deformity **B**. Shortening and external rotation

Meralgia parasthetica.

Pain anteriorly. Tender over medial aspect of superior anterior iliac spine (lateral cutaneous nerve of thigh).

Hernia

Anterior discomfort. Localised signs of hernia usually obvious. Femoral hernia may be difficult to define.

TYPICAL DEFORMITIES (Fig. 21.28)

1. Flexion deformity. Test with patient supine, flex other hip, affected leg rises off bed (Thomas's test).

2. External rotation deformity. Patient walks with foot externally rotated, no internal rotation on examination.

3. Shortening of leg (often with above two deformities). Measure from superior anterior iliac spine to medial malleolus, compare both sides. A common combination is hip arthritis with leg shortening and contralateral knee problems ('long-leg arthropathy' of knee).

THE ANTALGIC GAIT

Typical gait of hip pain. Patient often leans on a stick held in opposite hand. Pelvis lurches down on affected side on weight-bearing (Trendelenburg sign).

V The knee

SITES OF ORIGIN OF MUSCULOSKELETAL PAIN (Fig. 21.29)

Joints

Tibio-femoral joint

Diffuse pain, often worse on exercise. Tenderness along whole of joint line in affected compartments (medial, lateral or both). Pain with or without limitation of full flexion of the joint. Obvious effusions extending into supra-patella pouch or posteriorly are common.

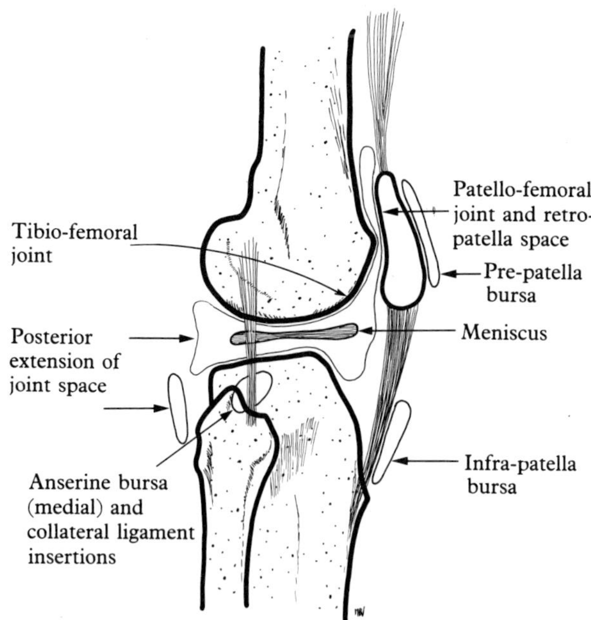

Fig. 21.29 Some possible sites of origin of pain in and around the knee joint

Patello-femoral pain

Anterior pain worse on using stairs or sitting with flexed knees. Pain and crepitus on grinding the patella onto the femur, or on pressure over patella when the patient contracts the quadriceps muscle.

Bursae

Pre-patella bursitis. Anterior pain. Localised pain and swelling over antero-inferior part of patella.

Infra-patella bursitis. Anterior pain. Localised pain and swelling over insertion of quadriceps tendon.

Anserine bursitis. Pain and localised tenderness over inferior part of medial joint line.

Posterior bursae. Ill-defined pain and tenderness in popliteal fossa. Difficult to differentiate from other sites of pain.

'Baker's cyst'. Posterior pain and palpable swelling due to extension of synovium into popliteal fossa. Often causes difficulty in flexing knee.

Ligaments

Collateral ligament pain

Isolated area of point pain and tenderness over inferior insertion of collateral ligament on lateral or medial side of tibia. May be exacerbated by testing for lateral instability (Fig. 21.30).

Menisci

Medial or lateral meniscus

Variable symptoms and signs. Pain usually localised to one compartment (medial or lateral). Clicking, locking or feeling of instability common. Tenderness and palpable clicks over joint line frequently found. Stress by fully flexing and extending knee with full rotation applied through the hindfoot (McMurray's test).

REFERRED PAIN

Hip pain. Often presents as pain in the knee only. Test hip movements.

L4 root pain. Pain exacerbated by back movements, coughing and sneezing. Anterior thigh and knee. Back movements often limited with or without scoliosis. Knee jerk may be reduced. Femoral stretch test positive.

TYPICAL DEFORMITIES (Fig. 21.30)

Flexion deformities

Develop quickly and easily in all knee disease. Associated with wasting and weakness of quadriceps apparatus. Knee often 'gives way' due to weakness.

Varus and valgus

Develop with serious tibio-femoral disease. Lateral (valgus) common in RA, medial (varus) in OA and RA. 'Windswept' knees (one valgus one varus) occasionally develop.

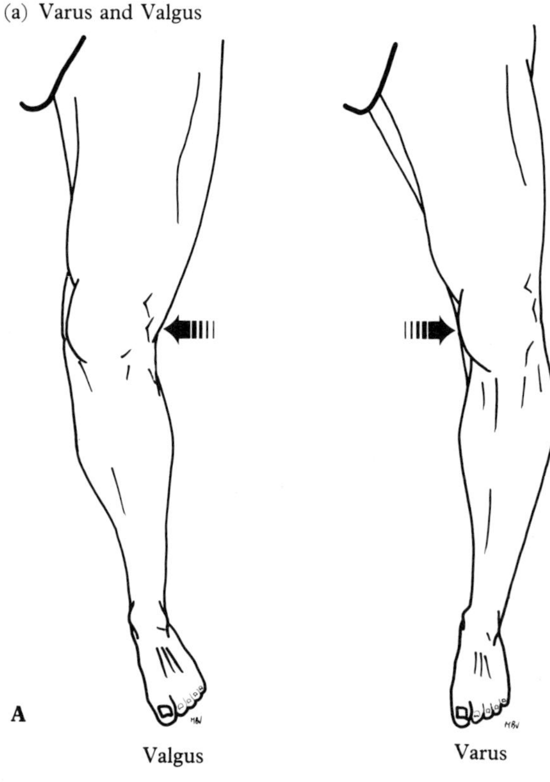

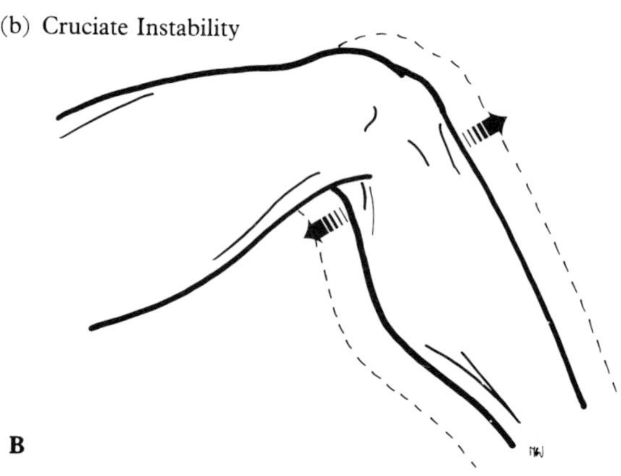

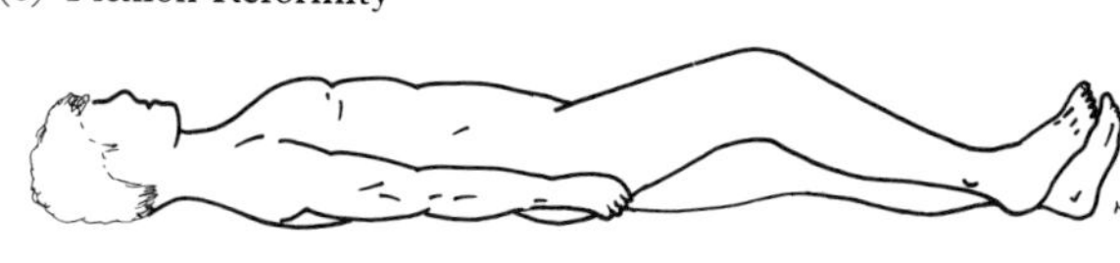

Fig. 21.30 Deformities of the knee joint **A**. Varus and valgus **B**. Cruciate instability **C**. Flexion deformity

VI The Ankle and Foot

SITES OF ORIGIN OF MUSCULOSKELETAL PAIN

Joints

True ankle joint

Synovitis in the ankle causes diffuse pain aggravated by standing and walking and may be associated with a diffuse anterior swelling. Pain is elicited by dorsi- and plantar flexion of the foot (Fig. 21.31A).

Subtalar joint

This causes diffuse pain which is aggravated by standing and walking, particularly on uneven surfaces, and is elicited by rocking the heel from side to side with the ankle flexed (Fig. 21.31B).

Midtarsal joints

Diffuse pain is felt midway down the foot and may be accompainied by swelling. Pain is elicited by twisting the forefoot with the hindfoot fixed (Fig. 21.31C).

Metatarsal joints

This pain is localised under the metatarsal heads and patients characteristically complain that it is like 'walking on marbles'. The toes may be pushed apart by the swelling, the so-called 'daylight sign'. Pain is elicited by transverse compression of the metatarsal arch or squeezing each joint individually (Fig. 21.31D).

Tendon sheaths and entheses

Peroneal tendons

Pain is localised behind the lateral malleolus and is often associated with a linear swelling along the tendon sheath. Pain is reproduced by plantar flexion and inversion of the foot (Fig. 21.31E).

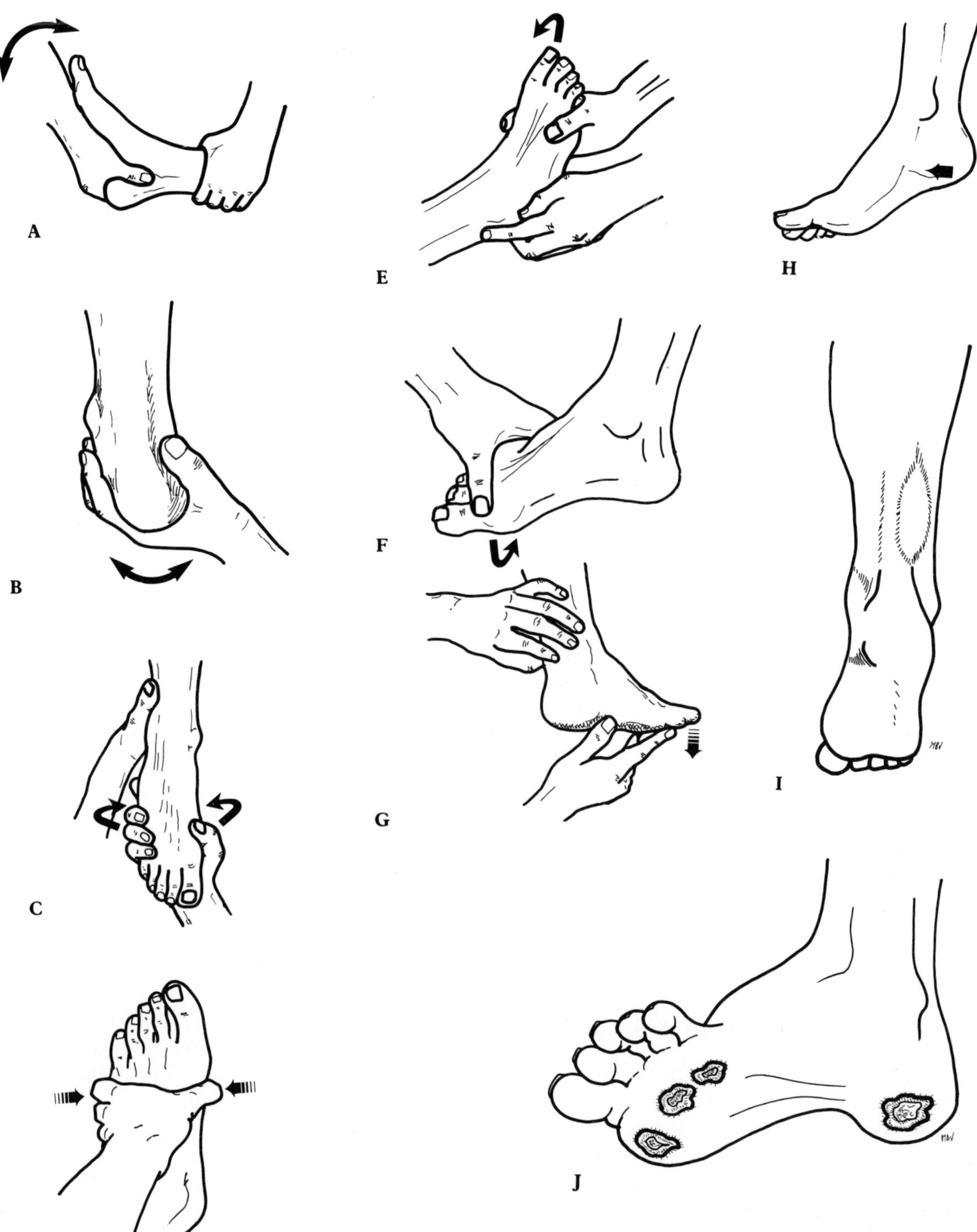

Fig. 21.31 Sites of origin of musculoskeletal pain in the ankle and foot **A**. True ankle joint **B**. Subtalar joint **C**. Midtarsal joints **D**. Metatarsal joints **E**. Peroneal tendons **F**. Tibialis posterior tendon **G**. Achilles tendon **H**. Plantar spurs **I**. Subachilles bursa **J**. Metatarsal bursae

Tibialis posterior tendon

Pain and linear swelling lies behind the medial malleolus and pain is elicited by plantar flexion and eversion of the foot (Fig. 21.31F).

Achilles tendon

Pain and diffuse swelling behind the ankle is made worse when walking and often aggravated by pressure from footwear. The symptoms are reproduced by resisted plantar flexion of the foot (Fig. 21.31G).

Plantar spurs

Sharply localised pain under the heel is made worse by standing. The site of origin is located by palpating the insertion of the plantar fascia on to the heel (Fig. 21.31H).

Bursae

Subachilles bursitis

This causes pain similar to that experienced in Achilles tendinitis except that the swelling bulges out on either side of the tendon (Fig. 21.31I). It is elicited by plantar flexion of the foot.

Metatarsal bursitis

Localised pain is associated with swelling over the metatarsal heads (Fig. 21.31J) and causes pain in the forefoot when walking.

REFERRED PAIN

First sacral nerve root (prolapsed disc)

This causes pain and paraesthesiae in the heel and lateral side of the foot and may be associated with some or all of the following signs: diminished pin-prick sensation over the sole, wasting of the calf muscle, weak resisted plantar flexion of the foot and absent or diminished ankle reflex. Pain is exacerbated by straight-leg raising.

Posterior tibial nerve (L5–S1) 'tarsal tunnel syndrome'

This is analogous to the carpal tunnel syndrome and causes painful burning in the foot particularly at night and diminished pin prick sensation on the sole. The symptoms can be reproduced by tapping behind the medial malleolus with a patellar hammer.

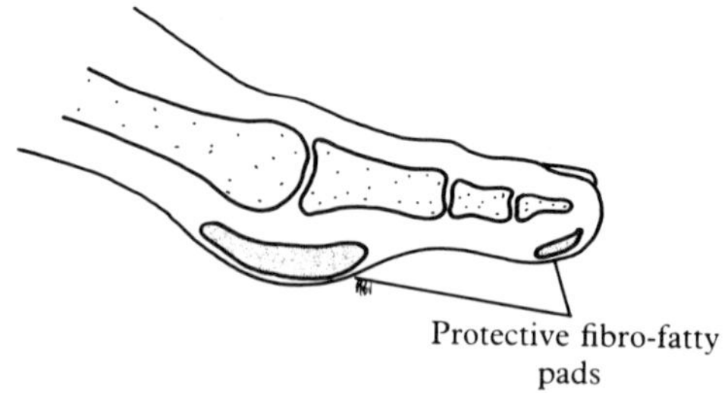

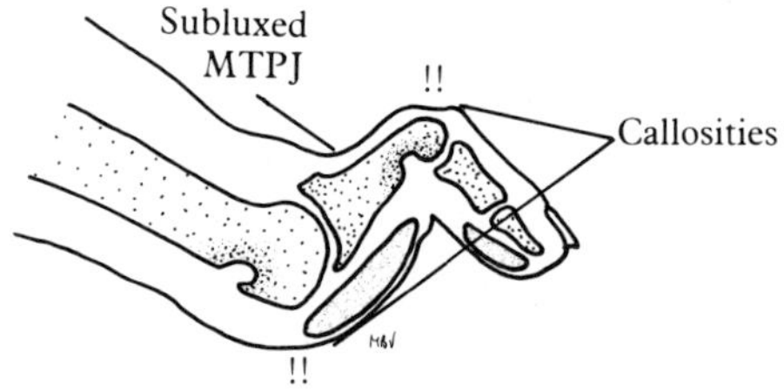

Fig. 21.32 Mechanism producing hammer toes

TYPICAL DEFORMITIES

Some common foot deformities are: the valgus ankle due to talonavicular disease collapse of the longitudinal arch due to midtarsal disease plus 'cock-up' toe deformity producing a 'rocker-bottom' foot. Cock-up toes (or hammer toes) are very common in the population generally and may be part of rheumatoid disease. The mechanism of this deformity is shown in Figure 21.32. The dorsal phalanx subluxes upwards, displacing the fibro-fatty cushion and exposing the unprotected metatarsal head to the full force of the body's weight on walking. Painful callosities develop as a consequence.

22 Differential diagnosis

I Peripheral Arthritis

INTRODUCTION

The first essential step in establishing the correct diagnosis in a patient complaining of joint pain is to ascertain that the symptoms are actually arising from the joints. Inflammation of bursae, tendon sheaths and ligamentous or capsular insertions may simulate acute arthritis, as may cellulitis and osteomyelitis in an adjacent bone. Psychosomatic illness often presents with multiple vague aches and pains which may be confused with chronic arthritis.

Synovitis such as occurs RA is characterised by pain at rest and during joint use, is accompanied by generalised joint swelling, tenderness around the joint and a capsular pattern of restricted movement and is associated with morning and inactivity stiffness. Inflammation in periarticular tissues is characterised by localised pain and tenderness which is aggravated by specific movements which stress that particular tissue. The pain of osteoarthritis is aggravated by joint use, relieved by rest and is accompanied by inactivity stiffness of an affected joint but without the generalised inactivity stiffness or morning stiffness experienced in more inflammatory joint disease. Internal derrangement of a joint from for example, a loose body, is associated with intermittent bouts of severe pain and locking with a specific movement.

PRESENTATION AND CAUSES

Arthritis can be grouped into three major divisions: acute and chronic polyarticular and monoarticular but there is a lot of movement between these artificial divisions which really just form a starting point for diagnosis. Chronic monoarthritis may, for example, have acute exacerbations and with time may become polyarticular. Diagnosis thus largely depends on recognition of a pattern of disease.

Acute arthritis

The common causes of acute arthritis in normal and previously damaged joints are listed overleaf. The circumstances surrounding the onset of the pain in a most important part of the history. An acute attack may be triggered by any infection, inoculation or intercurrent illness occurring within two or three weeks of onset: Reiter's disease may follow a bout of diarrhoea or non-specific urethritis, rubella and other viral infections may produce an arthritis; gout and pseudogout are commonly excerbated by surgery or intercurrent systemic disease; and rheumatic fever follows a streptococcal throat infection. Preceeding environmental factors may also be relevant as in, for example, acute SLE induced by sunbathing or precipitated by antibiotics.

The rate and time of onset may also be helpful. Gout characteristically starts at night and rapidly gets worse, with the intensity of the pain peaking within hours of onset. Septic arthritis gives rise to severe pain within 24–48 hours of onset as pus accumulates inside the joint. If trauma is significant, it generally preceeds the onset of pain by

Some common causes of acute arthritis in previously normal joints

Usually mono-articular but may be polyarticular

1. Gout
2. Pseudogout
3. Calficic periarthritis
4. Septic arthritis
5. Traumatic synovitis
6. Haemarthrosis
7. Foreign-body reaction

Usually polyarticular, but may be monoarticular

1. Reiter's disease
2. Gonococcal arthritis
3. Other reactive arthropathies
4. Rheumatoid arthritis
5. Psoriatic arthropathy
6. Other Seronegative spondarthropathies
7. Associated with neoplasia
8. Erythema nodosum
9. SLE
10. Rheumatic fever

Some common causes of acute arthritis in previously damaged joints

1. Bone disease
   a) Avascular necrosis
   b) Subchondral collapse or fractures
2. Cartilage problems
   a) Cartilage tears
   b) Cartilagenous detritus
3. Loose bodies
4. Haemarthrosis
5. Exacerbation of the underlying disease
6. Septic arthritis

1–3 days, since this is the time it takes to develop a haemarthrosis or a traumatic synovitis. Palindromic rheumatism which may preceed the onset of RA, is characterised by repeated attacks of pain in or near the joints, lasting hours to days and subsiding without disability. Periods of remission vary from days to months.

The site of acute arthritis, or the pattern of joint involvement if more than one site is affected, is also important. The common causes of acute monoarthritis show a preference for particular joints. About two thirds of attacks of gout, pseudogout and calcific periarthritis occur in the first MTPJ, knee and shoulder respectively. Haemarthroses are commonest in the elbows, shoulders, knees and ankles and foreign body reactions often occur in the small joints of the hands and feet or in the knees.

The pattern of acute polyarthritis may also be characteristic. The lower-limb distribution of Reiter's disease and other seronegative spondarthritides and the upper-limb preference of gonococcal disease may be helpful. Psoriasis may cause acute swelling of the whole digit ('sausage' finger or toe), hypertrophic pulmonary osteoarthropathy usually affects wrists and ankles and rheumatic fever tends to flit from one joint to another. Palindromic rheumatism commonly affects the knees, shoulders and small joints of the hands, although the pattern may vary from one attack to another.

Chronic arthritis

This is said to be present when the arthritis has persisted for more than 6 months. A list of causes with their relative frequencies is shown below. Many types of chronic arthritis have an acute onset which gradually settles into a chronic pattern. For example, recurrent attacks of acute gouty arthritis will lead to permanent, often polyarticular, joint damage with chronic pain and swelling. Once this happens the characteristic acute attacks tend to disappear. Conversely, patients with an established chronic polyarticular arthritis may have intermittent acute flares in one or two joints only which gradually settle again.

RA has a farily insidious onset in its typical form, usually affecting initially the small joints, often of the feet and then gradually spreads to other sites, particularly the hands, wrists, elbows, shoulders and knees. A disease like SLE may present with one feature such as pleurisy or pericarditis, followed by rash, then arthritis, in an additive pattern. The symptoms of many forms of chronic polyarthritis tend to follow an unpredict-

Somc causes of chronic polyarthritis

Common
1. OA
2. RA
3. 'Non-specific arthralgia'
4. Polymyalgia rheumatica

Uncommon
1. SLE
2. Reiter's syndrome
3. Psoriatic arthritis
4. Ankylosing spondylitis
5. CPPD
6. Gout

Rare
1. Juvenile chronic arthritis
2. Cancer, e.g. hypertrophic pulmonary osteoarthropathy
3. Metabolic arthropathy
4. Enteropathic arthropathy
5. MCTD
6. Scleroderma

Very rare
1. Polymyositis
2. SBE
3. Sarcoidosis
4. Multicentric reticulohistocytosis
5. Adult-onset Still's disease

able course, good days alternating with bad days for no apparent reason.

The distribution of joint involvement is also helpful. Generalised osteoarthritis has a predelection for the terminal interphalangeal joints of the fingers and the CMC joints of the thumbs, in contrast to RA which favours the proximal interphalangeal and metacarpal joints. Psoriatic arthropathy may affect the DIPJs and the MCPJs but, unlike OA or RA, tends to pick off individual joints in a random assymetrical fasbion. Assymetrical peripheral joint involvement, particularly of the lower limbs, together with stiffness and limitation of movement in the axial skeleton, or sacro-iliitis, is highly characteristic of a seronegative spondarthritis such as AS. Inflammation of the tendon sheaths is a major feature of SLE and may result in quite striking hand deformity with subluxation of the MTPJs, ulnar drift of the fingers and 'hitch-hiker's' thumbs, but in contrast to RA the underlying joints are not damaged and the deformity is usually reversible.

Monoarthritis

When a patient presents with apparently only one affected joint it is important to bear in mind that some causes of polyarthritis may have a predominantly monoarticular onset; patients may have a false monoarticular onset because lesser degrees of joint involvement have gone unnoticed and an apparent monoarthritis may in fact be due to a localised syndrome of para-articular tissues. Once it is established that the patient has a true monoarthritis, many causes need to be considered (Table 22.1). The joints favoured by the different causes of monoarthritis are shown in Figure 22.1. A major concern is to exclude a chronic infection or foreign body as the cause. Retrospective analysis has revealed that a quarter of cases of monoarthritis have degenerative joint disease and another

Polyarticular diseases with frequent (early) monoarticular component

Common
1. RA (small proportion but numerically common)
2. Psoriatic arthropathy
3. Reiter's syndrome
4. Ankylosing spondylitis
5. Pyrophosphate arthropathy
6. Juvenile chronic arthritis

Less common
1. Haemophilic arthropathy
2. Enteropathic arthritis
3. Whipple's disease
4. Sarcoidosis
5. Haemochromatosis
6. Scurvy
7. (Sepsis due to *N. gonorrhoeae* and *N. meningitidis* (may *follow* polyarticular onset)).

Table 22.1 Causes of chronic monoarticular arthritis

	Relatively common	Rare
'Non-inflammatory' disorders	Trauma Mechanical internal derangement Hypermobility Aseptic necrosis Osteochondritis dissecans	Charcot joint
'Inflammatory' disorders	RA Seronegative spondarthritides Pyrophosphate arthropathy Juvenile chronic arthritis Synovitis of unknown cause	Sarcoidosis Familial Mediterranean fever Relapsing polychondritis
Infections	–	TB, atypical mycobacteria Fungi Brucellosis, common bacterial pathogens, osteomyelitis, congenital syphilis
Foreign Bodies	–	Plant-thorn synovitis Sea-urchin spines Synovitis secondary to prosthesis
Proliferative disorders	–	Pigmented villonodular synovitis (PVNS), synovial chondromatosis/osteochondromatosis, joint neoplasma

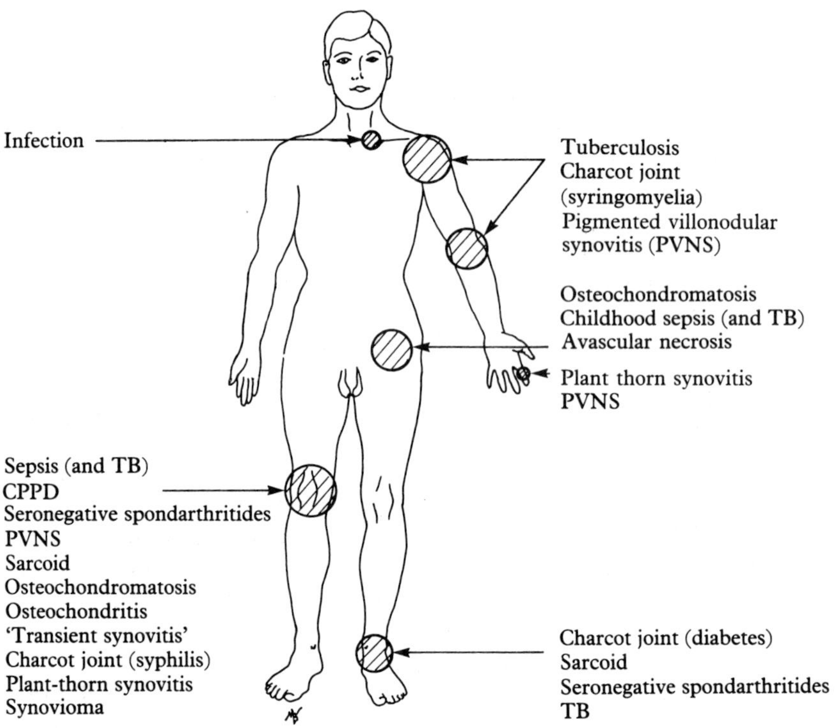

Fig. 22.1 Joints of predilection for diseases which cause chronic monoarthritis

Table 22.2 Guide to the age and sex distribution of the major causes of arthritis

	Male	Female	Both sexes
Children	Haemophilia		Osteomyelitis Traumatic synovitis Juvenile chronic arthritis Leukaemia Rheumatic fever Post-viral arthritis
Young adults	Reiter's AS	Gonococcal arthritis RA SLE	
Middle age	Gout	RA OA	
Later life			OA RA Gout Pseudogout Polymyalgia rheumatica Neoplasia

quarter are subsequently diagnosed as rheumatoid arthritis. Joint tumours, infection, osteochondritis dessicans and pyrophosphate arthropathy are less frequently diagnosed and in 30% of patients, expecially those with knee involvement, no cause is found for their synovitis. Some of them probably represent cases of intermittent hydroarthrosis, which is a recognised condition occurring in adolescence of both sexes. Relatively painless swelling regularly affects the same joint every 2–4 weeks and, in woman, may occur simultaneously with menstruation. The episodes last about 3–4 days and are characterised by relatively painless-effusions without other signs of inflammation. The knee is the common site, though involvement of elbows, hips or ankles has been described.

Influence of age, sex and race

Many forms of arthritis have an characteristic sex and age distribution (Table 22.2). A good example is gout, which virtually never occurs in premenopausal women and presents in men in middle age, and in old ladies, particularly if they are on diuretics. The influence of sex, age and occasionally race produces characteriestic patterns of arthritis which are the best guide to the correct diagnosis. Some typical examples of these patterns are shown in Figure 22.2.

ASSOCIATED FEATURES

Many very useful diagnostic clues can be found on careful examination. Some important ones are listed on page 398.

INVESTIGATIONS

A list of routine useful investigations is given (p 398). In acute arthritis the most important additional test is synovial fluid aspiration to exclude sepsis. In monoarthritis which has been present for more than 6 months without a clear diagnosis, synovium should be biopsied to exclude chronic infection such as tuberculosis. In chronic polyarticular arthritis, the diagnosis is usually made on the history and physical examination and investigations are carried out to confirm the clinical suspicion. It is important to realise that even after a host of tests, some patients elude precise diagnosis but need careful follow up in case useful clinical symptoms and signs should develop with the passage of time.

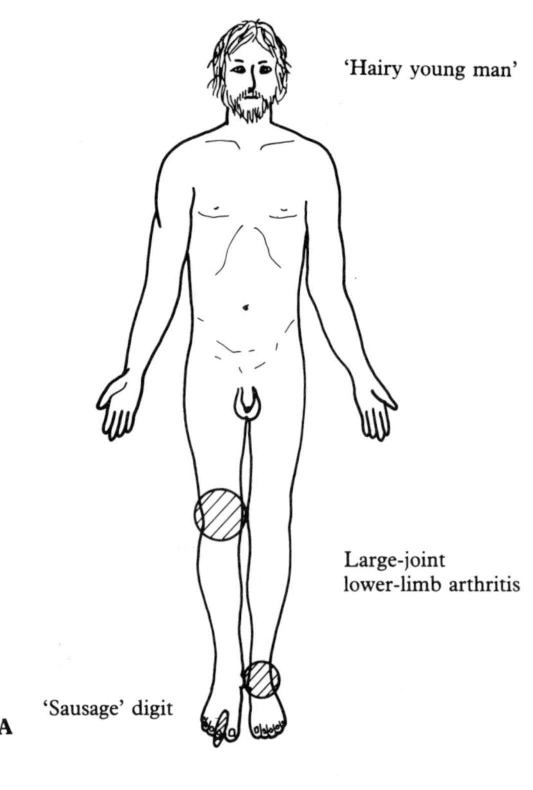
'Hairy young man'
Large-joint
lower-limb arthritis
'Sausage' digit
A

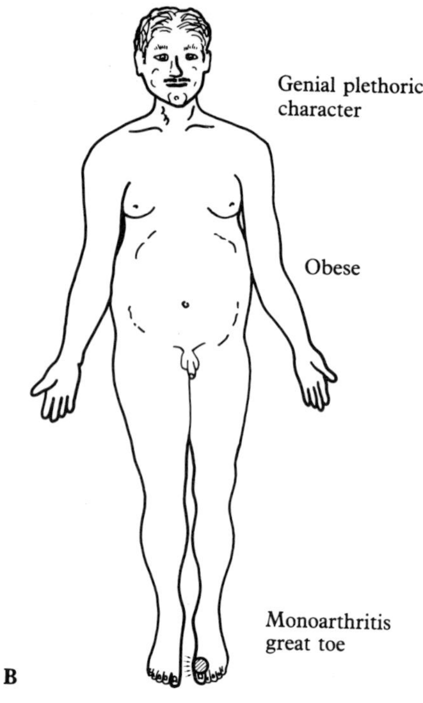
Genial plethoric
character
Obese
Monoarthritis
great toe
B

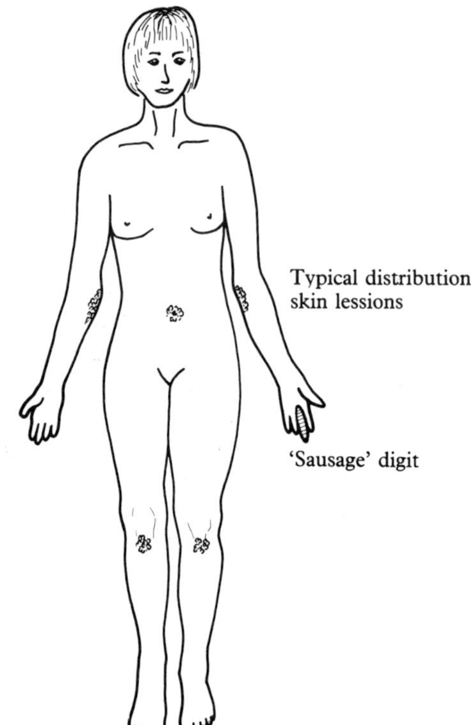
Typical distribution
skin lessions
'Sausage' digit
C

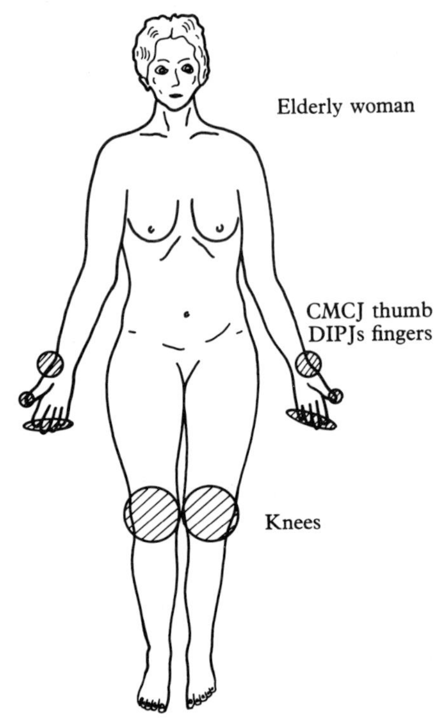
Elderly woman
CMCJ thumb
DIPJs fingers
Knees
D

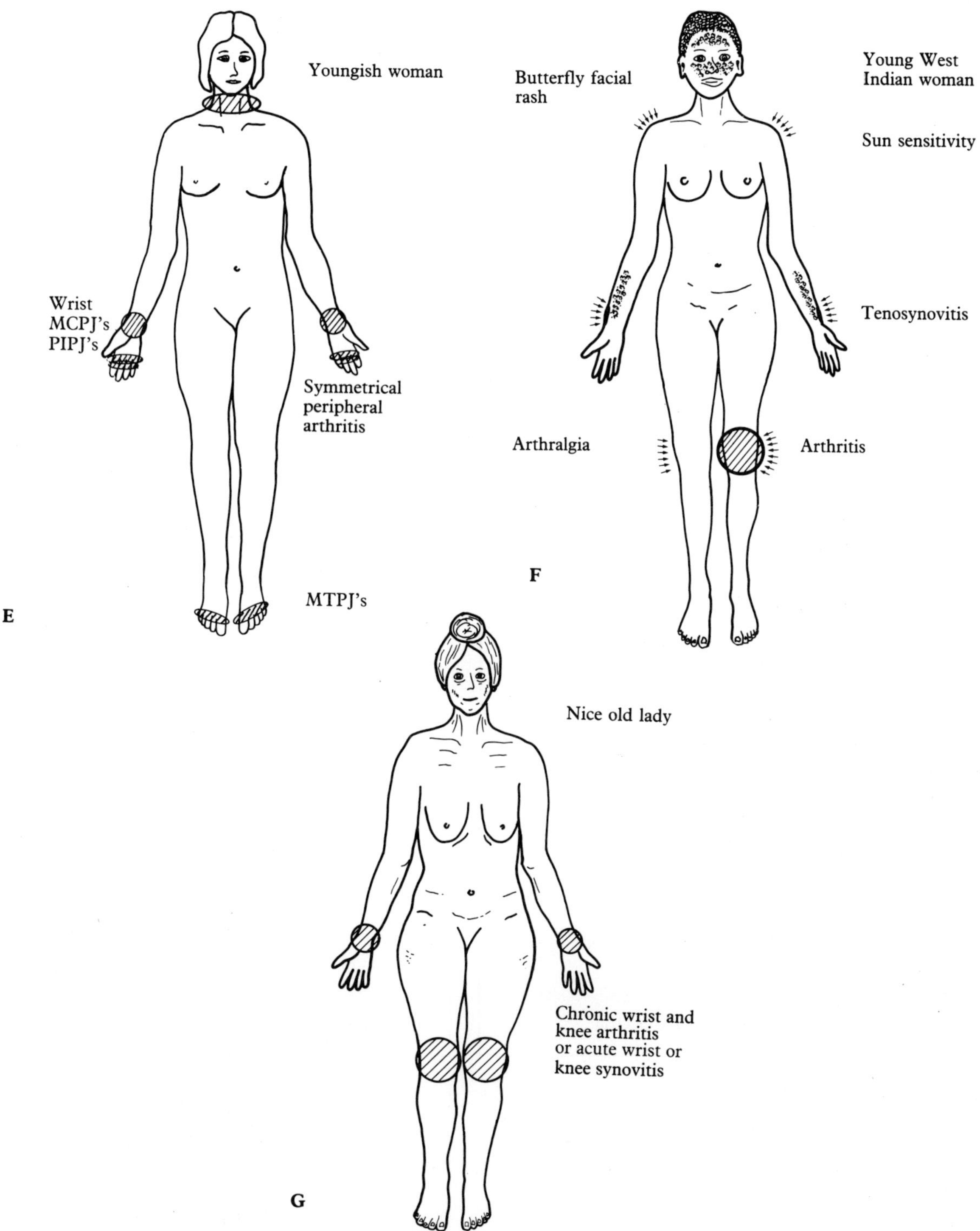

Fig. 22.2 Some typical diagnostic patterns of arthritis **A**. Reiter's syndrome **B**. Gout **C**. Psoriasis **D**. Generalised osteoarthritis **E**. Rheumatoid arthritis **F**. Systemic lupus erythematosus **G**. Pyrophosphate arthropathy

Clues to cause of arthritis

Skin and appendages	
Nodules	RA
Tophi	Gout
Heberden's nodes	OA
Psoriasis	Psoriatic arthritis
Onycholysis	Psoriatic arthritis, Reiter's
Raynaud's	SLE, scleroderma, MCTD
Butterfly rash	SLE
Oral ulcers	SLE, Reiter's, Behçet's
Calcinosis cutis	Scleroderma
Lividio reticularis	SLE
Sclerodactyly	Scleroderma, MCTD
Heliotrope discoloration	Dermatomyositis
Nasal ulceration	Wegener's
Keratoderma blenorrhagica	Reiter's
Fever	Rheumatic fever Still's disease Infection
Sensory loss	Charcot joint
Major organs	
Pericarditis	SLE, Still's, RA
Pleurisy	SLE, RA
Fibrosing alveolitis	Scleroderma
Mononeuritis	PAN
Asthma	PAN, Churg–Strauss
Glomerulonephritis	SLE, PAN, scleroderma

Aids to the diagnosis of arthritis

1. *History*
   a) When, why and how did it start?
   b) Any predisposing condition or associated disease?

2. *Examination*
   a) Joints
      (i) Articular or periarticular?
      (ii) Pattern of joint involvement
   b) Associated features
      Look for rashes, nodules, inflammation of mucous membranes, serositis, eye disease, urogenital inflammation and changes in other systems

3. *Investigations*
   a) X-RAY OF INVOLVED JOINTS (+ contralateral joint)
   b) Chest X-ray
   c) Haematology to include differential white cell count
   d) Consider blood cultures, serum uric acid, rheumatoid factor and A.N.A. (± other special investigations based on likely diagnoses)
   e) ASPIRATE INVOLVED JOINT IN ALL SEVERE CASES AND IF THERE IS DOUBT ABOUT THE DIAGNOSIS:
   f) Analysis of synovial fluid
      (i) Gram stain and culture (? infection)
      (ii) Polarised light microscopy (? crystals)
      (iii) Differential white cell count

4. *Think*
   a) What is likely? (age, sex, race and occupation of the patient)
   b) Could I be missing infection?
   c) Is it really arthritis?

II Pain in the Back and Neck

Back and neck pains account for about 6% of all medical consultations in the United Kingdom and are a major cause of lost work. Several specific disorders of the axial skeleton and joints are recognised (p 405), which between them account for a small percentage of those presenting with back pain. In the majority no precise anatomical or pathological diagnosis can be made ('non-specific' back pain). Several different clinical patterns are discernible: most patients present with acute self-limiting episodes of pain — it has been estimated that about 75% of the adult population will experience a significant event of this sort at some time; in some patients repetitive episodes occur; and an important minority develop severe, chronic symptoms. Management of 'non-specific' back pain is unsatisfactory as diagnosis is usually impossible, the available therapeutic measures are limited, empirical and often ineffective.

STRUCTURAL ASPECTS OF BACK PAIN

The vertebral column is a flexible supportive structure, which protects the spinal cord and segmental nerve roots (Fig. 22.3). Movement is provided by two types of joint: the synovial apophyseal joints and the fibrous intervertebral joints (Fig. 22.4).

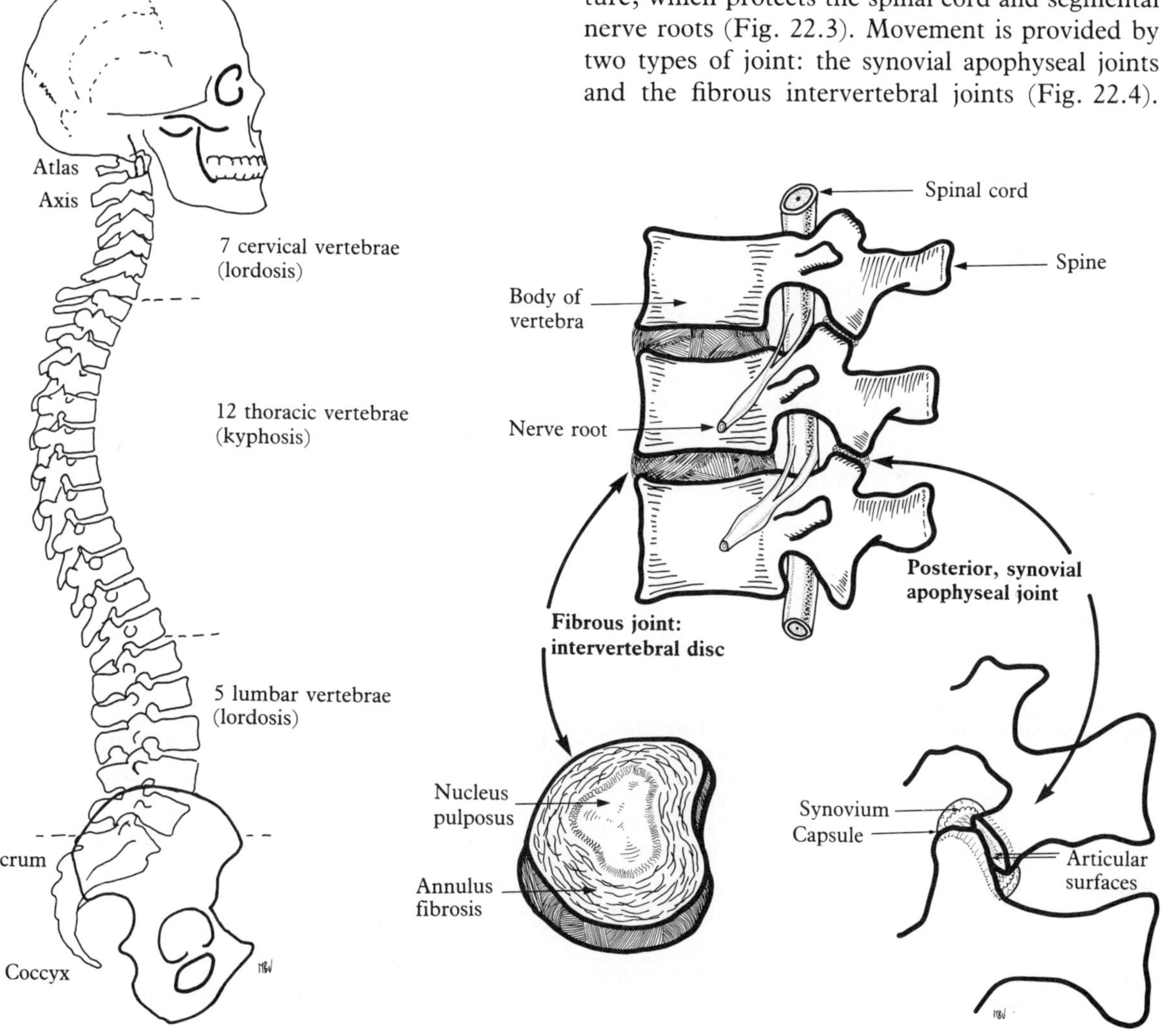

Fig. 22.3 The vertebral column

Fig. 22.4 The joints of the vertebral column

They are innervated through the capsule and long spinal ligaments respectively, and pain will only arise if these structures are stretched or irritated. Support is enhanced by the tone of the spinal muscles and by ligaments. Myofascial bundles are probably a common source of back pain, and the ligament–bone insertions (entheses) in the cervical, low lumbar and pelvic regions are also prone to localised, tender inflammatory lesions. The spinal cord and nerve roots are surrounded by a richly-innervated dural sheath, and inflammation or pressure on these neural structures is another source of pain. Disease of the bones may also cause back pain.

Although the clinical pattern may suggest one or other of these sites (Table 22.3), symptoms are usually poorly localised and often variable. Experimental injections of various structures in and around the vertebral column have resulted in diffuse pain which often radiates into distant areas such as the shoulder, arm, buttock or leg. It is therefore not surprising that the history and physical examination often fail to reveal which of these structures is the cause of pain.

Table 22.3 Some of the anatomical sites giving rise to back or neck pain (in most patients it is difficult to be sure of the site of origin of back pain)

Source of pain	Clinical features
Apophyseal joints	Pain exacerbated by extension (lumbar spine) or rotation (cervical and thoracic spine)
Intervertebral discs	Pain aggravated by flexion. Herniation may cause root pain
Pressure on nerve roots	Pain exacerbated by raising intra-thecal pressure (coughing, sneezing, straining), radiates in a dermatome, exacerbated by stretching the nerve root
Bone disease	Constant pain, worse on weight bearing, local bony tenderness
Ligament and tendon insertions (entheses)	Local soft-tissue tenderness

AETIOLOGICAL FACTORS

There are many possible causes of back pain, and several different classifications have been suggested. The list shown in Table 22.4 has the advantage of correlating to some extent with the clinical patterns of presentation outlined below. In a few cases inflammatory, metabolic, infective, neoplastic or referred causes of pain can be identified. In the majority the findings suggest a mechanical or

Table 22.4 Causes of back pain

Type of cause	Usual pain pattern observed
1. *Structural abnormalities* e.g. Intervertebral disc disease Spondylosis Fractures Spondylolisthesis Spinal Stenosis Osteochondritis	'Mechanical' pain pattern with or without neurological features.
2. *Inflammation* e.g. Ankylosing spondylitis and variants	'Inflammatory' pain pattern
3. *Infection* e.g. Discitis (pyogenic or TB) Epidural abscess	'Sinister' pain pattern
4. *Neoplastic* e.g. Myeloma Metastatic malignancy Lymphoproliferative disorders Primary bone/soft-tissue neoplasma	'Sinister' pain pattern
5. *Metabolic* e.g. Osteoporosis Osteomalacia Hyperparathyroidism Paget's disease	'Mechanical' or 'sinister' patterns
6. *Visceral* e.g. Pyelonephritis Peptic Ulcer Pancreatitis Pancreatic tumor Aortic aneurysm Retroperitoneal neoplasm	'Referred' pain
7. *Idiopathic* (*the majority*)	The majority of acute syndromes, mechanical and 'non-specific' back pain remain undiagnosed

structural cause — in some of these radiographs may show a specific congenital or acquired structural defect, but in most the cause is not apparent, and 'non-specific mechanical back pain' is diagnosed. In some patients with this label a degree of pain amplification through psychogenic factors may be present; total psychogenic pain with no organic basis is rare.

The causes of non-specific back pains are as difficult to identify as the anatomical structures involved. Most authorities stress three main aetiological factors: 1. specific traumatic events (e.g. sudden unaccustomed lifting of a heavy object); 2. the day-to-day mechanical stress applied to the back and 3. the structural integrity and strength of the spine. A balance between the forces applied in lifting, sitting, standing and moving and the resistance of the connective tissue of the intervertebral discs and ligaments must exist: excess forces or decreased resistance may result in a small structural change, and the development of back pain. The high incidence of disabling back pain in association with certain jobs illustrates the importance of mechanical stress.

HISTORY AND EXAMINATION

The history should include the patient's activity and factors which may exacerbate pain, such as driving or lifting, as well as an exact record of the mode of onset, chronology and distribution of the pain. The pattern of pain is often the most helpful feature: most non-specific pain is exacerbated by prolonged sitting and standing, inflammatory back pain is worst in the morning and associated with morning stiffness, nerve-root pain is exacerbated by movement and coughing or sneezing, bone pain is often constant and unrelated to activity. The patient's general health, and the effect of the pain on his or her life, are also important.

A general examination to exclude relevant disorders of another system (e.g. the breast lump which has metastasised to the spine) is essential. An abdominal check to exclude referred pain may need to include vaginal and rectal examinations. The neurological system must be covered to exclude damage to nerve roots or the spinal cord. Leg length should be measured and pulses should be checked.

The back itself should be examined with the patient stripped to underclothes. The contour and movement of the lumbar spine is best examined with the patient standing: the range of forward flexion, side flexion and extension can be assessed and, if need be, measured by use of a spirit level goniometer or tape measure. Movement can be roughly assessed by the examiner placing his fingers on two adjacent spinal processes and seeing how much they move apart on flexion. Rotation of the thoracic spine is examined with the patient sitting on the couch to immobilise the pelvis. The movements of the cervical spine (flexion, extension, side flexion and rotation) are also assessed with the patient seated, the passive as well as active range being elicited by the examiner. Palpation of the spine should include assessment of muscle tone, bone tenderness and a search for tender 'trigger spots'. Movements which exacerbate pain should be noted, for example back extension (possible apophyseal joint disease) or flexion (possible disc disease), and manoeuvres which stretch nerve roots such as the sciatic or femoral stretch tests (Fig. 22.5).

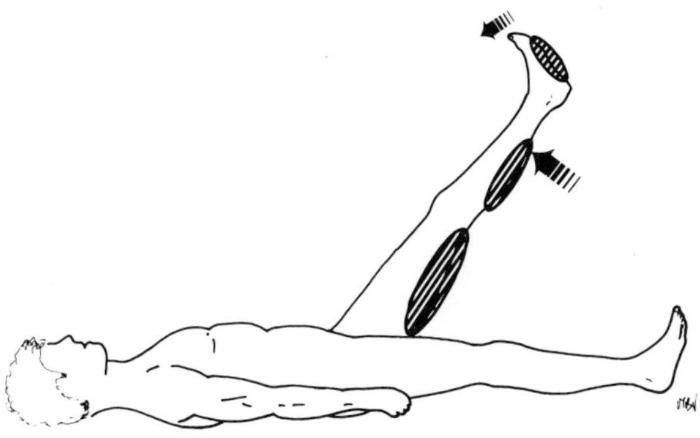

Fig. 22.5 Sciatic stretch test. The patient lies flat and the leg is raised with the knee straight. Further stretching of nerve roots may be achieved by dorsiflexion of the foot (arrows). In a positive test pain is felt down the back of the leg and into the sole of the foot in the L5 or S1 nerve root distribution (shaded areas). (For the femoral stretch test see Fig. 21.27.)

PRESENTATIONS

1. Acute pain in the neck or back

Sudden severe pain in a diffuse area around the neck or back is common; it often coincides with a sudden movement such as turning, bending or lifting. There is often immediate immobility, pain being exacerbated by the smallest movement. On examination the paraspinal muscles are in spasm, and there may be severe tenderness in the region of the apophyseal joints; other signs are usually absent. Attacks are self-limiting, subsiding over a period of days. Manipulation may produce sudden relief and return of painless movement. The aetiology of these attacks is unknown, although locking of apophyseal joints is often postulated. Radiation of pain in a root distribution sometimes occurs, suggesting disc disease with root compression as the possible cause. Many patients experience recurrent attacks requiring rest, time, manipulations ('putting my spine back in place') or other popular remedies to relieve them.

2. Chronic pain

Recurrent or chronic pain presents in a variety of ways and it is often impossible to make a logical deduction of the cause or anatomical problem from the history and examination. A few patterns are recognised, although patients do not always fit into the categories described:

a) Mechanical low-back pain

Patients are usually between 20 and 60 and the sexes are affected equally. There is often a long history of mild pain interrupted by severe exacerbations. Discomfort is related to activity, being exacerbated by prolonged sitting or standing and relieved by movement. Lifting is often difficult. On examination, movements, especially forward flexion, may be limited and there is sometimes a sudden 'block' to further movement. Tender spots around the pelvic brim are common. Signs of a mechanical cause are occasionally found — e.g. a step between vertebrae in spondylolisthesis, a leg-length inequality, scoliosis or kyphosis.

b) Recurrent or chronic neck pain

Patients are often middle-aged or elderly women, although other groups are affected. Mild neck discomfort on movement is punctuated by attacks in which the neck becomes rigid and painful for days or weeks on end. Muscle spasm and reduced movement are found on examination, the neck may 'creak' and there are often severe spondylitic changes on the radiograph.

c) Inflammatory back pain

This is characterised by morning stiffness of the spine, and relief of discomfort on mobilising or exercising the back. The pain may radiate from the lumbar region into the buttocks or thighs, and from the neck into the shoulders. It is a poorly-localised ache. Examination reveals a straightening of the spine and reduced movement. In young men ankylosing spondylitis should be suspected; early signs include loss of the lumbar lordosis, preferential loss of side flexion, pain on 'springing' the chest and stressing the sacro-iliac joints, and reduced chest expansion. In older people apophyseal joint OA or disc degeneration (spondylosis) can cause a similar presentation. Inflammation due to infection or other disorders occasionally presents in this way.

d) Neurological pain

The best established pattern of pain is that which starts in or around the spine and radiates into the arm, chest wall or leg in the distribution of a dermatome. Pain is often severe, it may develop suddenly or slowly, and is usually exacerbated by movements which stretch or irritate the nerve root, e.g. side flexion away from the pain, and by manoeuvres which raise intrathecal pressure, such a cough, sneezing or straining. The physical signs may include muscle spasm, a protective scoliosis (concave to the side of the lesion), reduced movement and exacerbation on nerve-root tension (e.g. the femoral or sciatic stretch tests). There may be sensory or motor signs in the appropriate nerve root distribution. Intervertebral disc prolapse is the best known and established cause, although nerve-root irritation can occur in spondylosis and patients sometimes present with these symptoms and signs without there being any definable disc disease or other cause. Hypertonic saline injections into facet joints can also reproduce 'radicular' or 'neurological'pain of this description, indicating the extent of our ignorance in explaining back pain.

e) 'Sinister' back pain

Recognition of the occasional patient with a sinister cause of back pain is crucial. Primary and secondary neoplasms, infections and metabolic bone disease can all present as pain in the neck or back which on initial enquiry may have no special features. Symptoms suggesting a serious cause include weight-loss, general malaise, pain unrelieved by rest or movement and progressive deterioration. Signs may include a clue on general examination (a lump, pleural effusion, heart murmur, fevers etc.) and an area of localised bone tenderness. These features warrant further investigation.

f) Referred pain

Back pain may arise from disorders of the kidneys, pancreas, stomach (posterior ulceration) and duodenum, large bowel or female genital tract. The pain is usually unrelated to activity, is diffuse, and may be altered by eating, defaecating, urinating or menstruating. The need for a careful systemic enquiry and general examination is obvious.

g) Pain amplification and psychogenic pain

Pain rarely has no organic cause, but back pain seems to be peculiarly prone to psychogenic amplification. Features of pain enhancement include a thick wad of medical notes, multiple consultations and investigations and unremitting symptoms in spite of many popular, conventional and fringe remedies. Physical signs often include variable loss of movement, a variety of tender spots and exaggerated descriptions and demonstrations of pain severity. A number of tests which help the diagnosis include pain on light pinching or stroking of the skin, pain on pressure on the top of the head and increased movement when the patient is distracted. Pain amplification may be a feature of depression or anxiety, may occur as part of the 'fibrositis syndrome' (p 360), and can develop as a result of chronic low-grade pain of organic cause. The prognosis is poor.

AGE, SEX AND RACE

Acute disc prolapse and spondylitis are disorders principally occurring in young working men; chronic disc disease, apophyseal joint OA and chronic non-specific pain are commoner in middle-aged women. Acute self-limiting syndromes can occur at any age, but the development of sudden pain in the very young or the elderly should alert suspicion of possible infection, bone disease or neoplasia. Mechanical and non-specific back pain seems to be particularly common in countries with a high standard of living, although good epidemiological data is lacking. It also shows a clear relationship with activities and the types of seating used (especially poorly-designed car seats and low, sagging chairs). Back pain is said to increase in response to dissatisfaction at work, stress in the home and other social factors, such as unemployment.

INVESTIGATIONS

Investigations are unhelpful and unnecessary in the majority of patients. Controversy exists as to the criteria for investigations and which tests should be performed, but any suspicion of 'sinister' pain, progressive neurological signs or symptoms and persistent, severe, incapacitating pain always require further tests.

Some of the available techniques are listed (Table 22.5). The ESR is a simple, useful screening test for general disease, and in older age groups screening for metabolic bone disease, intrapulmonary disease, myeloma, other tumours and infections is sometimes necessary. Plane radio-

Table 22.5 Some investigations available for back pain

Information required	Available techniques
1. Screening test for major abnormalities of spinal bone and joint anatomy	Plane radiograph AP view Lateral Obliques for facet joints Flexion/extension views
2. Screening tests for inflammatory, metabolic or neoplastic causes	Blood count and ESR Calcium and alkaline phosphatase Protein electrophoresis (possible myeloma) Acid phosphatase (in men) Chest X-ray Tc diphosphonate bone scans
3. Tests to aid visualisation of intervertebral discs	Radiculography and myelography Discography Venography
4. Other imaging techniques for bones, joints and soft tissues	Tomography CT scans Ultrasound scans

graphs produce the most controversy. They occasionally reveal unexpected bone or joint lesions but are more often useless or misleading — the very common spondylitic changes, for example, bear almost no relationship to the incidence or pattern of pain, and other findings (spina bifida occulta, Schmorl's noes, vertebral hyperostosis or old osteochondritis for example) may be unrelated to the pain and lead to unnecessary concern.

The indications for investigation of neurogenic pain are the same as those for possible surgery: persistent disabling symptoms of several weeks duration, motor signs or progressive neurological change of any sort. Radiculography is the standard technique used in most centres, although high resolution CT scanning may take over in the future. A variety of other imaging techniques are available, their usefulness depending on the degree of experience with the technique and the severity of the situation.

TREATMENT

A huge range of conventional, unconventional and bizarre remedies are available. Very few controlled trials have been carried out, but those published suggest that none of the conventional approaches are much better than placebo in most acute or non-specific pain syndromes.

The acute neck or back demands rest at onset. It usually resolves spontaneously. Corsets, collars and physiotherapy probably make little difference. Manipulation soon after onset can produce dramatic relief, resulting in good business for osteopaths and chiropractors.

Treatment of back pain (some of the techniques used)

1. Rest
2. Corsets and collars
3. Physiotherapy and Postural exercises
4. Manipulation and cheiropracty
6. Local injections
7. Drugs
8. Surgery

Chronic non-specific back pain may be aided by postural advice and other measures aimed at altering the mechanics of the spine. If particular environmental factors, stresses or physical anomalies, such as a leg-length inequality, are detected, correction may bring relief. Traction, physiotherapy, drugs and many other measures are often prescribed without any evidence that they help. Injection of local tender spots sometimes produces lasting relief. Extradural steroid injections may also speed up the rate of recovery in some patients with root symptoms.

Surgery can be essential in spinal stenosis, root or cord compression and an unstable spondylosis-thesis, but has little or no place otherwise. The laminectomy rate per head of population varies by over tenfold in Western countries, indicating a degree of confusion about the indications and benefit of back surgery. Interdisciplinary clinics specialising in back pain are blossoming in some countries and claim good results in chronic back pain via a combination of physical, psychiatric and other pain-relieving measures.

PROGNOSIS

Most acute attacks and acute-on-chronic exacerbations resolve. Recurrences are common, but only a minority of patients develop chronic symptoms of sufficient severity to lead to medical intervention. Once investigations and therapy have begun the outlook is probably bad except for the minority in whom an obvious, treatable organic cause is apparent. The available data suggests that conventional medicine makes little or no difference to the majority, harms an important group through over-investigation and treatment and only helps a small minority.

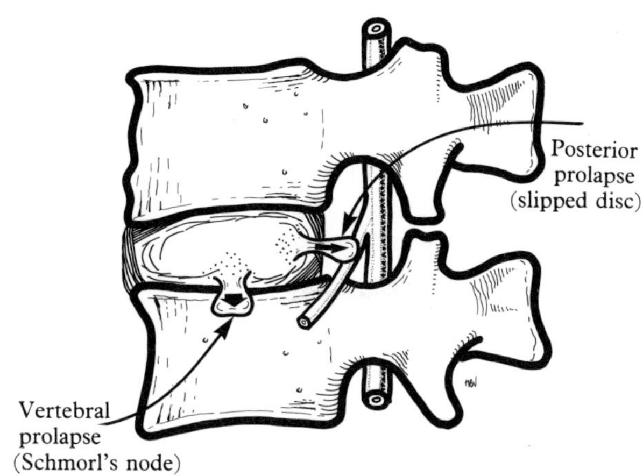

Fig. 22.6 Prolapsed intervertebral disc

SHORT NOTES ON SPECIFIC DISORDERS OF THE BACK

1. Prolapsed intervertebral disc

Vertical or posterior herniation of the contents of the intervertebral disc (Fig. 22.6). Usually L4–L5, sometimes L5–S1 or L3–L4, occasionally at other levels. Common in young adults. Often precipitated by lifting or bending. Vertical subluxation through bone end-plate results in a Schmorl's node. Posterior subluxation may press on nerve roots (posterior-lateral, common) or spinal cord (central, rare).

Causes acute pain in the back with paraspinal muscle spasm and sciatic scoliosis. Pain may radiate into nerve-root distribution. Stretching of involved nerve root then exacerbates pain (e.g. straight-leg raising test, Fig. 22.5). Radiographs usually normal; radiculography or other contrast media tests may show prolapse. 90% recover spontaneously after a few weeks.

2. Spondylosis

Degenerative changes in the intervertebral disc with loss of disc height and osteophyte formation. Usually accompanied by osteoarthritis of the apophyseal joints. Very common, age-related finding on radiographs of the lumbar and cervical regions. No relationship to back pain, which is as common in those without as those with spondylosis and is unrelated to the severity of the spondylosis (Fig. 22.7).

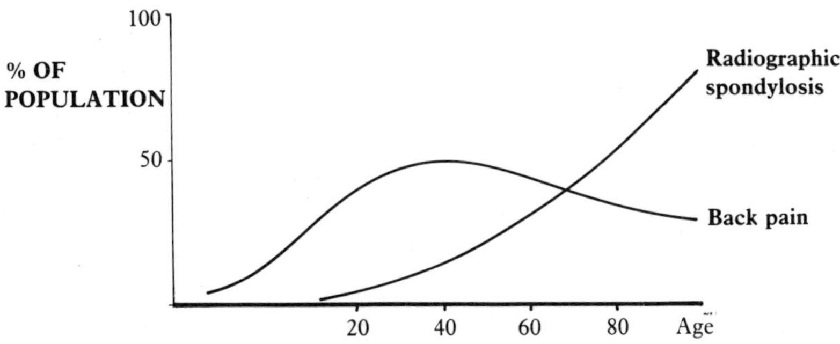

Fig. 22.7 Prevalence of back pain and radiographic spondylosis. Spondylosis on X-rays is age-related and eventually affects everyone. Back pain occurs in about half the population, mainly in young adults. There is no relationship between symptoms in the back and the incidence or severity of radiographic spondylosis.

3. Spinal stenosis

Uncommon condition occurring in the elderly. Usually associated with severe spondylosis and/or disc prolapse. Diameter of the lower part of the spinal canal is reduced. Congenital narrowing and a 'trefoil'-shaped canal confer increased susceptibility to the condition. (Fig. 22.9). Paget's disease and other conditions can also be the cause. Pain in the back and lower limbs may be aggravated by exercise and relieved by rest (pseudoclaudication) Pain is also relieved by flexion (as in riding a bicycle or going upstairs).

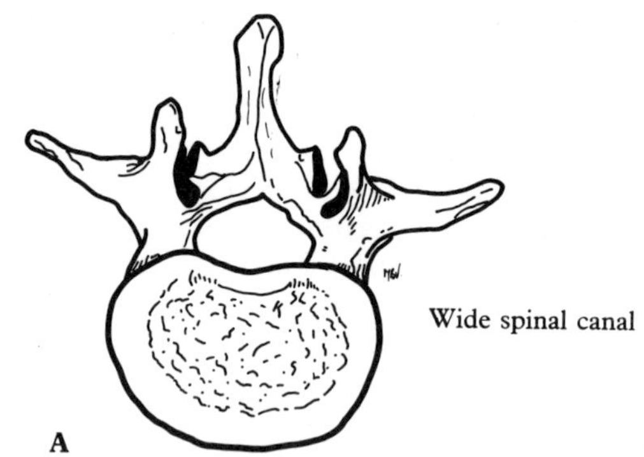

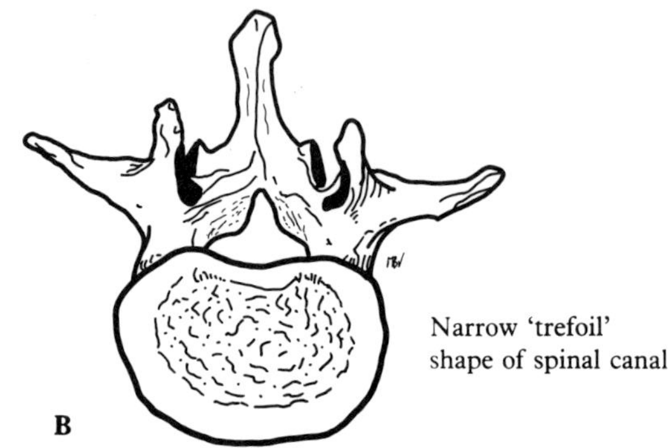

Fig. 22.9 Spinal stenosis **A**. Normal **B**. Spinal stenosis

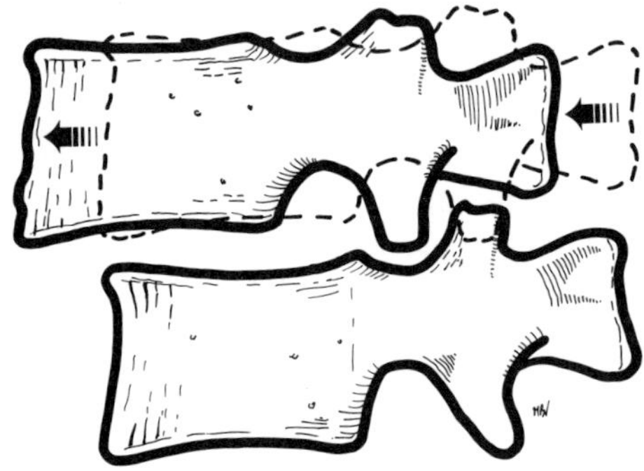

Fig. 22.8 Spondylolisthesis

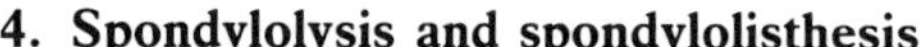

4. Spondylolysis and spondylolisthesis

Spondylolysis is a defect in the posterior elements of the vertebral canal detectable on oblique radiographs. May allow one vertebra to slip forward on the one below (spondylolisthesis) (Fig. 22.8). An uncommon cause of low-back pain which is sometimes accompanied by root or cord compression. If the slip is unstable (as shown on flexion/extension radiographs), the pain may respond to spinal supports or surgical fusion.

5. Scheuermann's osteochondritis

Osteochondritis of the vertebral end-plates in the thoracic and low lumbar spine. Common in adolescent males. Often asymptomatic, may cause mild pain and an exaggerated kyphosis. Secondary spondylosis develops in the elderly. Usually asymptomatic. May be accompanied by osteophytosis and osteoarthritis of peripheral joints (see also Chapter 8).

6. Diffuse idiopathic skeletal hyperostosis

A condition characterised by formation of exuberant 'dripping wax' osteophytes on the right-hand side of the thoracic spine, with preservation of disc height and leading to fusion. Common in the elderly. Usually asymptomatic. May be accompanied by osteophytosis and osteoarthritis of peripheral joints (see also Chapter 8).

7. Arachnoiditis

Chronic inflammation and thickening of nerve-root sheaths in the vertebral canal. Follows invasive procedures such as surgery and myelography.

Causes chronic severe low-back pain and restriction of movement.

8. Vertebral collapse

Compression fractures of the vertebral end-plates. Common in the elderly. Usual cause is osteoporosis. Myeloma, secondary deposits and metabolic bone disease must be considered. Often causes severe localised back pain with an acute onset. Resolves slowly over a period of several weeks.

9. Discitis

Inflammation in the intervertebral disc. Uncommon. Usually infective in origin, may be staphylococcal, tuberculous or caused by other organisms. May cause severe but poorly-localised back pain and systemic symptoms. The back pain is sometimes mild. Difficult to diagnose as radiographic changes take several days to develop.

FURTHER READING (BACK PAIN)

Grabias S L Mankin H J 1980 Pain in the lower back. Bulletin on the Rheumatic Diseases 30(8)

Grahame R G 1980 Low back pain. Clinics in Rheumatic diseases 6(1)

Jayson M I V 1976 The lumbar spine and back pain. Sector Publishing, London

23 Arthritis in specific groups

I Children

INTRODUCTION

Arthritis is rare in children and adolescents but musculoskeletal pain is a common clinical problem. The causes of joint pain in childhood are listed (right), with an indication of their relative frequency.

Children differ from adults in a number of ways which influence their susceptibility and reaction to rheumatic diseases. One of the fundamental physiological processes of childhood is skeletal growth which can proceed because of the presence of unfused epiphyses. Disturbance of the blood supply to the growing ends of bone may result in growth anomalies and inequality in the length of bones. Usually this takes the form of impaired growth but occasionally the increased blood supply resulting from inflammation accelerates growth. The epiphyses at the growing ends of bone are particularly susceptible to interruption of blood-supply causing a number of typical clinical syndromes which are grouped together as *osteochondritis* (p 348). The epiphyses may also dislocate — particularly at the femoral head, resulting in 'slipped femoral epiphysis'.

The articular cartilage is relatively thicker in children than in adults and seems better able to withstand erosive damage in inflammatory joint disease; this may be one reason why erosions are less often observed in JCA in the younger age groups.

Children's joints are much more mobile than

Differential diagnosis of musculoskeletal pain in children

Common

1. Limb pain syndrome (growing pains)
2. Trauma (including non-accidental injury)
3. Osteochondritis
4. Viral infections including vaccination
5. Psychogenic attention seeking
6. Henoch-Schönlein purpura

Uncommon

1. Juvenile chronic arthritis
2. Juvenile rheumatoid arthritis
3. Juvenile ankylosing spondylitis (and other seronegative arthropathies)
4. Acne arthralgia

Rare

1. Connective disease
2. Haemorrhagic disorders
3. Leukaemia
4. Rickets and scurvey
5. Rheumatic fever
6. Bone tumours
7. Caffey's disease
8. Sickle-cell disease

Very rare

1. Immunodeficiency syndromes
2. Neuroblastoma
3. Histiocytosis
4. Hypercholesterolaemia
5. Gout
6. Farber's disease

adult's. This hypermobility has been shown to decline steadily between the ages of 5 and 11 years and at the end of adolescence, with girls tending to be more mobile than boys at all stages. This ligamentous laxity seems to render some children more vulnerable to ill effects of physical activity and sport and may be a factor in recurrent acquired dislocation of the patella and hip and transient effusions in the knee. Some children, particularly girls, develop persistent arthralgia called the *hypermobility syndrome* (p 352) which is benign and improves with age. There is some evidence that hypermobility in childhood may predispose to osteoarthritis in later life.

Most of the significant pathogenic viruses and bacteria are encountered for the first time in childhood and many of these can cause arthralgias or arthritis. Vaccination may produce a transient serum-sickness-like illness with joint involvement and a post-rubella vaccination arthritis is not infrequent in adolescent girls.

The presentation of a rheumatic disease may be very non-specific particularly in the under-5s. Apathy and malaise may be the only early features and repeated falls, a limp or reluctance to use a limb should suggest joint disease. On the other hand, many features which would be considered highly significant in an adult carry less weight in the clinical assessment of a child. For example, fevers, lymphadenopathy, splenomegaly, high white counts and streptococci in the throat are common occurrences in childhood. The serum alkaline phosphatase in markedly elevated in children until growth has ceased.

COMMON MUSCULOSKELETAL SYNDROMES OF CHILDHOOD

Some of the common childhood musculoskeletal syndromes are listed below.

Common musculoskeletal syndromes of childhood

1. Growing pains
2. Hypermobility
3. Irritable hip
   a) Transient synovitis
   b) Perthes' disease
   c) Slipped femoral epiphysis
   d) TB
4. Painful knee
   a) Sinding-Larsen's syndrome (jumper's knee)
   b) Osgood-Schlatter's syndrome
   c) Chondromalacia patellae
   d) Recurrent dislocation of the patella
   e) Osteochondritis dessicans
5. Non-accidental trauma

Growing pains

It is no longer fashionable to talk about 'growing pains' but studies have shown that about 5% of school children, particularly the 8–12-year-olds, have limb pains which last more than 3 months and cause interruption of normal activities. These children tend to come from 'painful' families in which one or more member suffers from anxiety and pain syndromes — often of a rheumatic nature. The children themselves have a high incidence of associated pains, particularly in the head or abdomen ('little bellyachers'). The limb pain predominantly affects the legs and, to a lesser extent, the arms. Two-thirds of the children develop a 'heavy ache' in the daytime, usually after strenuous exercise. A quarter have nocturnal pain of the shins, calves and thighs which may wake them from sleep and cause crying. The pain is eased by rubbing and applying hot water bottles, and quickly passes off. Once organic disease is excluded therapy should be directed towards the family and school environment, since such factors as learning difficulties, compulsory games, a cold bed and faulty posture may precipitate attacks

Hypermobility

This has already been mentioned as a cause of arthralgia, recurrent dislocation and transient effusions, often occurring in girls who are keen on ballet or gymnastics. Once a hereditable disease of connective tissue such as Ehlers–Danlos syndrome has been excluded this condition is managed by reassurance. Unless the symptoms are significant there is no point in forbidding activities such as ballet or sport since the hypermobility often conveys significant advantage, allowing the patient to excel.

Irritable hip

A common problem is the child who presents with a limp, restricted movement and mild pain in the hip joint. The commonest cause is transient synovitis which is often preceeded by a history of mild trauma. On examination, hip extension and internal rotation are usually slightly restricted but there is no systemic disturbance and a normal ESR. The X-ray may show evidence of synovitis, but is usually normal. It is not necessary to aspirate the joint unless there is a real suspicion of infection. The hip usually settles after 4–6 weeks' bed-rest.

Perthes' disease (osteonecrosis of the epiphysis of the femoral head) presents as an irritable hip usually in boys between 8 and 11 years and X-ray changes are usually apparent by the time symptoms develop. This is treated by bed-rest, traction and occasionally surgical intervention. The outcome depends on the size of the infarcted area, but a significant number of these boys develop premature OA.

Slipped femoral epiphysis occurs in adolescent boys, usually, but not always, preceeded by trauma. Pain may be mild, presenting as irritable hip, or severe, making it impossible to walk. Internal rotation and abduction are restricted. The diagnosis is confirmed by a lateral X-ray and it is managed by surgical fixation. Osteonecrosis and coxa vara deformity may result in premature OA.

Tuberculosis of the hip is rare now but should still be considered, particularly in children from the Indian subcontinent who present with irritable hip. The pain is atypical in that it is constant, unrelieved by rest and disturbs sleep. There is a capsular pattern of restriction of movement and fixed flexion deformity is common. X-rays show rarefaction of the bones with widening of the joint space early on, later progressing to joint destruction. The diagnosis must be confirmed on synovial fluid is possible but if this is negative it is necessary to carry out a formal surgical synovial biopsy. If diagnosed early, tuberculosis of the hip may resolve with traction and anti-tuberculous chemotherapy. In more advanced cases there is joint destruction and bony ankylosis.

Painful knee

This is another common clinical presentation, often in adolescents. Osgood–Schlatter's and Sinding-Larsen's syndromes (jumper's knee) are examples of 'enthesitis' presenting with pain at the insertion of the patellar tendon into the tibial tubercle and lower pole of the patella respectively. Both conditions occur in boys between the ages of 10 and 15 who are sporting enthusiasts and both usually settle spontaneously after a year or so, although it may be necessary for the sufferer to give up sport for a while.

Recurrent dislocation of the patella is an affliction of hypermobile adolescent girls. The first episode is usually associated with trauma and produces severe pain. Subsequently the patella may dislocate with comparative ease and may become permanently displaced to the side of the knee. In severe cases, various surgical procedures may be performed to stabilise the patella.

Chondromalacia patellae is a condition of adolescent girls and young women in which the cartilage of the patella becomes soft, spongy and flaky. It presents with aching pain in the knee which is aggravated by quadriceps contraction such as in going upstairs and by patello-femoral compression. It is managed conservatively with rest and analgesia but severe cases may need to have the articular surface of the patella shaved or even require patellectomy to control pain. The natural history is not clearly established but the majority probably settle with only the unfortunate minority progressing to patello-femoral OA.

Osteochondritis dessicans is a form of osteonecrosis affecting the articular surface of the medial femoral condyle. It presents with pain, instability and occasional locking in young men between 10 and 20 years of age. The diagnosis is confirmed by tunnel radiography which may show the affected bony segment as a dense area surrounded by a clear halo (Fig. 17.15 p 350). This piece may become detached, forming a loose body and leaving behind a small crater on the femoral condyle. Early cases may settle with immobilisation, but surgical fixation of the loose fragment may be required.

Non-accidental trauma

Battered children may present with loss of use of a limb, or pain and swelling around a joint, suggesting arthritis. The presence of finger-sized discrete bruises, particularly on the neck, traumatic lesions in and around the mouth and previous fractures on X-ray are useful pointers to the correct diagnosis. Such children require urgent admission to hospital for their own protection while further enquiries are made into the family background.

Septic arthritis

Although rare, septic arthritis must always be excluded in a child presenting with an acute monoarthritis, since delay in diagnosis and treatment can lead rapidly to permanent joint damage or even death. Joint infection can occur in perfectly fit children but those on immunosuppressives or with leukaemia are particularly susceptible. If more than one joint is affected, hypogammaglobulinaemia or some other disorder of the immune system should be suspected. The commonest organism in the under-2s is *Haemophilus influenzae* and in older children *Staphylococcus aureus* and haemolytic streptococci. These organisms usually reach the joint via the bloodstream, although the source is not usually obvious. Infection may also spread from osteomyelitis of the adjacent bone, particularly in the hip.

SBE occasionally presents as a septic monoarthritis in children. Those over the age of 5 are usually obviously ill with fever, rigors and a hot tense, swollen, extremely painful joint which is held rigidly, but the under-5s may present diagnostic difficulty, since they often show little constitutional disturbance with minimal loss of joint function and yet may have more than one infected joint. The hip is the commonest site, followed by the knee. The joint should be gently palpated to see if the tenderness is confined to the joint margins or extends along the shaft of the bone, in which case osteomyelitis should be considered.

Joint fluid must be obtained in all cases of suspected septic arthritis and sent for urgent Gram stain, culture and sensitivity. Blood cultures should be taken at the same time. The synovial fluid is usually turbid and the sugar low. It is important to realise that the ESR and white blood count are no guide to the presence of infection in children since they are often markedly elevated in other causes of childhood arthritis. Treatment is commenced as soon as the samples have been sent to the laboratory. The pus should be completely aspirated by wide-bore needle or surgical drainage if necessary. The limb is splinted and antibiotics are started. A typical regime would be oral fucidic acid suspension and erythromycin stearate given according to the child's age and weight and continued for a minimum of 6 weeks. Once pain and spasm have subsided, gentle exercises are commenced. The joint should be re-X-rayed at intervals to assess the degree of damage.

Tuberculosis is now very rare but must still be considered, particularly in children with a chronic monoarthritis of the hip or knee, or synovitis in the tendon sheaths of the hands. The child may have a low-grade fever, weight-loss and evidence of tuberculous infection elsewhere, particularly in the lung or kidney. The ESR and white count may only be slightly raised with a relative lymphocytosis. The Mantoux test is usually positive. X-ray shows juxta-articular osteoporosis only in early cases. The organism is rarely isolated from the synovial fluid and biopsy of the synovial membrane is necessary. Tuberculous arthritis is managed with rest, splintage or traction and antituberculous chemotherapy.

Adolescents, particularly girls, are prone to gonoccocal arthritis which may be missed because it has an insidious, often periarticular, presentation. Characteristic pustular skin lesions on the fingers or toes or near an affected joint are useful diagnostic clues. The organism is hard to isolate and multiple blood, synovial, urethral and cervical swabs may be required. Fortunately, the majority of gonococci are still sensitive to penicillin.

Rheumatic fever

This is a multi-system disease affecting heart, joints, central nervous system, skin and subcutaneous tissues. It was once the commonest acute arthritis of children but has virtually disappeared in the developed world owing to a combination of improved living standards and use of antibiotics to treat childhood sore throats. Its importance as a disease rests on its effect on the heart, and throughout the world it is still the leading cause of death from heart disease among the 5–24-year-old age group. St Vitus' dance or chorea is its other less common but dramatic manifestation.

Rheumatic fever results from a delayed reaction to a group A streptococcal infection in the throat and may recur in an affected individual each time the organism is encountered. During epidemics of streptococcal infection about 3% of people will have a first attack of rheumatic fever but this figure rises to 50% amongst those previously affected. Cross-reactivity has been demonstrated between components of the streptococcus and the human sarcolemma membrane as well as between antibodies directed against heart tissue and the caudate and thalamic nuclei of the brain.

Pathologically there is exudative and proliferative inflammation in arterioles, fibrinoid degeneration of collagen and Aschoff's nodules in the heart. The arthritis is due to periarticular and articular inflammation with effusions but without pannus formation or erosion. Scarring and fibrosis of heart valves results in mitral regurgitation and stenosis and, less commonly, disease of the arotic and tricuspid valves.

Clinical features

The first attack occurs between the ages of 3 and 15 years, with a peak incidence around the age of 6. It presents with fever and joint pain on average 18 days after a sore throat, although the gap between may vary between 1 and 5 weeks. In one third of children there is no recollection of sore throat. The arthritis is migratory, flitting from one large joint to the next and never persisting for much more than 1 week at one site. The joints are characteristically red, hot, swollen and tender. In recurrent attacks the small joints of the hands may eventually become involved and, later still, periarticular fibrosis may cause mild hand deformity called Jaccoud's arthritis.

About half the children have cardiac involvement during the first attack and the younger ones under 5 are particularly susceptible. This is pancarditis affecting all layers of the heart. It appears within the first week or two of the onset of the illness. One of the earliest features is a raised sleeping pulse in an afebrile child. Rubs, murmurs, an enlarging heart on X-ray and cardiac failure may follow, depending on the severity of cardiac involvement. The commonest early murmur is mitral regurgitation, but it is important to distinguish this from the common systolic-flow murmur of childhood. Delayed AV conduction, detected as a prolonged PR interval on an ECG, is common but is not specific for rheumatic fever and alone does not indicate cardiac disease.

Chorea only occurs in about 10% of children with rheumatic fever and never in those with arthritis, although it frequently co-exists with carditis. After puberty it is only seen in girls, never in sexually-developed boys. It is characterised by involuntary, purposeless, non-repetitive, rapid movements, muscular weakness and emotional lability. Bizarre facial expressions are common and the protruded tongue may writhe like a 'bag of worms'. It usually persists for 8–12 weeks and then settles. It is one aspect of rheumatic fever which may occur with a normal ESR and CRP.

Other minor features which may be diagnostically valuable are a rash, called *erythema marginatum*, and subcutaneous nodules. The rash is non-irritant, non-indurated, red, spreads out in serpiginous rings and may come and go rapidly. The nodules occur over bony prominences, particularly the occiput, vertebrae, elbows and Achilles tendons.

An attack of rheumatic fever usually lasts about 3 months but may persist for as long as 6 months with carditis. Recurrences do not occur if streptococcal infections are prevented.

Investigations

There is no diagnostic test for rheumatic fever but

laboratory investigations are useful to look for evidence of antecedant streptococcal infection and in monitoring inflammation and response to treatment. Streptococci can only be isolated from the throat in under a quarter of children by the time rheumatic fever has developed. However, infection can be established in the majority by following the rise in streptococcal antibody titres. These are measured as extracellular products produced by the bacteria. The two most commonly measured are the anti-streptolysin O and anti-DNA-ase B titres. These peak at about 4–5 weeks, usually at the onset of arthritis and decline rapidly over the following few months. Titres of 200–300 units are common in normal children, so to be of significance there must be much greater rises than this. The anti-DNA-ase B has the advantage of staying elevated for longer than the ASO titre. A new slide agglutination test called the *streptozyme test* is proving reliable and sensitive.

The ESR and CRP are usually elevated except in a few children with only chorea and a normochromic normocytic anaemia is common.

An enlarging heart and prolonged PR interval with flattening of T waves signifies myocarditis.

Differential diagnosis

Diagnostic criteria for rheumatic fever are shown below. Rheumatic fever is diagnosed if two major or one major and two minor criteria are present, plus evidence of antecedant streptococcal infection. The main conditions to be considered in the differential diagnosis of the child with joint pain and fever are shown below.

Diagnostic criteria for rheumatic fever

Major
1. Carditis
2. Polyarthritis
3. Chorea
4. Erythema marginatum
5. Subcutaneous nodules

Minor
1. Fever
2. Arthralgia
3. History of rheumatic fever
4. Raised ESR and CRP
5. Prolonged PR interval

Plus evidence of recent streptococcal infection from positive throat culture or rising ASO titre

Differential diagnosis of rheumatic fever
1. Rubella
2. Hepatitis
3. SBE
4. Gonococcal arthritis
5. Sickle-cell disease
6. JCA/RA
7. Leukaemia/lymphoma
8. FMF

Management

The child should be rested in bed until fever and arthritis have resolved. The development of carditis is monitored by checking the sleeping pulse, ECG and chest X-ray and listening for murmurs. Streptococci are eradicated by a full course of penicillin which is then continued until adult life in a dose of 125 mg b.d. orally or monthly intramuscular injections of 1.2 Mu of benzylpenicillin. In adults who continue to be exposed to young children, e.g. school teachers or young mothers, the prophylaxis should be continued indefinitely. Salycilates are useful in lowering fever and relieving arthritis in doses of 70–100 mg/kg/day aiming for a serum level of 20–30 mg/dl. In severe cases which do not respond adequately to full doses of aspirin, prednisolone may be required (1–2 mg/kg/day) but it has no effect on the eventual outsome.

Erythema nodosum arthropathy

This syndrome is usually triggered by a haemolytic streptococcal infection in young children and by sarcoidosis in the adolescent age group. It characteristically causes acute synovitis of the knees and ankles associated with raised, indurated reddish-purple tender skin lesions on the shins, and resolves spontaneously with rest and analgesics.

Serum-sickness

This is an allergic type III reaction which may be triggered by ingestion of foreign protein, vaccination or drugs in a susceptible child. Symptoms usually appear between 8–12 days from contact and consist of an urticarial rash, fever and pain and swelling in the joints. Symptoms are usually mild, self-limiting and respond to antihistamines and analgesics. The offending agent should be avoided in future.

Acne arthritis

A severe form of necrotising, scarring acne — *acne fulminans* — occurring in adolescent boys is occasionally accompanied by systemic disturbance including fever, weight-loss and arthralgia. The joint symptoms are usually mild and resolve without residua. The condition is thought to arise from hypersensitivity to antigen derived from skin bacteria. Immunoglobulin levels may be elevated and C3 reduced and microscopic haematuria is occasionally detected. The symptoms resolve as the skin improves.

Viral infections

The viral illnesses which may be associated with an arthropathy in children are listed below. Rubella infection causes a polyarthritis which usually follows, but may precede, the rash. It affects the knees and hands. Tenosynovitis and carpal tunnel syndrome may be prominent features. Arthritis may also follow rubella vaccination in teenage girls and knees are the common site. The rubella virus has been isolated from the affected joints. Mumps causes a large-joint, flitting arthritis and periarthritis in teenage boys and may mimic rheumatic fever. Infectious mononucleosis may simulate Still's disease in children with arthritis lymphadenopathy and splenomegaly. The arthropathy of hepatitis-B virus infection usually preceded the onset of jaundice or bilirubinuria and is characterised by synovitis of the DIPJ's with marked morning stiffness, sometimes associated with an urticarial rash. *Mycoplasma pneumoniae* and cytomegalovirus may also caused a polyarthritis: erythema multiforme is common with *Mycoplasma pneumoniae* infection and, if there is considerable disturbance of liver function, cytomegalovirus should be considered.

Some viral causes of arthritis in childhood

1. Adenoviruses
2. Rubella
3. Chickenpox
4. Mumps
5. *Mycoplasma pneumoniae* infection
6. Cytomegalovirus infection
7. Epstein–Barr virus infection (infectious mononucleosis)
8. Rocky Mountain spotted fever

MAJOR RHEUMATIC DISEASES IN CHILDHOOD

Rheumatoid arthritis

Classic seropositive rheumatoid arthritis occasionally occurs in childhood, usually after the age of 10 and more commonly in girls than boys. It presents as a peripheral symmetrical small-joint arthritis, often associated with elbow nodules. Erosive changes appear on X-ray early and are often associated with periostitis. Vasculitis is a rare complication compared to the adult disease. The outcome is less favourable than JCA, with nearly a third having severe disability. Because of this bad prognosis these children warrant early aggressive therapy with second-line drugs such as gold or penicillamine.

Seronegative spondarthritides

Ankylosing spondylitis

This is one form of JCA occurring in children around the age of 10 years. Boys are affected five times more frequently than girls. The features of the classic adult disease — back pain, limitation of back movement and sacro-iliitis — are not seen very often at onset. Instead, the children tend to have a large-joint lower-limb arthropathy, not uncommonly a monoarthritis, and present with a limp. There is often a family history of AS and the patient is B27-positive. Some years from onset, changes of sacro-iliitis appear on X-ray, followed later still by back pain and limitation of movement. The complications are the same as in the adult disease and include iritis, aortitis and amyloidosis.

Psoriatic arthropathy

Nearly one-third of all cases of psoriasis start before the age of 15 years but psoriatic arthropathy in the same age group is rare. It occurs more commonly in girls with a peak around puberty. It presents as an acute pauci- or monoarticular arthritis of the lower limb in the majority, resulting in a limp, and the arthritis appears before the rash in about half the children. Nail changes are very common, even without the rash, and have a close relationship to the presence of arthritis. Involvement of the DIPJs and tendon sheaths similar to that in the adult disease is seen quite often. Growth anomalies indistinguishable from those of Still's disease occur, often affecting a single metatarsal or metacarpal bone. Radiological features of periostitis and erosion of the interphalangeal joints may develop but the bony dissolution so characteristic of the adult disease is rarely observed. The prognosis in terms of disability is very good compared to other forms of childhood arthritis, but the disease progresses into adult life.

Inflammatory bowel disease

This usually presents as a pauciarthritis affecting the large joints, lasting for a few weeks and resolving without residua although there is a tendency to recurrence. Inflammatory bowel disease should be considered in the differential diagnosis of any child with arthritis. In comparison with adults, children have a much higher incidence of mucocutaneous lesions, particularly erythema nodusum, pyoderma gangrenosum and mucosal ulceration. Fever is much more common and there may be significant stunting of overall growth. Acute iridocyclitis does not appear to occur and spondylitis is very rare. Children will often not admit to having diarrhoea and regard it as a 'secret' to be kept even from their mother.

Reactive arthritis

A syndrome of ocular, urogenital and joint inflammation may occur in children. This is often due to a specific bowel infection with *Shigella*, *Salmonella* or *Yersinia* organisms.

Gout

This only occurs in children who have an underlying disease, such as leukaemia or haemolytic anaemia, causing increased purine production, or an enzyme defect such as is seen in Lesch–Nyhan syndrome.

Connective tissue diseases

Systemic lupus erythematosus

Childhood lupus is uncommon, occurring in about 3% of all cases of SLE, usually in adolescent girls. Arthritis, skin rash and fever are the commonest presenting features. Some cases of childhood idiopathic thrombocytopenia eventually turn into lupus with time. Neurological involvement and severe lupus nephritis appear to be more common than in the adult disease. The course is unpredictable but spontaneous remissions are seen less often than in SLE presenting in adult life.

Dermatomyositis

The incidence of dermatomyositis shows a peak in childhood and is 10–20 times more common in children than polymyositis alone. It often presents with falls, malaise and back pain. The rash may precede or follow the onset of muscle weakness and may easily be overlooked in Black children. High fever, periorbital oedema heliotrope discoloration of the eyelids and calcinosis are common associated findings. The majority of children survive and regain normal function but treatment with corticosteroids is necessary during the acute phase. Widespread calcification in the muscles is common and may cause contractures and marked disability but there is a tendency for reabsorption to occur gradually over several years. There is no association between malignancy and childhood dermato- or polymyositis.

Progressive systemic sclerosis

Systemic sclerosis is a rare disease that is even rarer in children but it appears to mirror the adult disease when it does occur. Localised scleroderma and linear morphea are commoner in children than adults. The latter condition may affect the growth of a limb, causing such severe contractures and deformity that amputation is required.

Vasculitis

Henoch–Schönlein purpura. This is a common widespread vasculitis affecting the skin, joints, gastro-intestinal tract and kidney. Although described in adults, the peak age of onset is 5 years. The cause in uncertain but response to an infection seems likely. Pathologically it is characterised by IgA deposition in vessel walls. The rash occurs on the buttocks and extensor surfaces, starts as urticaria and then purpura, and finally fades after about 2 weeks. Recurring crops are characteristic. A mild bilateral symmetrical arthritis is present in about 50%, usually affecting the knees and ankles. Vasculitis of the gastro-intestinal tract causes colicky abdominal pain sometimes with melaena or rectal bleeding. Infarction, perforation and intussusception complicate severe cases. The renal lesion is a focal glomerulonephritis and although 40% of children have proteinuria and haematuria, only a few go on to develop frank nephritis with hypertension and oliguria. There is no one diagnostic test. The ESR is raised and platelet and clotting tests are normal. About 25% have haemolytic streptococci in the throat, but this is the same frequency as children in general. Immunofluorescent staining of renal and skin tissue shows IgA, complement and fibrin deposition. Mild cases respond to bed-rest and analgesia, but occasionally steroids and cytotoxic drugs are indicated. The prognosis depends on renal involvement and is generally good.

Polyarteritis nodosa. This presents in childhood with prolonged fever, leucocytosis, abdominal pain and rash. There is often a clear history of preceding mild upper-respiratory infection. Coronary arteritis is seen much more frequently in the childhood form of the disease.

Kawasaki's disease, also known as the *mucocutaneous lymph node syndrome*, is thought to represent a variant of childhood polyarteritis nodosa. The oriental races, particularly in Japan and Hawaii, appear particularly susceptible, although sporadic cases do occur elsewhere. The classical clinical features are fever, conjunctivitis, hand oedema and erythema of the fingertips, irregular red eruption elsewhere on the body, strawberry tongue and unilateral swelling of the lymph nodes in a boy under 2 years of age. Aneurysm of the coronary arteries and myocarditis lead to death from cardiac arrest in about 2% 2–4 weeks from onset. Those who recover may have persistent angiographic abnormalities in the coronary arteries and aorta.

HAEMATOLOGICAL DISORDERS

Leukaemia

Childhood leukaemia is usually of the acute type and may present with primary musculoskeletal symptoms at onset, during the course of the disease or as a result of treatment. Symptoms may arise as a consequence of the haematological abnormality, for example bleeding into the muscles or joints, or bacterial infection in the bone or joint. The joints may also be directly infiltrated by leukaemic tissue, causing a transient lower-limb arthritis which may be associated with muscle-wasting and subcutaneous nodules. Bone pain, swelling and tenderness around joints and sometimes over the sternum is due to infiltration of the marrow cavity by blasts. Bone lesions are often present on X-ray. A few children present with musculoskeletal symptoms, fever and hepatosplenomegaly without evidence of leukaemia in the peripheral blood, or even occasionally in the marrow, at onset, and they can easily be misdiagnosed as Still's disease. The picture may be further complicated by the appearance of rheumatoid-like nodules around the joints and a positive latex fixation test for rheumatoid factor.

Haemoglobinopathies

Sickle-cell disease causes episodes of acute bone and joint pain due to thrombosis. Bony infarcts are prone to infection, particularly with *Salmonella* organisms. There may be generalised and local growth effects and osteonecrosis of the femoral head is common. Any Black child who presents with bone or joint pain, particularly swelling and pain in the hands or feet should be screened for sickle cell disease. Thalassaemia causes characteristic radiological changes in the skeleton but does not present with musculoskeletal symptoms.

Bleeding disorders

The first episode of bleeding in haemophilia usually occurs in infancy, often into a joint or muscle. Unless further episodes are prevented by factor VIII injection, a chronic arthropathy will develop. Christmas disease may also cause haemarthrosis in childhood, as may acquired thrombocytopenia.

NUTRITIONAL DISORDERS

Rickets

This is the equivalent of osteomalacia occurring in children, and, owing to public health measures such as slum clearance, smokeless zones, adequate milk for children and education of mothers, it is now rare. The cause is vitamin D deficiency from either poor diet, inadequate sunshine exposure or malabsorption. Children with pigmented skins or those being reared in adverse social circumstances are vulnerable. Rickets presents between 9 months and 2 years. The baby often appears well-nourished but is flabby and fretful. There is often excess sweating around the head and abdominal distension. The child is reluctant to crawl or sit and is prone to episodes of diarrhoea and pneumonia. Tooth eruption is delayed. The growing ends of bones are tender and swollen — particularly the wrist and costochondral junction (the *rickety rosary*). In those under one year, the soft skull bones crackle under finger pressure like old parchment (*craniotabes*). In the older child, mechanical stresses of sitting and standing produce kyphosis of the spine and deformities such as bowing of the legs or knock-knees. Pelvic deformities in girls may cause difficulties in childbirth later on. The diagnosis is confirmed by X-ray of the long bones — the metaphysis becomes expanded and cupped with an irregular hazy outline (Fig. 23.1). The alkaline phosphatase is markedly elevated with a normal or low calcium and a low phosphate. Vitamin D should be given in therapeutic doses (25–120 μg/day) plus an ample supply of calcium either as a supplement or as milk. The best guide to healing is return to normal of the growing ends of the bones on X-ray. Thereafter, prophylatic vitamin D (10 μg or 5 ml cod-liver oil) and milk should be continued. Occasionally a case will be encountered which is resistant to ordinary doses of vitamin D and a renal tubular defect such as Fanconi's syndrome should be sought. Large doses of vitamin D, e.g. 1.25 mg strong calciferol, will be needed to effect healing.

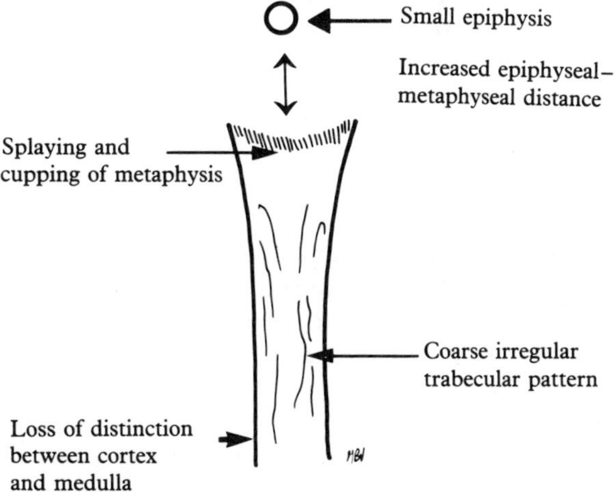

Fig. 23.1 Radiological features of rickets

Scurvy

Vitamin C (ascorbic acid) deficiency is due to lack of fresh fruit and vegetables. Once the curse of seafarers and prisoners, it now occurs at the extremes of life through ignorance, poverty or maternal neglect. Cow's milk is low in vitamin C and so those babies fed artificially without supplements are at risk. Major manifestations occur in the bones and joints because of subperiosteal bleeding. The child is pale, inert and lies with the hips and knees semiflexed and hips adducted in a 'frog-leg' posture. He may fret, cries most of the time and screams if touched or lifted. The joints are swollen and extremely tender. Perifollicular haemorrhages, petechiae and easy bruising are common and, if teeth have erupted, the classical scorbutic gingivitis with livid swelling and haemorrhage may be present. Confirmatory X-ray changes are best seen in the femur and tibia. There is porosis with loss of trabeculation, giving a 'ground-glass' appearance. A dense line of calcification is seen over the widened end of the metaphyses and in a ring around the epiphysis. Healing subperiosteal haemorrhages cause striking elevation of calcified periosterum (Fig. 23.2). There is usually anaemia and a low leucocye ascorbic acid level. Treatment with 100 mg/day of ascorbic acid abolishes pain in a few days but bony swelling may persist for months. Long-term deformity does not occur; prevention is achieved by giving infants fruit juices from about 4 weeks of age.

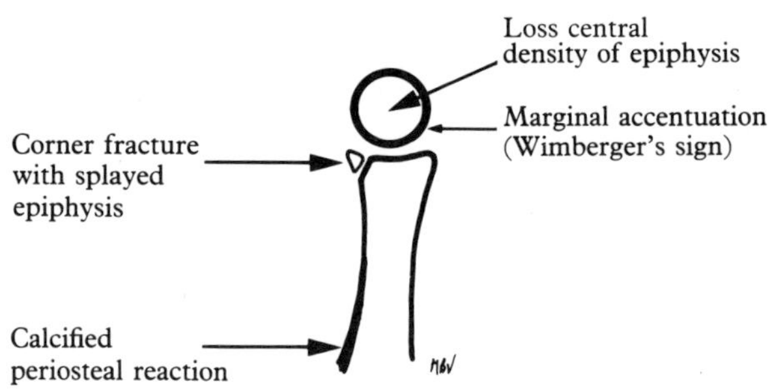

Fig. 23.2 Radiological features of scurvy

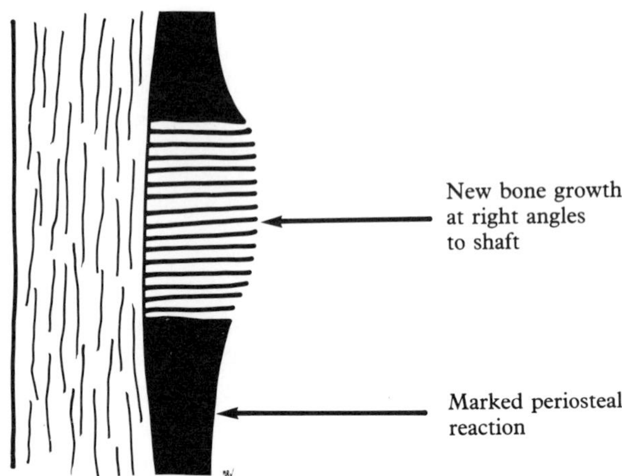

Fig. 23.3 Radiological features of osteosarcoma

BONE DISEASE

Malignant disease

Osteosarcoma

This is a malignant tumour of osteoblasts which often presents in childhood around the time of puberty. The femur is the commonest site, and the tumour usually present with pain and a limp. The characteristic radiological finding is periostitis associated with 'sun-ray' calcification due to bone formation by the spreading tumour (Fig. 23.3). Treatment is amputation, but the prognosis is not very good, with secondary spread occurring to the lungs.

Secondaries

Neuroblastoma is one of the commonest tumour of childhood and is derived from neural crest tissue from within the abdomen. Bone metastases are frequent and often widespread. The child may presents with a limp or refusal to walk, symptoms resembling childhood arthritis. Affected bones have a translucent, mottled, 'moth-eaten' appearance on X-ray, accompanied by marked periosteal new bone formation and occasional pathological fractures. The diagnosis is confirmed by finding a raised urinary VMA level, but the outlook is grim.

Ewing's tumour, lymphoma, rhabdomyosarcoma and malignant teratoma may also metastasis to bone in children.

Caffey's disease

This affects babies under the age of 1 year and causes pain, swelling and tenderness in one or several bones, usually the clavicle or mandible, accompanied by fever and malaise. X-ray shows swelling of bone with periosteal new bone formation. Osteomyelitis is the main differential diagnosis but if a limb bone is affected arhtritis may also be simulated. The condition is seldom severe and settles spontaneously after several months.

FURTHER READING (ARTHRITIS IN CHILDREN)

Ansell B M 1980 Rheumatic disorders in childhood. Postgraduate Series, Butterworth, London
Ansell B M 1983 Arthritis in young children. British Medical Journal 286: 1917–1918
Huskisson E C 1981 Musculoskeletal problems (adolescence). British Journal of Hospital Medicine Dec
Vaughan V C, McKay J R Jr, Behrman R E (eds) 1978 Nelson's textbook of paediatrics W B Saunders, Philadelphia

II The elderly

Rheumatic diseases are a major problem in the elderly. Some of the reasons for this are tabulated below.

Causes of disability from rheumatic disease in the elderly

1. Effect of ageing on normal connective tissues
2. High prevalence of chronic, non-fatal rheumatic diseases
3. Concurrent disease and failure of other systems
4. Social and psychological problems

Ageing of connective tissue results in loss of collagen and an alteration in the chemistry of cartilage proteoglycans, thin skin and bones, loss of muscle power, reduced joint mobility and a general loss of reserve and adaptability of the musculoskeletal system. There is also evidence of an alteration in immunological responses in the elderly, which may affect the expression of some rheumatic diseases and physiological changes which affect the handling of drugs.

Most of the major rheumatic diseases have a wide range in age of onset and many are chronic and progressive, but not fatal. The elderly therefore have an increased prevalence and severity of these diseases. Age is also associated with failure of other functions such as sight, hearing, balance and muscular co-ordination, which may make the disability much worse. Suffering and functional impairment may be further affected by social isolation, depression and other disadvantages of the elderly. Finally, dual pathology is common, so that elderly patients often have to contend with rheumatological problems in addition to some other major disorder. Multiple drug therapy often results, with further problems arising from toxicity and drug interactions.

AGEING AND RHEUMATIC DISEASE

Rheumatic diseases and age changes are related in several different ways. A few musculoskeletal conditions are a direct consequence of the ageing process. Many are more common in the elderly without being an inevitable part of growing old, whereas the onset of others is less frequent in older people. Finally, many of the major rheumatic diseases are expressed differently as age advances.

Ageing connective tissue

The ageing process includes several major changes in the structure and function of connective tissues. The skeleton loses calcium steadily from the age of about 50 onwards, women being affected much more severely than men. Articular cartilage also changes, losing volume and changing in its water content and in the biochemistry of the proteoglycans. Osteophytosis (but not osteoarthritis) appears to be an age-related phenomenon, and the incidence of chondrocalcinosis rises directly with age. Changes in the collagen and matrix of periarticular connective tissues contribute to the increasing prevalence of arthralgias and periarticular problems around the shoulder and elsewhere.

The relationship between ageing and musculoskeletal disease

1. *Rheumatic conditions related directly to ageing*
   a) Osteoporosis
   b) Chondrocalcinosis
   c) Osteophytosis
2. *Rheumatic conditions more common in the elderly*
   a) Paget's disease
   b) Polymyalgia rheumatica
   c) Giant cell arteritis
   d) Pyrophosphate arthropathy
   e) Osteoarthritis
3. *Rheumatic conditions less common in the elderly*
   a) Seronegative spondarthritides
   b) Connective tissue diseases
   c) Rheumatic fever
4. *Rheumatic conditions expressed differently in the elderly*
   a) Rheumatoid arthritis
   b) Systemic lupus erythematosus

Diseases which are common in the elderly

Many major rheumatic diseases are particularly common in old people. Paget's disease of bone, polymyalgia rheumatica, giant cell arteritis and pyrophosphate arthropathy are all very uncommon below the age of 50. Osteopaenic collapse of bone is common in the elderly, as is osteoarthritis, although the onset of OA peaks at about 60 and then subsides. Although related to age, none of these conditions are a direct consequence of ageing alone, other aetiological factors being necessary.

Diseases which are uncommon in old people

Ankylosing spondylitis and the reactive arthropathies rarely start in people over the age of 50. The onset of SLE is also uncommon in this age-group although it does occur. The reasons for these discrepancies are not known; perhaps the ageing process protects the body against certain reactions, just as it renders it more susceptible to others.

Diseases with a different expression in the elderly

Rheumatoid arthritis is thought by many authors to behave differently if it begins in old people. A high incidence of an acute onset, with a relatively benign course, has been reported by some but denied by others. The male–female ratio of RA reaches 1:1 in the elderly, and proximal joint involvement and increased peripheral oedema also appear to be more frequent than in younger patients. Systemic and extra-articular features are not prominent, although very high titres of rheumatoid factor are common.

SLE presenting in those over 50 is dominated by cutaneous, neuropsychiatric and pulmonary disease. The disease is often insidious and diagnosis may be made difficult by absence of conventional diagnostic aids such as antibodies to DNA. As with RA, the prognosis may be better than in those in whom the disease starts earlier.

Gout occurs in elderly women as often as men. Diuretics are often to blame and tophi may be prominent, whereas acute joint inflammation is often less obvious than in younger patients.

PRESENTATIONS

The major rheumatic diseases prevalent in the elderly are listed opposite. Three important presentations of these conditions will be described: exacerbation of a chronic musculoskeletal disorder, acute arthritis and arthralgia. In addition, rheumatological problems are frequently found to be contributing to suffering and disability in elderly patients admitted to hospital or presenting to the doctor with other types of health problems.

1. Exacerbation of chronic disease

Many rheumatic diseases are tolerated in people of all ages, being regarded as 'inevitable' or 'part of getting old', and with the attitude that 'nothing can be done'. Other patients remain fiercely independent of doctors and other help in spite of severe disease out of pride and self-respect.

Rheumatic diseases in the elderly

Common
1. Osteoarthritis and intervertebral disc disease
2. Rheumatoid arthritis
3. Pyrophosphate arthropathy
4. Polymyalgia rheumatica
5. Diuretic-induced gout
6. Osteopaenia
7. Ankylosing vertebral hyperostosis
8. Periarticular and soft tissue disorders

Uncommon
1. Rheumatological manifestations of neoplastic disease
2. Septic arthritis
3. Nutritional disorders

Rare
1. Sero-negative spondarthritides
2. SLE and other connective tissue diseases
3. Collagen and storage disorders, and other rheumatic diseases

Increasing age, with loss of ability in other systems and decreasing tolerance of long-standing problems, frequently results in patients with chronic disorders presenting for the first time at a stage when management may be difficult and therapy limited. Exacerbations of chronic rheumatic disease in the elderly may be part of the natural fluctuant history of a disease such as RA, or brought on by falls or intercurrent infection or disease. Age-related loss of function in the back of shoulder may also precipitate problems by preventing the patient from coping.

2. Acute arthritis in the elderly

Speedy diagnosis and treatment are essential to avoid prolonged inactivity which may lead to irrecoverable functional impairment. Of the listed causes, pseudogout is the commonest, but acute RA in the elderly and diuretic-induced gout are also frequently seen. Exacerbations of OA are sometimes quite severe, and may be induced by trauma. Rheumatological manifestations of neoplasia such as pulmonary osteoarthropathy, pancreatic arthropathy, dermatomyositis and carcinomatous arthritis are rare but important causes and are easy to miss. The signs of infection may be masked in the elderly, and joint sepsis, although uncommon, must always be excluded. Polymyalgia rheumatica is an important differential diagnosis, which may present with rapid onset of proximal myalgia, arthralgia and stiffness with prominent systemic symptoms.

Causes of acute arthritis in the elderly

Very common
Pseudogout

Common
1. Gout
2. Rheumatoid arthritis
3. Exacerbations of osteoarthritis
4. Polymyalgia rheumatica
5. Trauma

Uncommon
1. Neoplastic disease
2. Sepsis

Rare
Anything else

3. Arthralgia in the elderly

Old people often complain of severe musculoskeletal pain ('fibrositis', 'rheumatics', 'arthritis', 'the screws' etc). There is often no significant rheumatic disease to account for this. Common causes of both localised and generalised arthralgia are listed overleaf. Awareness of possible hypothyroidism, bone disease, neoplasia or Parkinson's disease is important, although pain is often based on minor articular or periarticular problems exacerbated by depression, loneliness with attention seeking, or the pain-amplification syndrome (syn 'fibrositis', see Chapter 19). Atypical polymyalgia rheumatica may also present as ill-defined arthralgia and drug toxicity must be considered, as many elderly patients are taking several different medicines.

Causes of arthralgia in the elderly

Generalised

1 Parkinson's disease
2. Hypothyroidism
3. Neoplastic disease
4. Depression
5. Pain-amplification syndrome
6. Osteopaenia
7. Polymyalgia rheumatica
8. Other rheumatic diseases

Localised

1. Soft-tissue disorders
2. Paget's disease of bone
3. Neoplastic disease
4. Osteopaenic bone collapse
5. Referred visceral pain
6. Referred root or peripheral nerve pain

DIAGNOSTIC PROBLEMS

Poor histories, difficulty in eliciting physical signs, confusing test results and multiple pathology are among the problems which may cause diagnostic difficulty in the elderly. Some physical signs and test results, all of which are often present in fit elderly people but would be considered abnormal in younger patients, are listed below.

Mild ulnar deviation, muscle-wasting and thin skin which easily bruises are common features of ageing, and may lead to the erroneous diagnosis of rheumatoid arthritis. Similarly, joint crepitus and a reduced range of movement, especially in the back, are common and normal in old people.

Investigations which may cause confusion include radiographic changes of OA. These are almost universal in the elderly, are often asymptomatic, and may have nothing to do with the symptoms and functional problems present. Chondrocalcinosis is present in about 25% of people over 75, and high ESRs, hyperuricaemia and low titres of a variety of auto-antibodies are also common in the elderly.

Tests, as well as the history and physical signs must be interpreted cautiously, and the chances of dual pathology are high in old people.

'Normal abnormalities' in elderly people

Physical signs and test results that may occur in elderly people without necessarily indicating the presence of rheumatic disease

Physical signs

1. Muscle-wasting
2. Joint subluxation
3. Ulnar deviation
4. Thin skin
5. Bruising
6. Reduced joint mobility
7. Joint crepitus

Investigations

1. Radiological osteoarthritis
2. Chondrocalcinosis
3. Vertebral hyperostosis
4. Hyperuricaemia
5. Rheumatoid factor
6. Anti-nuclear antibodies
7. Other auto-antibodies
8. Mild elevation of ESR

MANAGEMENT

The patient's social circumstances are crucial to management decisions. Home conditions, help available and functional requirements may alter the priority given to different therapeutic goals. Other factors which must be taken into account include the presence and prognosis of any intercurrent diseases and other therapy, as old people often find their way to huge numbers of drugs, clinics, doctors and paramedicals.

Some important management principles are outlined opposite. The biggest problems often arise from enforced immobility, which may lead to loss of function which can never be regained, and drug toxicity. Old people are particularly prone to fluid retention, neuropsychiatric disturbances and other side effects from anti-rheumatic drugs. Conversely, inflammatory diseases may respond particularly well to small doses of steroid (e.g. 7.5 mg nocte) which may be easier to justify than in younger people. The dose of many other drugs should be reduced in the elderly, as a combination of low

Management of rheumatic disease in the elderly

Priority aim

Maintain independence

Avoid

1. Bed-rest
2. Immobilisation
3. Too many drugs
4. Too much drug

Consider

1. Low-dose steroids for inflammatory disease
2. Local injections of steroid or radioactive colloids
3. Aids and appliances
4. Home physiotherapy and occupational therapy

serum albumin levels, reduced blood-flow to the liver and kidney and poor hepatic function can all increase free drug levels. Drug interactions, such as steroid-induced reduction of salicylate levels, may also be more common in the elderly.

Elderly patients are often unable or unwilling to get out of their houses for treatment, which may alter what can be attempted. Their expectations may be limited, and their acceptance of some degree of pain and immobility is often great. Common sense in the development of treatment goals is essential. Maintenance of functional independence, dignity and self respect, as well as reduction of symptoms, are the main aims of treatment. Aggressive therapeutic intervention with drugs or surgery should be avoided if possible. Many elderly people have enough to contend with, and tolerate doctors poorly. A team approach, with help being provided by social workers, occupational therapists, physiotherapists and chiropodists, is often needed.

III Pregnancy

Profound changes in cells of the immune system and of the connective tissues are produced during pregnancy. Although advantageous in preventing fetal rejection and in allowing accommodation and delivery of a sizeable infant, such changes may in addition influence the development and course of rheumatic disease. Though incomplete, knowledge of the factors involved is of obvious importance since:

1. Many of the major rheumatic diseases affect women of child-bearing age who need advice on possible effects of pregnancy on their disease and on effects of their disease and drugs on their pregnancy and baby
2. A pregnant woman with rheumatic symptoms may present a diagnostic and therapeutic dilemma
3. Investigation of disease modification by hormonal and non-hormonal factors may afford insight into pathogenetic mechanisms

Relevant normal physiological alterations in pregnancy will first be considered, and then known interactions between pregnancy and rheumatic disease will be described. The safety of anti-rheumatic drugs in pregnancy is discussed separately.

PHYSIOLOGICAL EFFECTS OF PREGNANCY

Major adaptations relevant to rheumatic disease are seen in connective tissues and in the inflammatory and immune response.

Connective tissues

Smooth muscle relaxation and generalised connective tissue extensibility result from increased progesterone levels and predispose to features such as varicose veins, skin hyperelasticity and ligamentous and joint laxity. Joint hypermobility (p 352) occurs throughout pregnancy, is independent of age and appears maximal during the second pregnancy. Further extreme relaxation of pelvic joints occurs around delivery and correlates well with circulating levels of relaxin: widening and instability of symphysis pubis and sacro-iliac joints may be particularly marked.

Calcium, utilised late by the fetus, is withdrawn from maternal long-bone trabeculae. If maternal stores are insufficient, preferential delivery to the fetus may occasionally result in maternal osteomalacia with maintained serum calcium levels and, in addition, contribute to osteoporosis in later life.

Inflammatory and immune response

There is ample evidence for suppression of the inflammatory response. Several animal models exhibit marked reduction of inflammation during gestation, and human pregnant serum is capable of depressing PMN phagocytosis, enzyme release, intracellular killing and chemotactic response *in vitro*.

Evidence suggesting depression of cell-mediated immunity in pregnancy

1. Depressed tuberculin reaction
2. Delayed skin graft rejection
3. More severe periodontal disease
4. Hastened dissemination of breast carcinoma
5. Increased severity of intracellular pathogens (viral, protozoal, fungal)
6. Diminished *in vitro* T lymphocyte response
7. ? altered T:B cell ratio

Serum factors implicated in depression of cell mediated immunity in pregnancy

1. Human chorionic gonadotropin (HCG)
2. Human chorionic somatomammotropin (HPL)
3. Oestrogens (oestriol, oestrone, oestradiol)
4. Progestagens
5. Adrenal corticosteroids
6. Alpha fetoprotein (AFP)
7. Circulating antibodies
8. Pregnancy-associated α_2-glycoprotein (PAG)

Maternal cell-mediated immunity has understandably received considerable attention, since blocking of the recognition or effector limbs of this response is vital in prevention of fetal rejection. Evidence for depression of CMI is impressive. The normal behaviour of washed lymphocytes from pregnant women strongly suggests that serum factors are responsible for this depression, and several pregnancy-associated factors have been implicated.

Although these factors inhibit lymphocyte and/or PMN function *in vitro*, their immunosuppressive role at physiological concentrations remains in question. HPL, first detectable at 6 weeks and rising to a plateau after the second trimester, shows definite *in vitro* lymphocyte suppression at physiological levels, but evidence for other hormones is unimpressive. An IgG blocking factor, which prevents production of lymphocyte migration inhibitory factor and which is absent from serum of recurrent aborters, has been identified, but its specificity and role in immunosuppression remain uncertain. Undoubtedly the single most promising candidate is PAG. Serum levels of this glycoprotein are detectable by 12 weeks and rise until 30 weeks — its half-life post-partum is 7 days. Serum levels appear genetically determined, being greatly raised in 75% of pregnant women, and correlate well with disease remission in RA. PAG demonstrates suppressive effects on inflammatory and immune cells *in vitro* at physiological concentrations and its detection on leukocyte surfaces suggests that it may act by masking surface receptors.

Clinical aspects of physiological adaptations

Alteration in connective tissues during pregnancy uncommonly results in peripheral joint problems due to benign hypermobility syndrome (p 352). Ligamentous and joint laxity, however, together with the bulk of a gravid uterus and the necessary alteration in locomotion ('waddling gait') may contribute to the common symptom of backache. Abdominal distension and water retention may both predispose to development of meralgia paraesthetica in late pregnancy.

INTERACTION BETWEEN PREGNANCY AND RHEUMATIC DISEASE

Information on such interaction is sparse, often being based on collected case reports, and largely relating to RA or SLE. In general, however, it would seem that pregnancy exerts an ameliorating effect on inflammatory synovitis, but connective tissue disorders usually fare worse.

Rheumatoid arthritis

75% of patients report a marked decrease in joint symptoms during pregnancy (Fig. 23.4). Improvement usually starts near the end of the first trimester, lasts through to the end of gestation, and appears independent of age, disease duration, disease severity or seropositivity. Objective evidence of improvement may be less striking and the effect on extra-articular features is unknown. Regardless of any improvement during pregnancy, almost all patients experience exacerbation, usually within 6 weeks and inevitably by 8 months, following abortion, miscarriage or delivery — the timing appearing unrelated to length of lactation or resumption of menstruation. Such exacerbation at a time when many healthy mothers experience considerable stress may result in major difficulties with the increased work load of child care.

Although 75% of patients undergo remission, pregnancy is not a panacea for RA: 25% will either not improve or deteriorate, and in a few the disease may actually appear for the first time in the second or third trimester. In any individual, however, whatever happens in one pregnancy will recur in others, suggesting a constitutional mechanism for pregnancy–disease interaction. Genetically controlled marked increases in PAG occur in those patients that improve; the levels correlating well with the timing of disease remission.

There is no evidence that pregnancy alters the subsequent course of RA. Observations on the effect of disease on fetal abnormality, abortion rate or incidence of obstetric complication are lacking. Some reports suggest decreased fertility in patients with RA and it seems likely that fecundity is lowered by the effects of chronic disease, depression, and hip involvement with limited hip abduction. Current low-dose oestrogen oral contraceptives appear perfectly safe in patients with RA, and there is recent evidence to suggest that use of the oral contraceptive may actually decrease the risk of developing RA.

SLE

In general, pregnancy in a patient with lupus is more likely to result in exacerbation than

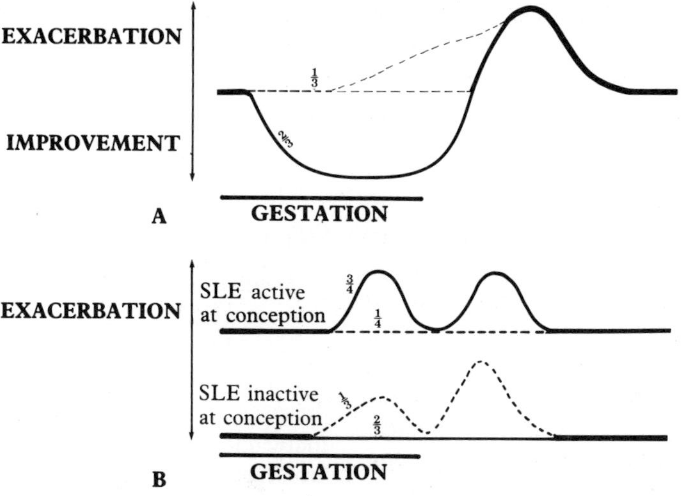

Fig. 23.4 Effect of pregnancy on patients with (**A**) RA and (**B**) SLE

remission, the likelihood of a flare being principally determined by disease activity at the onset of gestation (Fig. 23.4). If inactive at conception mild flares may occur at any stage, but particularly during the puerperium, in one-third of patients; but if the lupus is active at the outset then two-thirds of patients may expect exacerbation, occasionally severe, especially during the third trimester or puerperium. Unlike the situation in RA, the response in one pregnancy is not necessarily repeated in others. Patients with moderate or severe renal disease rarely become pregnant but in those that do deterioration in renal function occurs in less than 10%. Deterioration in such patients should be aggressively treated with steroids together, if necessary, with immunosuppressives after the first trimester.

A special problem may be the differentiation of acute lupus nephritis from pre-eclampsia, an immune-complex-mediated disorder particularly occurring in primigravidae after the twentieth week. Both conditions may give rise to hypertension, proteinuria, oedema, thrombocytopenia, confusion and seizures. In SLE, additional features may be present to aid in diagnosis (e.g. rash, alopecia) and hypocomplementaemia and positive ANA, both absent in pre-eclampsia, are usual. The two disorders may, however, occasionally occur together and if there is any doubt both should be treated simultaneously (magnesium sulphate for PET: steroids for SLE).

Fertility is probably unaffected by SLE except during active disease when amenorrhoea, altered libido and marital dysharmony are frequent. There is good evidence, however, that active lupus adversely affects fetal survival, patients with SLE showing increased incidence of spontaneous abortions, premature labour and stillbirths, and an increased perinatal mortality. The cause of the increased fetal wastage is unknown, though a variety of factors have been implicated, including circulating lupus anticoagulant, lymphocytotoxic antibodies which cross-react with trophoblast, decidual vasculopathy and lupus nephritis. Although IgG antibodies readily cross the placenta, neonatal SLE is uncommon, usually presenting with rash, splenomegaly, anaemia and thrombocytopenia, and undergoing spontaneous resolution within 4 months. Though congenital heart block may rarely occur, major organ involvement or death are unusual. The development of both neonatal lupus and congenital heart block as an isolated feature in the new-born is strongly associated with the placental transfer of a particular maternal autoantibody, namely anti Ro(SSA).

In general, therefore, patients with lupus who wish to become pregnant should be encouraged to do so if their disease is inactive and renal function normal — only 30% will experience a mild, easily controlled flare and delivered children will probably be normal. Initiating or increasing the dose of steroids at delivery may reduce the incidence of post-partum flares. Patients with active lupus, renal insufficiency or hypertension, however, should be discouraged from pregnancy until their disease has been controlled for at least 6 months. There is both animal and human data to suggest that oestrogens may exacerbate SLE so that if oral contraceptives are used the lowest oestrogen dose should be selected and the patient should be monitored carefully — any disease exacerbation should lead to prompt withdrawal.

Diseases that may be ameliorated by pregnancy

1. Peripheral psoriatic arthropathy (c. 30% improve)
2. Chronic sarcoid arthritis (two-thirds improve but relapse post-partum)
3. Palindromic rheumatism
4. Behcet's
5. Familial Mediterranean fever

Other rheumatic diseases

Though information is scant, inflammatory synovitis in general appears to be improved by pregnancy. The effect of pregnancy on other organ systems and the fetus in systemic connective tissue diseases, however, is more often deleterious, maternal renal function in particular being adversely affected e.g.:

1. Patients with scleroderma show increased fetal wastage (perhaps due to placental transmission

of an anti-endothelial cell factor), and development of hypertension during pregnancy carries a very high mortality.
2. PAN is almost uniformly fatal post-partum due to renal failure and hypertension.
3. Eosinophilic fasciitis and polymyositis may both first present in pregnancy: polymyositis may subsequently remit post-partum but a high infant mortality is usual:

It therefore seems sensible, as with lupus, to dissuade patients with connective-tissue diseases from pregnancy if their disease is active or if they show renal impairment. Further information on pregnancy–disease interaction, however, is badly needed and such advice must always be balanced by the situation of the individual patient.

PRESENTATION OF *DE NOVO* RHEUMATIC DISEASE

Diagnosis of rheumatic disease in pregnancy presents a difficult clinical problem. Backache is almost universal and may be considered a normal feature, though persistent, severe or asymmetrical back pain should always alert one to the possibility of renal infection or obstetric complication. X-rays and scans are obviously contra-indicated and biochemical tests of inflammation may be falsely misleading. Great reliance must therefore be placed on the history and physical examination.

Since any of the rheumatic diseases, including RA, may first start in pregnancy, they must still be considered, as appropriate, in the differential diagnosis of rheumatic problems in a pregnant woman. Certain conditions, however, appear particularly associated with the pregnant state and should therefore always be considered.

Alterations in haematological and biochemical indices in normal pregnancy that may be falsely interpreted as reflecting inflammation

1. Lowered haemoglobin ('anaemia of pregnancy')
2. Low serum iron and depleted iron stores (common)
3. Raised ESR (× 4), elevated viscosity
4. ↑ fibrinogen, ↑ β globulin
5. ↓ total protein, ↓ albumin, ↓ γ globulin (followed by ↑ in late pregnancy)
6. (↑ lipids and lipoproteins, particularly cholesterol)

1. Transient osteoporosis of the hip

This rare disorder of unknown aetiology may particularly occur in late pregnancy or around delivery. Presentation is typically with rapid onset of severe, progressive hip pain, worsened by movement and made better by rest. Movement of the affected hip is restricted by pain, and atrophy of pelvic girdle and quadriceps muscles may develop after several weeks. X-rays, if performed, are normal at the onset, but within 6–8 weeks the following typical appearance is usually present:

a) Diffuse osteoporosis of the femoral head and neck, and occasionally also of the acetabulum and adjacent iliac bone (i.e. regional osteoporosis)
b) A diffuse femoral head and acetabular cortical outline implying demineralisation of the calcified cartilagenous zone
c) Normal width of articular space
d) Absence of erosions or deformity

Early isotope bone scans in cases unassociated with pregnancy show increased activity in the absence of X-ray changes. The condition is inevitably self-limiting, with complete recovery and remineralisation within several months. Steroids or ACTH may hasten recovery but reassurance, initial rest and subsequent graded exercise are usually sufficient. In some cases, the condition may recur in the opposite hip.

Aseptic necrosis of the femoral head may present similar symptoms but X-ray changes are characteristic after several weeks (p 347). A similar clinical, X-ray and isotope scan appearance may occur in migratory regional osteoporosis (reflex sympathetic dystrophy, p 233) but in this condition hyperaemia, oedema, warm dry skin and causalgia-like tenderness are usually present.

2. Acute gonococcal arthritis

This is a notable exception to the general rule that synovitis is improved by pregnancy. Mechanical, hormonal and vascular changes in the third trimester particularly predispose to haematogenous dissemination of gonococci with resultant tendency to joint involvement (p 197).

3. Acute sarcoid arthritis

This classically may present, usually with erythema nodosum, in late pregnancy or during lactation (p 314). .

ANTIRHEUMATIC DRUGS AND PREGNANCY

For patients with rheumatic disease the principle that all drugs should be avoided in pregnancy unless absolutely necessary still applies. The risk from drug use, however, must always be weighed against the need for control of the mother's symptoms and disease.

The ethical impossibility of controlled drug trials on pregnant women and the understandable reluctance of drug companies to recommend anything other than total avoidance of their product during gestation means that information on toxic effects of drugs on the fetus is based on theoretical grounds alone or on isolated case reports, retrospective observation or extension from animal studies. Assessment of deleterious effects on the fetus is particular difficult since active rheumatic disease itself may result in increased fetal wastage and high incidence of low-birth-weight infants. Although potential toxic effects from drugs used in rheumatic disease are numerous, in practice their sensible and judicious use rarely results in problems.

Data on toxic effects of NSAIDs in pregnancy is lacking, except for aspirin where several studies suggest that the risk of fetal abnormality is not enhanced but that gestation and labour may be prolonged (but only by 1 week and 5 hours respectively): perinatal maternal bleeding may also be enhanced. Since these risks probably relate to prostaglandin synthetase inhibition they are likely to be shared by other NSAIDs and depend on continued drug use. In the absence of other data, therefore, it would seem sensible to use aspirin for women who require an anti-inflammatory agent in pregnancy, but to use as low and infrequent a dose as possible and to try to withdraw medication in the last month.

Glucocorticosteroids appear to be well tolerated in pregnancy and there is no convincing evidence for significant danger to the fetus. The teratogenicity of methotrexate, cyclophosphamide and chlorombucil, if used in the first trimester, is well

Potential effects of antirheumatic drugs on the fetus

Salicylates
1. Prolonged gestation and labour
2. Perinatal maternal haemorrhage
3. Neonatal haemorrhage
4. Fetal salicylism

NSAIDs
1. Premature closure of ductus arteriosus
2. Uteroplacental circulatory dysfunction

Penicillamine
1. Reversible cutis laxa
2. B6 deficiency
3. Neonatal myaesthesia

Gold
Teratogenicity (rats)

Hydroxychloroquine
Sensorineural hearing loss

Glucocorticosteroids
1. Intra-uterine growth retardation
2. Suppression of adrenocortical function
3. Suppression of fetal immunity
4. Congenital malformation

Azathioprine
Intra-uterine growth retardation

Methotrexate
Cyclophosphamide
Chlorambucil
Multiple fetal abnormality if given in first trimester

documented and such drugs should not be used. Azathioprine, however, appears relatively safe and is the cytotoxic of choice if such an agent is necessary, though avoidance of use in the first trimester is still advised (use of steroids may allow postponement of azathioprine introduction until the end of the first trimester in conditions such as active lupus nephritis).

Hydroxychloroquine, penicillamine and gold are generally avoided, though data on their effects during pregnancy is scant. Such agents should be stopped if pregnancy is confirmed.

Most drugs are excreted in breast milk but usually in very small amounts. The newborn metabolise and excrete drugs inefficiently and preterm infants are especially at risk: the risk decreases as renal and hepatic function mature. Where practicable all drugs should be avoided during breast feeding, but unfortunately the postpartum period is the time that most rheumatic diseases flare. Paracetamol and aspirin are safe for occasional use: aspirin dosage exceeding 3 g/day may, however, result in metabolic acidosis in the infant. Codeine and dihydrocodeine in high doses should be avoided for fear of infant CNS depression. Of the anti-inflammatory analgesic agents naproxen, ibuprofen, ketoprofen and fenbufen, which appear only in minute amounts in the milk, are to be preferred. There is no evidence that glucocorticoids damage the suckling infant, but cytotoxic and 'second-line' agents are to be avoided.

FURTHER READING (PREGNANCY)

Cecere F A, Persellin R H 1981 The interaction of pregnancy and the rheumatic diseases. Clinics in Rheumatic Diseases 7(3): 747–768

Persellin R H 1981 Inhibitors of inflammatory and immune responses in pregnancy serum. Clinics in Rheumatic Diseases 7(3): 769–780

IV Racial and Geographic Groups

INTRODUCTION

Complete data on the prevalence of rheumatic disorders throughout the world is not available; nevertheless from epidemiological surveys that have been done on selected populations, it is clear that there is considerable variation in the prevalence and severity between peoples. Many factors may account for these differences including genetic defects, as in FMF and sickle-cell disease; climate; sanitation; nutrition; prevalence of infecting agents; and cultural influences.

GEOGRAPHIC VARIATION IN THE MAJOR RHEUMATIC DISEASES

Rheumatoid arthritis

Although RA was once thought to be a disease of the wet northern areas, it is now known that it occurs worldwide and that there is no relation with latitude, humidity or hours of sunshine. The highest prevalence recorded so far for RA is in the Yakima Indians in Washington state, USA, and the lowest in Japan, where 0.2% of the population are affected and the disease is virtually unknown in men. There is a marked variation in disease severity throughout the world: progressive erosive disease with extra-articular features such as vasculitis and complications such as amyloidosis are commoner in Western Europe, particularly in the United Kingdom.

Black races tend to have benign seronegative RA and one theory postulated to explain this is that malaria may exert a suppressive effect. Many black Africans are also chronically iron-deficient from hook-worm infestation and this may diminish their ability to mount a sustained inflammatory response. There is, on the other hand, a five- to tenfold increase in the incidence of positive latex fixation tests for rheumatoid factor in Central Africa compared to Europe and again the high prevalence of parasitic infection, particularly malaria and filariasis, may cause this.

The distribution of joint involvement also varies in different racial groups. For example, Jamaicans have synovitis primarily of the knees, ankles and feet, with prominent erosions in the feet, which has been related to their habit of going barefoot and is supported by the converse finding of a very low incidence of erosions in the feet of people who wear clogs.

Osteoarthritis

There are some striking geographical differences in the prevalence of generalised nodal osteoarthritis (GOA). It is rare in the Black population and amongst the Pima Indians. When it does occur in the latter group it is far commoner in men than in women, which is the reverse situation to that in Europeans. GOA is rare in the black people of Jamaica but thoracic spinal OA is frequently seen and is thought to be due to the habit of carrying heavy loads on the top of the head. OA of the hip is rare in Chinese and cultural factors have again been suggested as the reason, in particular the national habit of squatting at rest rather than sitting in a chair. Ankylosing hyperostosis of the spine (Forrestier's disease) is common in the Pima Indians and may be related to the high fluoride level in the water which stimulates new bone formation and the high incidence of diabetes which is known to be associated in other populations.

A particularly severe and crippling form of OA is endemic in children and young adults in Eastern Siberia, Northern China and North Korea and is called Kashin–Beck disease after the people who described it. There is arrested epipheseal maturation, avascular necrosis and disturbance of growth affecting the fingers, large joints and spine, which progresses causing marked disability with arthritis mutilans and shortening of the limbs. This disease is of considerable theoretical importance since it appears to be due either to toxic destruction of cartilage and bone caused by eating cereal grain contaminated with the fungus *Fusaria sporotrichiella*, to an abnormal amino acid present in strains of cereal grain which are adapted to grow in these cold areas, or to a high iron content in the drinking water.

SERONEGATIVE SPONDARTHRITIS

Ankylosing spondylitis affects about 1% of the white male population but in male Haida Indians there is a 10% incidence of sacro-iliitis, and there is also a high prevalence of HLA-B27 in this racial group. The American Black on the other hand has a low carriage rate for B27 and only about 0.25% of the men have sacro-iliitis. Reiter's syndrome is common in many of the Third World countries but the antecedent infection is much more likely to be dysentery than a venereal disease.

SLE AND THE VASCULITIDES

SLE is a common disease in black American and West Indian women as a cause not only of arthritis and skin rash but also of severe neuropsychiatric disturbance. The reason for this is not clear, but it cannot be entirely genetic since SLE is rare in African women. The disease generally follows a typical clinical course but the skin manifestations are influenced by skin colour and hyperkeratotic scarring and depigmentation are common.

People of oriental extraction, particularly the Japanese, are prone to two special variants of arteritis. Kawasaki's disease is a form of infantile PAN with a predilection for the coronary arteries which is discussed further earlier in this chapter. Takayasu's disease (aortic arch syndrome or pulseless disease) occurs in young women and is characterised by occlusion of the major vessels arising from the aorta, resulting in syndromes of vascular insufficiency, including transient cerebral ischaemia, strokes, blindness, myocardial infarction and peripheral gangrene. There is often a 'pre-pulseless' stage associated with Raynaud's phenomenon, a variable arthritis, skin rash, pericarditis, iritis, arterial tenderness and bruits, and a raised ESR. Aortography confirms the diagnosis. Steroids, anticoagulants and arterial surgery may be required. The course is chronic and relapsing and arterial occlusion may be fatal.

Gout

This is a common disease amongst the Pacific Polynesian people and the Maoris of New Zealand. This may partly be explained by its association with obesity and high alcohol intake but it is probably also genetically determined.

Paget's disease

This disease has a striking geographical distribution, being common in Anglo-Saxon populations but rare in Africa, India, China and the Middle East; and it is unheard-of in North American Indians. The prevalence varies also within countries and in the United Kingdom there is a marked concentration around the old cotton-mill towns of Lancashire, for unknown reasons.

Osteoporosis

Women of Anglo-Saxon origin are prone to develop osteoporosis much more frequently than women of a similar age in the Third World. A comparison between Bantu women and women of European extraction in South Africa showed that the European women had 25 times the risk of osteoporotic fracture. Whether this relates to the economic necessity for Bantu women to continue hard physical work into old age is not known, and genetic factors may also be involved.

INFLUENCE OF NUTRITION

Over two-thirds of the world's population is half-starved so that in certain parts of the world nutritional musculo-skeletal diseases such as rickets, osteomalacia, scurvy and stunted growth are rife. Malnutrition also lowers resistance to disease generally, particularly infection which in turn may cause permanent joint damage. Unfortunately even when useful sources of food are available, cultural traditions may prohibit their use. On the other hand, gout is the disease of plenty and its declining prevalence may be due to a reduction in the gluttony practised by those people fortunate enough to have access to limitless amounts of food and drink. Obesity is still a common finding in patients with gout and may also accelerate osteoarthrits of the weight-bearing joints.

Rickets and scurvy are due to deficiency of vitamins D and C respectively, occur in children and are discussed fully in the first part of this chapter. Women and children from the Indian subcontinent who migrate to areas where there is no shortage of vitamin-D-containing foods continue to have a high incidence of osteomalacia and rickets. The cause is a combination of a diet poor in vitamin D, usually vegetarian, and a lack of skin production of vitamin D due to racial skin pigmentation, total concealment of the body by clothing and a housebound existence. An extreme version of the last is seen in the Moslem world where the cultural tradition still imposes strict *purdah* on its women which, coupled with constant child-bearing and poor diet, can result in severe osteomalacia. Death in childbirth from obstructed labour secondary to pelvic disproportion was a common occurrence in harems.

Tropical polymyositis is an entity well-recognised in the tropics to be associated with malnutrition. It presents with fever, malaise and painful indurated muscles usually of the lower limbs and culminates in suppuration and abscess formation. Streptococci and staphylococci are frequently isolated, but it is not clear if these are primary or secondary infecting organisms.

INFECTIOUS FACTORS

Climate, prevalence of organisms, suitable insect vectors or intermediate hosts and public health facilities such as sewers and clean water supply will influence the type of infectious disease occurring in people living in different parts of the world. Some organisms are ubiquitous and are capable of causing outbreaks of disease if the natural balance is altered in their favour. In times of war and deprivation typhoid fever, dysentery, tuberculosis and rheumatic fever quickly surface even in the most advanced societies. Brucellosis, for example, is only controlled by eradication of the organism from cattle by pasteurisation of milk. In countries where these measures are not so stringently carried out, such as in Spain, brucellosis is a not uncommon cause of severe back pain and sacroiliitis.

Ross River epidemic polyarthritis and Lyme arthritis are examples of diseases occurring in a limited geographical area because they require a specific tick for transmission to occur. Major infectious diseases such as leprosy, tuberculosis, syphilis, brucellosis and the fungal infections are described fully in the chapter on infection and arthritis and rheumatic fever earlier in this chap-

Some infectious causes of joint and bone disease common outside Europe

1. Bacterial
   a) Leprosy
   b) TB
   c) Yaws
   d) Brucellosis
   e) Salmonellosis
   f) Rheumatic fever
   g) Syphilis
   h) Bacillary dysentery
2. Viral
   a) Dengue fever
   b) Lymphogranuloma venerum
3. Protozoal
   Guinea worm
4. Fungal
   a) Histoplasmosis
   b) Coccidioiodomycosis
   c) Blastomycosis

ter. Some aspects of these and other more exotic causes of musculoskeletal pain will be discussed in this section.

Tuberculosis

This is said to be 30 times commoner in Asians and Africans and three times commoner in Irish and West Indians than in Western Europeans generally. This is not due to environmental factors alone, although poor social circumstances are an added risk, since these people transport their increased susceptibility with them when they move to areas where tuberculosis is rare. Non-pulmonary tuberculosis is frequently encountered and multiple infections of hips, knees, spine and tendon sheaths without an obvious primary focus are frequently encountered. Systemic features such as fever, sweats and weight-loss are often pronounced in Asians but the ESR may be normal and the Mantoux test unhelpful. The diagnosis must be confirmed by aspiration of pus if possible and culture of the bacillus, since many tropical strains of mycobacteria are resistant to standard chemotherapeutic agents.

Salmonellosis

In countries where sanitation is primitive, enteric fever is common. Elsewhere it is rare but occasional outbreaks, such as that caused by contaminated Argentinian corned beef in Aberdeen in the early 1960s, do occur and people travelling abroad may also become infected. Arthritis due to direct spread to joints occurs in 0.25% of all cases but 2.5% of cases caused by *Salmonella cholerasuis*. This is usually monoarticular and affects the large joints, particularly the knee. Diarrhoea is often absent. The organism can be cultured either from the synovial fluid or from the stool. A post-*Salmonella* reactive lower-limb arthritis occurs in 2.5% of cases of *Salmonella typhimurium* infections, usually 2 weeks after the onset of diarrhoea and fever, and follows a chronic course with remissions and relapses over several months; however, it usually resolves completely. Rising titres of antibodies can be detected in the blood. The organism can be isolated from the stools but not the joints. *Salmonella* organisms have a predilection for the bony infarcts in sickle-cell disease where they are a common cause of osteomyelitis.

Bacillary dysentry

This is caused by the *Shigella* organism and is endemic throughout the world. Outbreaks occur wherever there are crowded conditions with poor sanitation. In the tropics, dysentery is spread by flies and elsewhere by unwashed hands and contaminated food, particularly in institutions such as schools or hospitals for the subnormal. The illness is characterised by diarrhoea, tenesmus and colicky abdominal pain. About 1.5% of patients develop a Reiter's-type reactive arthritis but this figure rises to 20% in those who possess HLA-B27. Sulphonamides and ampicillin are effective in treating *Shigella* infection.

Dengue fever

This disease is common along the coast in tropical and subtropical countries and is caused by an airborne virus transmitted by the *Aedes* mosquito. About 5 days following a bite, there is onset of malaise followed by fever and severe generalised arthralgia in many joints. The fever classically subsides after a week only to recur several days later ('saddle-back fever') often accompanied by a morbilliform rash on the extremities. The disease is self-limiting and recurrent infection confers a degree of immunity. The diagnosis is confirmed by rising titres of viral antibodies. There is no specific treatment but aspirin or paracetamol are symptomatically helpful. Mosquito nets and abolition of stagnant water breeding sites are the most useful measures against this disease.

Lymphogranuloma venereum

This is caused by a ricketsial virus related to the organism of trachoma and psittacosis. It is a venereal infection common in the sexually promiscuous who visit foreign ports. 1–4 weeks after exposure, a small lesion appears on the penis or vulva, followed by massive enlargement of the inguinal lymph nodes which may become necrotic and form numerous small skin sinuses; fistulae between rectum and urethra or vagina; and lymphatic obstruction. A polyarticular arthritis of large joints can occur at any stage. The diagnosis is confirmed by the response to an intradermal injection of killed virus (Frei test). Tetracyclines are effective but a large number of infected nodes may require surgical clearance.

Yaws

This is caused by *Treponema pertenue* which is morphologically and serologically indistinguishable from syphilis. It is common in people living in isolated primitive communities. The organism is transmitted by close bodily contact — most often from mother to child. The primary lesion is a cutaneous sore, like a syphilitic chancre, often on the leg or buttock, followed by a formidable generalised papillomatous eruption. The metacarpal, phalangeal and carpal bones are the site of intense periosteal inflammation, causing 'sausage-digit', swollen nasal bones and sabre tibia. These early lesions usually heal. 5–10 years later, tertiary yaws may develop, characterised by deep, penetrating cutaneous ulcers, periostitis and osteitis. Lesions on the face and scalp, collapse of the bridge of the nose and palatal perforation may lead to hideous deformities. Contraction of joints and bony collapse from rarefaction of bone are common musculoskeletal features. Penicillin is highly effective in eradicating the organism.

Guinea worm

The female guinea worm (*Dranunculus medinensis*) is a thin nematode about 1 m long which lives in the intestines and subcutaneous tissues of men. Infection is acquired by ingesting the intermediate host, a crustacean — *Cyclops* (water flea), which lives in ponds and wells. Once fully mature, the gravid female seeks the surface of the skin in order to lay her eggs externally in a site likely to be inhabited by *Cyclops*. Occasionally, the female discharges her larvae into a joint, causing a severe monoarthritis usually of the knee. There is often considerable systemic disturbance with fever, pruritis and a marked eosinophilia. The worms may grow to maturity in the joint. Exploration via arthrotomy or arthroscopy is needed to remove the worms and larvae under cover of niridazole given for a week prior to the procedure. Antibiotics may be needed to treat secondary infection, and tetanus is a well-described complication. Calcified remains of worms may be seen in the soft tissues or on X-ray.

REFERENCES (RACIAL AND GEOGRAPHIC GROUPS)

Lawrence J S Heinemann J S 1977 Rheumatism in populations

Wright F J, Baird J P 1971 Tropical diseases, 4th edn. Supplement to: Davidson S, MacLead J The principles and practice of medicine. Churchill Livingstone, Edinburgh.

24 Investigations

I Disease Assessment

In any chronic disease it is vital to be able to assess the activity, progression and therapeutic response of the patient. A variety of clinical, haematological, biochemical and imaging techniques have been developed to assess rheumatic diseases. Many of these methods are used most widely to assess treatment, particularly in drug trials. No measurement is perfect, most vary considerably and many have a large subjective element. Rheumatologists therefore often use composite charts which correlate several different clinical and laboratory assays to follow the progress of their patients.

CLINICAL MEASUREMENTS

Some of the clinical measurements used are categorised below. Subjective assessment of the patient's or physician's opinion of change with time is unsatisfactory and numerical indices to measure specific aspects of the symptoms (e.g. pain), activity (e.g. evidence of inflammation) or functional impairment have therefore been developed.

Categories of clinical measurement used to assess rheumatic diseases

1. Subjective assessment of change (better or worse)
2. Measurement of pain, pain relief or stiffness
3. Measurement of joint tenderness
4. Measurement of inflammation and disease activity
5. Measurement of joint movement
6. Assessment of function

Clinical measurements of disease activity

Pain
Simple descriptive scale (none–mild–moderate–severe)
Visual analogue scale

Stiffness
Severity of morning or inactivity stiffness
Duration (min) of stiffness

Joint tenderness
Articular index (summation of tenderness scored as none–mild–moderate–severe in individual joints)

Inflammation
Joint size/circumference e.g. PIP 'ring' size; Knee circumference
Grip strength

Function
20-yard walking time
Timed tasks
Functional index of disability (e.g. Steinbocker Index)
Range of movement

Symptoms

Pain is the major symptom of most disorders, but is difficult to measure. Simple descriptive scales, None–Mild–Moderate–Severe for example, may be useful; visual analogue scales may improve discrimination and are widely used. Patients are asked to mark a point representing their pain on a 10 cm line between 'no pain' and 'pain as bad as it could be' (Fig. 24.1A). The scale is non-linear and the figure obtained has no absolute value, but the technique is useful when measuring treatment responses in a given patient. Stiffness is another symptom which can be charted on a descriptive scale or assessed in terms of duration: the time it takes to loosen up in the morning is a rough measurement of the activity of inflammation in many diseases.

Joint tenderness

Joint tenderness, like pain and stiffness, may reflect inflammation, but can have other causes. Local tenderness can be recorded as absent, mild, moderate or severe, and a summation of the score obtained from all the major joints can provide a relatively quick and easy numerical assay of disease activity. The Ritchie articular index is one such score often used to assess rheumatoid arthritis.

Inflammation

Joint swelling can be measured and used to assess changes in inflammation (Fig. 24.1C). Proximal interphalangeal joint diameter is used in RA, and knee-joint circumference can also be followed. Grip strength of the hand also reflects inflammation and can be measured with a modified sphygmomanometer (Fig. 24.1D). When these techniques are used by a single skilled observer errors are reduced, and if combined with measurements of morning stiffness, pain and articular index, a useful clinical assessment of disease activity can be obtained.

Joint movement

Normal joint motion varies with age, sex and race. Figure 24.2 outlines the normal ranges of some of

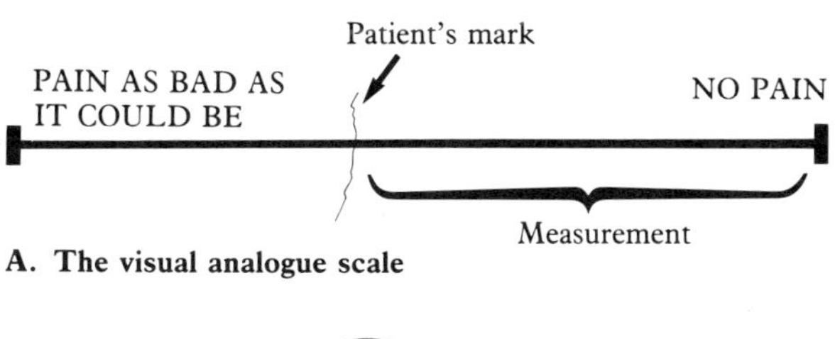

A. The visual analogue scale

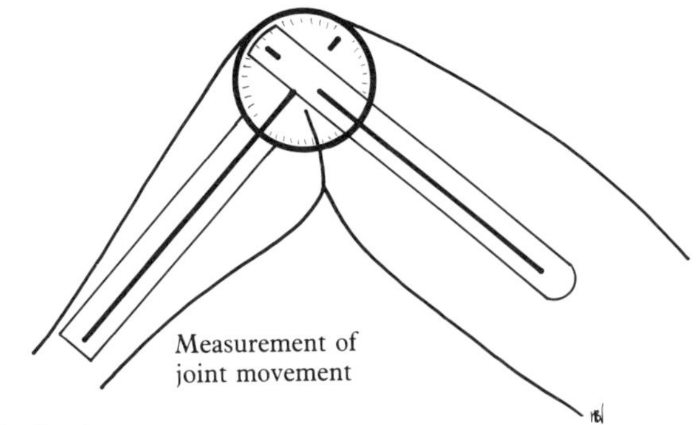

B. Goniometer

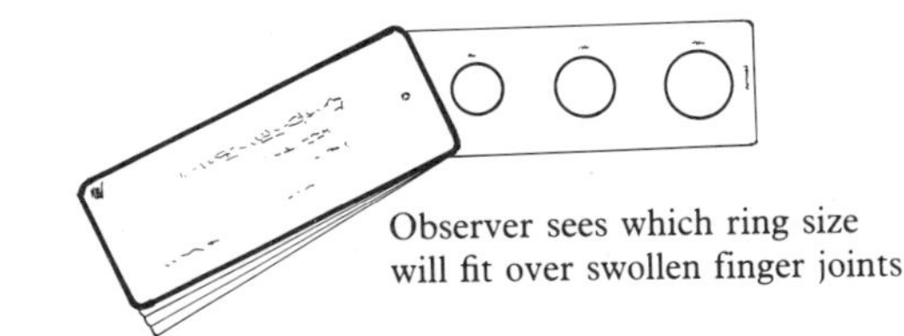

C. Measurement of 'ring size'

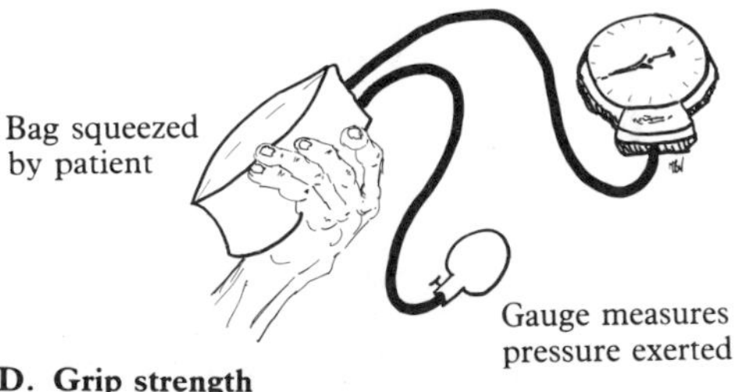

D. Grip strength

Fig. 24.1 Examples of some techniques used to measure joint disease.

the major joints. Accurate measurements can be made with a goniometer (Fig. 24.1B), and change with time can be recorded.

Function

Function is probably both the most important and the most difficult parameter to measure. A variety

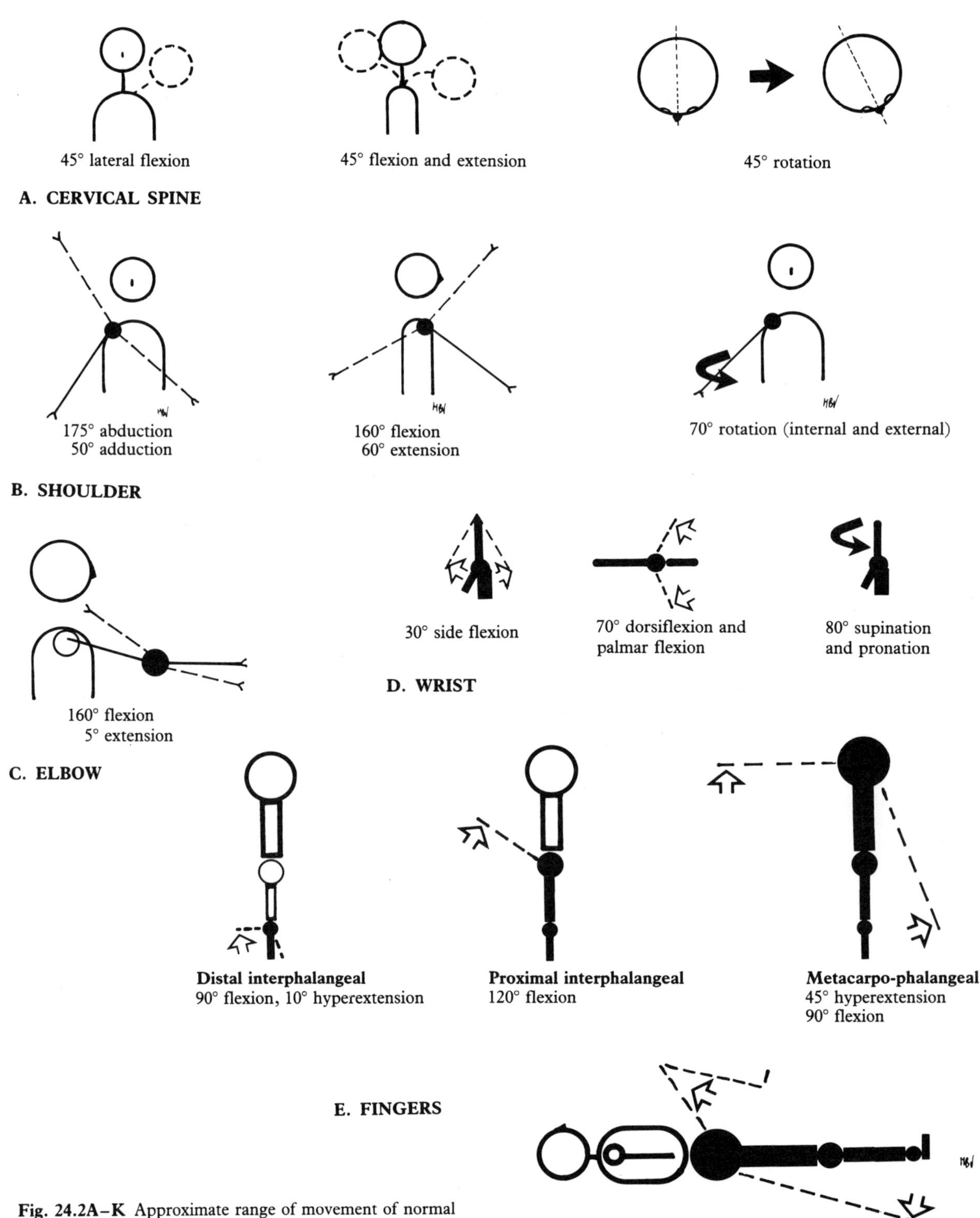

Fig. 24.2A–K Approximate range of movement of normal joints (normal movement varies with age, sex and race of the individual)

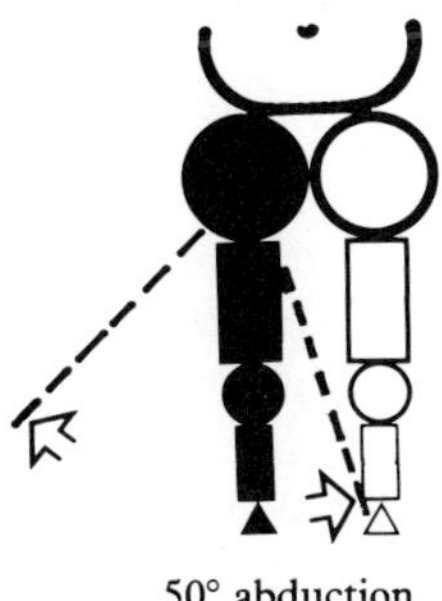

50° abduction
30° adduction

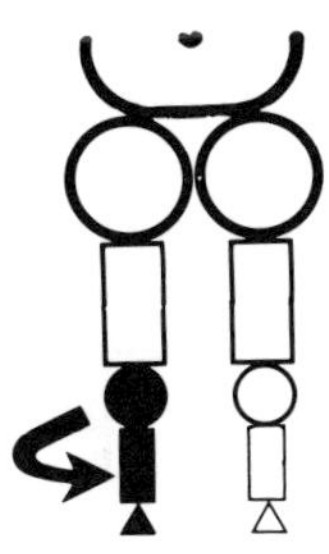

45° rotation (internal and external)

F. HIP

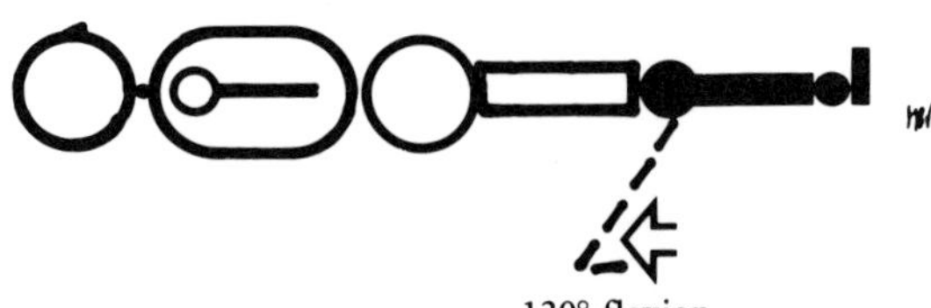

130° flexion

G. KNEE

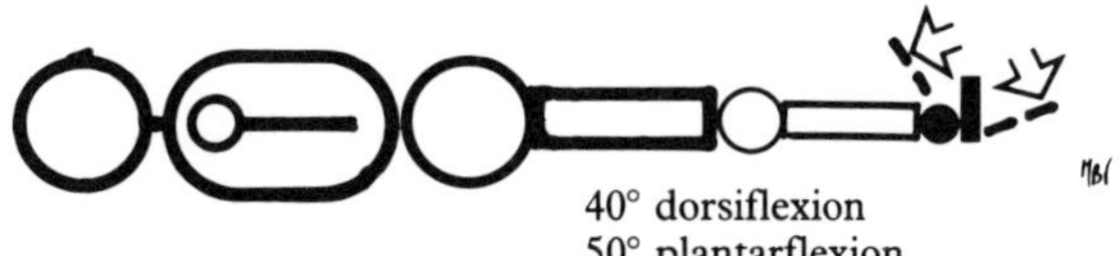

40° dorsiflexion
50° plantarflexion

H. ANKLE

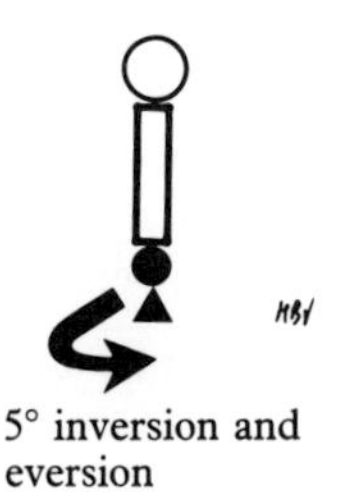

5° inversion and eversion

I. SUB-TALAR

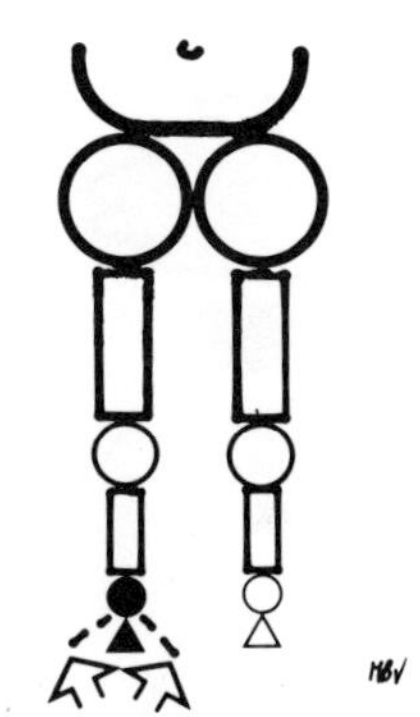

30° inversion and eversion

J. MID-TARSAL

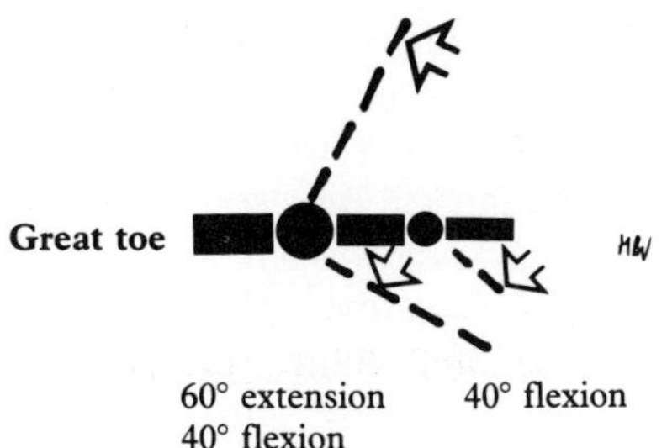

60° extension
40° flexion

40° flexion

Little toes

40° extension
40° flexion

40° flexion

50° flexion

K. TOES

of indices are available to record the degree of dependency or handicap, and measurements of the time taken to walk a given distance or perform a set task are sometimes used. These methods are extremely variable and difficult to interpret; it is often more useful to enquire about changes in ability to perform certain every-day tasks.

LABORATORY MEASUREMENTS

A variety of specific biochemical or haematological assays may provide diagnostic information or aid the assessment of a rheumatic disease: changes in the serum uric acid level in gout or the ASOT in suspected rheumatic fever are examples. In inflammatory joint disorders the systemic response to local inflammation results in other changes that can be measured and used to assess disease activity.

The systemic response to local injury is summarised in Figure 24.3. Changes in blood cells include a fall in haemoglobin with or without an increase in leucocytes or platelets. The ESR or plasma viscosity rises due to alteration in the balance of fibrinogen, albumin and globulin, and the liver produces increased quantities of several specific 'acute-phase' proteins. The haemoglobin and ESR are usually measured to assess disease activity and acute-phase protein concentrations are being increasingly investigated. Patients with connective-tissue diseases such as scleroderma and SLE do not mount the normal response, but in RA and the seronegative spondarthritides acute-phase changes such as C-reactive protein levels may provide a useful guide to prognosis as well as to disease activity. These values are most useful when used in conjunction with clinical assessment.

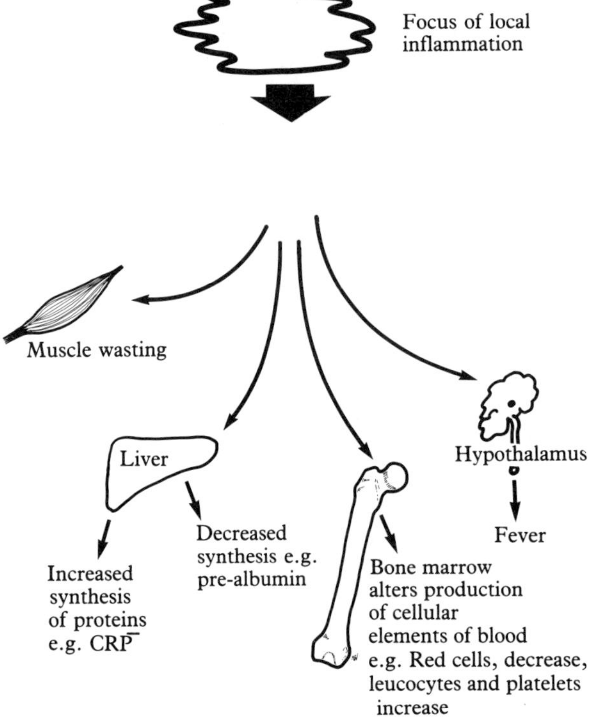

Fig. 24.3 Aspects of the systemic response to inflammation used to measure disease activity

IMAGING TECHNIQUES

The plain radiograph is one of the most useful means of following disease progression in many cases. Imaging techniques can also be used to provide a numerical index of disease activity. Thermography, which measures infra-red heat emission from joints, can be quantified and is useful in following joint inflammation and its response to treatment. Scintigraphy (see p 447) can be used in a similar way.

THERAPEUTIC TRIALS

Trial methodology has become an area of special interest in its own right. Trial design and the measurements made depend on both the disease being treated, and the type of agent being used. If an analgesic is being tested pain relief is the most important assessment, but if an anti-inflammatory agent is used other clinical indices such as ring size, grip strength and articular index may be useful. If gout or muscle disease is being treated special biochemical assays such as uric acid or muscle enzymes (creatine phosphokinase or aldolase) may be important. In inflammatory arthropathies assessment of the acute phase response is useful. Some of the usual methods used in drug trials on some different rheumatic diseases are shown opposite.

Some typical measurements made to assess treatment of rheumatic diseases
PAIN SCORE (visual analogue scale)
PATIENT RESPONSE OR DRUG PREFERENCE

Rheumatoid Arthritis
1. Duration of early morning stiffness
2. Ritchie articular index
3. PIP ring size
4. Grip strength
5. Haemoglobin
6. ESR or viscosity
7. Acute-phase proteins
8. Rheumatoid factor and immunoglobulins
9. Radiographic erosions
10. Quantified thermographs or scans

Osteoarthritis
1. Severity/duration of inactivity stiffness
2. Osteoarthritis articular index
3. Range of joint motion
4. Pain on joint movement
5. Radiographs
6. Thermography or scans

Ankylosing spondylitis
1. Range of motion of lumbar spine
2. Fingertip-to-floor distance
3. Tragus-to-wall distance
4. Early morning stiffness
5. Haemoglobin
6. ESR or viscosity
7. Acute-phase proteins
8. Imaging of sacro-iliac joints

Gout
1. Pain
2. Uric acid
3. Number of attacks

FURTHER READING (DISEASE ASSESSMENT)

Jayson M I V 1976 Diagnosis and assessment. Clinics in Rheumatic Diseases 2(1)

Wright V 1982 Measurement of joint movement. Clinics in Rheumatic Diseases 8(3)

II Imaging Techniques

A variety of techniques are available for visualising the bones and soft tissues of the joints.

Imaging techniques used in rheumatology
1. Plain x-ray
2. Radioisotope scanning
3. Contrast radiography
   a) Arthrography
   b) Myelography
   c) Angiography
   d) Sialography
4. Computer-assisted axial tomography
5. Thermography
6. Ultrasound

PLAIN X-RAY

A plain X-ray is probably the single most useful investigation in joint disease. It will give a vast amount of information about the state of the articular components and distribution of lesions and will often enable the correct diagnosis to be made. Although a plain film is a static record of past events, serial films allow the progress of the disease to be assessed and may also reveal clinically quiescent lesions. A single view is usually sufficient for most joints, although views at different angles can sometimes be helpful (e.g. AP and lateral views of the knee). A single AP view of the pelvis and a lateral view of the lumbar or thoracolumbar spine are sufficient to detect most back disorders. It is useful to X-ray a number of joints at presentation to serve as a baseline for future reference but, in the peripheral arthropathies, serial views of the hands and feet are most helpful. In some situations, particularly back and neck pain, the value of a routine plain X-ray is open to question since symptoms usually arise from the soft tissues rather than the osseous elements and the patients can be screened for serious pathology by attention to the history, physical examination and a sedimentation rate.

Differential diagnosis of plain X-ray findings

The abnormalities that may be seen on a plain radiograph are listed below. There may be a widespread increase or decrease in bone density or local radiolucent lesions. A periosteal reaction (a thin line of new bone formation often lying alongside the metaphysis of a long bone) may be seen in a variety of different conditions. Calcification may be present in the soft tissues and cartilage in a number of conditions. Other findings, e.g. erosions, joint space narrowing, sclerosis and new

What a plain X-ray will show

1. Soft-tissue swelling
2. Increased bone density
3. Decreased bone density
4. Radiolucent lesions
5. Periosteal reaction
6. Joint erosion
7. Joint-space narrowing
8. New bone formation (osteophytes , sclerosis)
9. Bone cysts
10. Soft-tissue calcification
11. Intra-articular loose bodies
12. Deformity

Causes of increased bone density

1. Osteopetrosis
2. Myelofibrosis.
3. Paget's disease
4. Metastases (particularly prostate and breast)
5. Bone islands
6. Osteoid osteoma

Causes of decreased bone density

1. Senile osteoporosis
2. Disuse
3. Cushing's syndrome and steroid therapy
4. Osteogenesis imperfecta
5. Myeloma, leukaemia
6. Infection
7. Inflammatory arthritis
8. Sudeck's atrophy
9. Rickets, osteomalacia
10. Vitamin C deficiency
11. Hyperparathyroidism

Causes of radiolucent lesions

1. Inflammatory arthritis (erosions)
2. Infection
3. Bone cysts
4. Myeloma
5. Osteochondromata
6. Osteogenic sarcoma
7. Metastases (breast, kidney, lung, thyroid)
8. Histiocytosis X

Causes of periosteal reaction

1. Tumour
2. Trauma
3. Infection
4. Hypertrophic pulmonary osteoarthropathy
5. Scurvey
6. Seronegative spondarthritis

Causes of calcification

Soft-tissue

1. Systemic sclerosis
2. Polymyosisitis
3. Cysticercosis
4. Gout
5. Calcific periarthritis
6. Renal dialysis

Cartilage

1. Calcium pyrophosphate deposition disease
2. Ochronosis (spine)
3. Haemochromatosis (larger joints)
4. Hyperparathyroidism

bone formation which result from a specific type of arthritis will be discussed further under specific disease headings.

Plain X-ray features of the major rheumatic diseases

Rheumatoid arthritis

Radiological changes usually appear after a latent period of 2–3 months and almost never in the absence of symptoms. The earliest feature is fusiform soft-tissue swelling around the MCP and PIP joints and the carpus. This is commonly accompanied by juxta-articular osteoporosis which develops prior to the onset of erosions. Erosions are the hallmark of rheumatoid disease and first appear on the joint margin at the site of synovial insertion (Fig. 24.4). There are initially small, discrete, well-defined areas of bone resorption which may gradually increase to considerable size. Early erosions tend to develop on the radial side of the second and third MCP joint, in the carpus and wrist (particularly the ulnar styloid) and the fifth MTP joint. The joint space may be wide in early disease owing to the presence of a synovial effusion but narrows and is lost as the spreading pannus destroys the cartilage. Large cysts or geodes may appear in the subarticular bone particularly in patients who use their hands in heavy work (called 'typus robustus' RA). As the disease progresses into its destructive phase, subluxation, angulation, secondary osteoarthritis and bony anklyosis may occur (Fig. 24.5). Occasionally there is marked resorption of bone, particularly at the phalangeal joints, resulting in shrinking of the digits which is termed *arthritis mutilans* and corresponds to the clinical appearance of *main-en-lorgnette*.

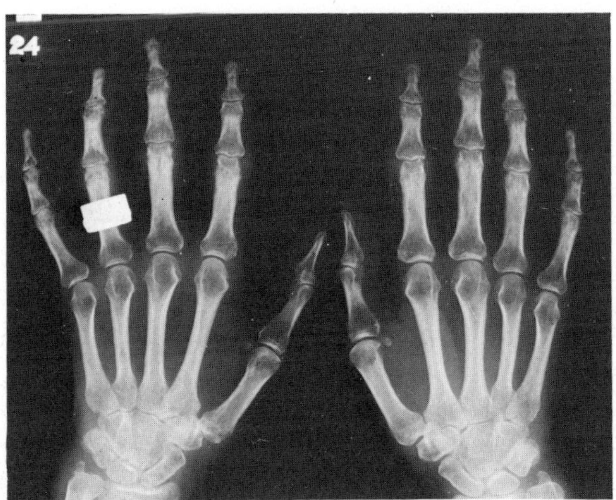

Fig. 24.4 Early rheumatoid arthritis of the hands showing symmetrical soft tissue swelling, juxta-articular osteoporosis, and early erosions

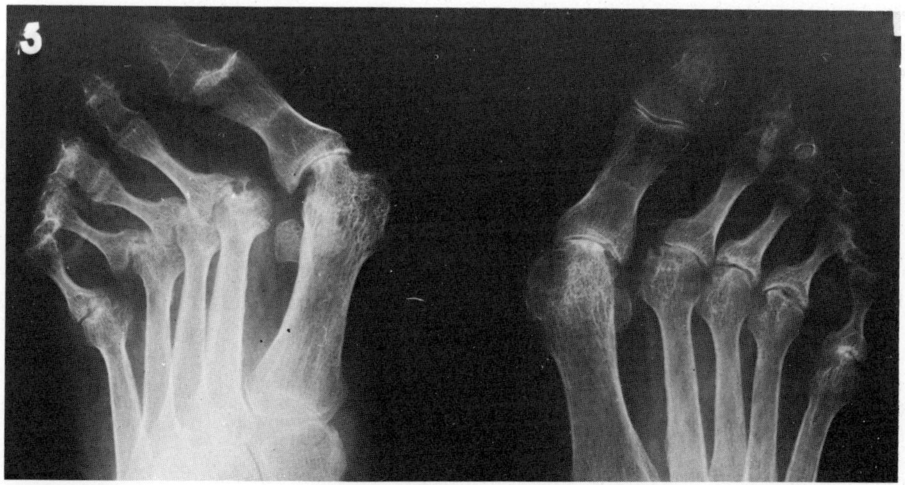

Fig. 24.5 Long-standing rheumatoid arthritis of the feet showing large erosions, cartilage destruction, subluxation and deformity

Characteristic radiological features in the hip joint are protrusio acetabuli, in which the head of the femur pushes into the pelvis, and secondary degenerative change with loss of joint space and sclerosis of the opposing joint margins but with little butressing of the femoral neck or osteophytosis. Avascular necrosis and disintegration of the femoral head are often seen in patients who have been on long-term steroid therapy.

Characteristic signs of early disease in the shoulder are cephalic migration of the humeral head relative to the glenoid fossa with excavation and eburnation of the acromion.

The only part of the axial skeleton to be significantly involved in RA is the cervical spine. Atlanto-axial subluxation is present when the gap between the posterior surface of the anterior arch of the atlas and the anterior surface of the odontoid peg is greater than 4 mm. This is best assessed by flexion and extension lateral views of the cervical spine. The odontoid peg is often eroded and can best be seen by a Townes view (through the mouth) or, if very ill-defined, by tomography. Subaxial subluxation may be seen at one or more levels, giving a step-ladder effect. It is most commonly present at the C3–C4 interspace. Spondylodiscitis may be observed usually at a single level as gross erosive change with obliteration of the disc space unaccompanied by soft-tissue swelling. Destruction and fusion of the apophyseal joints may occur causing loss of disc space and sharpening of the spinous processes due to impingement on each other.

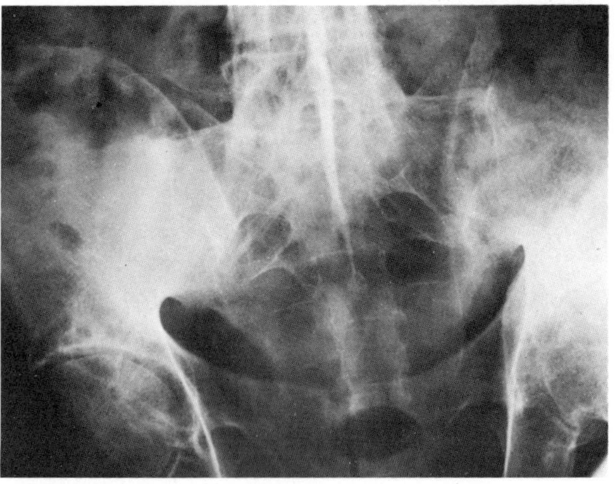

Fig. 24.6 Fusion of the sacro-iiliac joints and lumbar vertebrae in ankylosing spondylitis

Ankylosing spondylitis

The radiological hallmark of this disease is sacroiliitis. Early changes are sometimes difficult to detect on the straight AP projection of the pelvis and tomography or stereoscopic views may be helpful. There is blurring of the normal outline followed by absorption of the subarticular bone accompanied by osteoporosis. The joint space appears widened initially due to the loss of bone. Later, the joint space narrows and there is patchy sclerosis of bone. These changes are bilateral and symmetrical. Eventually there may be bony ankylosis of part or all of the joint (Fig. 24.6). Early sacroiliitis is particularly difficult to detect in adolescents whose healthy SIJs are wide, have a serrated edge and lack an articular cortex.

Spinal changes occur initially at the spinal flexures, particularly at the dorsolumbar junction and in the neck, and are best seen on a lateral view. Ill-defined superficial erosions develop at the superior and inferior end-plates of the vertebral bodies accompanied by reactive sclerosis and laying down of new bone anteriorly which produces a 'squared-off' appearance, most striking in the lumbar vertebrae which normally have quite a markedly concave anterior border. Repair of these erosions results in the formation of symetrical syndesmophytes which fuse above and below with the adjacent end-plate and may spread up and down the spine resulting in the classic fused bamboo spine (Fig. 24.7). If fusion occurs early, the disc spaces are preserved, but if fusion occurs at a level already affected by degenerative disc disease, the syndesmophytes may be seen to encase a bulging disc or buckled ligaments. Occasionally, a segment of the spine, particularly in the neck, remains mobile between two fused segments and this level is often the site of striking disc degeneration.

Peripheral joint involvement occurs in about 20% and usually affects the large joints, particularly the hip. There is juxta-articular osteoporosis

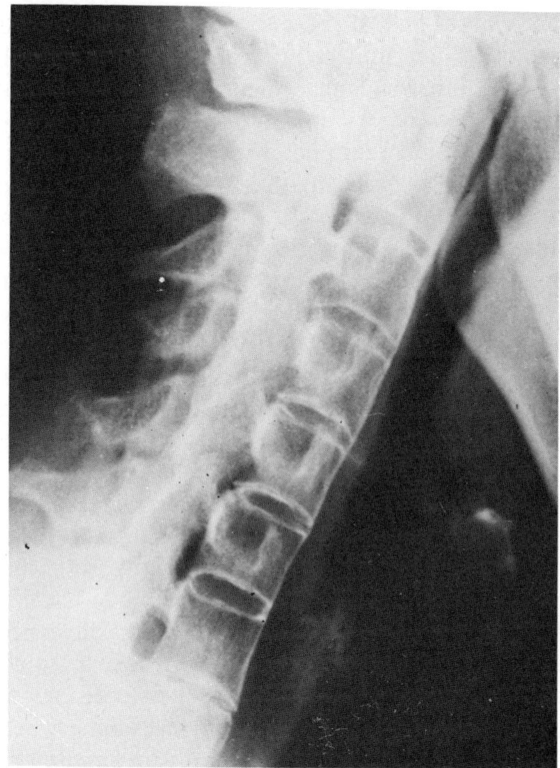

Fig. 24.7 'Bamboo' cervical spine in ankylosing spondylitis

and erosive change. Bony fusion may occur with apparent preservation of the joint space.

Ligamentous attachments are frequently the site of erosion and repair which results in fringes of new bone, particularly on the outer borders of the ileum and ischium and on the plantar surfaces of the calcaneum.

Psoriatic arthropathy

The radiological features of PA can be distinguished from RA (Table 24.1). Four patterns of skeletal lesions may be observed:

1. Interphalangeal joints and wrist
2. Arthritis mutilans with sacro-iliitis
3. A rheumatoid-like arthropathy which is more asymmetrical and also associated with sacro-iliitis
4. A spondylitic arthropathy with occasional large-joint involvement.

Table 24.1 Contrasting radiological features of psoriatic and rheumatoid arthritis

Psoriatic	Rheumatoid
Asymmetrical	Symmetrical
Less marked juxta-articular osteoporosis	Pronounced juxta-articular osteoporosis
Periosteal reaction common	Periosteal reaction rare
Bony ankylosis common	Bony ankylosis rare
Prominent new bone formation	Little new bone formation
Spinal lesions common	Spinal lesions rare (except cervical spine)

The small joints show periarticular erosions accompanied by marked new bone formation at the sites of erosion and a periosteal reaction along the shaft of involved long bones. The lesions are asymmetrical, with little juxta-articular osteoporosis and there is a predeliction in the hands for the distal interphalangeal joints. Bony dissolution associated with new bone formation is a feature of PA and gives rise to the radiological arrow-head deformity at the DIPJ and the 'pencil-in-cup' appearance at the MCP and PIP joints. It is not uncommon for the joint space to be preserved despite considerable destruction, but eventually bony ankylosis occurs in some joints.

The spinal lesions are less symmetrical than in AS and single syndesmophytes may appear which do not form bridges with the adjacent vertebral body. The sacroiliitis is also patchy and asymmetrical.

Reiter's syndrome

Radiological features are similar to those seen in psoriasis, with a tendency to bony dissolution and prominent, often fluffy, new bone formation, particularly along the metacarpal and metatarsal bones, along one or two vertebrae and at the os calcis forming a bony spur, and in the posterior joints of the spine. Sacro-iliitis is usually asymmetrical and patchy and total fusion is uncommon.

Osteoarthritis

The radiological features of OA are loss of joint space, osteophytes at the joint line, subcortical sclerosis and subchondral cysts with a sclerotic rim. Periosteal new bone formation is not a feature except along the medial aspect of the femoral neck, and osteoporosis is not seen. Subluxation may occur in the interphalangeal joints causing angulation deformity of the fingers and at the carpometacarpal joints of the thumb and the hip (Fig. 24.8). Loose bodies formed from detached osteophytes and periarticular ossicles are occasionally seen.

The distribution varies acoding to the type of OA. The primary form has a predilection for the terminal interphalangeal joints of the fingers associated with large dorsal osteophytes (Heberden's nodes), CMC joint of the thumbs, knees and hips. Secondary OA may result from another arthropathy and the pattern of involvement will reflect that of the underlying disease.

Typical features in the hip and knee are shown in Figures 24.9 and 24.10. Collapse of the head of the femur with lateral subluxation are seen in more severe cases of hip OA. Protrusio acetabuli rarely occur and, if present, should suggest the existence of an underlying condition, particularly RA. An inferior displacement of the femoral head is often present in cases of slipped femoral epiphysis, and a mushroom deformity with shortening of the femoral neck is suggestive of old Perthes' disease. Rapid collapse of the femoral head with increasing areas of bone density and a relative lack of osteophytes of femoral neck buttressing suggests avascular necrosis. The knee may show sharpening of the tibial spines (intraarticular osteophytes), with joint-space narrowing which is more marked in the medial compartment. Large subchondral cysts may be present in the tibia and there are often marked changes in the patello-femoral joint.

Secondary OA occurs in the cervical and lumbar spine as the result of degeneration of the intervertebral discs. Radiological signs of disc degeneration are present in most people by the fifth decade of life. The earliest feature is loss of vertical height of the disc, followed by marginal osteophytes on all sides of the end-plates (seen best in a lateral view) and at the apophyseal joints, where they may encroach on the neural exit foramina.

OA is rare in the throacic spine except where it is secondary to Scheuermann's disease, old tuber-

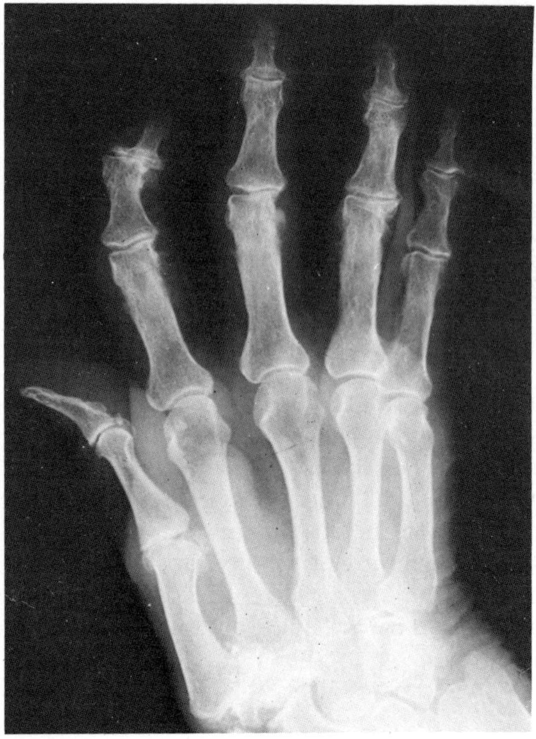

Fig. 24.8 Osteoarthritis of the hand affecting the carpometacarpal joint of the thumb and the interphalangeal joints

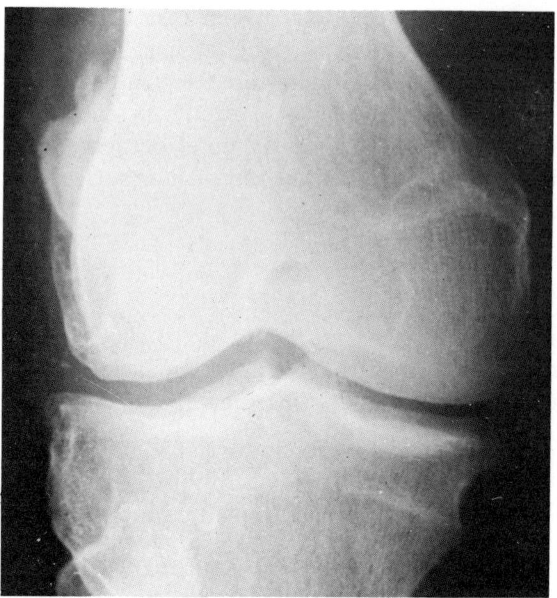

Fig. 24.9 Osteoarthritis of the knees showing loss of joint space, bony sclerosis and osteophyte formation

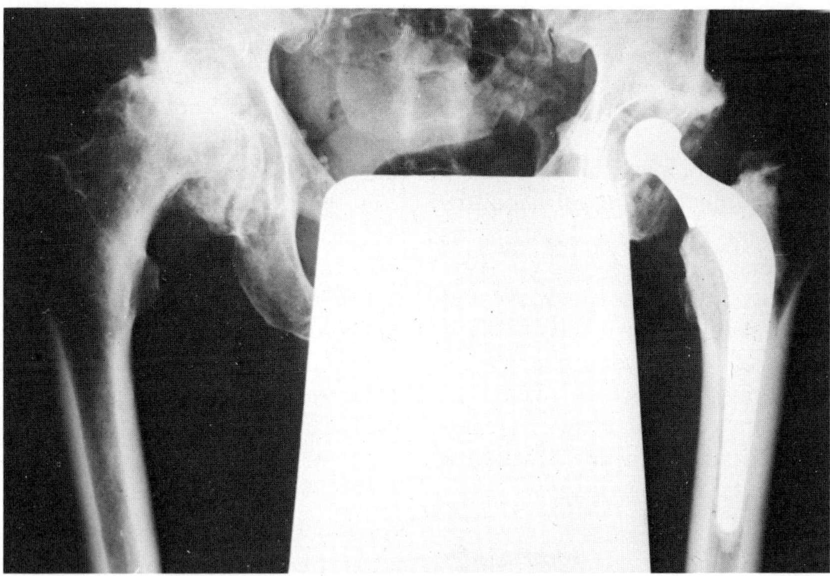

Fig. 24.10 Osteoarthritis of the right hip with a Charnley hip prosthesis on the left side

culosis or trauma. A hyperostotic spondylitis (Forrestier's disease) is described with extensive marginal osteophytes which may form bridges between the vertebrae, more frequently on the right side of the spine. The disc spaces may be fairly well preserved. This condition is often seen in association with diabetes and obesity.

A Charcot joint radiologically shows an exaggerated form of osteoarthritis with severe loss of joint space, fragmentation of the articular surface, intra-articular calcified loose debris and pathological intra-articular fractures. Spinal changes are an advanced form of degenerative disc disease with end-plate destruction, florid sclerosis and osteophytes.

Gout

In acute gout, the only radiological feature is soft tissue swelling of the affected joint, with little juxta-articular osteoporosis. The radiological hallmark of chronic tophaceous gout is a punched-out, round or oval erosion occurring along the shaft of the bone rather than on the articular surface, particularly around the interphalangeal joints of the hands and feet. They are usually assymetrical and often multiple. Adjacent lesions may coalesce forming a honeycomb area leading to subchondral collapse. These lesions are due to the presence of tophi which also excite a periosteal reaction, resulting in the formation of an overhanging hook of bone (Martel's hook) (Fig. 24.11). Soft-tissue swelling may be present and corresponds to the

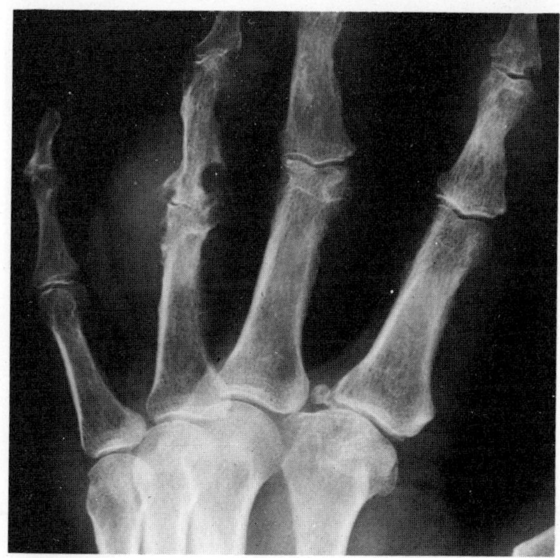

Fig. 24.11 Gout showing gross asymmetrical soft tissue swelling corresponding to tophi and typical para-articular punched-out erosions (Martel's hook)

distribution of tophi which may rarely become calcified or even ossified.

Pyrophosphate arthropathy

Deposition of calcium pyrophosphate in hyaline and fibrocartilage results in radiological chondrocalcinosis, commonly in the knee, wrist, symphisis pubis, shoulders and intervertebral disc. (Fig. 24.12). Its frequency increases with age and is present an incidental finding in nearly 40% of patients over the age of 80. In some patients, a rapidly destructive form of osteoarthritis is associated with pyrophosphate deposition involving primarily the knees and wrists and in this situation is probably not an incidental finding (p 175).

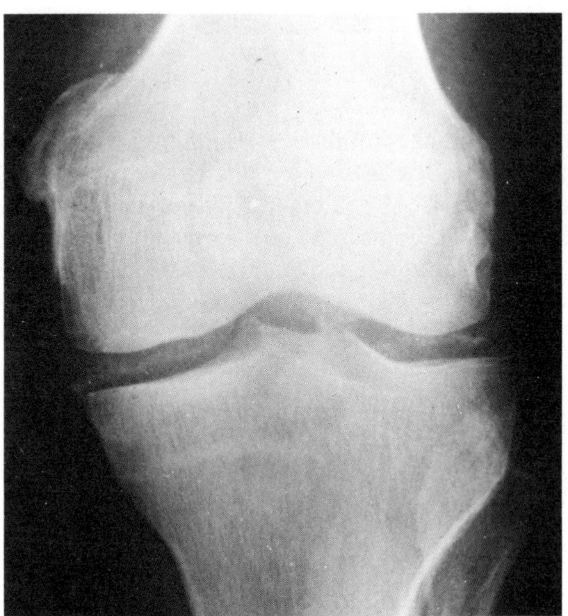

Fig. 24.12 Pyrophosphate arthropathy showing calcification in the meniscal cartilage of the knee

Juvenile chronic arthritis

In early disease there is non-specific soft-tissue swelling around affected joints with little juxta-articular osteoporosis. Accelerated development followed by early closure of the epiphyses may result in growth disparity, particularly in the fingers, toes and jaw. A generalised retardation of bone growth occurs during exacerbations of disease, resulting in multiple Harris's lines in the metaphyses and short stature. A small proportion go on to develop florid periosteal reaction in the phalanges. There is a tendency to late bony ankylosis, particularly in the carpus and CMC joints and the cervical spine. The odontoid peg is frequently eroded, with atlanto-axial subluxation. A few children have a severe destructive arthropathy, often involving the hips with intense osteoporosis, erosions, collapse of the femoral epiphysis and protrusio acetabuli.

Connective-tissue diseases

Skeletal X-ray changes are less common in the connective-tissue diseases. In SLE, juxta-articular osteoporosis, soft-tissue swelling and deformity may be seen particularly in the hands, but there is a striking lack of erosion or destruction. Extensive para-articular soft-tissue calcification is often present in dermatomyositis, particularly on the extensor surfaces. In scleroderma there is often fusiform soft-tissue swelling of the digits and obliteration of the skin creases and in established disease there may be obvious flexion contractures and amputations as the result of vascular disease. The tufts of the terminal phalanges are absorbed and there may be prominent subcutaneous calcification. A small proportion of patients develop an erosive rheumatoid-like arthritis.

CONTRAST INJECTION TECHNIQUES

Arthrography

The soft tissues of a joint can be visualised by the injection of positive (aqueous iodine solutions) or negative (air) contrast media. This is usually perfomed under local anaesthetic using screen control. Almost every joint can be examined in this way, including the disc spaces, and there is a very low complication rate. In practice the knee is the most common joint to be thus visualised. (Fig. 24.13). Some common indications for arthrography are given opposite.

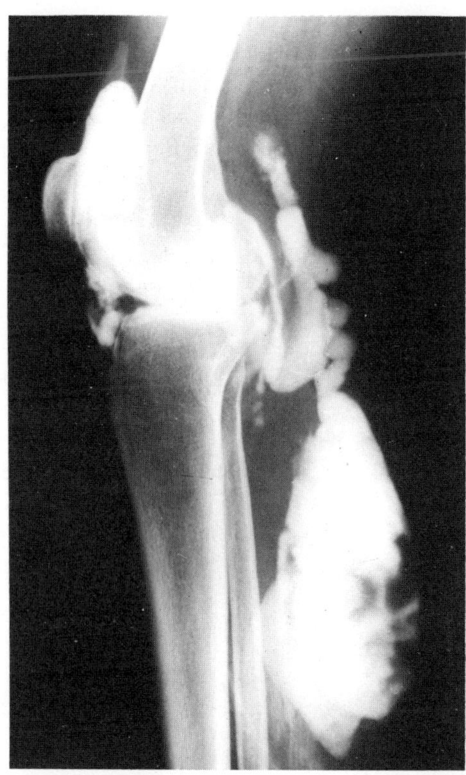

Fig. 24.13 Arthrogram of the knee showing extravasation of contrast medium in the calf from a ruptured popliteal cyst

Some indications for arthrography
Diagnosis of:
1. Meniscal injuries in the knee
2. Rupture of:
   a) Popliteal cyst
   b) Triangular ligament of the wrist
   c) Cruciate ligament of the knee
3. Radio-opaque loose bodies (e.g. osteochondromatosis)
4. Pigmented villonodular synovitis
5. Tears of rotator cuff and adhesive capsulitis

Myelography

This technique is used to outline the soft tissues of the spinal canal and the nerve roots. Contrast medium is injected into the subarchnoid space via a lumbar or cisternal puncture depending on the level of the lesion. The progress of the column of contrast is tracked along the subarachnoid space. Myelography is indicated in is indicated in the pre-operative diagnosis of spinal cord or nerve root compression and to establish the level and extent of a lesion. Cervical myelography is most commonly performed in rheumatological practice in severe cervical spondylosis and rheumatoid myelopathy. A radioculogram is the same technique confined to the lumbosacral region and is useful in the investigation of prolapsed intervertebral disc and lumbar canal stenosis.

Other contrast techniques

Sialography is useful in the investigation of the sicca syndrome and will differentiate this form an obstructed salivary duct. Angiography is occasionally used in the investigation of polyarteritis nodosa where characteristic lesions have been described in the coeliac axis and occasionally in the other vasculitides, particularly Takayasu's disease. Ascending lumbar venography is very occasionally useful in delineating a lateral disc prolapse.

RADIO-ISOTOPE IMAGING

This is most commonly performed using ^{99}Technitium labelled diphosphonate, which is taken up by the skeleton and occasionally ^{67}Gallium which binds to intracellular lysosomal enzymes and seeks out tumours and pus. The isotope emits gamma rays which are detected by a gamma camera. It is a cheap technique and delivers only a small dose of irradation, less than is received in a conventional plain X-ray. An early image shortly after injection will show abnormal perfusion, a delayed image at about 3 hours will show abnormal calcium turnover, and a late image will show abnormal retention. High activity occurs at sites of increased vascularity, over freshly-mineralised osteoid, at sites of fracture and over inflamed joints in RA and over active osteophytes in OA. A particular advantage of the isotope scan is that it reflects the current state compared to the plain X-ray which is really a historic record. Some indications for an isotope bone scan in the rheumatic diseases are shown below.

Some indications for radioisotope bone scan

1. To exclude metastases and bone tumours
2. To delineate the extent of Paget's disease and osteomalacia
3. To diagnose difficult cases of sacro-iliitis
4. To detect occult joint sepsis
5. To aid diagnosis of hypertrophic pulmonary osteoarthropathy
6. As a research tool in assessing activity of RA and OA
7. To detect early osteonecrosis
8. To reassure doctor and patients in psychogenic rheumatism

COMPUTER-ASSISTED AXIAL TOMOGRAPHY

This technique produces high-resolution cross-sectional images of the body. Its use in the investigation of the lesions of rheumatic diseases has not yet been fully explored. So far it has a place in the investigation of spinal-canal stenosis and in detecting prolapsed intervertebral discs where other conventional techniques, such as radiculgraphy, have produced results which do not agree with the clinical situation.

ULTRASOUND

High-frequency sound waves (1540 m/s) penetrate the soft tissues and are reflected off interfaces of a different acoustic impedance and this technique is particularly useful in differentiating between solid and cystic masses and for detecting fluid. It is used for the investigation of pericardial effusion in patients with pericarditis, a common feature of RA and SLE. The fluid appears as an echo-free space between the chest wall and the heart wall. It has also been shown to be useful in detecting popliteal cysts and measuring the size of the lumbar spinal canal.

THERMOGRAPHY

This technique measures infra-red heat emission on the surface of bones and joints and produces colourful temperature-related pictures. It is a useful means of assessing active synovitis and quantifying response to treatment. It is also helpful in the investigation of Raynaud's phenomon, Paget's disease (particuarlarly of the tibia), and possibly in sacro-iliitis.

FURTHER READING

Forrestier D M, Brown J C, Nesson J W 1978 The radiology of joint disease. W B Saunders, Phildelphia

Simon G S 1973 Principles of bone X-ray diagnosis. Butterworth, London

Sutton D 1983 A textbook of radiology and imaging, 2nd edn. Churchill Livingstone, Edinburgh

Watt I, Middlemass H 1980 Radiology of joint disease. In: Diagnosis and assessment. Clinics in Rheumatic Diseases. W B Saunders, Philedelphia

III Examination of Synovial Fluid

Most joint diseases alter both the volume and contents of the synovial fluid. The findings in crystal synovitis and septic arthritis are diagnostic, and fluid analysis is an essential investigation if either condition is suspected. In other diseases the changes are usually non-specific, but may contribute to diagnosis and assessment. Samples should be examined by gross inspection and ordinary and polarised light microscopy. The total and differential white cell count should be estimated, and bacteriological examinations should include gram stains and culture on suitable media. The lactic acid level is helpful if sepsis is suspected, but other assays rarely help in the clinical situation.

Analysis of synovial fluid

Routine analysis

1. Gross Inspection
   a) Colour and volume
   b) Viscosity
   c) Opacity
   d) Presence/absence of blood
   e) Clot formation on standing
2. Microscopy
   a) Total and differential white cell
   b) Presence of cartilage fragments and other particles
   c) Presence/absence of crystals (polarised light)
3. Bacteriology
   a) Gram stain of fluid and centrifuged deposit
   b) Culture of fluid on suitable media

Other assays

1. Lactic acid level
2. Glucose
   — May aid the diagnosis of septic arthritis
3. Rheumatoid factor/ANA and complement levels
   — Occasionally useful in assessing immune synovitis
4. Protein and enzyme content
   — Reflect the activity of synovitis
5. Analytical electron microscopy
   — Reveals the presence of minute particles (e.g. apatite crystals)

OBTAINING SYNOVIAL FLUID

The indications and contra-indications for joint aspiration are listed below. Most synovial joints can be needled with little discomfort, and complications are rare. The basic procedure used is the same for all joint sites, and identical whether the arthrocentesis is being performed to obtain fluid for diagnostic purposes, or to allow injection of diagnostic or therapeutic agents (Chapters 19 and 26). Joint aspiration is a safe procedure which can

Indications for examination of synovial fluid

1. Absolute
   a) Suspected septic arthritis
   b) Suspected crystal synovitis

2. Relative
   a) Undiagnosed and atypical arthropathies
   b) When puncturing joints for other diagnostic or therapeutic purposes (e.g. arthrography, steroid injection etc)

CONTRAINDICATIONS

1. Bleeding disorder
2. Sepsis overlying the puncture site

be performed in surgeries, out-patient departments or the patient's home, provided that suitable precautions are taken to reduce the risk of sepsis.

The patient should lie on a couch in a relaxed position allowing easy access to the site of joint entry. The skin is carefully cleaned, and local anaesthetic is usually used. A 'no-touch' technique is essential. After penetrating the skin and subcutaneous tissue, the operator usually feels the resistance of the joint capsule; a twinge of pain may be felt as the needle then slips into the joint space. Gentle aspiration will usually result in fluid entering the syringe, although the needle may be blocked by synovial fronds, fibrin bodies or other particles in the joint space. If fluid is not obtained (the 'dry tap') it is still worth trying to expel the contents of the needle on to a glass slide for examination, as a minute amount of fluid is often sufficient to identify crystals or pathogenic organisms. The technique used for each individual joint is best learnt by observing and working with an experienced operator. Some of the common approaches used to major joints are shown in Figure 24.14.

Complications of arthrocentesis are rare, but include pain, a haemarthrosis or septic arthritis. It has been estimated that less than 1/10 000 aspirated joints will become infected.

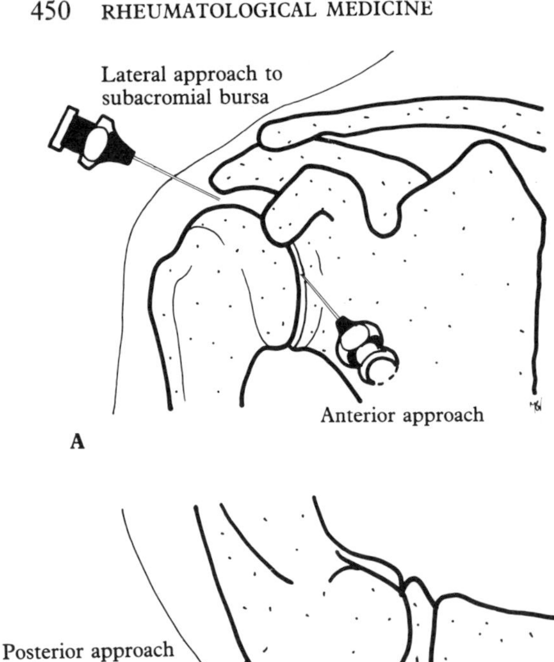
Lateral approach to
subacromial bursa
Anterior approach
A

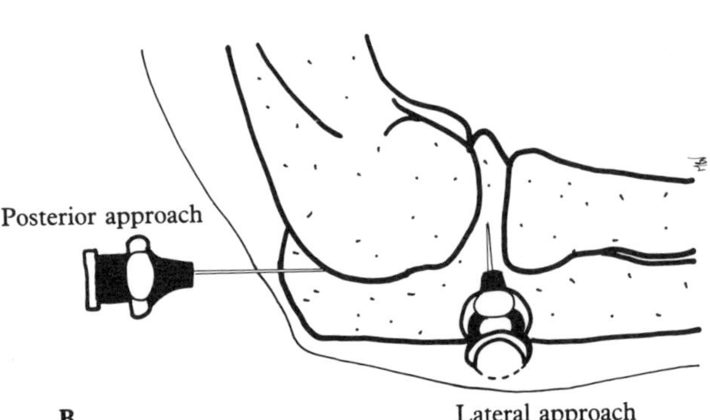
Posterior approach
Lateral approach
over head of radius
B

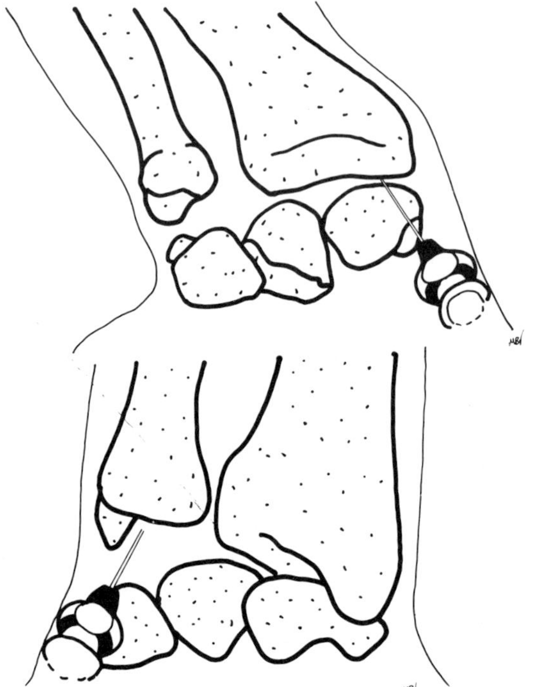
C

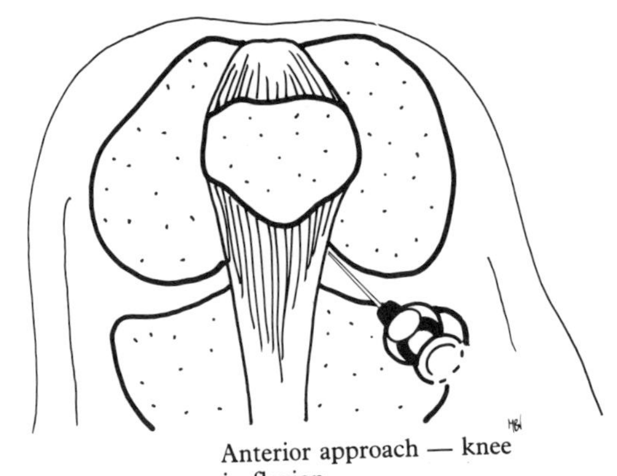
Anterior approach — knee
in flexion

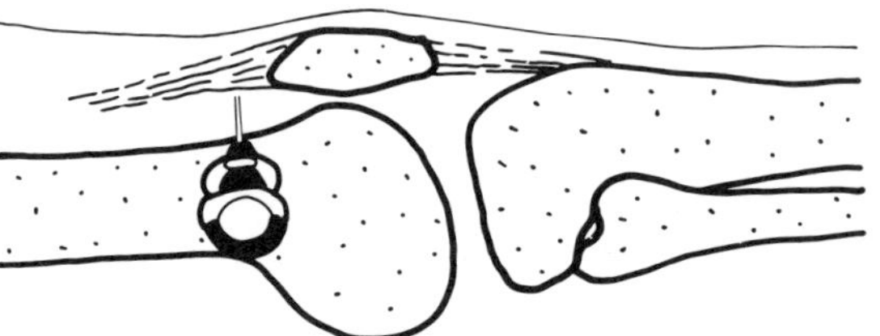
Lateral approach via supra-patella extension

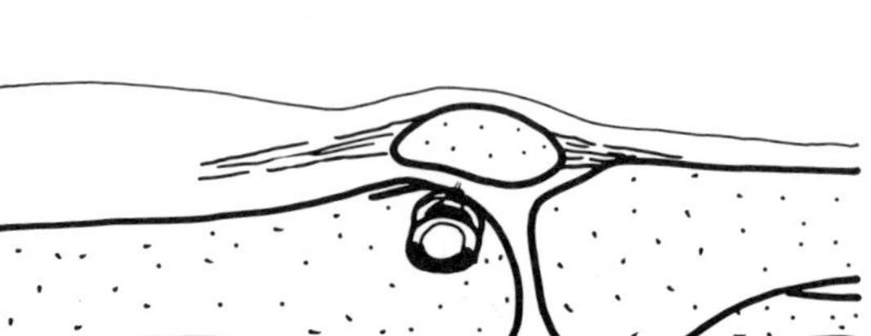

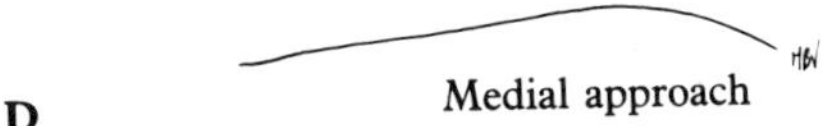
Medial approach
D

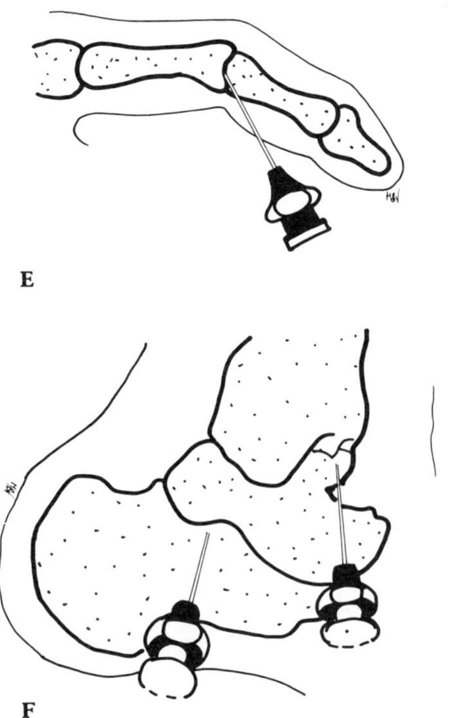

Fig. 24.14 Arthrocentesis: some of the approaches used **A**. Shoulder **B**. Elbow **C**. Wrist **D**. Knee **E**. Interphalangeal joints **F**. Ankle and subtalar joints

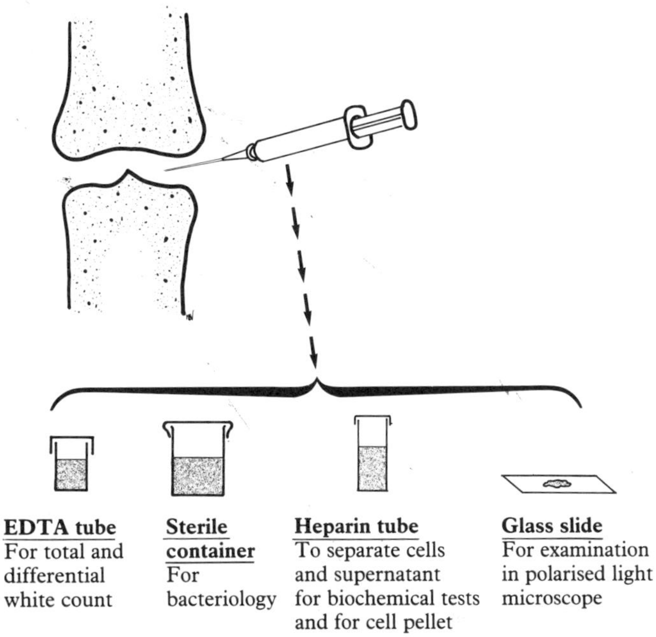

EDTA tube
For total and differential white count

Sterile container
For bacteriology

Heparin tube
To separate cells and supernatant for biochemical tests and for cell pellet

Glass slide
For examination in polarised light microscope

Fig. 24.15 Handling synovial fluid. Apart from those illustrated, other containers which may be used are 1) Oxalate tubes (glucose) 2) Special transport media (unusual organisms) 3) Blood culture bottles and culture plates (direct innoculation to aid bacteriological isolation) and 4) Containers with oil (avoids air contact and pH change)

Complications of joint puncture

1. Exacerbation of arthritic pain and inflammation
2. Haemarthrosis
3. Septic arthritis (approximate incidence 1:10 000)

HANDLING SYNOVIAL FLUID

The volume of fluid obtained varies from the contents of the needle to several 100 ml. The priorities among the different assays vary in different clinical situations, influencing the way in which smaller quantities will be processed, but polarised-light microscopy of a drop of fresh fluid and bacteriological examination by Gram stain and culture are usually the most important investigations to perform. If only a drop is available it should therefore be smeared on clean glass slides for microscopy and Gram stain, and used to innoculate a culture dish. When several millilitres are obtained the fluid should be distributed in different bottles for the various assays, as shown in Figure 24.15.

Most of the examinations are best done as soon as possible after joint puncture. A search for crystals should be made on a fresh drop of fluid placed directly on a clean glass microscope slide. Close liaison with bacteriologists will aid the processing of fluids for isolation of infective agents; immediate transport of a sterile container to the laboratory is often the best option, although in some centres or at difficult times, the use of transport medium, the direct innoculation of fluid into culture plates or blood culture bottles, or Gram stain of a centrifuged deposit by the operator, may be advised. Cell counts can be done on EDTA samples using either an automatic counter or a haemocytometer. Differential white cell counts are usually done on fluid smears washed in Wright's stain. If cell diluents are used acetic acid must be avoided, as it causes synovial fluid to clot (this is the basis of the now redundant mucin clot test). Biochemical assays are only valid if the cells and supernatant are separated soon after joint aspiration.

Routine analysis of synovial fluid

The examination begins as soon as fluid enters the syringe. The viscosity, cloudiness and presence or absence of blood and visible particles provides useful information. Other points of interest on gross examination include volume, colour and clot formation on standing. The fluid is then examined by microscopy, in the bacteriology laboratory, or by use of the special assays listed if required (p 449). All fluids should be examined to determine the presence or absence of blood, crystals and infectious agents, and to estimate the degree and type of inflammatory response occurring in the joint. The use and interpretation of these findings is outlined below.

Four important questions relating to synovial fluid analysis

1. Is the fluid blood stained? If so, why?
2. What is the nature and intensity of the inflammatory response in the joint?
3. Is the joint infected?
4. Is the patient suffering from a crystal-induced synovitis?

1. Bloodstained fluid

Bloodstaining often results from trauma during joint puncture; this is usually obvious to the operator; fluid and blood are not evenly mixed and there is no free pigment in the synovial fluid. However, if fluid is then mixed in a sample tube and sent to the laboratory it may be difficult to differentiate traumatic staining from a haemarthrosis.

Conditions often associated with bloodstained synovial fluid

1. Traumatic joint puncture
2. Traumatic arthritis
3. Fractures communicating with joints
4. Pigmented villonodular synovitis
5. Other joint tumours
6. Pyrophosphate arthropathy
7. Neuropathic joints
8. Haemophiliac arthritis
9. Other bleeding disorders
10. Resolution of a septic arthritis
11. Severe destructive arthritis of any cause

Some of the conditions which cause a true haemarthrosis are listed above. Heavy blood contamination may follow trauma, and occurs in the bleeding disorders such as haemophilia, but blood never clots in synovial fluid, allowing a distinction to be made from inadvertent puncture of a blood-vessel. In the majority of the other listed conditions bloodstaining is moderate, usually visible but sometimes microscopic, and only occurs in a proportion of cases with the disorder.

2. Assessing inflammation in the joint

Inflammation of the joint lining (synovitis) results in a leucocytic infiltrate spilling over into the synovial fluid, and in the production of products such as lysosomal enzymes which break up hyaluronate aggregates and change the fluid's contents. Unfortunately, these changes are non-specific and only indicate the intensity of the reaction, not its cause.

Gross examination of the opacity, viscosity and clot formation of fluid reflect the inflammatory reaction (Fig. 24.16 and Table 24.2).

Normal fluid is clear, but a cellular infiltrate makes it appear cloudy, and very high cell counts result in thick, yellow fluid — i.e. pus. Pus in the joint should always alert one to the possibility of a septic joint, although other diseases associated with intense synovitis can cause the same sort of exudate (see above), and cholesterol crystals

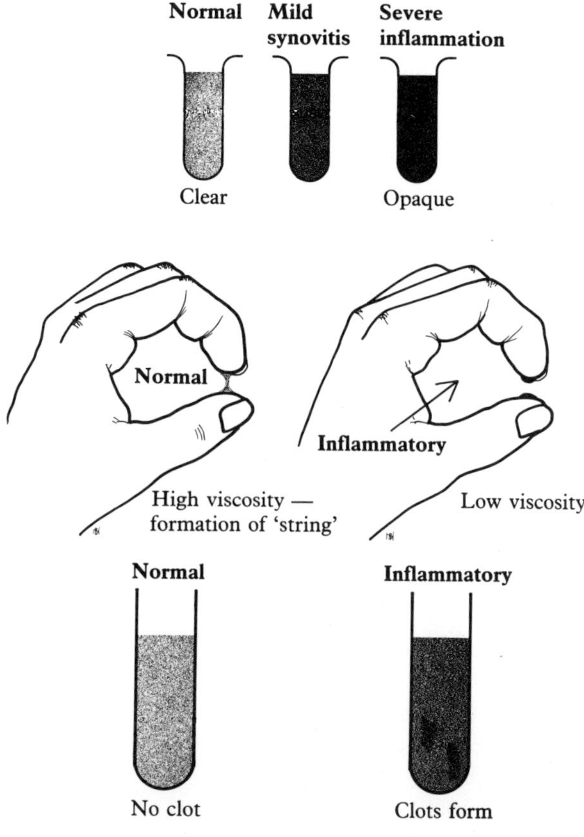

Fig. 24.16 Appearance of normal and inflammatory synovial fluid

> **Causes of 'pus' in the synovial fluid**
>
> *Common*
> 1. Septic arthritis
> 2. Crystal synovitis
>
> *Uncommon*
> 1. Very active RA
> 2. Very active seronegative spondarthritis (e.g. acute Reiter's syndrome)

occasionally appear in the synovial fluid, giving it a similar creamy appearance. The viscosity of fluid is also a guide to the cellular exudate, as products of the phagocytic cells in synovial fluid break up its hyaluronate aggregates, reducing normal viscosity; this is easily assessed by rubbing a small drop between finger and thumb and then trying to draw it out into a thin 'string' (Fig. 24.16). Clot formation never occurs in normal fluid, but fibrinous exudates may result in the formation of ragged masses of fibrin and cells if the fluid is left without anticoagulant.

The total and differential white cell counts are the most useful guide to the type and degree of synovitis in a joint (see above). The cell count in normal fluid is very low, consisting in part of cells derived from the lining. The mild reaction of OA,

Table 24.2 Typical synovial fluid findings in some different rheumatic diseases

Diagnosis	Intra-articular inflammation	Viscosity	Opacity	Clot formation	Total leucocyte count ($<10^9$/l)	% polymorphs
1. Normal	None	High	Clear	–	100 (10–200)	10 (0–40)
2. Osteoarthritis and related conditions	Less inflammatory			–	1000 (400–4000)	25 (0–60)
3. Connective-tissue diseases				–	2000 (1–5000)	25 (10–60)
4. Seronegative spondarthritides			Cloudy	+/–	5000 (1–20 000)	60 (30–90)
5. Rheumatoid arthritis				+	10 000 (1–50 000)	75 (30–95)
6. Crystal synovitis				+	15 000 (5–50 000)	85 (50–100)
7. Joint sepsis	More inflammatory	Low	Purulent	+	50 000 (10–100 000)	95 (80–100)

connective tissue diseases and early or mild forms of polarthritis cause a modest rise in cell count, often with a predominance of mononuclear cells. RA and other diseases causing an active synovitis cause a more substantial polymorphonuclear (pmn) cell infiltrate, and acute crystal synovitis and sepsis result in very high counts. The differential is often more helpful than the total count: OA fluids hardly ever have more than 50% pmns, whereas the converse is true of RA, and in sepsis the pmn. ratio is generally 95% or more.

Many other fluid assays reflect synovial inflammation. They include the now redundant mucin-clot test (fluid clots on addition of acid in inflammatory conditions), protein concentrations, and levels of a variety of enzymes such as LDH and β glucuronidase, derived largely from phagocytic cells. These tests do not help in the routine diagnosis or assessment of joint disease.

3. Bacteriological examination

If there is any suspicion of joint sepsis fluids must be sent for bacteriological examination and the lactic acid level should be assayed if possible. Infection does not always make the fluid look like pus, and can coexist with other conditions including RA and crystal synovitis so a high index of clinical suspicion is required.

The investigations performed will depend on the type of infection suspected, emphasising the need for rheumatologist and bacteriologist to liaise directly over individual cases. The best screening investigations are a Gram stain of a spun deposit of synovial fluid and the lactate level in the supernatant. Very high levels of lactic acid are very suggestive of infection, but do not indicate the type of organism involved; normal or low levels make sepsis unlikely but not impossible. Gram stains may reveal the common Gram-positive rods or diplococci helping in the immediate choice of treatment before cultures are available (see Chapter 10). ZN staining for tubercle bacilli and special culture media for anaerobes and other organisms may be used in addition to standard culture plates. Glucose levels are lower in the synovial fluid than in serum in infections, but this is not a specific finding and is rarely useful diagnostically.

In general the isolation of organisms in synovial fluid should lead to immediate treatment with antibiotics. However, occasional bacteria in an otherwise innocuous-looking fluid may be a contaminant so the results must always be interpreted in the light of the clinical situation and other findings.

4. Looking for crystals and other particles

Synovial fluids contain fragments of articular cartilage and occasional clumps of cells or fibrin. In destructive joint disease the amount of 'joint debris' increases and in inflammatory disorders clumps of fibrin and fibronectin may form into particles of varying diameter (rice bodies). In addition a range of specific crystals may be found (Chapter 9.)

Examination of a drop of fresh fluid in an ordinary light microscope will show cartilage fragments, cell clumps and fibrin deposits. A drop of alizarin red added to the synovial fluid will stain hydroxyapatite and bone fragments and allow clumps of apatite crystals to be detected. Detection of urate and pyrophosphate crystals is best done by polarised-light microscopy, visualisation of other crystals may be improved by electron microscopy.

The basis of polarised-light microscopy is described in Chapter 9.I. All fluids should be examined with this technique, looking for crystals, which appear light against a dark background when crossed polars are used, and then establishing the sign of birefringence using a first-order red compensator. In acute arthritis the finding of several crystals, many of which may be attached to or inside polymorphonuclear cells, is diagnostic of gout or pseudogout (Chapters 9.II and 9.III). Urate crystals are only found in gouty patients, although occasionally they exist in asymptomatic joints in the intercritical period. Pyrophosphate crystals are common in synovial fluid in the elderly and in association with OA, as well as occurring in pseudogout. Apatite crystals are also common in OA and are not disease specific.

OTHER INVESTIGATIONS

When rheumatologists first began the systematic study of synovial fluid in the 1950s, it was assumed that changes in the exudate might reflect disease-specific changes in the synovium. The hope that fluid analysis could therefore lead to easy diagnosis has largely been dashed by the lack of specificity of the various assays attempted. In clinical practice the investigations outlined above are the only useful ones. Other findings of interest include:

1. Immunological assays

Cells in the synovial membrane synthesise antibodies such as rheumatoid factor, and immune complex deposition and complement consumption occur in the membrane and the fluid itself in immune synovitis. Rheumatoid factor and ANA are sometimes found in the synovial fluid before they can be detected in the serum, but unfortunately this is neither a reliable nor a disease-specific finding. Complement levels are often low in the fluid, but again this occurs in most inflammatory arthropathies and does not aid diagnosis. Several new immunological techniques are now being used to study synovial fluid further.

2. Cellular morphology

Joint tumours may result in malignant cells appearing in synovial fluid, but this is so rare that there is no point in looking on a routine basis. In the past inclusion bodies in the phagocytic cells of synovial fluid have received considerable attention — 'ragocytes' (cells with numerous visible inclusions) were thought to be a marker of RA, but are found in many disorders. Immunoflorescent staining may detect immune complexes in these inclusions in RA and SLE, but the exact nature of inclusions in other disorders is not clear.

3. Enzymes and enzyme inhibitors

Lysosomal enzymes including collagenase may be found in synovial fluid. Inhibitors such as α_2 macroglobulin are also present, and the balance of active enzyme-v-inhibitor in free fluid and on the joint surface is of considerable theoretical interest, although difficult to measure.

4. Analysis of protein content

The total protein and hyaluronate content of synovial fluid reflects the inflammatory reaction in the synovium. Separation of the different proteins and products of cartilage is now being carried out in an attempt to look for disease-specific markers and to provide better assays of the activity of joint destruction as well as inflammation.

5. Characterisation and quantification of joint particles

A variety of sophisticated analytical techniques are being used to extract and analyse joint particles in synovial fluid. This may help crystal identification and provide an assessment of joint destruction. Particles can be extracted by cyto-centrifugation or ferrography, and analysed by electron microscopy or infra-red spectroscopy.

FURTHER READING (SYNOVIAL FLUID)

Revell P A 1982 Examination of synovial fluid. Current Topics in Pathology 71: 1–24

Currey H L F, Vernon-Roberts B 1976 Examination of synovial fluid. Clinics in Rheumatic Diseases 2: 149–177

Ropes M, Bauer W 1953 Synovial fluid changes in joint disease. Harvard University Press, Cambridge, Mass

IV Histopathology

Histopathology has a limited role to play in the diagnosis and management of rheumatic diseases. A few rare multi-system disorders and all joint tumours require tissue biopsy for diagnosis. In some of the connective-tissue diseases and in a few other joint disorders biopsies may also be helpful in the diagnosis or management of the condition. However, in the majority of the common rheumatic diseases histology is either unnecessary or unhelpful, and biopsy of joint tissues is surprisingly unrewarding in most cases.

BIOPSY OF ARTICULAR TISSUE

The cartilage, synovium capsule or periarticular tissues of synovial joints can all be biopsied relatively easily. In clinical practice only the synovium is worth examination, and even then only a minority of biopsies will reveal helpful information.

Obtaining and handling synovial tissue

Synovial tissue can be obtained by blind biopsy, at arthroscopy or during an arthrotomy. Some of the advantages and disadvantages of these methods are outlined in Table 24.3.

1. *Percutaneous biopsy* of the synovial lining of large accessible joints is possible using special instruments such as a Parker–Pearson biopsy needle. In practice only the knee is easily biopsied this way; small fragments of the lining of the infrapatella extension of the joint can be obtained via the lateral approach (see Fig. 24.14). The technique is simple, and relatively non-invasive, but limited in the amount of tissue obtained and sites at which it can be used.

2. *Arthroscopy* is a technique which has become very popular in recent years, particularly in orthopaedic practice. Sophisticated instrumentation and flexible fibreoptics allow the insertion of arthroscopes into many joints, both large and small. In large joints, such as the knee, operations can be carried out by use of small surgical instruments inserted into the joint cavity and observed through the arthroscope. Most other joints can be visualised and biopsies can be taken through the arthroscope itself under direct vision. The ability to see all the internal structures of the joint, and take biopsies from suspect areas without a formal arthrotomy, has obvious potential in rheumatological and orthopaedic practice; to date its use is mainly confined to the knee joint, and the major applications are the diagnosis and treatment of internal derangements. Many rheumatologists use knee arthroscopy to assess the synovial lining and articular cartilage and to take samples under direct vision. A limited procedure of this sort can be carried out under local anaesthetic, but it does require operating theatre conditions to minimise the risk of infection.

3. To obtain synovial tissue from most joints other than the knee an *arthrotomy* is required. The obvious disadvantage of surgical opening of a joint cavity is countered by the ability to see the pathology, obtain large amounts of tissue for the histopathologist, and perform any surgical correction necessary at the time of biopsy.

Synovial tissue is delicate, easily crushed, and needs careful handling. For most purposes it is fixed in formal saline, routinely processed and stained with standard reagents such as haematoxylin and eosin. Special procedures are necessary

Table 24.3 Methods of obtaining synovial tissue for histopathology

Method	Advantages	Disadvantages
Percutaneous biopsy	Simple Relatively non-invasive Few complications	Limited number of joints (mainly used at the knee) 'Blind', and may be unrepresentative Small fragments of tissue
Arthroscopy	Can be done with local anaesthetic Very small incision needed Biopsy under direct vision Joint contents can be examined visually	Full sterile operative conditions required Expensive equipment and skilled operator necessary Limited number of joints (mainly used at the knee) Small fragments of tissue obtained
Arthrotomy	Any joint can be biopsied Full examination of joint contents possible Adequate samples of all joint tissues can be obtained Surgeon can proceed to other things (e.g. meniscectomy or synovectomy) if necessary	Full-scale operation required Increased risk of joint damage, sepsis and other peroperative complications

for the histological diagnosis of certain diseases. ZN staining may detect tubercle bacilli, and culture of the synovium sometimes aids diagnosis of tuberculosis and other chronic infections. Congo Red or other amyloid stains, and iron stains for haemachromatotic tissue, may be helpful. Urate and other crystals are easily dissolved, especially in acid media, and all crystal deposits may be dislodged by sectioning the tissue; limited use of aqueous and acid media, thick sectioning and calcium stains may help detect crystal deposits. Immunofluorescent stains may detect immune-complex deposition in SLE and other conditions, and electron microscopy can reveal special aspects of cellular morphology or apatite crystals, but these and other special techniques are rarely useful in diagnostic rheumatology.

Interpretation of synovial biopsies

Normal synovium consists of a superficial layer of lining cells, only one or two cells thick, on top of a well-vascularised, loose connective-tissue stroma (see Chapter 1). Most joint disease is accompanied by changes in this structure, but they are usually non-specific because the tissue reacts in a small number of stereotyped ways to a variety of different insults. Biopsies are usually small and may not be representative of the whole joint reaction because synovial changes are often patchy and vary greatly in quantity, if not in quality, in different parts of the joint.

Non-specific changes

These include hypertrophy, inflammation, hyperaemia, fibrosis and the formation of splits. Hypertrophy of the lining cells results in an increased area of the membrane — reflected by formation of fronds or folds in the synovium — and in an increase in the number of cells in the layer lining the joint cavity. Inflammation is reflected by a cellular infiltrate. In rheumatoid arthritis plasma cells and lymphocytes are numerous and nodules occasionally form; in acute synovitis of other causes polymorphonuclear leucocytes are often prominent; and in osteoarthritis a patchy, mild mononuclear cell infiltrate is common. However,

'Non-specific' synovial changes seen in most joint diseases

1. Hypertrophy of lining cells
2. Inflammatory cell infiltrate
3. Hyperaemia
4. Fibrosis
5. Splits in synovial lining.

inflammatory findings at synovial biopsy are patchy, non-specific and correlate poorly with clinical findings; plasma cell infiltrates can occur in OA and other 'non-immunological' diseases, for example. Fibrosis and hyperaemia are equally variable and non-specific findings, although the latter is more prominent in chronic low-grade synovitis as in OA, whereas hyperaemia is often very prominent in bacterial and other types of acute synovitis. Splits are often seen in the lining of pathological synovial tissue, but have no disease specificity.

Specific synovial histology

This may be found in the diseases listed below.

Diagnoses which may be made by synovial biopsy

Joint diseases which require biopsy for diagnosis

1. Pigmented villonodular synovitis
2. Synovial chondromatosis
3. Synovial sarcoma

Joint diseases in which synovial biopsy may contribute to diagnosis

1. Joint tuberculosis
2. Primary amyloidosis
3. Low-grade bacterial and fungal infections
4. Sarcoidosis
5. Ochronosis
6. Haemochromatosis
7. Crystal deposition diseases
8. Multicentric reticulohistiocytosis

Synovial tumours can only be diagnosed by biopsy, as discussed in Chapter 13.III. In the other diseases listed diagnosis is often made from biopsies of other sites, or from other investigations, but synovial findings are disease-specific and may clinch the diagnosis. The use of special stains or other techniques may help, and liaison between clinician and pathologist is required if one of these unusual arthropathies is suspected.

Other articular-tissue samples

Samples of capsule, cartilage, subarticular bone or periarticular tissues are sometimes available at operation, particularly when arthroplasty is being performed. This is very rarely of any help in the diagnosis or assessment of joint disease, although the study of resected cartilage has aided the understanding of osteoarthritis and related disorders, and often shows evidence of clinically unsuspected crystal deposition. Occasionally it is only when the tissues of an operated joint are examined that the definitive diagnosis of one of the rarer arthropathies is made.

BIOPSY OF EXTRA-ARTICULAR TISSUES

Numerous tissues may be biopsied to aid the diagnosis or management of rheumatic diseases. Below are listed some sites of biopsy and the conditions which may be apparent on examination of the tissues obtained. Of those listed, the skin

Extra-articular tissues sometimes biopsied in rheumatology practice, and diseases which may be apparent on histopathology of biopsy

1. Skin
   a) Scleroderma
   b) SLE
   c) Vasculitis
   d) Psoriasis
   e) Sarcoidosis
2. Subcutaneous tissue/nodules
   a) Rheumatoid arthritis
   b) Gout
   c) Calcinosis
   d) Sarcoidosis
   e) Xanthomatosis
   f) SLE
   g) Granuloma annulare
   h) Multicentric reticulohistiocytosis
   i) Eosinophilic fasciitis
   j) Amyloidosis
3. Liver
   a) Amyloidosis
   b) Haemochromatosis
   c) Granulomatous disease of the liver
   d) Wilson's disease
4. Rectal mucosa
   a) Amyloidosis
   b) Vasculitis
   c) Ulcerative colitis
5. Bowel mucosa
   a) Ulcerative colitis
   b) Crohn's disease
   c) Whipple's disease
   d) Amyloidosis
   e) Coeliac disease
6. Lymph nodes
   a) Lymploma
   b) Tuberculosis
   c) Sarcoidosis
7. Kidney
   a) SLE
   b) Amyloidosis
   c) Wegener's granulomatosis
8. Muscle
   Polymyositis
9. Salivary glands
   Sjögren's syndrome
10. Temporal artery
    Giant cell arteritis
11. Bone
    a) Osteoporosis
    b) Osteomalacia
    c) Bone tumours
    d) Osteomyelitis
    e) Hyperparathyroidism

and subcutaneous tissues and rectal mucosa are perhaps most often looked at for diagnostic purposes. Renal biopsy is helpful in managing SLE and the labial glands, temporal artery and skeletal muscle are each obtained for a specific diagnostic purpose. Liver samples or gut mucosa may be necessary to make a diagnosis of certain gastrointestinal disorders, and bone biopsy is often helpful in assessing osteopaenia.

Some of the rheumatic diseases in which it may be helpful to obtain biopsy material are listed below. In addition to the disorders listed above, which require synovial biopsy, a few rare systemic disorders which may present with arthritis, or affect the joints, can only be diagnosed by histopathology. Biopsies may contribute to several other, more common, rheumatic diseases, although in the majority of individual cases it is unnecessary. The histological findings and their significance are dealt with in the sections describing the individual diseases and will not be repeated here.

Multisystem diseases which require diagnosis by histopathology, and sites from which biopsy material can be taken to make a diagnosis

1. *Amyloidosis*
   Rectum, liver or kidney, subcutaneous fat, synovium and carpal tunnel
2. *Sarcoidosis*
   Skin, lymph nodes, synovium
3. *Whipple's disease*
   Bowel mucosa, lymph nodes, synovium
4. *Haemachromatosis*
   Liver, synovium
5. *Multicentric reticulohistiocytosis*
   Skin, subcutaneous nodules, lymph nodes, synovium
6. *Leukaemias and lymphomas*
   Lymph nodes, bone marrow (synovium)
7. *Eosinophilic fasciitis*
   Skin and subcutaneous tissue

Multisystem diseases in which histopathology may contribute to the diagnosis, and sites from which biopsy material can be taken

1. *Rheumatoid arthritis*
   Nodules, synovium
2. *SLE*
   Skin, kidney
3. *Scleroderma*
   Skin
4. *Polymyositis*
   Muscle
5. *Polyarteritis nodosa*
   Muscle, skin, and subcutaneous tissue, kidney testes
6. *Wegner's granulomatosis*
   Nasal mucosa, lung, kidney
7. *Giant cell arteritis*
   Temporal artery
8. *Sjögren's syndrome*
   Lip gland, salivary glands
9. *Ochronosis*
   Synovium, cartilage
10. *Crystal deposition diseases*
    Nodules, synovium
11. *Psoriasis*
    Skin
12. *Inflammatory bowel disease*
    Bowel mucosa

FURTHER READING (HISTOPATHOLOGY)

Berry C L 1982, Bone and joint disease. Current Topics in Pathology 71. Springer, Berlin

Gardner D L 1972 The pathology of rheumatoid arthritis. Williams & Wilkins, Baltimore.

Goldenberg D L, Cohen A S 1978 Synovial membrane histopathology. Medicine 57: 239–256

V Diagnostic Immunology

Immunological abnormalities are found in many rheumatic diseases and have been studied in an attempt to understand the underlying pathogenesis of these disorders. Another major aim of studying these abnormalities has been to identify tests which will be helpful in clinical practice in one or more of the following ways:

1. As a sensitive screening test
2. As a specific and reliable diagnositic aid
3. As a marker of disease activity
4. As a indicator of prognosis

Tests which are helpful in the diagnosis and management of patients with rheumatic diseases are shown below. As will be seen, they all have their drawbacks and are not intended to stand alone but should be interpreted in conjunction with a careful history and physical examination, and other investigations.

Immunological tests used widely in rheumatology

1. Screening tests
   a) Rheumatoid factor
   b) ANA
2. Diagnosis and disease classification
   a) Anti-DNA
   b) Precipitating anti-tissue antibodies, e.g. anti-Sm
   c) Lupus band test
3. Prognosis
   a) Rheumatoid factor
   b) Anti-DNA
   c) Anti-nRNP
4. Disease activity
   a) Complement
   b) Anti-DNA

RHEUMATOID FACTOR

Rheumatoid factor is a term applied to any antibody that reacts with the Fc fragment of human or animal IgG. The classical rheumatoid factor is a 19s IgM molecule, but it is now clear that rheumatoid-factor activity can be detected in all the immunoglobulin classes. Assays commonly used in diagnostic laboratories have not changed much in the last 30 years and employ agglutination or flocculation of IgG-coated cells or particles which primarily detect IgM rheumatoid factor because of its multiple valency. An example is the RA latex test which uses latex beads passively coated with human IgG which are cross-linked by rheumatoid factor to produce a visible flocculation (Fig. 24.17). Another widely-used technique is the Rose–Waaler test in which rheumatoid factor interacts with sheep red cells coated with subagglutinating doses of rabbit IgG to cause haemagglutination. Since the presence of heterophile antibodies which react directly with sheep red blood cells can give rise to false-positive results, sera are usually tested in parallel with both coated and uncoated sheep cells and the difference in titres is expressed the differential agglutination titre (DAT). Alternatively the test serum is incubated with untreated sheep red cells prior to testing with immunoglobulin-coated cells. This is the SCAT technique. The titre is expressed as the greatest serum dilution to cause agglutination. This test detects rheumatoid factor which cross-reacts with rabbit IgG. Rheumatoid factor of this specificity is highly characteristic of RA and the DAT tends to be less sensitive but more specific for RA. Recently the technique of laser nephelometry has been more widely used to detect rheumatoid factor and

Diseases commonly associated with rheumatoid factor

1. Rheumatoid arthritis (75%)
2. Other rheumatic diseases — SLE, PSS, Sjogren's
3. Acute viral infections — mononucleosis, hepatitis, influenza, etc, after vaccination
4. Parasitic infections — trypanosomiasis, malaria, schistosomiasis, etc
5. Chronic inflammatory diseases — TB, leprosy, syphilis, SBE, etc
6. Neoplasms — after irradiation or chemotherapy
7. Other hyperglobulinaemic states — hypergammaglobulinaemic purpura, sarcoidosis, chronic liver disease, cryoglobulinaemia

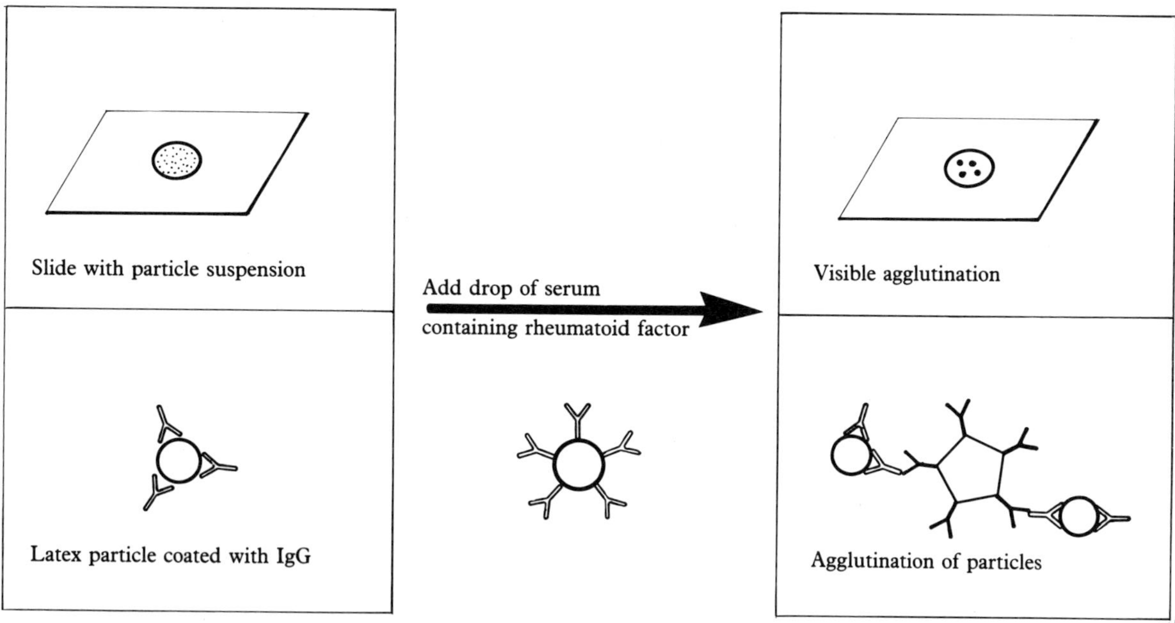

Fig. 24.17 The RA latex test

appears to have the advantage of being more reproducible than other methods.

Tests for IgM rheumatoid factor have some value as screening tests for rheumatoid disease. Rheumatoid factor is present in 75% of RA patients and a positive DAT in a titre greater than 1:32 supports the diagnosis of RA in the appropriate clinical setting. However, it is not specific for RA and, as can be seen from the list opposite, it can be found during the course of certain infections, in a proportion of patients with other diseases and in 15% of the population over the age of 65.

The presence of rheumatoid factor in RA indicates a poorer prognosis, with more severe joint disease and a higher frequency of systemic manifestations. The presence of high titres of IgG rheumatoid factor is also associated with severe systemic complications, such as vasculitis. IgG rheumatoid factor can only be measured at present in specialised centres using techniques such as solid-phase radio-immunoassays, illustrated in Figure 24.18.

ANTINUCLEAR ANTIBODIES

The discovery of the lupus erythematosus (LE) cell by Hargreaves in 1948 led to the first serological test used in the diagnosis of SLE. The LE cell test has now been replaced by the technique of indirect immunofluorescence (IMF) to detect

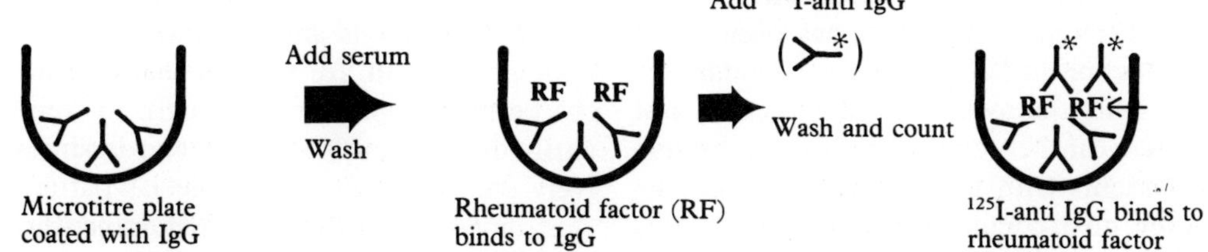

Fig. 24.18 Radio-immunoassay for IgG rheumatoid factor

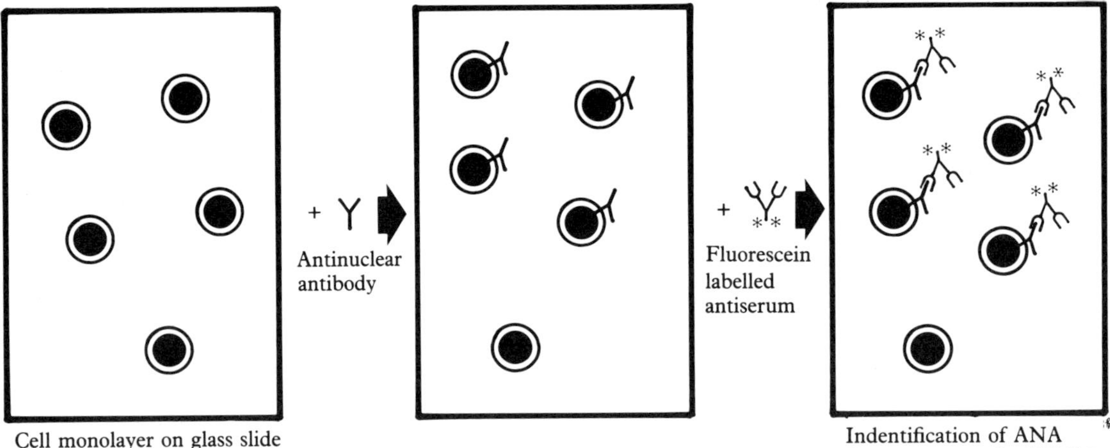

Fig. 24.19 Indirect immunofluorescence technique to detect antinuclear antibodies

ANA. This technique is more sensitive, simpler to perform, and easier to interpret.

The IMF test is illustrated in Figure 24.19. A preparation of mammalian nuclei on a glass slide is incubated with the patient's serum. At one time thin sections of tissue, e.g. rat kidney or mouse liver, were used as the substrate, but now there is a trend towards using human cell lines from tumours or fibroblasts grown as a monolayer on the glass slide. The advantage here is the large nuclei which are easier to visualise and the presence of cells in all stages of cell division which present nuclear antigens either absent or only in small quantities in resting nuclei. After incubation, which allows ANA to fix to nuclear antigens the serum is washed off and replaced by a solution containing fluorescein-conjugated antibody to human gammaglobulin. The fluorescent antiglobulin attaches to the ANA and is visualised when the slide is examined under the fluorescence microscope. The incidence of ANA depends upon the assay system and the titres chosen to separate positive and negative sera, and uniformity of this test between different laboratories has been aided by the introduction of WHO positive standards.

This represents the most helpful screening test for SLE. ANA can be detected by this technique in 95% of patients with this disease. It is important, however, to recognise the limitation of this test. It is diagnostically non-specific and ANA can be detected by fluorescence not only in other connective tissue diseases but also in other disorders, as shown in Table 24.4. Furthermore, althought the titre of ANA may fluctuate during the course of SLE it is not a predictable indicator of disease activity.

Table 24.4 Antinuclear antibodies in various diseases

Disease	Pos ANA (%)	Titre > 1/1000 (%)
RA	61	1
Scleroderma	90	30
Polymyositis	22	0
PAN	18	0
JCA	33	8
Lupoid hepatitis	100	50
Myaesthenia gravis	50	0
Waldenstrom's	13	2

Different patterns of nuclear fluorescence can be visualised and are presumed to reflect the predominant specificity of ANA present in the serum. The major patterns are illustrated in Figure 24.20, and to some extent the interpretation of these patterns can increase the diagnostic specificity of this test. The homogeneous and speckled patterns are very non-specific and are seen in many disorders, but the peripheral pattern is thought to correspond to antibodies directed to DNA and is almost exclusively seen in SLE. The nucleolar pattern and the centromere pattern are predominantly seen in systemic sclerosis, the latter being associated with the CREST syndrome (Table 24.5).

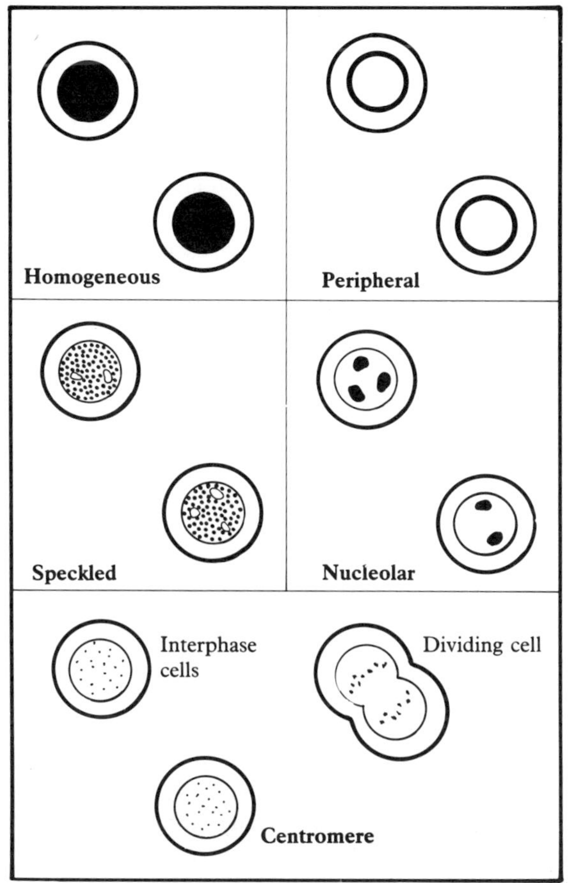

Fig. 24.20 Patterns of nuclear immunofluorescence produced by antinuclear antibodies

ANTI-DNA

Tests to detect antibodies to DNA are valuable in the diagnosis and the management of patients with SLE. Antibodies may be formed to a number of different antigenic determinants on the DNA molecule. It is convenient, however, to divide these antibodies into two categories: those that react with native or double-stranded DNA (nDNA) and those that react only with denatured or single-stranded DNA (ssDNA).

1. Antibodies to nDNA

Antibodies to nDNA are highly specific for SLE. They are present in two-thirds of patients with active, untreated SLE and are only rarely found in other disorders. Titres of anti-DNA often fluctuate with disease activity and may be used in conjunction with complement levels to help assess the disease activity. Chapter 2 describes how these antibodies are almost certainly involved in the pathogenesis of this disease. There are two assays which are commonly used to detect anti-nDNA.

a) Radioimmunoassay (Fig. 24.21)

In this technique radio-labelled nDNA is incubated with the serum. If antibody to nDNA is present, antigen-antibody complexes containing ^{125}I-labelled nDNA are formed and are subsequently separated from the free radio-labelled DNA by precipitation with either 50% ammonium sulphate or an anti-human immunoglobulin serum. The precipitate is then counted in a gamma counter. The limitation of this test is the difficulty of obtaining purely native DNA. Most substrates contain regions of denatured DNA and antibodies reacting only with ssDNA may also be detected. Antibodies to ssDNA have less specificity (Table 24.6) but titres can still be used to monitor disease activity.

Table 24.5 Immunofluorescence patterns of ANA in different connective-tissue diseases

	SLE (%)	RA (%)	Scleroderma (%)	MCTD (%)	Polymyositis (%)
Homogeneous	60	70	10	10	50
Peripheral	5*	0	0	0	0
Speckled	30	25	45	85	20
Nucleolar	5†	5†	15*	5†	30†
Centromere	0	0	30*	0	0

* pattern with greater disease specificity
† often low-titre; high titre anti-nucleolar antibodies characteristic of systemic sclerosis

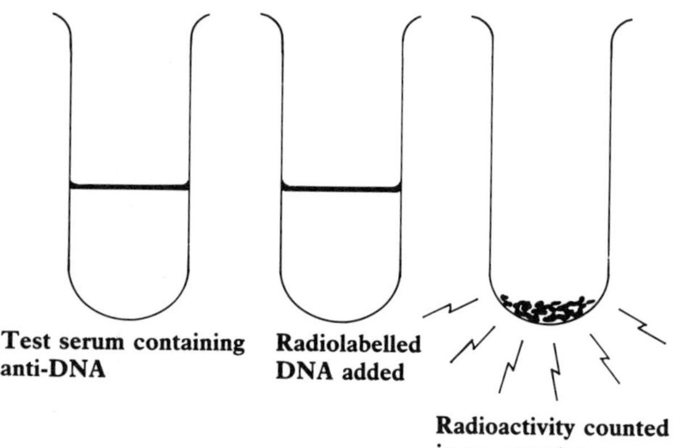

Fig. 24.21 Demonstration of anti-DNA antibodies using a radioimmunoassay

Table 24.6 Incidence of antibodies to native and single-stranded DNA

Disease	Anti-n DNA (%)	Anti-ss DNA (%)
SLE	60	90
Drug-induced LE	0	50
Lupoid hepatitis	2	60
RA	3	50
PBC	0	15
'Normals'	0	5

b) Immunofluorescence using Crithidia luciliae (Fig. 24. 22)

Crithidia luciliae is a haemoflagellate which contains a kinetoplast located near the flagellum and contains a large amount of nDNA. In this test the serum is incubated with organisms which have been layered and fixed on a microscope slide. The slide is developed with fluoroscein-conjugated anti-human globulin and a positive test is indicated by fluorescence of the kinetoplast. The advantage of this technique is that it is possible using appropriate reagents to detect complement-fixing antibodies to DNA since these correlate well with disease activity and particularly with the presence of lupus nephritis.

2. Antibodies to ssDNA

Antibodies to ssDNA react with purine and pyrimidine bases and other sites revealed by denaturing DNA. As shown in Table 24.6, they have less specificity and are found in a variety of disorders. However, they are found in the majority of SLE patients and since these antibodies also have a role in the pathogenesis of tissue lesions such as nephritis, titres may be used to help monitor disease activity. Radioimmunoassay techniques are used using DNA denatured by methods such as boiling.

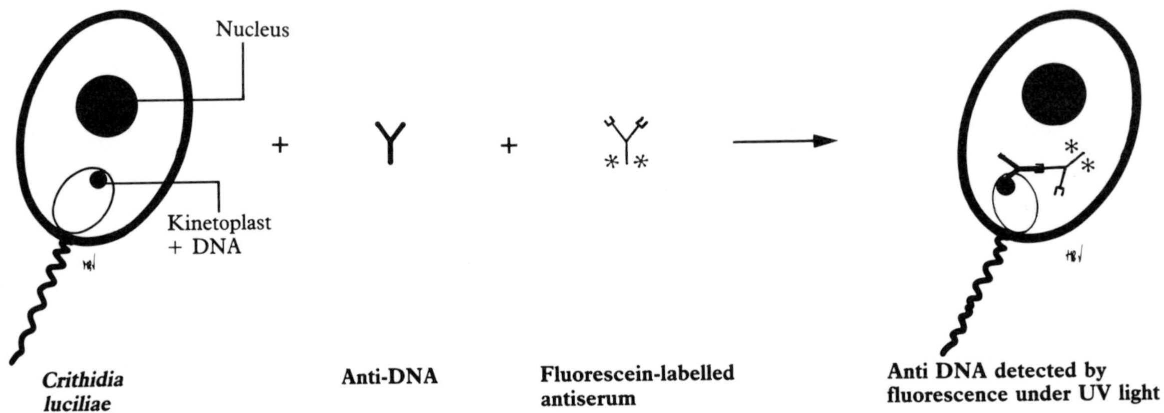

Fig. 24.22 Demonstration of anti-DNA antibodies by immunofluorescence using *Crithidia luciliae*

PRECIPITATING ANTIBODIES TO SOLUBLE ANTIGENS IN TISSUE EXTRACTS

Certain specialist laboratories use immunodiffusion to detect auto-antibodies to a variety of nuclear and cytoplasmic antigens present in tissue extracts. These auto-antibodies are commonly found in the sera of patients with various connective tissue diseases (Table 24.7). The technique of double immunodiffusion is commonly used in which test and reference sera are allowed to diffuse in agarose gels against a source of antigen, usually a saline extract of mammalian tissue such as calf thymus extract (CTE) or human spleen extract (HSE). The presence of antibody which reacts with a component of the tissue extract results in a precipitin line (Fig. 24.23). If this antibody system is identical to a reference serum which contains a defined antibody system, the precipitin lines will fuse to form a line of identity. If not, the precipitin lines will cross.

Some laboratories use the technique of counter-immunodiffusion which makes use of the acidic properties of many of these tissue antigens. Serum is placed in the cathodal well and extract in the anodal well. During electrophoresis, antibody and antigen migrate towards each other to form a precipitin band (Fig. 24.24). This test is more sensitive than double immunodiffusion but comparisons with prototype sera are more difficult.

Antibodies to the four antigens nRNP, Sm, Ro (SSA), and La(SSB) are commonly found in the sera of lupus patients Table 24.8) and their presence helps to support the clinical diagnosis. Anti-Sm is rarely found in conditions other than SLE but the other autoantibodies are found in other connective tissue disease. Their potential value lies in identifying patients with various patterns of clinical manifestation and this is described in further detail on p. 110.

Table 24.7 Auto-antibodies characterised by precipitin reactions in connective-tissue diseases

Antigen	Disease
Sm	SLE
nRNP	SLE, MCTD
Ro(SSA)	SLE, Sjogren's
La(SSB)	SLE, Sjogren's
Ma	SLE
RAP	RA
Scl-70	Systemic sclerosis
Jo-1	Polymyositis
Mi	Polymyositis
PM-1	Polymyositis-scleroderma overlap
Ku	Polymyositis-scleroderma overlap

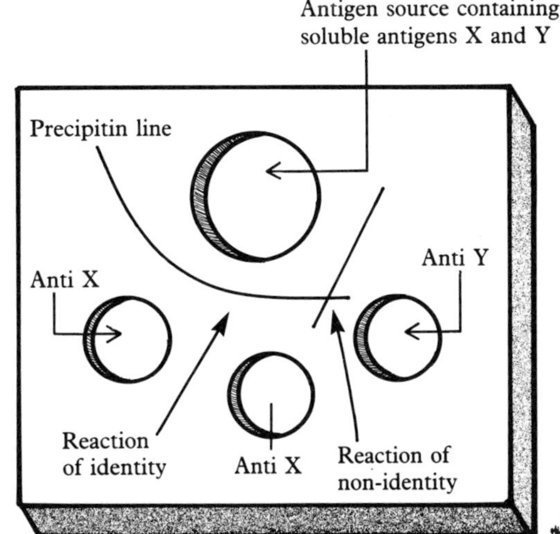

Fig. 24.23 The technique of passive immunodiffusion to detect precipitating antibodies to soluble antigens

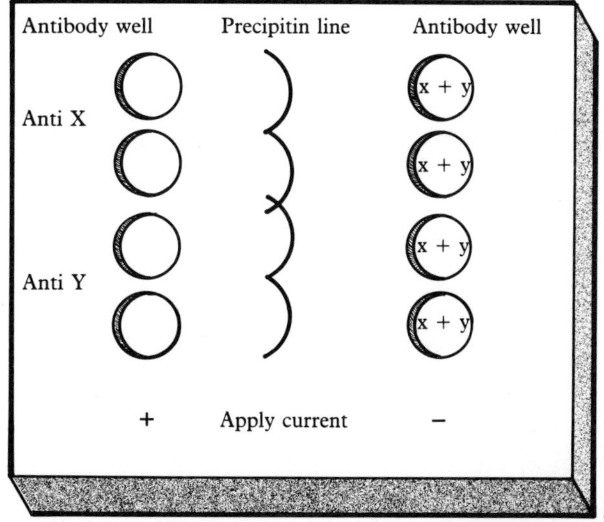

Fig. 24.24 The technique of counter-immunoelectrophoresis

Table 24.8 Frequency of precipitins to soluble antigens in connective-tissue diseases

Disease	Frequency of precipitins (%)	Predominant precipitin	
SLE	75	Anti Ro	40%
		Anti nRNP	30%
		Anti La	20%
		Anti Sm	10%
PSS	65	Anti Scl-70	20%
Polymyositis	55	Anti Jo-1	30%
Sjögren's	60	Anti-Ro	50%
		Anti La	20%

Precipitating auto-antibodies to other soluble antigens are found in the sera of patients with systemic sclerosis and polymyositis but their clinical relevance is not yet well defined.

COMPLEMENT

The standard method of complement measurement has been the total haemolytic complement level (CH50) which is measured by determining the greatest dilution of the patients serum that will cause 50% haemolysis of sensitised sheep red blood cells. Methods are also widely available to measure the level of individual complement components such as C3, C4 and Factor B using the technique of single radial immunodiffusion. This is illustrated in Figure 24.25, and for C3, anti-human C3 antiserum is incorporated into an agarose gel and wells cut to contain the patient's serum. C3 diffuses into the agarose forming a precipitin ring. The diameter of the ring corresponds to the concentration of C3 in the serum.

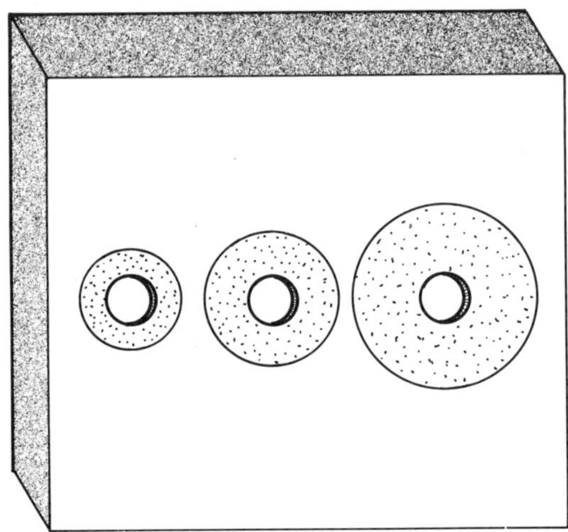

Fig. 24.25 Single radial immunodiffusion. Antibody is incorporated into the gel and the diameter of the precipitin ring is proportional to the concentration of antigen in the well.

Causes of depressed and elevated complement levels

Elevated complement levels — Any stimulus, e.g. inflammation causing an acute phase response

Depressed complement levels

1. Complement consumption
   a) Rheumatic diseases — SLE
      — RA with extra-articular features, e.g. vasculitis
      — Systemic vasculitides
   b) Glomerulonephritis — Post-streptococcal
      — Membranoproliferative
   c) Infections — SBE
      — Hepatitis B surface antigenaemia
      — Gram-negative sepsis
   d) Deficiency of control proteins — CI esterase inhibitor deficiency
      — C3b inactivator deficiency
2. Specific complement component deficiency
3. Severe hepatic failure and malnutrition (hyposynthesis)

Specialised complement laboratories have the capability to measure other complement components and inhibitors of the complement pathway such as C1-esterase inhibitor.

Causes of depressed and elevated complement levels are shown opposite. Depressed complement levels suggest complement consumption during active immunologically-mediated tissue injury and occurs most commonly in active SLE. It may also occur in patients with RA who develop systemic vasculitis. In these cases, complement levels are valuable in helping to assess the state of disease activity and the response to treatment. Inherited selective deficiences of complement components or inhibitors are a rare cause of low CH50 and are described in Chapter II. High complement levels are not so helpful and occur as part of the acute phase response to inflammation. High levels of C3, for example, are seen frequently in Reiter's syndrome, RA and gout.

IMMUNOFLUORESCENCE OF SKIN BIOPSIES

1. Direct immunofluorescence of skin lesions in SLE and DLE

Direct immunofluorescence examination of lupus skin lesions employing fluorescein-conjugated antisera virtually always demonstrates deposition of immunoglobulin and complement in a granular pattern along the basement membrane of the diseased skin. The diagnosis should be questioned in the absence of such deposits.

2. Direct immunofluorescence of uninvolved skin in SLE: the lupus band test

Granular deposits of immunoglobulin and complement can be demonstrated at the basement membrane of uninvolved skin in the extensor surface of the upper third of the forearm in two-thirds of SLE patients. This finding strongly suggests the clinical diagnosis of SLE, since it is rarely found in other conditions. These immunofluorescent deposits tend to appear and disappear with fluctuating disease activity and correlate with anti DNA titres and complement levels.

MISCELLANEOUS TESTS

Multiple auto-immune phenomena are seen in patients with SLE, and a positive Coomb's test and a biological false-positive WR help to support the clinical diagnosis of lupus. A number of other tests including those to detect circulating immune complexes and HLA-typing are more relevant to the pathogenesis of certain rheumatic diseases than to their diagnosis and clinical management.

1. Circulating immune complexes

The role of circulating immune complexes in the pathogenesis of rheumatic diseases such as SLE and RA is discussed in Chapter 2. More than 20 methods have been developed for detection of immune complexes. Some of these are shown below and are based on various physicochemical and biological properties of immune complexes. Physicochemical methods are based on size separation, diminished solubility at 4°C and differential solubility in solutions such as polyethylene glycol. Immunological methods are based on complement-

Examples of methods to detect immune complexes

1. Physical methods
   a) Analytical ultracentrifugation
   b) Sucrose density gradient ultracentrifugation
   c) Gel filtration
2. Interaction with C1q
   a) Precipitation in gels with C1q
   b) Precipitation in polyethylene glycol of radio-labelled C1q with complexes
   c) C1q coated polystyrene tubes
   d) C1q deviation test
3. Interaction with Fc and complement receptors on cells
   a) Raji cell assay
   b) Platelet aggregation
4. Interaction with rheumatoid factor
5. Histamine release from perfused guinea-pig lung preparations

binding and activation, immunoglobulin content, and on interaction with cell surface receptors for complement components and the Fc region of IgG. Each assay appears to have a differential sensitivity for immune complexes of certain sizes and composition and this probably accounts for why there is such a poor correlation between the different assays. For example, on one hand the fluid phase Clq assay is more sensitive in detecting immune complexes formed at equivalence to relative antigen excess, and on the other the Raji-cell assay is more sensitive in detecting immune complexes formed at equivalence to relative antibody excess. These assays correlate poorly with disease activity and a major direction for the future will be to clarify the composition and properties of the complexes being detected and to develop assays that can be directly related to particular disease manifestations.

2. Immunogenetics

In recent years there has been considerable progress in elucidating the relationship between HLA antigens and certain rheumatic diseases. This association is described in Chapter 2. The most striking relationship to date is the association between HLA B27 and ankylosing spondylitis. This has greatest relevance to the study of immunopathogenesis of these diseases and HLA typing does not have a role in routine clinical management.

FURTHER READING (IMMUNOLOGY)

Jeffery M S, Carson Dick W 1983 The role of the laboratory in rheumatology. Clinics in Rheumatic Diseases 9: 1

Synkowski D R, Mogavero H S, Provost T T 1980 Lupus Erythematosus: laboratory testing and clinical subsets in the evaluation of patients. Medical Clinics of North America 64: 921–940

VI Electromyography in the Investigation of the Rheumatic Diseases

Electomyography is helpful for investigation of lower motor neurone lesions and in muscle disorders.

Nerve conduction time can be measured by applying an electrical stimulus at two points along a nerve and measuring the motor response at a distal muscle via a needle electrode, or the sensory impulse arriving at a distal branch of the nerve via a surface electrode. The time taken for the impulse applied at each of these points to evoke a response is called the *latency* and the nerve conduction time is calculated by dividing the distance between the two points by the latency at each point (Fig. 24.26). The normal motor conduction velocity is 50–60 m/s in the median and ulnar nerve and 45–50 m/s in the lateral popliteal nerve.

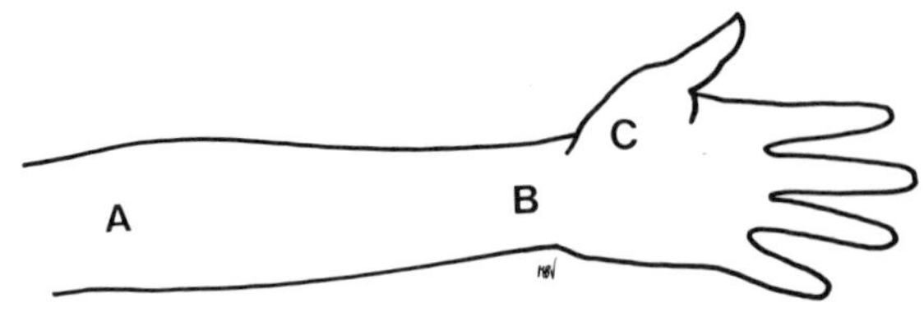

Fig. 24.26 Calculation of nerve conduction time. **A** and **B** = points stimulated; **C** = muscle electrode. Nerve conduction = (Latency from **A**) – (Latency from **B**)

The electrical activity of muscle is investigated by measuring action potentials produced at rest and on contraction of the muscle. The evoked responses are displayed on an oscilloscope and a paper record can be taken. Normal muscle is electrically silent at rest. On slight contraction, motor-unit potentials of 500–1000 μV in amplitude and 4–8 ms in duration are recorded. On maximal contraction, as many motor units as possible are recruited and interference pattern develops.

Some indications for electromyography in the rheumatic disorders are shown below.

Some common indications for electromyography in rheumatic disorders

1. Peripheral entrapment neuropathy particularly carpal tunnel syndrome
2. Polymyositis
3. Peripheral neuropathy (particularly RA, PAN)

The diagnosis of carpal tunnel syndrome is confirmed by showing that motor nerve conduction in the nerve is normal in the forearm but slowed across the wrist. Prolongation of sensory conduction can also be demonstrated and is usually present before motor nerve impairment. It is essential to show that conduction velocity is normal in another peripheral nerve in the limb, usually the ulnar, to exclude a peripheral neuropathy. Nerve conduction may also help in: 1. the diagnosis of ulnar nerve compression at the elbow and differentiation from a peripheral neuropathy; C8/T1 root compression in the neck; brachial plexus compression in the thoracic outlet syndrome; syringomyelia; and motor neurone disease; 2. differential diagnosis of weakness of the small muscles of the hand; 3. diagnosis of common peroneal nerve lesions; (and differentiation of this from a sciatic nerve-root lesion, and a peripheral neuropathy).

In polymyositis, there may be a diagnostic triad of electromyographic abnormalities: 1. spontaneous fibrillation; 2. short duration action potentials in a polyphasic disorganised outline; 3. repetitive bouts of high-voltage oscillations produced by contact of the diseased muscle with the needle.

It is important to realise that in a clinically obvious case of polymyositis, the electromyogram may be entirely normal. Serial tests at intervals of about 6 weeks are useful to assess progress of the disease and response to therapy.

In the distal sensory neuropathy of rheumatoid arthritis, the sensory nerve conduction is slowed due to segmental axonal demyelination. The more serious mixed sensorimotor neuropathy that may arise from vasculitis of the vasa vasorum is characterised by axonal degeneration and, consequently, nerve conduction is normal but there is a denervation pattern (multiple fibrillation potentials in the muscle).

FURTHER READING (ELECTROMYOGRAPHY)

Walton J N 1977 Brain's diseases of the nervous system. Oxford University Press, Oxford

SECTION SIX

Treatment

25 An introduction to therapy of rheumatic disease

AIMS OF THERAPY AND PATIENT ASSESSMENT

Therapeutic aims include the relief of musculoskeletal symptoms, preservation of function, and the control of rheumatic disease. Pain is often the most important symptom, although stiffness, immobility, anxiety or depression may dominate the clinical picture. Preservation of function may involve the use of local treatment such as splints, injections and physiotherapy, as well as altering the patient's environment to adjust to his or her disability. Control of the disease process should help prevent further disability or complications of the condition, as well as relieving symptoms. Several different types of treatment may be applicable to each of these aims.

Therapeutic aims and techniques available in the management of rheumatic diseases

Aims

1. Relief of symptoms
2. Maintenance and restoration of function
3. Specific treatment for a disease process or complication

Techniques

1. Education and advice
2. Physiotherapy and manipulation
3. Occupational therapy
4. Splints, footwear, walking aids
5. Other aids and appliances
6. Drugs
7. Intra- or periarticular injections
8. Surgery
9. Experimental therapy
10. Alternative medicine

Construction of an effective management plan and correct use of these measures for the individual patient, depend on clear delineation of the most important problems. Factors that must be taken into account include the patient's present circumstances and his or her fears and aspirations for the future, as well as the activity, symptoms and functional problems caused by the disease. The physician is unlikely to make good long-term decisions without some idea of the personality, life-style and expectations of the patient.

CO-ORDINATED MANAGEMENT AND PATIENT EDUCATION

Priorities in patient managment vary in different diseases. The development of an acute emergency (Table 25.1) must take preference over all other issues. Some rheumatic disorders are quickly put right, and lengthy explanations or use of ancillary services may be quite unnecessary. In others chronic problems are likely to develop and effective therapy is limited; these are the most difficult situations and the ones in which the skill of the physician in assessment, choice of therapy and general patient management are fully tested.

When a 'cure' is not available, and chronic symptoms or some disability are inevitable, some

Table 25.1 Some acute emergencies in rheumatology

Condition	Presentation	Susceptible patients	Chapter
Joint or bone sepsis	Acute monoarthritis	Immunosupressed patients, rheumatoid arthritis	4, 10
Temporal arteritis	Visual disturbance, blindness	Elderly people, polymyalgia rheumatica	12
Other forms of vasculitis	Mononeuritis multiplex, gangenous extremity, severe abdominal pain	Connective-tissue disorder	7(V)
Iritis	Painful red eye	Seronegative spondarthritis	5, 15
Scleritis		Rheumatoid disease	4, 15
Gout, Pseudogout	Acute monoarthritis	Elderly, hyperuricaemic, diuretics, with surgery or intercurrent illness	9(II), 9(III)
Vertebral collapse	Severe back pain	Steroids, Osteoporosis	17, 22(II)
Cervical subluxation, spinal compression	Weakness, long tract signs	Rheumatoid arthritis	4, 15(IV)
Acute adrenal insufficiency	Hypotensive collapse	Steroids	26
Acute joint rupture	'Deep venous thrombosis' in the calf	Any active synovitis	4, 15(IV)
Acute bone marrow failure	Oral ulceration, infection, bleeding and bruising	Patients on gold, penicillamine and immunosuppressive drugs	26
Cardiac tamponade	Hypotensive collapse	Rheumatoid arthritis	4, 15(V)
Perforation or acute GI bleed	Collapse, haematemesis, severe abdominal pain	Steroids, non-steroidal drugs, especially in rheumatoid disease	4, 15(VIII), 26
Lupus crisis	Fever, bleeding, collapse, fits, and severe neuropsychiatric disturbance	Systemic lupus erythematosus	7(II)

patients and doctors get disheartened. Many patients still report that their doctor dismissed them saying that 'nothing could be done' and that they must 'learn to live with it'. The patient usually needs a more optimistic approach, but it must be a realistic, honest and genuinely helpful one. Informed advice, an understanding approach and caring atmosphere can themselves be of major benefit. More specific therapy requires a careful assessment of need and the ability to orchestrate and co-ordinate the different treatments indicated. The physician may need help and advice from a variety of ancillary specialists, and needs a good knowledge of the help available both in the health system and the community.

Education and advice

Most patients with rheumatic problems are frightened about the future, and concerned that they may have a serious, crippling form of joint disease. Many need advice about rest and exercise, about food, drink, drugs, sex and many other aspects of life.

Reassurance about the correct diagnosis, and advice that normal activity will not wreck joints and that food won't make much difference, may be all that is necessary. Counselling about employment, sexual problems, housing and other aspects of adjustment to a chronic disabling disease may require a good deal of time and expertise. Several patient booklets and advice sheets are available to supplement the doctor's advice, and patient self-help groups can be helpful.

SEQUENTIAL STAGING OF THERAPY IN CHRONIC RHEUMATIC DISEASES

Patients who contract a disease such as rheumatoid arthritis pass through several different stages in the evolution of their illness. The physical condition often has an insidious onset, an early inflammatory phase and then a later stage in which destructive changes may be present but the disease is less active. Phases in the psychological reaction to the condition may include shock, rejection, anger, depression and finally acceptance of the disease.

Table 25.2 Sequential approach to the treatment of rheumatic disease

Stage of disease	Therapy
Early disease, minor symptoms	Advice, joint protection, little or no use of drugs
Early disease with active inflammation	Rest splints, general rest, non-steroidal anti-inflammatory drugs
Continuing active disease in spite of above	Physio to maintain muscles and movement, full anti-inflammatory drugs, consider use of specific drugs
Chronic disease with joint damage	Physiotherapy as above, aids and appliances, surgery
Applicable at all times	Education, advice and support and injection therapy for local problems

Therapy must be geared to the physical and mental stage reached by an individual patient (Table 25.2). In the early phases education, rest to reduce inflammation and psychological support for the family as well as the patient are often most useful. Resting splints, maintenance of movement and muscle bulk and non-steroidal anti-inflammatory drugs are often used. If disease activity continues other drugs, local injections, other physical therapy or surgery may be helful. In the chronic phase aids, appliances and other rehabilitation measures may be more useful.

SOME SPECIFIC THERAPEUTIC MEASURES AVAILABLE

1. Physiotherapy

The physiotherapist can help relieve musculoskeletal symptoms, improve joint motion and muscle power and re-educate co-ordinated function of the back and limbs. In some conditions, such as ankylosing spondylitis, physical therapy is the single most important aspect of therapy, and in many others it is a useful adjunct to other measures.

Heat, ice-packs, wax baths and other local external applications may cause temporary relief of symptoms and induce muscle relaxation, but do little else. Their main role is to help the physiotherapist to improve movement and muscle activity, although they are sometimes overused or abused in lieu of more active and effective treatment.

Educating patients to maintain a full range of joint motion and contract muscles to maintain their bulk and power is often very important. Early training of this sort can, for example, prevent patients developing flexion deformities of the knee or weakness and contractures of other joints.

Various manipulative techniques are used by physiotherapists and may help improve the range of movement of joints in the back, the shoulder and elsewhere. Re-education of posture and movement may be an essential part of rehabilitating the disabled patient who, due to pain or deformity, has lost function.

Hydrotherapy also has an important role in rehabilitation, allowing muscles and joints to relax and move freely in a warm, pain-relieving environment without the constraints of normal gravity. Many disabled patients are able to walk again by first taking steps in a hydrotherapy pool. Some local conditions such as osteoarthritis of the hip may also respond well to pool exercises.

Appropriate full use of these skills requires close co-operation between the physician and physiotherapist.

2. Splints and orthoses

Splints may be used to rest joints, to prevent deformity or to aid power and function in a limb. Rest is an important part of treatment in active synovitis, and resting hand, wrist or leg splints may help treat acute arthritis. They should not be used for too long, and daily exercises to maintain joint motion and muscle bulk are necessary. Splints may also be useful in chronic disease: back splints for the knees, for example, may stop the development of flexion contractures, which often appear due to an unconscious tendency to flex the knees at night. Wrist splints may aid power and movement of the fingers where these are being inhibited by pain, deformity or inflammation in the wrist. These and other splints are often very helpful, but must be avoided in ankylosing spondylitis and other conditions where the risk of joint ankylosis is particularly great.

Orthoses are more permanent appliances used to prevent instability and movement. They need skilled manufacture and individual tailoring to each patient. Examples include irons and T-straps to control ankle instability, knee orthoses, spinal supports and braces and working wrist splints. Orthoses can be particularly useful for severely disabled patients in whom a surgical option is inappropriate.

3. Aids, appliances and occupational therapy

In many chronic rheumatic diseases permanent joint deformity and damage prevent normal function. It may then be necessary to change the environment to suit the patient, rather than trying to restore irrevocably damaged joints to normal usage.

A variety of simple aids and applicances may transform the lives of disabled patients; allowing dignified, independent living instead of soul-destroying dependency on others. Common examples include long handles on taps (wrist and hand disease often prevents patients turning taps on and off); toilet-seat raisers (hip or knee disease may prevent one from getting up from the normal low seat); long-handled combs, shoe horns and sock or stocking holders; wide rubber handles on cutlery for those without finger flexion; kettle stands; and velcro fasteners (Fig. 25.1).

Occupational therapists assess the difficulty encountered in daily tasks such as washing, dressing, cooking, housework and shopping; they can then give advice so that the patients can help

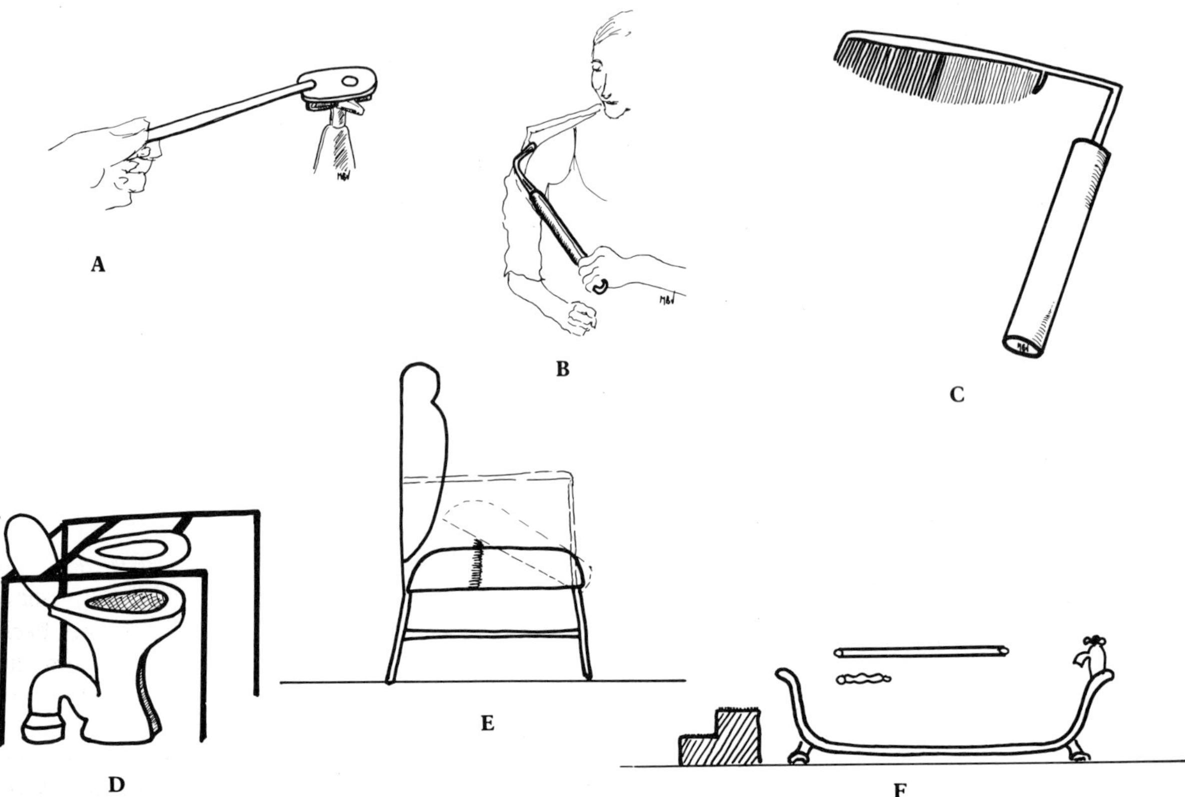

Fig. 25.1 Examples of some aids and appliances used to help disabled patients **A**. Tap-turner **B**. Dressing stick **C**. Handle on comb **D**. Raised toilet seat **E**. High-backed chair with spring-loaded 'ejector' **F**. Bath equipped with steps, bath seat, hand rails and non-slip material

themselves, and make suggestions about any 'aids to daily living' (often called the *ADL assessment*).

4. Drugs

Large numbers of drugs are available. They can be divided into symptomatic, anti-rheumatic and ancillary groups (see Chapter 26). In chronic disease they provide partial relief of symptoms, and may help to slow or stop the progression of the disease. Most neither cure nor provide complete relief, and they can have serious side-effects. Drugs must be used sparingly in conjunction with the other approaches outlined in this chapter.

5. Local injection therapy

Local injections may be anti-inflammatory or ablative; they are used to treat synovitis, intractable pain or local, tender periarticular lesions.

Local injections of long-acting corticosteroids with or without local anaesthetic are very useful for treating lesions at tendon and ligament insertions, such as tennis elbow, plantar fasciitis, rotator cuff lesions and some tender ligament spots in the back. They also relieve tenosynovitis in lesions like de Quervain's and trigger-finger (see Chapter 19).

Intra-articular steroids produce a transient local anti-inflammatory effect, lasting a few days or weeks, but may be of prolonged benefit in early synovitis of small joints. Radioactive colloids are used to induce a 'medical synovectomy', short half-life isotopes of limited penetration producing death of the synovial lining cells only. The synovium usually regrows after 2–3 years, and the benefit is largely symptomatic rather than disease-modifying (Chapter 28).

Other more specialist injection techniques that may be of benefit to patients with rheumatic disease include extradural injections to relieve root pressure and sclerosing injections to produce damage to peripheral nerve roots in intractable pain.

The main risks of injections are infection and unwanted tissue damage. Infection is a rare but a very serious complication of intra-articular injections; tendon ruptures are one of the commoner problems with extra-articular therapy. A good knowledge of local anatomy and a scrupulous technique are essential (Chapters 19 and 28).

6. Surgery

Synovectomy, tendon repair, osteotomy, arthrodeses or arthroplasty are all used in the management of rheumatic disorders (see Chapter 27). Surgery has an important part to play in the management of chronic disabling diseases provided that it is used as part of an integrated plan that takes into account all other aspects of the patient, his or her disease, needs and prognosis. Isolated operations for local problems that take no account of the whole patient are often disastrous.

7. Miscellaneous

A variety of special or experimental procedures are applicable to difficult rheumatic problems or disease complications: plasmaphoresis, for example, may cause temporary help in immune complex disease, and total body irradiation is now being used for some chronic immunological diseases (Chapter 29).

8. Alternative medicine

Several surveys have shown than most patients with a chronic rheumatic disease resort to some form of alternative medicine at some stage of their illness. Rubefacients, local heat and other local applications are commonly used and provide temporary symptomatic relief. Osteopaths and chiropractors treat many local problems, and have a particularly good reputation in the management of back pain. Dietary therapy is always popular, although the type of diet recommended by the popular press and journals varies regularly. Herbal and traditional folk remedies such as copper bracelets are also widely used. Acupuncture is available in many hospital pain clinics to relieve chronic suffering, and is also used widely by non-medical practitioners. Hypnotists, faith healers and many other fringe groups can number several patients with rheumatic disease among their clients.

ACUTE EMERGENCIES IN RHEUMATOLOGY

Several acute situations can develop in patients with rheumatic diseases, and may require prompt diagnosis and immediate treatment to prevent mobidity or mortality. Table 25.1 lists some of these conditions, which are dealt with more fully elsewhere in this book. A good knowledge of these situations and a high degree of clinical suspicion are required if they are not to be overlooked in the pursuance of total patient care.

26 Drug therapy

INTRODUCTION

For descriptive purposes, drugs used in rheumatic diseases may conveniently be divided into the following categories:

1. Analgesics
2. Non-steroidal analgesic anti-inflammatory drugs (NSAIDs)
3. Long-acting drugs with apparent 'anti-rheumatic' activity (e.g. gold, penicillamine)
4. Non-specific immunomodulatory and cytotoxic agents (e.g. azathioprine, levamisole, cyclophosphamide)
5. Corticosteroids
6. Miscellaneous and ancillary drugs (e.g. colchicine, allopurinol, muscle relaxants, iron, antidepressants)

The mechanism of action of most of these compounds is unknown; many are toxic or have significant side-effects; and interaction with other drugs is common. Therefore, as a general rule, the least number of drugs necessary, the least toxic drug available and the lowest dose required should be used to achieve the therapeutic aim of maximum benefit with minimal toxicity.

Both therapeutic and toxic effects of a drug depend on its concentration at receptor sites, and the major variable that governs this is dosage. The majority of adverse drug reactions are dose-related rather than idiosyncratic, and are therefore avoidable. Since most drugs have a narrow therapeutic ratio it is important to adjust the 'standard' dose for each individual by adequate consideration of both pharmacokinetic and pharmacodynamic factors. For example, hypoalbuminaemia due to chronic disease will increase the free fraction of many acidic, highly-bound drugs and necessitate reduction in dosage; administration of several acidic drugs may result in interaction from competition for serum albumin binding and active transport sites in the kidney; penicillamine chelates iron so that concurrent administration will reduce absorption of both drugs, and subsequent withdrawal of iron may lead to penicillamine toxicity; special care should always be exercised when prescribing to the elderly.

Drug administration should be an attempt to achieve an attainable therapeutic goal and this, of course, implies an element of reversibility. Judgements on efficacy are best made if only one drug is introduced and tried out at a time with specific goals in mind, e.g. pain or stiffness relief. Although many possibilities for toxicity and drug interaction exist, it is nevertheless important to ensure that an adequate dose is given for an appropriate length of time before deciding that a drug is ineffective: if such a decision is made the drug should be withdrawn. The time course for trial periods varies greatly between different agents — analgesics, for example, show benefit within hours, NSAIDs 1–2 weeks, antirheumatic agents 3–6 months. There is seldom a need to use more than one agent with a similar action, though a common exception to this is the use of one NSAID for daytime symptoms and one for night pain and morning stiffness. The commonest errors in rheumatological prescribing are undoubtedly: 1. inappropriate use of drugs e.g. chronic, regular use of symptomatic agents regardless of symptoms, iron for patients without iron deficiency; 2. multiple use of similar agents, e.g. two or three analgesics, two or three NSAIDs. Patient education and critical reassessment of current medication at each review should, however, help to reduce such errors.

In this chapter the drugs commonly encountered in rheumatological practice will be described, and the diseases in which they are of use will be listed. The clinical indications for drug treatment in individual diseases are dealt with in the specific disease sections.

ANALGESICS

Since pain is a purely subjective sensation the physician must accept the patient's assessment of pain magnitude and the extent to which it has been relieved by the drug prescribed. 'Pain behaviour' and the relation between pain and the patient's environment and psychological state are clearly relevant, and both psychological rehabilitation and adequate explanation of the disease process must be allocated time in the physician's counselling programme. Attention to altered sleep patterns and recognition of 'pain-amplification syndrome' (p 360) are important, and for certain individuals behavioural modification by a variety of 'counter-irritation' methods may prove more effective than conventional analgesics.

Recognition of the inflammatory element in OA and of the peripheral analgesic effect of NSAIDs has led to a general reduction in the use of pure analgesics. They may, however, provide a useful adjunct to treatment where structural changes not amenable to mechanical aids or surgery are a major cause of symptoms.

For chronic use drugs relatively free of CNS or gut side-effects (e.g. paracetamol, Distalgesic (paracetamol + dextropropoxyphene)) are recommended, but in practice each patient tends to find their own favourite, whether it be low-dose aspirin, pentazocine, codeine or one of the many variants or combinations. Such patient preference, as with NSAIDs, should be respected. It should be remembered, however, that constipation with codeine or dihydrocodeine may be paticularly troublesome, especially in the elderly. A sudden increase in analgesic intake is a frequent sign of clinical deterioration or intercurrent illness.

The short-term use of potent narcotic agents such as pethidine, or newer, safer agonist-anatagonist agents such as buprenorphine is only occasionally warranted, e.g. for acute bleed in a haemophiliac.

NON-STEROIDAL ANALGESIC ANTI-INFLAMMATORY DRUGS (NSAIDs)

The chemical classification of these drugs is shown in Figure 26.1. The large number of NSAIDs on the market not only reflects the high population

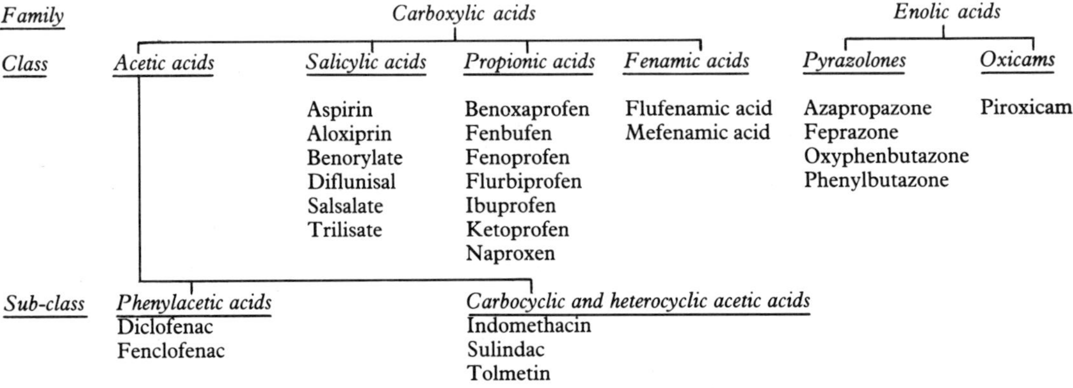

Fig. 26.1 Non-steroidal analgesic anti-inflammatory drugs

incidence of musculoskeletal disorders but also attests to the fact that, despite manufacturer's claims, there is no single 'best' NSAID.

Although these drugs may produce a variety of biological effects their mode of action remains unclear with no 'unifying hypothesis' to explain their activity. Interruption of the arachidonic acid pathway by prostaglandin synthetase or cyclo-oxygenase inhibition (p 14) has been proposed as a major mode of action (Flower & Vane 1974) but effects can also be demonstrated on oxidative phosphorylation; lysosomal and cell membranes; granulocyte and macrophage chemotaxis, mobility and function; and many other membrane and protein systems (e.g. kinins). The antiinflammatory effects of NSAIDs are generally deemed to be beneficial, but there is some, as yet unsubstantiated, evidence, predominately from animal and *in vitro* studies, suggesting that chronic use of these agents may be detrimental to cartilage and other tissues.

The clinical assessment of NSAID efficacy is difficult and imprecise and, for trial purposes, usually involves the monitoring of a large number of variables, e.g. pain, duration of morning or inactivity stiffness, grip strength, PIP ring size, articular index, standard distance walking time etc, (p 434). Careful trial design and selected emphasis on only some of these variables will allow any NSAID to compare favourably with accepted drugs such as indomethacin. In practice, patient preference and compliance are probably the best indices of therapeutic success and take into account adverse as well as beneficial effects. An interesting but unexplained observation in all trials comparing NSAIDs is the marked within patient and interpatient variation even for chemically similar drugs, and failure with one drug due to toxicity or lack of efficacy does not preclude success with another drug of the same chemical class.

Gastro-intestinal side-effects

A major drawback of the NSAIDs is their high incidence of GI side-effects, the most important being mucosal ulceration and haemorrhage. Multiple gastric erosions or single 'giant' pre-pyloric ulcers (particularly with indocid) are produced by a predominantly local effect and may present as acute or chronic bleeding or with pain. Interestingly, there is often little correlation between the patient's symptoms and the endoscopic findings. NSAIDs appear to exacerbate acute peptic ulcers but their relationship to chronic ulceration is less certain. It is likely, but not proven, that patients with systemic disease, particularly RA, have increased susceptibility to drug-induced mucosal damage, as do patients with hypovitaminosis C or chronic alcohol intake. Several attempts have been made to overcome gastric irritability caused by these drugs:

1. Enteric coating of tablets or combination with antacids — particularly used, with success, for salicylate preparations
2. Rectal administration of suppository — indomethacin, for example, is frequently given by this route, but local irritation (proctitis) may still occur. Such administration may present physical or social difficulties.
3. Formulation of 'prodrugs', i.e. drugs given in inactive, theoretically less irritant, form and then converted to the active form at a site distant from the stomach e.g. sulindac, fenbufen, benorylate.

Parenteral administration of NSAIDs, however, still causes gastric damage, suggesting that factors other than local irritation are important. Although the above measures reduce the incidence of gastric bleeding they unfortunately do not abolish the problem altogether.

Faced with the difficult, but not uncommon, clinical situation of which NSAID to give to a symptomatic patient with co-existant mucosal ulceration it seems sensible to:

1. Ensure that local measures such as splints or i.a. injections are receiving adequate attention
2. Consider addition of cimetidine/ranitidine, if not already being used
3. Consider use of second-line therapy, e.g. penicillamine, to reduce the need for symptomatic relief by NSAIDs. Such drugs, however, will take time to be effective.
4. Ensure that the patient is not smoking or taking other irritant, avoidable drugs

All NSAIDs have the potential to cause and exacerbate mucosal ulceration, and there is no convincing evidence to favour one particular drug.

Prescribing NSAIDs

When prescribing NSAIDs the following general advice may be given:

1. Make a small selection from each chemical class and get to know them well — familiarity probably improves usage. Propionic acids have a low incidence of side effects and are useful drugs to try first.
2. Prescribe one NSAID at a time — there is no evidence for synergism or reduced toxicity if two or more are used. An exception to this rule is to use one NSAID for day symptoms and another (usually indomethacin) for night pain/morning stiffness
3. Prescribe an adequate dose for a limited period (c. 2 weeks) before deciding on therapeutic success or failure.

The main side-effects and recommended dosages of the commonly used NSAIDs are briefly outlined in Table 26.1 Rash, GI disturbance and hypersensitivity (asthma, eczema) can occur with almost any NSAID.

LONG-ACTING DRUGS WITH APPARENT ANTI-RHEUMATIC ACTIVITY

Drugs included in this group appear to have a fundamental action on disease and do not just suppress manifestations. Although such drugs relate particularly to RA, the action of hydroxychloroquine in SLE may be regarded similarly. There is no general agreement on nomenclature and since the mode of action is unknown it is impossible to classify according to any fundamental property. The terms 'specific', 'remission-inducing', 'slow-acting', 'penicillamine-like' or 'second-line' are frequently used, though each has its disadvantages.

Drugs with an accepted slow-developing, long-lasting effect in RA include penicillamine, gold, hydroxychloroquine, immunosuppressive or cytotoxic agents and levamisole (the latter are particularly non-specific and are regarded separately in the next section). Their beneficial action on joints appears to be accompanied by the following:

1. Improvement in extra-articular features
2. Reduction in viscosity or ESR
3. Reduction in rheumatoid factor
4. Normalisation of other serological markers for active RA including:
   a) Elevated acute-phase proteins
   b) Lowered serum sulphydryl groups
   c) Lowered serum histidine
   d) Lowered serum free tryptophan (high protein-bound tryptophan)
   e) Lowered albumin, raised α globulin
   f) Elevated γ GT, alkaline phosphatase

Evidence, however, for alteration of radiological progression, regarded by many as the definitive test for disease modification, is less clear. Radiological assessments are difficult to standardise and great variability in disease requires large numbers of patient and non-treatment controls to be followed for some years before significant differences between groups can be demonstrated. At present, therefore, there is no hard evidence for true alteration of the natural history of the disease, though their action is obviously different from that of the NSAIDs. All unfortunately possess potentially serious side-effects which make them truly 'second-line' drugs.

D-penicillamine ($\beta\beta$-**dimethylcysteine**)

This component of the penicillin molecule differs from cysteine by the presence of two methyl groups in the α position. It is effective in treatment of Wilson's disease, cystinuria, heavy-metal poisoning, RA and palindromic rheumatism, and in addition may be of benefit in scleroderma, primary biliary cirrhosis and chronic active hepatitis.

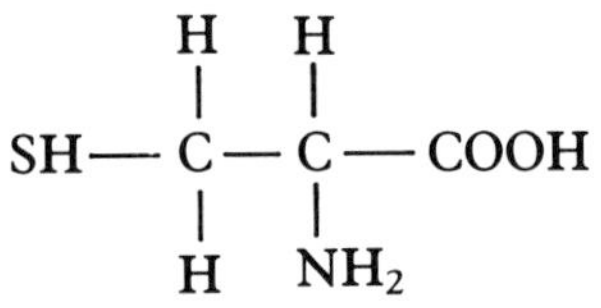

```
       H   H                    CH3   H
       |   |                     |    |
SH — C — C — COOH        SH — C  — C — COOH
       |   |                     |    |
       H   NH2                  CH3   NH2
     Cysteine                 Penicillamine
```

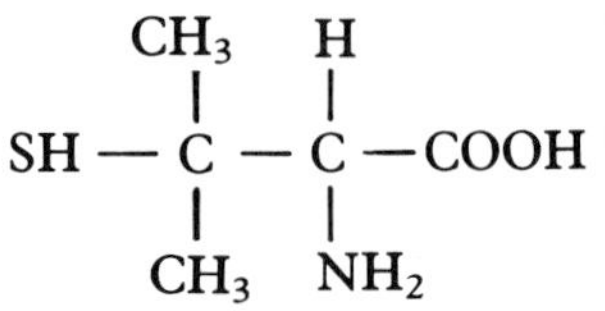

Table 26.1 NSAIDs: an outline of dosages and side-effects (of those available in the UK)

		Side-effects		
Drug	Dose	Common	Less common	Addition comments
Diclofenac	50 mg b.d./t.d.s. 100 mg nocte (Sp)	GID, headache, dizziness	Rash, oedema	Safe with AC/AD
Fenclofenac	600 mg b.d.	Rash, GID	Severe skin rash	? specific effect in RA May interfere with TFTs
Indomethacin	25 mg t.d.s. 75 mg (SR) nocte/b.d. 100 mg nocte (Sp)	GID, GI bleeds Headache, confusion depression	Peripheral neuropathy bleeding disturbance fluid retention	Avoid in elderly due to fluid retention and CNS effects
Sulindac	200 mg b.d.	GID	Rash, CNS disturbance	A 'pro-drug' — metabolised to active sulphide in liver. Safe with AC/AD
Tolmetin	400 mg t.d.s./q.d.s.	GID, CNS disturbance	Rash, oedema	Relatively safe with AC/AD
Aspirin	600–900 mg × 6/day			
Aloxiprin	1200 mg q.d.s.	GID		Toxicity is frequent but lower for EC compounds and antacid preparations
Benorylate	1.5 mg t.d.s.	Drug displacement and interaction		
Diflunisal	10 ml b.d.	Hypersensitivity		
Salsalate	500 mg b.d.	Bleeding disturbance		
Trisalicylate	1–1.5 g b.d.	Tinnitus		
	1–1.5 g b.d.	Renal effects and hepatitis		
Benoxaprofen	600 mg nocte	GID, photosensitivity nail dystrophy	Liver toxicity	Withdrawn due to toxicity
Fenbufen	600 mg nocte ± 300 mg daily	GID, rash		A 'pro-drug' with low gut toxicity
Fenoprofen	600 mg q.d.s.	GID	Rash	Highly protein bound (displaces AC/AD)
Flurbiprofen	100 mg t.d.s.	GID	Rash	
Ibuprofen	400–800 mg q.d.s.	GID	Rash	Very safe and widely used drug with low toxicity
Ketoprofen	50–100 mg b.d. 100 mg nocte (Sp)	GID	Rash	
Naproxen	500 mg b.d.	GID	Rash	
Flufenamic acid	200 mg q.d.s.	GID, diarrhoea, rash	LFT disturbance	Use limited by high frequency of diarrhoea
Mefanamic acid	500 mg q.d.s.	Diarrhoea, rash	Haemolysis	
Azapropazone	600 mg b.d.	GID	Rash, oedema	Highly protein bound (displaces AC/AD). Induce microsomal enzymes. Useful uricosuric action
Feprazone	200 mg t.d.s.	GID, rash, headache		
Oxyphenbutazone	200–300 mg daily	GID, rash, fluid retention, headache	Hepatitis, goitre, lymphadenopathy Aplastic anaemia (elderly on chronic dosage) Agranulocytosis (any age after short use)	Oxyphenbutazone is active metabolite of PBZ. Long half-lives, highly protein bound. Induce microsomal enzymes. Potential serious toxicity should limit use.
Phenylbutazone	100 mg q.d.s.			
Piroxicam	20 mg daily	GID	Oedema, rash	

GID = gastrointestinal disease; EC = enteric coated; Sp = suppository; AC = anticoagulants; AD = antidepressants

Penicillamine is well absorbed from the gut but may react with dietary constituents and other drugs, so it should be given at least 2 hours away from food and other medication. It shows high affinity for collagen-containing or protein-rich organs such as skin, tendon, pancreas, testis. Although a high proportion undergoes renal excretion, mainly as oxidised products, in the first 24 hours, urinary metabolites are still detectable 3 months after stopping the drug, perhaps accounting for persistance of drug effect and toxicity following cessation of therapy.

Penicillamine is neither cytotoxic nor anti-inflammatory in man. Although its mode of action in RA is unknown, several biological effects of interest have been demonstrated in man, including:

1. *Chelation of divalent cations*. Similar chelation with trien is without effect in RA.
2. *SH-SS interchange*. This reaction with cysteine produces penicillamine -cysteine which is more soluble than cystine and can result in cystine stone dissolution
3. *Thiazolidine formation*. This reaction with aldehyde cross-links of Type I collagen produces the dermolathyrogenic effect utilised in scleroderma. (Wound healing involves Type III, the keto links of which do not react with penicillamine.) Similar reaction with pyridoxal phosphate produces an anti-B6 effect particularly in children and malnourished adults (B6 supplementation does not reduce clinical efficacy or incidence of side-effects).
4. Dissociation of macromolecular complexes, including rheumatoid factors

Many side effects have additionally been observed *in vitro*, including an antimicrobial action and effects on lymphocyte transformation.

Although penicillamine is toxic, clinical experience has shown that side-effects may be reduced and compliance increased, without loss of efficacy, by introducing the drug at a low dose and allowing 4–6 week intervals between each increment — 'go low, go slow' policy.

In adults it is usual to start with 125 or 250 mg daily and to increase in increments of 125–250 mg until a clinical response is obtained or a daily dose of 500 mg is reached. By 5 months most patients who will benefit from the drug will have shown evidence of improvement, but, if necessary, the dose may be increased to 750 mg for a further 8–12 weeks, and occasionally even up to 1000 mg, preferably in a single dose. A satisfactory response is obtained in 75% of patients but shows no relation to age, sex, disease-duration or seropositivity, making selection of likely responders impossible. If a response is achieved penicillamine is continued indefinitely at the lowest possible maintenance dose. Since relapse may not occur for several months after stopping treatment, it seems wise to allow 4–6 months between any reductions in dose.

Toxicity

The major side effects of penicillamine are shown in Table 26.2. Patients starting on penicillamine should be seen every 3 weeks and a full blood (+ platelet) count and urinalysis should be performed at each visit. Most side effects occur in the first few months and are less likely after 18 months when the interval can be increased to 6–8 weeks. Patients should be warned to report any unusual symptoms at once.

Haematological toxicity is certainly the most serious and usually follows an increase in dosage. Those over 60 years appear most susceptible. The rate of change in cell count, rather than just the absolute number, is important, and a rapid fall from a high to a low normal count should alert one to underlying toxicity. Although thrombocytopenia usually recovers following temporary cessation and reinstitution at a lower dose, many regard any evidence of marrow suppression as an absolute contraindication to further treatment.

The other major cause of anxiety is renal damage. This usually manifests as minor, non-progressive proteinuria which is self-limiting. Less commonly, progressive proteinuria, nephrotic syndrome or haematuria demonstrates advancing renal toxicity that requires cessation of therapy. Non-selective proteinuria results from an immune complex, membranous glomerulopathy: renal biopsy is usually normal by light microscopy but EM and immunofluorescent staining may reveal

Table 26.2 Main side-effects of penicillamine (Pen) in patients with RA

Peak incidence	Problem (frequency)	Action	Likely outcome
1st month	Maculopapular rash ± pruritis (10%)	Stop Pen: restart low dose when better. Anti-histamines may be useful.	Transient even if Pen continued. Usually does not recur.
	Nausea/anorexia (20%)	No further dose increase	Usually settles
	Vomiting (uncommon)	Stop Pen: restart low dose when better	Usually possible to continue Pen
6 weeks	Blunting/loss of taste (20%)	Continue Pen	May last 1–3 months but recovers whether Pen stopped or not
3–6 months	Mouth (± genital) ulcers (5%)	Stop Pen if severe: use local therapy	Less severe cases may resolve with continued therapy: if severe do not rechallenge
4–18 months	Proteinuria (< 5 g/24 h) (10%)	Continue Pen. Check renal function weekly at first, then monthly; 24 h urinary protein every month.	May last up to 15 months but improves eventually whether Pen stopped or not
	Proteinuria + oedema (uncommon)	Stop therapy	Recovers slowly. Rechallenge may not lead to recurrence.
6–18 months	Late rash: raised, itchy, demarcated, scaly, indolent lesions	Stop Pen. Anti-histamines and topical steroids of no use.	Usually recovers slowly
Any time	Thrombocytopenia (10%)	Stop Pen if $< 50 \times 10^9$/l. (Frequent counts if falling) . Restart low dose when better.	Often possible to continue Pen at lower dose
	Pancytopenia (uncommon)	Frequent counts if WBC or platelets falling. Stop Pen when trend is clear.	Usually recovers. Do not rechallenge.
Late	Drug-induced lupus reaction (1%)	Stop Pen	Recovers rapidly
	Myasthenia gravis reaction (rare)	Stop Pen. May need anticholinesterases	Usually recovers
	Pemphigus reaction (rare)	Stop Pen	Usually recovers
	Goodpasture-like syndrome (rare)	Stop Pen	Often fatal

smooth subepithelial deposits containing IgG, sometimes IgM or IgA, and occasionally complement. Proliferative changes and fibrosis are minimal or absent, and renal function is usually normal. Patients who develop gross proteinuria on penicillamine should undergo renal biopsy since amyloid or coincidental renal disease may present similarly.

Congenital connective tissue syndromes may occur in infants born to mothers on penicillamine, and pregnancy is normally taken as a contraindication to its use.

Gold compounds

Gold was introduced therapeutically for treatment of tuberculosis and then tried in RA in the 1920s on the mistaken assumption that RA and TB were linked. Subsequently gold compounds were shown to be effective in RA, palindromic rheumatism, some cases of JCA and possibly also peripheral psoriatic arthropathy. Sodium aurothiomalate is used in the UK: elsewhere aurothioglucose, aurothiosulphate and other salts are additionally available. Colloidal gold is rapidly cleared by the RE system and is ineffective in RA.

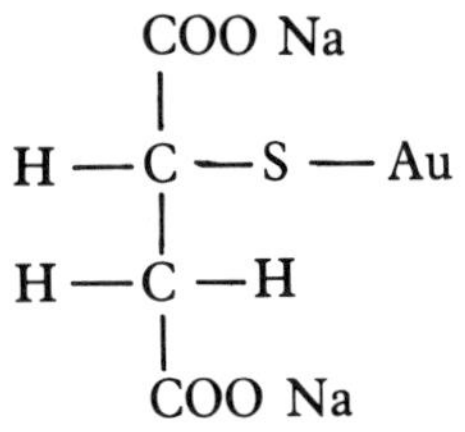

$$
\begin{array}{l}
\quad\;\; \mathrm{COO\ Na} \\
\quad\;\;\; | \\
\mathrm{H-C-S-Au} \\
\quad\;\;\; | \\
\mathrm{H-C-H} \\
\quad\;\;\; | \\
\quad\;\; \mathrm{COO\ Na}
\end{array}
$$

Sodium aurothiomalate — containing 50% gold by weight. It is water soluble and therefore poorly absorbed orally.

Gold given by IM injection reaches peak plasma levels within hours and is then cleared by first order kinetics with a $T\frac{1}{2}$ of 5–6 days. Two-thirds is excreted via the kidneys, one-third via the faeces. Due to avid protein binding, up to 50% of a single dose is still present in body tissues 180 days after injection: frequent administration will therefore result in progressive accumulation.

Although its mode of action is unknown, gold produces a wide variety of biological effects, including:

1. Inhibition of lysosomal enzymes (not their release)
2. Inhibition of PMN and macrophage phagocytosis
3. Inhibition of monocyte function and subsequent T-cell activation
4. Inhibition of complement components
5. Decrease in serum concentration of trace metals normally elevated in RA
6. Antimicrobial activity
7. Displacement of tryptophan from its binding site on albumin

Recent interest has focused on the possible role played by the sulphydryl component of the molecule (sodium thiomalate, without gold, has been claimed to be effective in RA) and it is of interest that penicillamine, azathioprine and levamisole are also sulphydryl compounds suggesting the possibility of a common chemical reaction. Auranofin is a lipid soluble, orally absorbed gold agent currently under investigation — it differs from sodium aurothiomalate in several respects, including its ability to inhibit lysosomal enzyme release and its lack of potent sulphydryl reactivity.

The conventional dosage schedule is empirically derived. An initial test dose (10 mg) is given in case of hypersensitivity, and thereafter 50 mg is given weekly until the patient responds, usually about 3 months later, after a total dose of c. 500 mg. The interval between injections is then increased to 2, and subsequently 3 or 4, weeks. As with penicillamine, relapse may take several months so that intervals should not be increased more than once every 4–6 months. If relapse does occur injections are again given weekly until a good response is achieved, following which the intervals may again be increased. If recurrence occurs after cessation of treatment further 'courses' may be less effective and side-effects more likely — therefore, if a patient responds, injections are continued at an average maintenance does of 50 mg every 3–4 weeks.

25% of patients fail to respond after 4–5 months of the above regime. Increasing the dose to 100 mg weekly for 6 weeks may be tried but this produces only a few extra responders. If a patient responds to penicillamine they tend also to respond to gold, and vice versa: as with penicillamine, response appears unrelated to sex, age, seropositivity or disease-duration.

Toxicity

Side effects of gold treatment are shown in Table 26.3. A FBC (with platelets) and urinalysis should be performed before each injection, the skin should be examined and the patient should be questioned about untoward effects. Side-effects occur with the same order of frequency as those seen with penicillamine, but are generally more serious and more likely to lead to treatment withdrawal. Efficacy and toxicity appear unrelated to serum or urinary levels of gold.

Mucocutaneous lesions are the commonest side-effects encountered. Most rashes last 1–2 months, are discrete and confined to the extremities, but almost any lesion may occur including severe exfoliative dermatitis. Rash is frequently accompanied by pruritis and eosinophilia, and other symptoms of toxicity, e.g. metallic taste.

Proteinuria, microscopic haematuria and nephrotic syndrome occur particularly if high, frequent doses are being used. Increasing protein-

Table 26.3 Main side-effects of gold

Peak incidence	Problem (frequency)	Action	Likely outcome
2–6 months	Dermatitis (30%) — may mimic any lesion and may proceed to exfoliation. ± pruritis, eosinophilia.	Stop therapy	May take up to 18 months to recover Retreatment usually leads to recurrence and is therefore avoided
	Stomatitis (common) — often painless, occurring alone or with dermatitis	Stop therapy	Full recovery. Although rechallenge may not lead to recurrence it is best avoided.
4–8 months	Proteinuria and nephrotic syndrome (5%)	Stop therapy	Usually recovers after 12–18 months. Avoid rechallenge.
Any time	Thrombocytopenia (2%)	Stop therapy	Potentially fatal but usually recovers
	Leukopenia (uncommon)	Stop therapy	Potentially fatal but usually recovers
Usually late	Aplastic anaemia (rare)	Stop therapy	High mortality, c. 60%

uria or a concentration exceeding 50 mg/dl requires treatment cessation. Renal biopsy findings are similar to those found in penicillamine-induced membranous glomerulopathy, implying an immune complex pathogenesis. In addition, particulate matter consistant with gold has been demonstrated in glomeruli, tubules and interstitium. There is no information available on the effects of continuing with gold. Full, though delayed, recovery usually follows its withdrawal.

The majority of deaths attributable to gold are due to marrow toxicity. Thrombocytopenia is not dose related and may occur early in treatment or even following its cessation. The latter is also true of aplastic anaemia. Deaths may result from haematological complications even when they are detected promptly and gold is withdrawn.

Less common side-effects include vasomotor reactions following injections, cholestatic jaundice, diffuse pulmonary infiltrates and peripheral neuropathy. Various drugs have been tried in patients with serious toxicity affecting kidneys, marrow, skin or lungs, including dimercaprol and penicillamine to increase renal excretion, and high-dose steroids. Evidence for their efficacy, however, is unconvincing.

The spectrum of toxicity with auranofin is apparently narrower and less severe — the main side effect being diarrhoea and GI upset.

Hydroxychloroquine

Chloroquine and hydroxychloroquine possess similar actions to other aminoquinolines but are less toxic. They demonstrate 'anti-rheumatic' activity in RA and are effective in treating skin and joint manifestations of SLE. Hydroxychloroquine is the less toxic of the two and is therefore used preferentially.

Hydroxychloroquine is readily absorbed, quickly cleared from plasma and bound largely unchanged to tissue mucopolysaccharide, nucleic acids and melanin. Degradation and excretion is slow and the drug may be detected for more than a year following cessation of therapy. Possibly significant biological actions include:

1. Lysosomal 'stabilisation'
2. Inhibition of DNA and RNA synthesis
3. Stimulation of interferon production
5. Impairment of lymphocyte responsiveness
6. Inhibition of disulphide-sulphydryl interchange

The initial dose of hydroxychloroquine is 200 mg b.d. If a satisfactory response is obtained, usually after 2–4 months, the dose is decreased by 100 mg increments every 8 weeks to a usual daily maintenance dose of c. 200 mg. If no response occurs after 4 months at 400 mg daily the drug is discontined.

Toxicity

Although many side-effects have been reported, the main problem that has undoubtedly limited use of quinine derivatives has been fear of retinal toxicity. Selective accumulation of both chloroquine and hydroxychloroquine occurs in the eye due to binding to melanin, and this may lead to pigment epithelium and retinal photoreceptor damage. Severe damage may eventually result in

Possible side-effects due to hydroxychloroquine

SKIN
1. Pruritis, rash
2. Increased pigmentation
3. Bleaching of hair.

GUT
1. Nausea, anorexia
2. Diarrhoea, weight loss

CNS
1. Peripheral neuropathy
2. Confusion, fits

BLOOD
Leukopenia, agranulocytosis

EYES
1. Subjective
   a) Impaired reading ability
   b) Poor distant vision
   c) Night blindness
2. Objective
   a) Decreased colour vision
   b) Scotomata with or without pigment changes at fundus
   c) Arterial constriction
   d) Retinal oedema, optic disc pallor
   e) Macular pigmentation
   f) 'Bull's-eye' lesion, retinopathy
   g) Loss of corneal reflex
   h) Corneal deposits

the classical 'bull's eye' maculopathy associated with severe, usually irreversible impairment of vision. Although various screening tests have been tried, e.g. electro-oculogram, colour vision and visual-field testing, there is no certain way of detecting early retinopathy, and even the classical maculopathy may be confused with senile macular degeneration. Such difficulties have made the use of hydroxychloroquine highly contraversial and opthalmological opinion has been sharply divided, partly due to the work load imposed and partly due to difficulty in early detection. It seems, however, that retinopathy has predominantly been reported in patients receiving chronic high doses of chloroquine, and evidence incriminating hydroxychloroquine is inconclusive. Until this difficult issue is resolved it would seem sensible to:

1. Avoid use of hydroxychloroquine in the elderly
2. Limit use to 10 months of each year, or for a maximum of 2 years
3. Restrict dosage to 400 mg a day or less
4. Seek regular 6 monthly ophthalmological supervision

Other drugs with possible anti-rheumatoid activity

A variety of other drugs have been claimed to show anti-rheumatoid activity with accompanying amelioration of serological abnormalities. Since all existing proved anti-rheumatoid drugs have been discovered by chance or by empirical testing such claims merit careful consideration and further study. Included amongst the more likely contenders are:

1. Dapsone. Clinical improvement associated with slow reduction in ESR and acute-phase proteins, but no change in rheumatoid factor, has been demonstrated for this drug. A major, frequent, and therefore limiting side-effect, however, is haemolytic anaemia, particularly in slow acetylators of the drug.

2. Sulphasalazine. This is not dissimilar in structure to dapsone and shares its immunosuppressive properties. In addition, however, it has anti-inflammatory and anti-microbial actions. It has been shown to produce an early onset anti-rheumatoid effect comparable to penicillamine. Advantages include: a) oral administration; b) lack of renal toxicity; c) lack of dose-related thrombocytopenia and extreme rarity of aplastic anaemia (regular blood and urine checks therefore probably unnecessary). Disadvantages, however, include reversible azoospermia in males and occasional late-onset macrocytic anaemia responsive to folate supplementation. GI intolerance is the main practical side-effect and occurs more frequently in RA than in ulcerative colitis — it is not always ameliorated by use of enteric-coated tablets or by slow introduction of the drug. The usual maintenance dose is 500 mg q.d.s

3. *NSAIDs*. Reports that fenclofenac exhibits a moderate, slow-onset anti-rheumatoid action awaits confirmation. Similar claims for alclofenac and benoxaprofen are now clinically irrelevant following withdrawal of these drugs.

4. *Captopril*. This thiol-containing compound, marketed as an antihypertensive, has a spectrum of side-effects similar to penicillamine and has recently been shown to produce clinical and biochemical improvement in RA.

5. *Analogues of D-penicillamine*. 5-thiopyridoxine appears to be a slower acting alternative to penicillamine. Patients withdrawn due to side effects with penicillamine do not necessarily develop the same problems with 5-thiopyridoxine. Pemphigus, however, only rarely seen with penicillamine, is a characteristic major side-effect. Pyrithioxine and thiopronine are alternative analogues which have not been reported to cause marrow toxicity.

IMMUNOMODULATORY DRUGS

Far from correcting a recognised immunological abnormality, the use of immunomodulatory drugs, as with gold or penicillamine, remains empirical. Most 'immunosuppressive' drugs are cytotoxic agents which affect the immune system by interfering with proliferation or differentiation of lymphocytes — none of these drugs are specific, however, and their ameliorating effect on rheumatic disease may well be produced by actions other than those on immune cells.

In practice, for each patient the physician must balance the potential risks of immunomodulatory therapy against the possible clinical improvement one hopes to achieve. Such a decision is made particularly difficult by: 1. uncertainty over the natural history of many of the conditions involved; 2. lack of adequate long-term controlled trials; 3. marked individual variability in response; 4. frequent and often impressive side-effects of the drugs available.

The principle toxicities of commonly used immunosuppressive drugs are summarised in Table 26.4. Marrow suppression and predisposition to infection are acute effects common to all such drugs, and alkylating agents may additionally produce infertility. A particularly worrying long-term effect is predisposition to malignancy which appears to result not from immunosuppression *per se* but from the variable carcinogenetic potential of the agents used. The relative risk of this complication in the context of rheumatic diseases requires clarification, but certainly appears to be significant. The decision to use 'immunomodulatory' treatment is therefore a major one that must be accompanied by detailed knowledge of the agent used and by careful patient monitoring.

Azathioprine

This thiopurine is for many the immunosuppressive of choice since it is less toxic and easier to use than cyclophosphamide or methotrexate. Its main use is in Wegener's, dermatomyositis, uveitis, RA and SLE, being frequently used in the latter situations for its 'steroid-sparing' effect.

The drug is well absorbed orally and undergoes hepatic conversion by xanthine oxidases to the active metabolite 6-mercaptopurine and subse-

Table 26.4 Main toxic effects of commonly-used immunosuppressive drugs

	Azathioprine	Methotrexate	Cyclophosphamide	Chlorambucil
Major marrow toxicity	+	+	+	++
Liver damage	+	+++	0	+
GI ulceration	0	++	0	0
Azoospermia	0	0	+++	++
Anovulation	0	0	+++	++
Teratogenecity	0	+++	++	++
Alopecia	0	+	+++	0
Bladder toxicity	0	0	+++	0
Carcinogenicity	++	0	++	++

quently to thiouric acid.The usual dose for 'immunosuppression' is 2.5 mg/kg/day: this is built up gradually over several weeks on a t.d.s. regime. Concommitant use of allopurinol requires a 75% reduction in dose.

Nausea may be troublesome but can usually be avoided by gradual introduction of the drug taken with food. Marrow toxicity is the major concern that requires weekly blood counts, extending to three weekly when the maintenance dose is established. Leukopenia is more common than thrombocytopenia or major anaemia, though red cell aplasia, which may respond to cyclophosphamide, may complicate long-term therapy. Sepsis due to common or opportunist organisms is the other major concern and may occur in the absence of leukopenia. Allergic hepatitis is a rare complication: recovery usually follows cessation of therapy but continuation may result in fatal hepatitis.

Although fetal abnormalities may occur, in the majority of recorded cases azathioprine administered during pregnancy has resulted in normal infants. Lymphoreticular malignancies are markedly increased in renal transplant recipients receiving purine analogue immunosuppression: epithelial tumours, particularly of skin or cervix, are also increased. The relative risk in rheumatic disease is unclear, though leukaemia and reticulum cell sarcoma have been reported in patients with RA and SLE who received azathioprine.

Methotrexate

This folic-acid analogue inhibits DNA synthesis in actively dividing cells by competitive binding to dihydrofolate reductase. It is of particular use in dermatomyositis and psoriatic arthropathy.

Only about 60% is absorbed after oral administration and most of the drug is excreted unchanged in the urine within 24 hours. Renal impairment or probenecid may greatly enhance serum levels.

Vomiting, diarrhoea, stomatitis, alopecia, leukopenia, thrombocytopenia and marrow aplasia can all occur and may be reduced by administration of folinic acid. Infertility is a further problem and the drug is strongly teratogenic in early pregnancy. The major complication of chronic daily treatment, however, is hepatic fibrosis. This requires regular, usually annual, liver biopsy for its detection since liver function tests are of no value. High doses may cause transient interstitial pneumonitis. Ultra-violet treatment should be avoided in patients on methotrexate because of risks of photosensitivity.

Intermittent weekly administration is less toxic and less likely to produce liver damage than daily regimes. Adult dosages range from 5–40 mg given as a single parenteral dose, or orally as three divided doses separated by 12 hours, each weekend. Methotrexate is the one cytotoxic agent that has not been associated with carcinogenicity in man.

Cyclophosphamide

This alkylating agent, arguably the most effective though most toxic immunomodulatory agent, has proved to be particularly effective in Wegener's, RA, SLE and steroid-responsive nephrotic syndrome.

It is well absorbed from the gut and is metabolised in the liver to its active alkylating metabolites which then undergo renal excretion. Mixed function oxidase-inducing drugs and renal impairment both increase its effectiveness and toxicity. In addition to its immunosuppressive action the drug also possesses anti-inflammatory properties. The usual daily dose is 100–150 mg (i.e. 1.5 mg/kg/day in divided doses).

Toxicity is common but may be reduced by combined use with steroids. Marrow suppression, manifested primarily by leukopenia, and alopecia are largely dose-related and usually recover on reducing or stopping the drug. Uroepithelial toxicity, presenting as haemorrhagic cystitis, requires immediate withdrawal since continuation may lead to bladder fibrosis and carcinoma: prophylactic increase in fluid intake and frequent bladder emptying should always be encouraged to avoid this complication. Other forms of malignancy, particularly lymphoma and leukaemia, have also been reported.

Amenorrhoea and impaired ovarian function are common and almost all men develop azoospermia, which may be permanent. Marked teratogenetic potential requires strict avoidance in pregnancy. Large, particularly i.v., doses may produce cardiac and pulmonary toxicity and an ADH-like effect: nausea and vomiting are common if prophylactic anti-emetics are not used.

Chlorambucil

This alkylating agent has been used extensively in Europe as an alternative to cyclophosphamide for Wegener's, RA, SLE and renal disease. Advantages include lack of bladder toxicity or alopecia and preferential lymphopoietic inhibition at low doses.

Side-effects include nausea, infertility, mutagenecity and allergic hepatitis, but the major clinical problem is marrow suppression, usually manifesting as leukopenia or thrombocytopenia. Rapid recovery following cessation of therapy is usual though persistent marrow failure can occur. The drug has been incriminated in subsequent development of lymphoreticular malignancy, especially acute leukaemia. The usual oral dose is 0.05–0.20 mg/kg/day (i.e. 4–12 mg/day) in divided doses.

Levamisole

This anti-helminthic agent has weak anti-inflammatory properties but can also stimulate differentiation of precursor T cells to mature forms, acting as an 'immune enhancer' or 'thymomimetic agent'. Among its many demonstrated actions is an anti-rheumatoid effect.

Side-effects include nausea, vomiting, fatigue, fever and urticarial skin rash. Agranulocytosis, however, appears to be particularly frequent in patients with rheumatic disease, especially those who are B27-positive, and this has severely limited its use. The frequency of side effects may be reduced by using a single weekly dose of about 150 mg.

Thymosin and thymopoietin

Thymosin is an extract of bovine thymus, thymopoietin a synthetic pentapeptide: both have complex actions on precursor and mature T and B cells, acting in general as 'immune enhancers'. Despite problems of purification, antigenicity and frequent parenteral administration, there have been claims for a possible beneficial effect in RA and other rheumatic diseases, and future controlled trials with these or related compounds may well prove to be of interest.

FUTURE DRUGS

Many other drugs are capable of altering immune function and may prove to be of interest in future treatment of the rheumatic diseases. Frentizole, for example, has been produced in an attempt to obtain immunosuppression without toxicity and preliminary trials in SLE appear promising. Bredinin is a fungal metabolite that suppresses rat adjuvant arthritis but has not yet been tried in man. Cyclosporin A, interferon, androgens and other drugs may also influence immune responses and would be theoretically attractive therapeutic agents in disease states such as lupus. The major toxicity of presently available agents demands that other potentially safer treatments are sought and investigated.

CORTICOSTEROIDS

Marked therapeutic benefit may be obtained from the impressive anti-inflammatory and immunosuppressive activity of corticosteroids, and these agents are particularly of use in conditions such as the granulomatous and necrotising vasculitides, dermatomyositis, polymyalgia rheumatica and relapsing polychondritis, and for treatment of major complications of RA and SLE. However, because almost all tissues possess receptors for corticosteroids (bladder, uterus, prostate and seminal vesicles are notable exceptions) the effects of these hormones are widespread and potentially devastating. Apart from the many systemic side effects there is the worrying possibility that steroids may in addition hasten joint destruction and influence the distribution of rheumatic disease.

Potential side-effects of corticosteroids

IMMUNOLOGICAL
Susceptibility to infection
Suppression of delayed hypersensitivity
↑ neutrophils ↓ monocytes, lymphocytes
Possible reactivation of old TB.

ENDOCRINE/METABOLIC
Growth suppression in childhood
Truncal obesity, moon facies, buffalo hump
Acne, hirsutism
Impotence, menstrual irregularity
Hyperglycaemia
Hyperlipoproteinaemia
Negative nitrogen, calcium, potassium balance
Sodium retention, metabolic alkalosis
Secondary adrenal insufficiency

MUSCULOSKELETAL
Myopathy
Osteoporosis
Avascular necrosis

GASTROINTESTINAL
Peptic ulcer disease
Pancreatitis

CARDIOVASCULAR
Hypertension
Congestive heart failure

CNS
Alteration in mood, personality
Psychosis
Benign intracranial hypertension

OCULAR
Posterior, subcapsular cataracts
Glaucoma
Exophthalmos

SKIN
Facial erythema, telangiectasia
Thin skin, easy bruising
Striae, impaired wound healing

In practice, once the use of steroids has been deemed necessary the main considerations are: 1. the avoidance or minimsation of steroid toxicity; 2. the development of secondary adrenal insufficiency; 3. the reactivation of disease on cessation of therapy

Toxicity of corticosteroids

Since steroid toxicity is in general a function of dosage and treatment duration, side effects may be kept to a minimum by careful consideration of the following factors:

1. Choice of corticosteroid

The important differences between available compounds (with regard to ACTH suppression) are duration of action and relative mineralocorticoid potency (Table 26.5). Prednisolone is the drug most commonly used and offers the advantage of fine dose adjustment — particularly useful when tailing patients off of steroids. Prednisone, active after hepatic conversion to prednisolone, is equally satisfactory. With potent drugs such as betamethasone or dexamethasone fine dose adjustment is impossible and there is a strong tendency towards overdosage. Cortisone and hydrocortisone should be avoided due to their mineralocorticoid activity. Enteric coated preparations offer some advantage in reducing gastric side-effects.

2. Dosage

The lowest dose necessary to control disease should be used. This usually involves an initial high, suppressive dose which is quickly reduced down until there is clinical or serological evidence of reactivation — a slightly higher dose is then used. Although there is considerable individual variation, major side-effects are unlikely with daily prednisolone doses of 7.5 mg or less: there is a strong clinical impression that patients with RA are more susceptible to side effects at low dosages than patients with other disease such as polymyalgia. Elderly patients often respond to lower doses, and reduced dosages should be used in patients with hypoalbuminaemia.

3. Timing of administration

A once-daily dose at 8.00 a.m. is preferable, as far as adrenal axis suppression is concerned, to a

Table 26.5

Drug	Relative glucocorticoid potency	Equivalent anti-inflammatory dose (mg)	Mineralocorticoid activity
Short-acting			
Hydrocortisone	1	20	+
Cortisone	0.8	25	+
Prednisone	4	5	0
Methylprednisolone	5	4	0
Paramethasone	5	2	0
Triamcinolone	5	4	0
Long-acting			
Betamethasone	25	0.6	0
Dexamethasone	30	0.75	0

single dose at night or divided doses through the day — contrary to popular belief there is no evidence for better symptomatic relief by the latter regimes. Alternate-day therapy offers the lowest incidence of side-effects but may not adequately control florid inflammatory disease such as temporal arteritis: it should always be considered, however, especially in children in whom growth retardation is a major concern. Pulse intravenous therapy with high dose methylprednisolone has been advocated for some conditions (e.g. rheumatoid vasculitis, early RA), but long-term efficacy and complications compared to other forms of administration have not been determined.

4. Additional therapy

The use of supplementary agents (e.g. azathioprine, penicillamine) should always be considered to minimise the dose and duration of steroid treatment. In many instances steroids are used to obtain rapid disease suppression while other agents are taking effect.

5. Patient education

Adequate explanation of the nature of steroid therapy, and of the need to increase the dose for intercurrent illness or stress in chronic treatment, is obviously essential. All patients should carry steroid cards so the dose and duration of their therapy is never in question. Because of the marked anti-inflammatory effects of steroids, patient 'dependency' and dosage manipulation remain potential problems.

Suppression of the hypothalamic-pituitary-adrenal axis (HPA)

Adrenal suppression can occur in chronic therapy on prednisolone doses as low as 3 mg/day, or within 7–28 days on daily doses of 20–30 mg. There is marked individual variation, and dose, duration and timing of administration are obviously important. The adrenocortical response to a short or long synacthen test is a useful guide to the presence or absence of significant adrenal suppression. Recovery may take up to 12 months following total cessation of therapy and during this period steroid cover may be required for the stress of intercurrent illness or surgery. When weaning patients off steroids the first step is conversion to a single morning dose: gradual reduction in dose will then encourage recovery of adrenal responsiveness.

Reactivation of disease

This remains a problem when steroids have been instituted for chronic disease states. When there is a possibility that the underlying disease may flare up, glucocorticoids must be withdrawn gradually, over intervals of weeks or months, with frequent reassessment of the patient. Concommitant use of alternative suppressive therapy should always be considered as a means of reducing the duration of steroid therapy. There is a strong clinical impression that activity in RA develops particular dependency to even small doses of steroids: withdrawal from patients with RA is inevitably extremely difficult compared to patients with inactive polymyalgia rheumatica or other steroid sensitive disease.

Apart from reactivation of underlying disease, steroid withdrawal may rarely precipitate the steroid withdrawal syndrome (p 328) or nodular panniculitis. The latter occurs almost exclusively in children with rheumatic fever and is characterised by painful, pruritic nodules over flexor surfaces of the limbs, the cheeks and the trunk.

Corticosteroids or ACTH?

Although disorders that respond to glucocorticoids may also respond to ACTH therapy, there is no evidence that the latter offers superior therapeutic activity in any of the rheumatic diseases. Its main advantage over oral steroids, when alternate-day therapy is not feasible, is lack of adrenal axis suppression. ACTH is therefore used particularly in situations that require marked anti-inflammatory activity for a limited period e.g. severe acute Reiter's, or during introduction of second line therapy in active RA.

Oral prednisolone, however, is generally preferable for therapeutic purposes since it can be given orally, the dose can be regulated precisely, effectiveness is independent of adrenal response (important particularly in patients who have previously received steroids), greater and more rapid anti-inflammatory activity may be achieved, and certain side-effects such as acne, hypertension and pigmentation are less common. It is a fallacy to assume that intermittent ACTH injections during prednisolone therapy counteract the tendency to adrenal atrophy: in fact, increased suppression occurs.

POLYPHARMACY AND DRUG INTERACTIONS

There is a rapidly expanding literature on interaction between drugs used for rheumatic disease, some of which are unwanted, some of which may be beneficial. Careful distinction, however, must always be made between interaction in the pharmacokinetic sense, of which there are many examples, and the clinical relevance of such interaction, of which there are few.

Most data relates to interaction between one NSAID and another, or between antirheumatic drugs and drugs used for other conditions, e.g. anticoagulants, antidepressants. Since there is no evidence for beneficial synergism between NSAIDs, and the possibility of adverse reaction always exists, polypharmacy with these agents should be avoided. Whenever a drug is prescribed the possibility of interaction should always be considered.

Combination therapy is of proven advantage in the treatment of many malignant conditions, but possible potentation of action through use of two or more 'second-line' agents in rheumatic disease has only recently been considered. Reluctance to use more than one agent at a time appears sensible when the spectrum of side-effects is similar — indeed, accumulation of side-effects has been demonstrated with sequential use of gold and penicillamine in RA. Increasing availability of drugs with a 'second-line' action, however, allows choice of drugs where side-effects do not overlap and future studies of combination therapy may well prove of interest. Currently, however, the only combination therapy proven to be of advantage is that of steroids with cyclophosphamide.

FURTHER READING

Bird H A, Wright V 1982 Applied drug thrapy of the rheumatic diseases. John Wright, Bristol

27 Surgical management of arthritis

INTRODUCTION

Surgery has a very useful place in the overall management of patients with arthritis but a successful outcome depends as much on correct selection of patients as performing the appropriate operation. For this reason it is customary for the orthopaedic surgeon and rheumatologist to have a combined clinic where a thorough assessment can be made. Many non-operative factors need careful consideration. The patient may have unrealistically high expectations of what can be achieved and be very disappointed unless he is fully informed. There is often a prolonged postoperative period of rehabilitation which may be uncomfortable and exhausting so that it is necessary to ensure that there is sufficient motivation to see this through. Overall general health, disease activity and quality of bone are also important, as is the state of other joints, since, for example, it is no use embarking on a hip or knee replacement if the patient's upper-limb disease precludes the use of crutches or painful foot deformity still makes walking difficult. Many patients with arthritis, particularly RA, are on drugs which reduce healing or predispose to infection so that medical therapy may need to be adjusted to reduce these effects. There are also a number of specific complications of rheumatic diseases which may be relevant to an anaesthetist, such as cervical spine subluxation in RA, cervical fusion in AS and JCA, micrognathia in JCA and reduced chest expansion in AS. A list of factors to consider before operating on a patient particularly applicable to RA is given.

Some important factors to consider prior to surgery in RA

1. Has the patient been on steroids?
2. Is there anaemia?
3. What is the state of the cervical spine?
4. Are there nodules over pressure areas?
5. Can the patient use crutches?
6. What is the state of the skin?
7. Is there generalised osteoporosis?
8. Are there any sites of sepsis?
9. Has the patient got Felty's syndrome?

SURGICAL PROCEDURES

The traditional aims of surgery are to relieve pain, improve function and correct deformity when conservative corrective measures and medical management have failed. There is also a small place for preventative operations, for example, synovectomy to preserve hand extensor tendons in RA, or cervical fusion in atlanto-axial subluxation to prevent quadriplegia. The types of operation used in arthritis are listed overleaf.

Synovectomy

Excision of inflamed synovium in RA will often relieve pain and swelling, although it does not influence joint mobility, and, contrary to earlier expectations, does not halt the progress of the disease. Persistent synovitis of the wrist and

Some operations available to treat arthritis

Soft-tissue procedures

1. Synovectomy
2. Repair of ruptured tendons
3. Release of entrapped nerves
4. Soft-tissue release

Bone and joint procedures

1. Osteotomy
2. Arthrodesis
3. Excision arthroplasty
4. Joint replacement

extensor-tendon sheath of the hand in association with a prominent ulnar head commonly leads to rupture of the extensor tendons and dropped fingers, which can be prevented by wrist synovectomy combined with tendon clearance and excision of the ulnar head. Small nodules of proliferating synovitis in the flexor tendons on the volar aspect of the palm may cause impairment of grip, which can be relieved by clearing the flexor tendons. Persistent knee synovitis with recurrent effusions, stretching of ligaments, popliteal cyst formation and pain can be relieved by synovectomy, which should ideally be performed before there is evidence of articular damage. Synovectomy is also indicated in the management of PVNS, osteochondromatosis and occasionally in haemophilic arthropathy under Factor VIII cover, since it may substantially reduce the number of bleeds into a joint. A synovectomy of a joint can also be achieved without surgery by intraarticular injection of a radioactive colloid such as ^{90}Yttrium, which locally irradiates the diseased tissue.

Tendon repair

In RA the extensor tendons of the hand are particularly prone to rupture. The little and ring fingers are usually affected first, probably because of their proximity to the prominent ulnar styloid, but they may quickly be followed by the middle and index finger, causing severe functional impairment. The frayed ends of the tendon retract up the forearm, making an end-to-end repair difficult. For this reason it is preferable to transfer a slip of tendon from an adjoining finger, or, if all the tendons have ruptured, to transfer extensor indices proprius at the wrist. Pending surgery, the MCPJs should be splinted in extension to prevent subluxation. It is also advisable to carry out a synovectomy and excision of the ulnar head where appropriate, with a view to preventing recurrence.

Soft-tissue release

Carpal tunnel syndrome can be relieved by incising the transverse carpal ligament of the wrist which reduces the pressure on the median nerve caused by carpal synovitis. Other nerve entrapment syndromes (p 281) can also be treated surgically. In all cases it is advisable to confirm the diagnosis by nerve conduction studies.

Restriction of joint movement may sometimes be due to, or aggravated by, constriction of the soft tissues, particularly tendons and muscles. This is most commonly seen in the knee and can be helped by surgical release either on its own, or when there is severe articular damage, in combination with a knee arthroplasty. Trigger fingers can be relieved by removing nodules of proliferating synovium from the flexor tendons of the hand.

Osteotomy

This procedure can be used to correct deformity and relieve pain, particularly in OA, but its use has declined with the development of joint replacement. High tibial osteotomy is successful in osteoarthritis of the knee, particularly in the younger patient with valgus or varus deformity due to unicompartmental disease but with good ligamentous stability. Femoral osteotomy is occasionally indicated in the younger patient with hip disease since it often gives several years of pain relief without precluding hip replacement at a later date (Fig. 27.1). The mechanism by which osteotomy relieves pain is not clear, but it may be due to reduction in interosseous venous pressure or operative denervation.

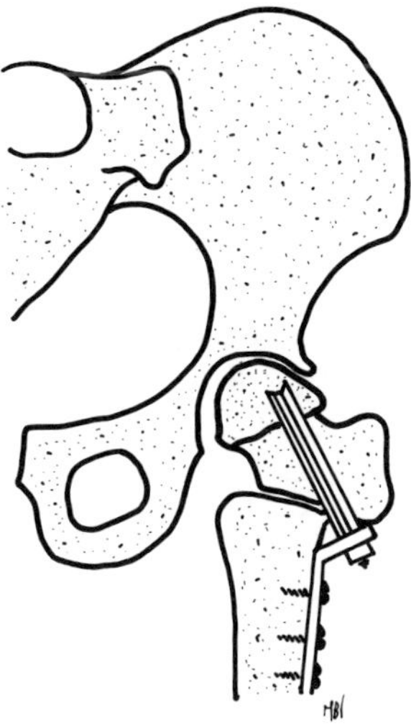

Fig. 27.1 Osteotomy of the hip for osteoarthritis

Excision arthroplasty

This was a common operation prior to the development of artificial joints and offered a combination of pain relief and reasonable preservation of movement. The affected articular surfaces are removed and the space left is allowed to fill with scar tissue, forming a pseudarthrosis. There are a number of situations in which primary excision arthroplasy is still indicated (Table 27.1). Secondary excision arthroplasty is occasionally used to salvage a failed replacement and can be surprisingly successful. Common examples are hip excision arthroplasty (Girdlestone) which often gives a pain-free result with good range of movement, although at the expense of considerable shortening of the leg, which may be unstable; and excision of the trapezium in OA of the CMCJ of the thumb, and removal of the radial head to relieve pain at the elbow in RA.

Table 27.1 Primary excision arthroplasty

Bone resected	Main indication
Patella	Patellofemoral OA
Radial head	Superior radio-ulnar RA
Trapezium	OA of first CMCJ
Lateral end clavicle	OA, RA acromioclavicular joint
Metatarsal heads	Dorsal subluxation of MTPJs in RA
Proximal phalanx	Hallux valgus

Arthrodesis

Fusing a joint will render it pain-free and stable but imposes considerable functional restriction. With the advent of joint arthroplasty the frequency of this rather drastic procedure has declined. Nevertheless, it is still indicated in certain selected joints where stability is more important than movement and is very successful for unilateral wrist disease in RA and for controlling the hindfoot and relieving symptoms from a valgus ankle. Arthrodesis is the usual salvage procedure when a knee prosthesis has to be removed. It is occasionally still the operation of choice in a young, physically-active person with disease confined to one knee whose level of activity would place too much strain on a prosthetic joint. Nevertheless, a stiff straight leg can be a liability, particularly sitting in confined places such as a car or cinema, and it makes climbing stairs or rising out of a chair awkward and obvious.

Joints amenable to arthrodesis

1. Atlanto-axial and subaxial cervical spine
2. Wrist
3. Ankle and subtalar
4. DIPJ thumb
5. 1st MTPJ
6. DIPJs fingers

Joint replacement

The development of artificial joints has been a major advance in the management of inflammatory and degenerative arthritis. Greatest success has been achieved with total hip replacement, pioneered by Sir John Charnley, but prosthetic knees, elbows, wrists, ankles, shoulders, elbows, wrists and finger-joints are also being developed and used, although with a less predictable outcome.

In a total joint replacement, both articulating surfaces are excised and replaced by artificial components. These are commonly made of stainless-steel, metal alloy or hard plastic material such as high-density polyethylene. The implants are held in place by special methylmethacrylate cement. Since foreign material is being left in the body it is essential that the operation is carried out under ultrasterile conditions which should ideally include laminar-flow operating theatre ventilation to reduce bacterial contamination of the operative field.

The selection of prosthesis is the prerogative of the orthopaedic surgeon and his choice will be influenced by the state of the bones and soft tissues as well as his own particular experience and preference. In some cases, for example hip replacement, the low friction metal-on-plastic type developed by Charnley (Fig. 27.2) is so outstandingly successful in 90% of patients that this would be the usual operation performed today for osteoarthritis and rheumatoid arthritis of the hip. In other joints, for instance the knee, the results of arthroplasty are less predictable, with a much higher morbidity than hip replacement. As a result many different types of prostheses have been designed (Fig. 27.3), testifying to the fact that no one is entirely satisfactory for every situation. The early knees prostheses were simple hinges but, because of their rigidity in all directions except flexion and extension, they easily worked loose. The more recent knee protheses generally have a contoured tibial component and a metal femoral condylar component. Some are unconnected and rely on the ligaments of the knee and geometric configuration to maintain stability. Others are hinged together but also allow a little rotation and lateral movement, reducing the tendency to loosening.

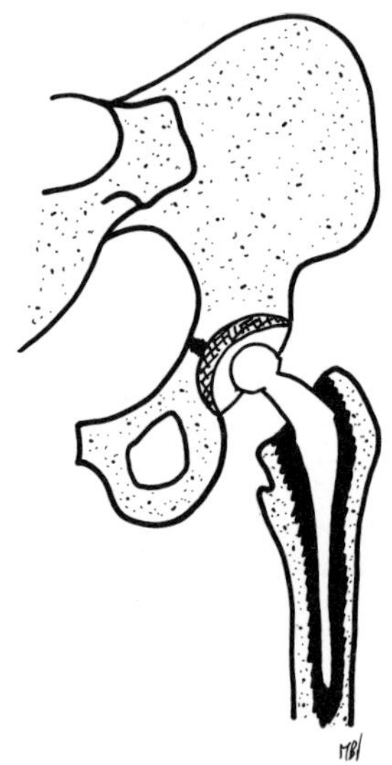

Fig. 27.2 Charnley hip arthroplasty

The main indication for joint replacement is severe pain which is uncontrolled by conservative means. Extremes of age are no bar and many thousands of old and very old people are enjoying the benefits of hip replacement. Artificial joints are also being used cautiously in young people, particu-

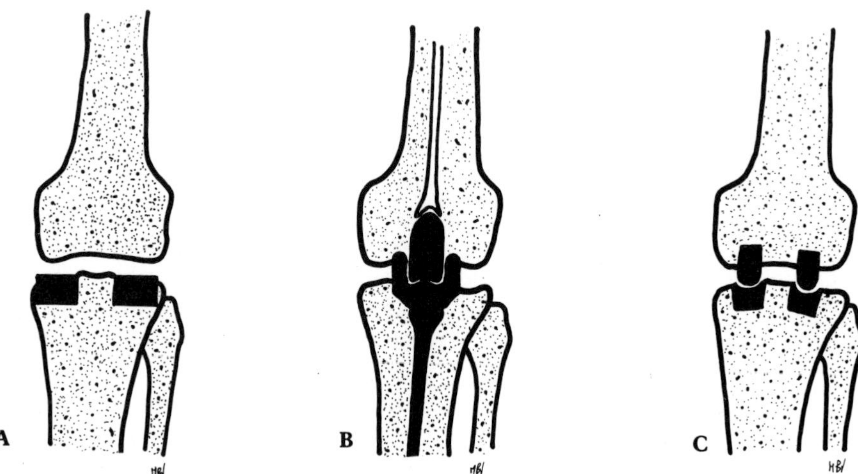

Fig. 27.3 Types of knee arthroplasty **A**. Surface replacement **B**. Fully-constrained hinge **C**. 'Hinged' by geomatric configuration

larly those severely disabled by juvenile chronic arthritis, although long-term questions about wear are not yet answered. The main causes of failure of artificial joints are shown below. This usually necessitates removal of the implant, so as a general rule no patient should be offered an artificial joint unless he would still be better off with an excision arthroplasty or arthrodesis should a salvage procedure be necessary. About 10% of hip arthroplasties fail but the figures for knee replacements are as high as 20–30% The failure rate for other prosthetic replacements is not yet known and use of these should probably be still regarded as somewhat experimental.

Complications of joint arthroplasty
Early
1. Thromboembolic disease
2. Infection
3. Haematoma
4. Dislocation
5. Metal allergy

1. Infection
2. Loosening
3. Fracture
4. Wear
5. Heterotopic bone formation

Many patients, particularly those with rheumatoid arthritis, may have several artificial joints. Since each offers a place of concealment for bacteria, these patients are at risk during episodes of bacteraemia, for example following dental treatment or various endoscopic examinations. There is a valid arguement for regarding them in the same way as patients with artificial heart valves and giving prophylatic antibiotic cover on such occasions. For the same reason, any episode of infection must be treated quickly and adequately.

SPECIAL SITUATIONS

The hand

Hand function is highly complex and depends on the integrated action of joints, tendons, muscles and ligaments. Any imbalance may result in quite disastrous functional incapacity. Also disease or deformity at one site may adversly affect function elsewhere in the hand, for example, radial deviation at the wrist promoting ulnar diviation of the fingers, or hyperextension of the PIPJs (swan-neck deformity) forcing the DIPs into flexion. RA may progress slowly in the hand without causing much pain, so it is important to watch actively for the signs of impending trouble in order that remedial action can be taken before permanent fixed deformity results. Remedial action does not necessarily mean only surgery, since splinting and careful injection of steroid into the joints and tendons may be useful, but there are a number of operations that, if used for the right indication, have a reasonable chance of success.

Useful operations in the hand
1. Wrist fusion
2. Synovectomy of the extensor and flexor tendons
3. Excision of the ulnar styloid
4. Fusion of the DIPJ of the thumb
5. MCPJ arthroplasty
6. Extensor loop operation for ulnar deviation

The object of surgery in the hand in RA is the preservation or restoration of function. Secondary to this, the appearance of the hand may be improved, but as a general rule, operating for cosmetic reasons alone is not justifiable. The major functions of the hand are lifting, pinching and gripping, and these can be assessed by asking questions about everyday activities such as carrying saucepans, holding cutlery, using a key, writing and personal hygiene and observing the patient carrying out these ordinary daily tasks.

In early disease, prophylatic removal of proliferating synovium in the extensor tendons may prevent subsequent rupture of the tendons. This also balances the stronger pull of the flexor tendons which tend to cause loss of extension at the MCPJs. Poor extension may also result from synovitis in the flexor-tendon sheaths blocking the

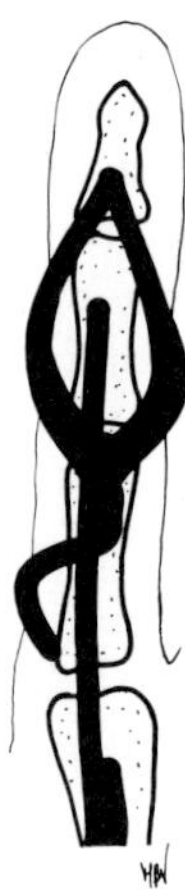

Fig. 27.4 Extensor tendon loop operation for ulnar drift

full excursion of the flexor tendons, again resulting in finger flexion. This may be considerably improved by clearance of the flexor-tendon sheaths. Ulnar deviation or the fingers is due in part to synovitis of the MCPJs causing dislocation of the extensor tendons into the ulnar grooves between the fingers. There are a number of operations disigned to correct this, including cutting the dorsal interossei (Littler's intrinsic release) and the extensor-tendon loop operation, in which the extensor tendon is split longitudinally and half is detached proximally and passed through a small hole drilled in the base of the proximal phalanx (Fig. 27.4) Swan-neck deformity results partly from tightening of the intrinsic tendons combined with ulnar diviation and can be corrected by removal of the tight lateral extensor band. A boutonniere deformity is caused by stretching of the central slip of the extensor tendon, which inserts into the base of the middle pahlanx and can be corrected by repositioning this central slip surgically.

In later stages of RA when joints are damaged and pain often severe, the surgeon really only has the choice of arthroplasty or arthrodesis. Hand function can be severely impaired by pain and subluxation at the wrist and this is amenable to treatment by arthrodesis. It is advisable to fix the wrist for which an arthodeesis is contemplated in a temporary splint to make sure preoperatively that the patient can manage. It is not possible to carry out the activities of daily living with two rigid wrists and, when both warrant surgery, it is usual to fix one and replace the other with a flexible implant.

Poor grip and limitation of rotation at the wrist can result from pain at the inferior radio-ulnar joint and may be greatly eased by resection of the ulnar styloid, an operation which is frequently combined with synovectomy of the extensor tendons to prevent rupture.

Arthroplasty is the treatment of choice for disorganisation at the MCPJs using silastic hinge-joints which are placed between the resected ends of the bones. Although there is a high frequency of fracture of these prostheses, they still continue to function well when this happens by acting as spacers between the bone ends which are held together by fibrosis around the implant.

The decision whether to fuse or replace damaged PIPJs depends largely on the state of the adjoining joints. If the DIPJs are fused then the PIPJs should be replaced by flexible implants, but if the MCPJs are replaced by implants, the PIPJs should be fused. The DIPJs are usually fused in slight flexion, since here stability is more useful than movement. Fusion of the DIPJs has the added benefit of helping function at a more proximal level, for instance correcting a mild swan-neck deformity. The same principles apply to the thumb. An unstable DIPJ should be fused in slight flexion to control pinch but the MCPJ should be replaced by an implant. The carpometacarpal joint is also frequently destroyed and, since motion is also essential at this level, is treated by resection of the trapezium which can be replaced by an implant inserted into the base of the first MCPJ (Fig. 27.5).

The foot

More operations are done to relieve pain and deformity in arthritis of the foot than at any other site in the body. The small joints of the forefoot are a common site of involvement in early RA, which results in splaying of the foot, subluxation of the MTPJs, cock-up toes, hallux valgus and callosities, which may ulcerate and become infected. The MTPJs can be treated by partial

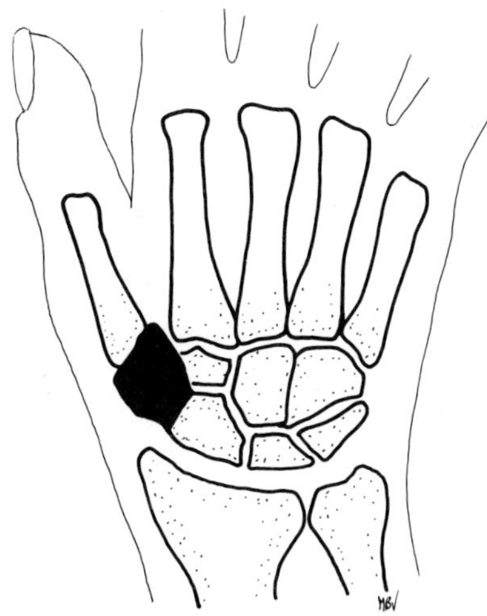

Fig. 27.5 Excision arthroplasty of the trapezium

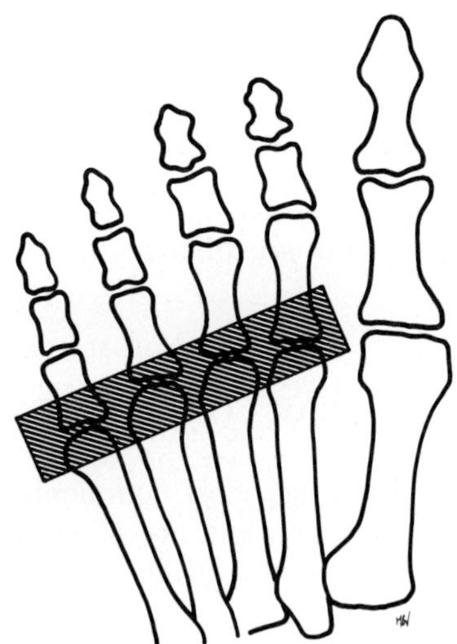

Fig. 27.6 Excision of metatarsal heads and bases of proximal phalanges (Fowler's operation)

phalangectomy of the toes combined with resection of the metatarsal heads if these are dislocated (Fig. 27.6). Hallux valgus is relieved by excision

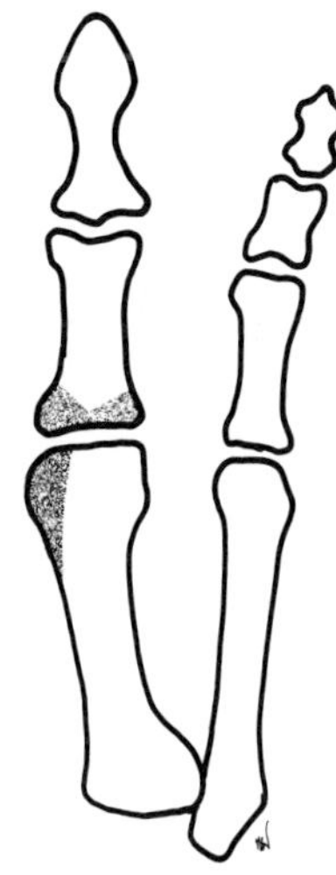

Fig. 27.7 Bone excised in Keller's operation for hallux valgus

of the proximal third of the proximal phalanx and removal of the medial prominence of the first metatarsal (Fig. 27.7). RA in the hindfoot is a common cause of ankle pain and valgus deformity which makes walking difficult. Provided there is a good movement in the true ankle joint and forefoot, this can be remedied by subtalar fusion or a triple arthrodesis if the talo-navicular and calcaneo-cuboid joints are involved. Severe pain in the ankle joint may also be relieved by fusion but this should only be done in the presence of flexible uninvolved lower hindfoot joints, since there is a slight risk of precipitating or worsening symptoms in these joints.

FURTHER READING

Bulgen D G, Hazleman B L 1975 Surgery in the rheumatic diseases. Hospital Update, August

Vainio K 1975 Orthopaedic surgery in the treatment of RA. Annals of Clinical Research 7: 216

28 Intra-articular therapy

Intra-articular therapy with a variety of compounds, particularly steroids, forms a useful adjunct to treatment. Although this technique offers the possibility of localised response, most materials injected into a joint are efficiently cleared by bulk flow through lymphatics, the rate of clearance reflecting: 1. properties referable to the drug itself, such as molecular weight, lipid solubility and charge; and 2. variables in the joint involved, such as surface area of synovium, effective blood- and lymph-flow, volume of effusion, hydrostatic and osmotic pressure relationships and histopathology of the disease process.

To overcome the problem of rapid elimination from the joint, chemical modification of the drug or attachment of the drug to one of several carrier systems has generally proved necessary. Avoidance of vigorous use of the joint for 24 hours after injection will further reduce drug clearance.

Before considering compounds administered by the intra-articular route, it must be emphasised that certain obvious precautions should always be observed whenever intra-articular injections are performed:

1. Never inject when the diagnosis is in doubt or when the condition is unlikely to respond
2. Do not inject in the presence of local or systemic infection
3. Be careful to use an aseptic technique that involves single dose ampoules, pre-packed disposable equipment and domestically clean, dry hands. Clean overlying skin with alcohol or similar antiseptic and do not guide needle with finger.
4. Be sure the needle is in the synovial space — confirmed by aspiration of fluid and/or ease of injection
5. Do not inject if aspirated fluid is heavily bloodstained or suggestive of infection
6. Always send aspirated fluid for culture

Suggested injection sites for commonly injected and aspirated joints are briefly outlined on page 449.

INTRA-ARTICULAR CORTICOSTEROIDS

Steroids are the drugs most commonly given by intra-articular injection and are potentially of use in any condition with an inflammatory component. Possible advantages of local steroid therapy include: 1. rapid reduction in synovitis with relief of pain and stiffness within c. 12–48 hours; 2. possibility of accelerated and effective mobilisation when used in combination with physiotherapy; 3. possible avoidance of systemic therapy for a local problem. Circumstances in which intra-articular steroid injection should be considered are outlined opposite. The speed of onset and duration of response varies with the steroid used, the underlying condition, the joint injected and, as with oral administration, with the individual patient. Commonly used steroids are outlined opposite; addition of complex side-chains to the

Circumstances in which intra-articular injection may be considered

1. Clinical evidence of active synovitis
2. Condition not amenable to simple local or systemic treatment
3. Definite diagnosis known

Commonly used intra-articular steroid preparations

* *Short-acting (2–7 days)*

1. Hydrocortisone acetate
2. Prednisolone acetate
3. 6-methylprednisolone acetate
4. Dexamethasone acetate
5. Triamcinolone diacetonide

* *Intermediate (c. 14 days)*

1. Hydrocortisone t-butyl acetate
2. Prednisolone t-butyl acetate
3. Dexamethasone t-butyl acetate
4. Triamcinolone acetonide

* *Long-acting (c. 21 days)*

Triamcinolone hexacetonide

* N. B. Many factors govern the duration of response in any one joint

steroid nucleus generally decreases solubility and prolongs steroid response. For triamcinolone hexacetonide, one of the least soluble and longest-acting agents, symptomatic improvement usually ranges from 1–4 weeks, but in some instances may last for many months, thus far exceeding any theoretical rationalisation. There is no concensus concerning the volume that should be injected, but for most preparations c. 1 ml is suitable for knees, shoulders or ankles, c. 0.5–1 ml for elbows and wrists, and c. 0.1–0.5 ml for small joints of hands and feet. In general, non-weight-bearing joints such as PIP, sterno-clavicular or temporomandibular joints, show more prolonged improvement than weight-bearing joints (e.g. knees, hips, MTPs). Some physicians regularly inject a small amount of local anaesthetic with the steroid in the same syringe.

Possible complications of intra-articular steroid injection

1. Iatrogenic infection
2. Enhancement of joint damage — 'steroid arthropathy'
3. Local-tissue atrophy and fat necrosis
4. Avascular necrosis
5. Impairment of adrenal axis
6. Postinjection flare

Although many side effects have been attributed to local steroid injection, in practice major complications are rare.

If simple precautions are observed, the incidence of iatrogenic infection is very low: nevertheless, this should be suspected in any troublesome joint that has recently been injected. Intra-articular steroids may damage cartilage in some animal models, though primate joints appear to respond differently: evidence for cartilage damage in man is inconclusive and may be offset by reduction in synovitis. A varying proportion of any injected steroid will be cleared from the joint, and thus be able to exert a systemic effect — this is often evident clinically by improvement in joints distant from the one injected. Repeated injections may compromise the HPA axis and result in complications such as osteonecrosis.

Poor technique may result in capsular or periarticular damage, and local atrophy around the injection site is not uncommon. Post-injection flares are thought to represent a form of crystal-induced synovitis (p 188): they develop within a few hours of injection and may last up to 48 hours.

The question of how often a joint may be injected remains unanswered. Although side-effects are remarkably uncommon, if a joint appears to require frequent injections to control symptoms it seems sensible to consider alternative approaches to treatment, especially in a young patient.

For many soft-tissue lesions steroid injection is the primary treatment (p 365). Good technique is all-important if tendon rupture, muscle atrophy or local skin and subcutaneous changes are to be avoided.

INTRA-ARTICULAR RADIOCOLLOIDS

Following initial trials with colloidal gold (^{198}Au), several radioactive isotopes have been used locally to procure 'medical synovectomy' or '*synoviorthèse*' in conditions such as RA, synovitis of chronic haemophilic arthropathy, chronic pyrophosphate arthropathy and PVNS. To minimise whole-body irradiation through penetration and leakage metal or metalloid β emitters with a short half life are preferable (Table 28.1).

Table 28.1 Commonly used radio-isotopes

Isotope	Half-life (days)	Type of radiation	Tissue penetration
^{90}Y	2.7	β	3.6–11 mm
^{169}Er	9.5	β,γ	0.3–1 mm
^{186}Rh	3.7	β (γ rare)	1.2–3.7 mm

Yttrium (^{90}Y) is commonly used for large joints such as the knee (c. 3–5 mCi): erbium (^{169}Er) has low tissue penetration and is more commonly used for small joints of the hand (0.5–1.0 mCi); rhenium (^{186}Rh) shows intermediate penetration and is occasionally used for wrist, elbow and other joints (c. 1–2 mCi). The use of colloids with a diameter of c. 100 nm allows good distribution within the joint but reduces extra-articular spread: autoradiography has demonstrated that shortly following injection radioactivity is concentrated within the synovium, due to phagocytosis by synoviocytes, and that the cartilage surface is relatively free.

Reported side-effects include fever, malaise, burns due to needle-track leakage and possible predisposition to joint instability. Shortly following injection chromosomal damage in circulating lymphocytes has been demonstrated, though the clinical significance of this is not known. Although theoretical considerations suggest that a significant association with malignancy is unlikely, the use of radiosynovectomy is usually reserved for those over 60. Meticulous technique, concommitant injection of steroid and subsequent splinting all reduce the risk of leakage and elimination from the joint.

Before considering use of radiocolloids, in general a good but temporary benefit from intra-articular steroid should first be demonstrated. The duration of response to *synoviorthèse* varies with the underlying condition, but can last from 6 months to several years: as with surgical synovectomy, however, the synovium eventually recovers. Beneficial response following repeat injection into the same joint has been reported.

CHEMICAL AGENTS

Chemical necrosis and subsequent fibrosis of inflamed synovium — 'chemical synovectomy' — is usually attempted with a 1–2% aqueous solution of osmium tetroxide. This agent is inexpensive and easy to prepare, and is still used widely in many European countries, particularly France.

The treatment is usually well tolerated. Pain in the hours following injection may be reduced by concommitant use of steroid and lignocaine. Osmium causes radiological opacities in injected joints and the reduced metal is eliminated in the urine, causing dark-brown discolouration but no renal damage. The chemical can produce severe cartilage damage in certain animal models and although the evidence in man is inconclusive, the risk of cartilage damage has deterred many from its use.

OTHER AGENTS

Intra-articular use of cytotoxic agents has generally been limited because of local and systemic toxicity, and has met with little success. Thiotepa, for example, initially reported to be of benefit in small joints of the hand in RA, was subsequently shown to be no better than intra-articular steroid; and methotrexate was found to be ineffective in psoriatic arthropathy, even when given by repeated injection with oral leucovorin to prevent systemic toxicity. There may, however, be a role for intra-articular rifamycin which has been reported to be of benefit in RA knees, and study of other cytotoxic agents is currently in progress.

Orgotein, a metalloprotein with superoxide dismutase activity, has been claimed to be of benefit in both RA and OA. Interestingly, this drug provokes a severe synovitis in experimental OA and its usefulness in man awaits confirmation.

Although trials of intra-articular aspirin have given conflicting results, the possible local action of NSAIDs, given appropriate formulation, may be worthy of further study, though rapid clearance from the joint is likely to be a problem.

LIPOSOMES AND OTHER CARRIER SYSTEMS

A liposome is a hollow sphere the wall of which resembles a cell membrane in consisting of polarised phospholipid molecules which present a hydrophilic and a hydrophobic surface. Drugs may be incorporated into either the aqueous or non-aqueous region and several layers can be added to form onion-like structures up to several microns in diameter. The drug remains largely encapsulated until released by degradation within a cell thus offering the potential advantages of drug direction towards a particular tissue, decreased metabolism of the drug prior to reaching its target, and decreased systemic toxicity. Using this delivery system intra-articular steroids have already been shown capable of producing a beneficial response in RA at 1/25th the conventional injected dose, and future use of liposomes certainly promises to be a major advance in intra-articular and oral drug administration.

Other potential carrier systems include entrapment within erythrocytes and linkage to monoclonal antibodies. These, however, although already in use in other branches of medicine, remain relatively unexplored in treatment of rheumatic disease.

29 Experimental forms of therapy

A theory that has figured prominently to explain the pathogenesis of rheumatoid arthritis and other rheumatic diseases is that a persistent immune response to an as yet unidentified antigen results in the perpetuation of inflammatory reactions that destroy articular cartilage and are responsible for other clinical disease manifestations. This theory provides the basis for treating these diseases with immunosuppressive drugs, and as a logical extension of this line of thought, clinicians have sought other ways of modifying the patient's immune response. A number of biological agents and physical methods presumed to modify immunoregulation have therefore been tested under experimental conditions in small numbers of patients, especially those with severe rheumatoid arthritis unresponsive to other forms of therapy, and those with other connective-tissue diseases.

BIOLOGICAL IMMUNOREGULATORY AGENTS

1. Anti-lymphocyte serum

The use of specific antisera to remove lymphocytes is very successful in suppressing experimental models of autoimmune disease. In man, the IgG fraction of anti-lymphocyte serum (ALG) is used in order to minimise the risk of serum-sickness, and ALG has been used extensively in recipients of renal allografts with good results. Experience of its use in rheumatic diseases is limited, but ALG has been shown to be a helpful adjunct to immunosuppressive drugs and prednisolone in inducing remissions in severe forms of connective-tissue disease. With the development of monoclonal antibody technology the future may see the use of monoclonal antisera to remove specific lymphocyte subpopulations.

2. Pulse therapy with high-dose methylprednisolone

Large doses of methylprednisolone given intravenously in pulses are effective in treating renal transplant rejection, and this has been the basis for its use in rheumatic diseases. This form of treatment has been used with success in both renal and non-renal manifestations of SLE, and in suppressing joint inflammation in RA. In combination with cyclophosphamide, pulse therapy with methylprednisolone has been used to control systemic vasculitis. The mode of action of large doses of methylprednisolone given in this way is not known. The absolute numbers of both T and B lymphocytes are reduced following a dose and there may be an effect on the immune response. However, the efficacy of this treatment may lie in its potent effect on the inflammatory response, both in impeding the access of inflammatory cells to the site of inflammation, and in suppressing the humoral component of inflammation.

3. Other biological substances

Biological substances such as interferon and thymopoetin are capable of modifying autoimmune disease in animals, and this is the basis for the trials of these substances in man. Their efficiency in the treatment of diseases such as RA and other connective-tissue diseases, however, is still to be established.

PHYSICAL METHODS TO REMOVE HUMORAL FACTORS AND CELLS

1. Plasmapheresis

The technique of plasmapheresis was first described in 1914 and involves the physical removal of the patient's plasma and replacing it with equal volumes of physiological iso-oncotic solutions such as fresh frozen plasma or albumin solutions. Modern experience of this technique dates from the early 1950s when it was used to remove the abnormal paraprotein in multiple myeloma. Subsequently it was used as an effective treatment of hyperviscosity in Waldenstrom's macroglobulinaemia. More recently it has been applied to the treatment of auto-immune diseases thought to be mediated by humoral factors: antibody, circulating immune complexes and other humoral mediators of inflammation.

Auto-immune diseases treated with plasmapheresis

1. Auto-immune thrombocytopenic purpura
2. Auto-immune haemolytic anaemia
3. Myaesthenia gravis
4. Goodpasture's syndrome
5. Rheumatoid arthritis
   (a) Joint disease
   (b) Extra-articular manifestations
6. SLE
7. PAN
8. Raynaud's phenomenon
9. Systemic sclerosis

With the introduction of cell separators to remove plasma via continuous flow centrifugation plasmapheresis is now safe and rapid, and up to 4 litres of plasma can be replaced in a 2-hour period with little risk to the patient.

A typical regimen of plasmapheresis involves replacement of 2 litres of plasma per session, three to five times a week, usually for 2 weeks, after which the great majority of native plasma has been exchanged. Regimens of this sort have been successful in treating active SLE, suppressing systemic vasculitis in rheumatoid disease and, to a lesser extent, rheumatoid synovitis. The favourable clinical response is accompanied by a fall in the serum levels of auto-antibody and immune complexes and, in addition, there is evidence that the function of the reticulo-endothelial system in clearing immune complexes is improved by plasmapheresis.

Trials have involved small numbers of patients so far and further experience is required before critical appraisal of plasmapheresis in the treatment of rheumatic diseases is possible. A problem of this treatment has been identified, however, in the rapid rebound of antibody production and immune complex levels accompanied by clinical deterioration after cessation of plasmapheresis This rebound has been abrogated by combining plasmapheresis with immunosuppressive drugs such as cyclophosphamide.

2. Thoracic duct drainage

Thoracic duct drainage is an effective way of removing large numbers of circulating lymphocytes. Up to 50×10^9 lymphocytes, predominantly T cells, can be removed per day with this technique. It has been used to a limited extent in the treatment of rheumatic diseases, but has produced marked improvement in both joint and systemic manifestations in patients with severe RA and SLE. However, it is a cumbersome and expensive in-patient procedure with serious potential complications, especially infection, and discontinuation of the treatment soon results in disease exacerbation.

3. Leukopheresis

The introduction of continuous cell separators offers a technique to remove as many lymphocytes as thoracic duct drainage, but without the same disadvantages. Preliminary results in severe RA are favourable, though short-lived.

4. Radiotherapy

20 years ago X-ray irradiation was a popular treatment for ankylosing spondylitis and was claimed to produce relief of pain and stiffness. It was often given on a repetitive basis and resulted in a cumulative dose of radiation in excess of safety. This form of treatment for ankylosing spondylitis has fallen into disrepute because of the subsequent increased risk of acute leukaemia and of developing cancer at sites within the field of radiation.

Regimens of total lymphoid irradiation as used in the treatment of Hodgkin's disease and non-Hodgkin's lymphoma, which are associated with a low incidence of serious side-effects have recently been examined in patients with severe rheumatoid arthritis unresponsive to other forms of treatment. Preliminary results have been favourable, with reports of long-lasting improvement in the disease.

Like thoracic drainage and leukopheresis, lymphoid irradiation produces lymphopenia, but the effect on immune regulation has not yet been defined.

The measures described in this chapter have not been demonstrated to be much more superior to established forms of treatment in these diseases. Furthermore, they are expensive and often need sophisticated equipment only available in specialised centres. If they have a role, it appears to be as adjunctive therapy in combination with other immunosuppressive agents in the treatment of severe disease manifestations.

FURTHER READING

Dosa S, Lawler W, Mallick N P et al 1978 The treatment of lupoid nephritis by methylprednisolone pulse therapy. Postgraduate Medical Journal 54: 628–632

Calabrese L M, Clough J D, Krakauer R S, Hoeltge G A 1980 Plasmapheresis therapy of immunologic disease. Cleveland Clinical Quarterly 47: 53–72

Kotzin B L, Stroker S, Engleman E G et al 1981. Treatment of intractable rheumatoid arthritis with total lymphoid irradiation. New England Journal of Medicine 305: 969–976

Karsh J, Klippel J M, Plotz P M et al 1981 Lymphopheresis in rheumatoid arthritis. Arthritis and Rheumatism 24: 867–871

Index